Neurology and Pregnancy

SERIES IN MATERNAL-FETAL MEDICINE
Published in association with the *Journal of Maternal-Fetal & Neonatal Medicine*

Edited by:

Gian Carlo Di Renzo and Dev Maulik

Howard Carp, *Recurrent Pregnancy Loss*,
ISBN 9780415421300

Vincenzo Berghella, *Obstetric Evidence Based Guidelines*,
ISBN 9780415701884

Vincenzo Berghella, *Maternal-Fetal Evidence Based Guidelines*,
ISBN 9780415432818

Moshe Hod, Lois Jovanovic, Gian Carlo Di Renzo, Alberto de Leiva, Oded Langer,
Textbook of Diabetes and Pregnancy, Second Edition,
ISBN 9780415426206

Simcha Yagel, Norman H. Silverman, Ulrich Gembruch, *Fetal Cardiology, Second Edition*,
ISBN 9780415432658

Fabio Facchinetti, Gustaaf A. Dekker, Dante Baronciani, George Saade, *Stillbirth: Understanding and Management*,
ISBN 9780415473903

Vincenzo Berghella, *Maternal–Fetal Evidence Based Guidelines, Second Edition*,
ISBN 9781841848228

Vincenzo Berghella, *Obstetric Evidence Based Guidelines, Second Edition*,
ISBN 9781841848242

Neurology and Pregnancy
Clinical Management

Edited by

Michael S. Marsh, FRCOG, MD
Department of Obstetrics and Gynaecology
King's College Hospital
London, U.K.

Lina A. M. Nashef, MBChB, FRCP, MD
Department of Neurology
King's College Hospital
London, U.K.

Peter A. Brex, FRCP, MD
Department of Neurology
King's College Hospital
London, U.K.

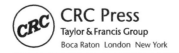

CRC Press
Taylor & Francis Group
Boca Raton London New York

CRC Press is an imprint of the
Taylor & Francis Group, an **informa** business

CRC Press
Taylor & Francis Group
6000 Broken Sound Parkway NW, Suite 300
Boca Raton, FL 33487-2742

First issued in paperback 2018

© 2012 by Taylor & Francis Group, LLC
CRC Press is an imprint of Taylor & Francis Group, an Informa business

No claim to original U.S. Government works

ISBN-13: 978-1-84184-652-1 (hbk)
ISBN-13: 978-1-138-37247-4 (pbk)

This book contains information obtained from authentic and highly regarded sources. While all reasonable efforts have been made to publish reliable data and information, neither the author[s] nor the publisher can accept any legal responsibility or liability for any errors or omissions that may be made. The publishers wish to make clear that any views or opinions expressed in this book by individual editors, authors or contributors are personal to them and do not necessarily reflect the views/opinions of the publishers. The information or guidance contained in this book is intended for use by medical, scientific or health-care professionals and is provided strictly as a supplement to the medical or other professional's own judgement, their knowledge of the patient's medical history, relevant manufacturer's instructions and the appropriate best practice guidelines. Because of the rapid advances in medical science, any information or advice on dosages, procedures or diagnoses should be independently verified. The reader is strongly urged to consult the relevant national drug formulary and the drug companies' and device or material manufacturers' printed instructions, and their websites, before administering or utilizing any of the drugs, devices or materials mentioned in this book. This book does not indicate whether a particular treatment is appropriate or suitable for a particular individual. Ultimately it is the sole responsibility of the medical professional to make his or her own professional judgements, so as to advise and treat patients appropriately. The authors and publishers have also attempted to trace the copyright holders of all material reproduced in this publication and apologize to copyright holders if permission to publish in this form has not been obtained. If any copyright material has not been acknowledged please write and let us know so we may rectify in any future reprint.

A CIP record for this book is available from the British Library.

Library of Congress Cataloging-in-Publication Data available on application

Typeset by MPS Ltd, Delhi

Visit the Taylor & Francis Web site at
http://www.taylorandfrancis.com

and the CRC Press Web site at
http://www.crcpress.com

Foreword

This volume is most timely. If non-neurologists approach our specialty with trepidation, most neurologists and neurosurgeons confront obstetrics and its many neurological aspects with equal uncertainty. The reasons are obvious. In pregnancy we are dealing not with a single patient, but with a woman, her unborn (or newborn) child, and a complex web of relationships surrounding them.

Thus a text that provides an assessment that is clear, scholarly, yet common sense and evidence-based (where evidence exists), of the interactions between science and clinical practice across the spectrum of neurological and neurosurgical challenges in pregnancy, is sure to find a wide and grateful readership. The editors have succeeded in welding into a coherent and authoritative whole a somewhat fragmented but vitally important and rapidly evolving field of clinical science.

Neurologists who work in a general hospital setting will wish to have this text to hand, as will obstetricians. All those who train neurologists and obstetricians will wish to ensure that this volume is readily available to their trainees. In practical terms, this enterprise will surely help to improve the care of people in whom pregnancy is complicated by neurological problems and the care of those with pre-existing neurological disorders who become pregnant. All these individuals and families require advice and care supported by sound evidence to ensure a safe and happy pregnancy, delivery and post-natal period. Towards this goal, *Neurology and Pregnancy* represents a landmark in clinical neurosciences and in obstetrics.

Nigel Leigh
Professor of Neurology
Brighton and Sussex Medical School
Trafford Centre for Biomedical Research
University of Sussex
Falmer, UK

Foreword

Neurological disease in pregnancy is now the second commonest cause of maternal death in the United Kingdom. Many of the pregnant or puerperal women who have died from epilepsy, subarachnoid haemorrhage and other neurological disease have done so without the benefit of pre-pregnancy counseling, appropriate multidisciplinary care, or timely involvement of neurologists. Therefore the development of a specific text addressing the issues of management of neurological disease in pregnancy is timely.

This authoritative reference brings together experts in the field of neurology, fetal medicine, obstetrics, genetics and psychiatry. The general chapters cover important issues such as pharmacokinetics of drugs in pregnancy and breast-feeding and neuroimaging, an understanding of which is a prerequisite to optimising management of pregnant women with neurological problems.

Part II covers pre-existing as well as new-onset neurological disease presenting in pregnancy, and includes chapters on common clinical problems such as blackouts, headaches and epilepsy, as well as dealing with less common problems such as peripheral nerve disease, myasthenia and stroke, which are also comprehensively covered.

Many of the chapters are the result of multidisciplinary collaboration reflecting the teamwork that should accompany optimal management of neurological disease in pregnancy. This book will provide a useful reference for all those who manage women of childbearing age with neurological disease as well as for obstetric care providers faced with common and less common neurological conditions complicating pregnancy.

Catherine Nelson-Piercy
Consultant Obstetric Physician
St Thomas' Hospital
London, UK

Preface

Dear Colleague

The management of neurological disorders in pregnancy is based on a good knowledge of the woman's medical and social history, available evidence and previous pregnancy outcomes, as well as an appreciation of her attitudes, beliefs, concerns and priorities. It calls for knowledge, judgement and experience and is as much an art as it is a science. It often requires balancing conflicting interests and supporting the patient and her partner in making potentially far-reaching decisions, sometimes based on insufficient evidence. It requires sharing the decision making process, aimed at ensuring the best outcome for both mother and child, so that the woman does not feel she alone carries the burden.

Advising a pregnant woman with a neurological presentation is by its nature a multidisciplinary process. No one specialist can do this alone and it is only by combining our skills and knowledge that we can provide the best care. This truly multidisciplinary book provides much of the background knowledge-base needed, both within and across specialties. Few volumes cover its scope. Moreover, where evidence is limited, authors have not shied away from giving sound clinical guidance.

We are enormously grateful to our contributing authors for generously sharing their expertise and for our publisher's patience in what has been a longer gestation than first envisaged. Our hope is that you, our reader, will explore sections in your field as well as other disciplines, and in doing so value this volume and learn from it as much as we have.

Michael S. Marsh
Lina A. M. Nashef
Peter A. Brex

Editorial Note on the FDA Classification of Drugs and Pregnancy

Many of the following chapters refer to the US FDA pregnancy category ratings for the teratogenicity of a drug, which are currently set out as follows:

Category A
Adequate and well-controlled studies have failed to demonstrate a risk to the fetus in the first trimester of pregnancy, and there is no evidence of risk in later trimesters.

Category B
Animal reproduction studies have failed to demonstrate a risk to the fetus, but there are no adequate and well-controlled studies in pregnant women.

Category C
Animal reproduction studies have shown an adverse effect on the fetus: there are no adequate and well-controlled studies in humans, but potential benefits may warrant use of the drug in pregnant women despite potential risks.

Category D
There is positive evidence of human fetal risk based on adverse reaction data from investigational or marketing experience or studies in humans, but potential benefits may warrant use of the drug in pregnant women despite potential risks.

Category X
Studies in animals or humans have demonstrated fetal abnormalities and/or there is positive evidence of human fetal risk based on adverse reaction data from investigational or marketing experience; the risks involved in use of the drug in pregnant women clearly outweigh potential benefits.

However, this classification has been proposed for review as some feel it is potentially misleading, and the reader is therefore advised to consult their pharmacists for the latest safety information when considering the use of a drug during pregnancy or during breastfeeding.

Contents

Contributors

Rustam Al-Shahi Salman Division of Clinical Neurosciences, Western General Hospital, University of Edinburgh, Edinburgh, U.K.

James Arden Department of Anaesthesiology, King's College Hospital, London, U.K.

Simon J. B. Aylwin Department of Endocrinology, King's College Hospital, London, U.K.

Iskandar Azwa Infectious Diseases Directorate, Faculty of Medicine, University of Malaya, Kuala Lumpur, Malaysia

Anish Bahra National Hospital for Neurology and Neurosurgery and Whipps Cross University Hospital, London, U.K.

Dave Berry Medical Toxicology Unit, Guy's Hospital, London, U.K.

David P. Breen Cambridge Centre for Brain Repair (Barker Group), Department of Clinical Neurosciences, University of Cambridge, Cambridge, U.K.

Peter A. Brex Department of Neurology, King's College Hospital, London, U.K.

Neil G. Burnet Neuro-Oncology Unit, Oncology Centre, Addenbrooke's Hospital, and Department of Oncology, University of Cambridge, Cambridge, U.K.

Katherine E. Burton Neuro-Oncology Unit, Oncology Centre, Addenbrooke's Hospital, Cambridge, U.K.

K. Ray Chaudhuri Institute of Psychiatry, London, U.K.

Matthew Crocker Department of Neurosurgery, King's College Hospital, London, U.K.

Jayaram K. Dasan Department of Anaesthesia, King's College Hospital, London, U.K.

Robert Delamont Department of Neurology, King's College Hospital, London, U.K.

William Dennes Department of Maternal-Fetal Medicine, King's College Hospital, London, U.K.

Dorota Dworakowska Department of Endocrinology, King's College Hospital, London, U.K.

Nicholas Gall Department of Cardiology, King's College Hospital, London, U.K.

Robert D. M. Hadden Department of Neurology, King's College Hospital, London, U.K.

Thomas W. Hale Department of Pediatrics, Texas Tech University Health Sciences Center, School of Medicine, Amarillo, Texas, U.S.A.

Fiona Harris Neuro-Oncology Unit, Oncology Centre, Addenbrooke's Hospital, Cambridge, U.K.

Peter Haughton School of Medicine, King's College London, London, U.K.

David A. Hawkins Directorate of Genitourinary and HIV Medicine, Chelsea and Westminster Hospital, London, U.K.

Jozef Jarosz Department of Neuroradiology, King's College Hospital, London, U.K.

Sarah J. Jefferies Neuro-Oncology Unit, Oncology Centre, Addenbrooke's Hospital, Cambridge, U.K.

Rajesh Jena Neuro-Oncology Unit, Oncology Centre, Addenbrooke's Hospital, Cambridge, U.K.

Dragana J. Josifova Department of Clinical Genetics, Guy's Hospital, London, U.K.

Catharina J. M. Klijn Department of Neurology, University Medical Center, Utrecht, The Netherlands

Sara Lailey Epilepsy Nurse Specialist, King's College Hospital, London, U.K.

Michael S. Marsh Department of Obstetrics and Gynaecology, King's College Hospital, London, U.K.

Victoria A. Mifsud Department of Neurology, King's College Hospital, London, U.K.

Nicholas Moran Department of Neurology, King's College Hospital, London, U.K.

John Moriarty Department of Psychological Medicine, King's College Hospital, London, U.K.

Lorraine Muffett Neuro-Oncology Unit, Oncology Centre, Addenbrooke's Hospital, Cambridge, U.K.

Yogini Naidu National Parkinson Foundation Centre of Excellence, King's College Hospital, London, U.K.

Lina A. M. Nashef Department of Neurology, King's College Hospital, London, U.K.

Fiona Norwood Department of Neurology, King's College Hospital, London, U.K.

Clemens Pahl Division of Intensive Care Medicine, King's College Hospital, London, U.K.

Prashanth Reddy Department of Neurology, University Hospital Lewisham and King's College London, London, U.K.

Mark P. Richardson Institute of Epileptology, Institute of Psychiatry, London, U.K.

Paul Riordan-Eva Department of Ophthalmology, King's College Hospital, London, U.K.

David N. Rushton Frank Cooksey Rehabilitation Unit, King's College Hospital, London, U.K.

Trudi Seneviratne Section of Perinatal Psychiatry, Institute of Psychiatry, London, U.K.

Pauline Shaw Nurse Specialist, King's College Hospital, London, U.K.

Roy A. Sherwood Department of Clinical Biochemistry, King's College Hospital, London, U.K.

Nicholas Thomas Department of Neurosurgery, King's College Hospital, London, U.K.

Hannah Turton School of Medicine, King's College London, London, U.K.

Daniel Walsh Department of Neurosurgery, King's College Hospital, London, U.K.

Francessa Wilson Department of Neuroradiology, King's College Hospital, London, U.K.

Neurogenetics and pregnancy

Dragana J. Josifova

INTRODUCTION

Neurogenetics has been one of the most intensively researched areas in medicine over the last few decades, a time which has seen an exponential growth in our knowledge of the molecular basis of health and diseases. A number of genes associated with neurological disorders have been identified and we are beginning to understand the complex network of molecular pathways involved in the development, function and maintenance of the nervous system. Diagnostically useful genetic tests for some paediatric and adult-onset neurological disorders have become readily available. Pre-symptomatic and prenatal tests can now be offered and, for some conditions, pre-implantation genetic diagnosis has become possible. This chapter outlines basic principles as well as many illustrative examples.

Genetic Code

There are approximately 25,000 genes in the nucleus of a human cell. Each gene is represented by a unique DNA code. Individual genes are strung by repetitive DNA sequences into condensed stretches of DNA called chromosomes. There are 46 chromosomes in the human genome arranged in 23 pairs, with one member of the pair coming from each parent (Fig. 1.1). One set of 23 chromosomes constitutes the haploid number; the normal chromosome complement is diploid.

The first 22 pairs are autosomal chromosomes (numbered from 1 to 22) and the 23rd pair comprises the sex chromosomes, X and Y. Males are hemizygous for the genes on the X chromosome (they have only one copy of these genes). In females, one of the X chromosomes is randomly inactivated to preclude over expression. Each chromosome carries hundreds of genes. The genes, like chromosomes, come in pairs with the exception of the genes on the X and Y chromosomes in males. Males inherit their X chromosome genes from their mothers and their Y chromosome genes from their fathers.

CHROMOSOME REARRANGEMENTS

The normal chromosome complement may be altered in number or individual chromosome structure. Regardless of the mechanism, a chromosome rearrangement may lead to a gain or loss of genetic material. This is frequently associated with phenotypic consequences: from mild learning difficulties to a complex picture including restricted intrauterine and post-natal growth, unusual physical features (dysmorphic features), structural abnormalities of organs and systems, epilepsy and significant disability. Pregnancies affected with chromosomal abnormalities are at increased risk of miscarriage.

1. *Rearrangements affecting chromosome number*
   a. *Aneuploidy*
      Aneuploidy means that the chromosome complement does not equal a multiple of the haploid number of chromosomes. Common aneuploidies are the triso-mies: Down syndrome (trisomy 21), Patau syndrome (trisomy 13), Edward syndrome (trisomy 18). Aneuploidies involving other autosomal chromosomes are not viable and usually result in early miscarriage. Aneuploidies involving the sex chromosomes are relatively common. With the exception of Turner syndrome (45,X), they are not associated with early pre- and post-natal recognisable phenotype.
   b. *Polyploidy*
      Polyploidy implies that there are more than two full haploid sets of chromosomes, for example, triploidy (69 chromosomes) or tertraploidy (92 chromosomes). These are usually associated with early miscarriage; however, live birth is possible if the polyploidy is in a mosaic pattern with a cell line which has a normal chromosome complement.

2. *Structural chromosome rearrangements*
   a. *Chromosome translocations, deletions and duplications*
      When portions of two or more chromosomes exchange places, but the total amount of genetic material remained unchanged, the rearrangement is called a balanced translocation (Fig. 1.2). About 1 in 500 healthy individuals carries a balanced chromosome rearrangement. Carriers of balanced chromosome rearrangements, although healthy, are at risk of passing the rearrangement on to their offspring in an unbalanced fashion. Unbalanced chromosome rearrangements are characterised by a deficit or excess of genetic material. Pregnancies affected with structural chromosome rearrangements have an increased risk of miscarriage.

      If both parents have normal chromosomes, a chromosome rearrangement identified in their offspring is considered to be de novo. The risk of recurrence of a de novo rearrangement in future pregnancies is low, approximately 1%, due to the possibility of germline mosaicism.

      Germline mosaicism means coexistence of gametes with normal and abnormal chromosome complement or normal and mutated single gene. Somatic mosaicism, however, concerns tissues other than the reproductive ones. Both, germline and somatic mosaicism arise as a result of a post-zygotic event. Somatic mosaicism may sometimes be identified in the DNA extracted from peripheral lymphocytes, but it is more likely to be found in chromosomes/DNA from solid tissue, for example, skin.

      If one parent carries a balanced translocation, the risk of miscarriage and the risk of having a child with unbalanced chromosome rearrangement vary depending on the nature of the rearrangement. De novo, apparently balanced translocations identified at prenatal diagnosis (PND) carry a risk of abnormalities up

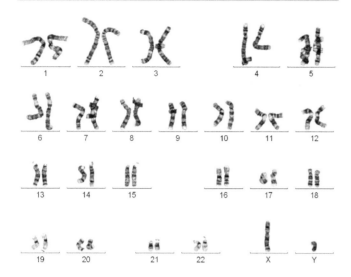

Figure 1.1   Normal male chromosome complement.

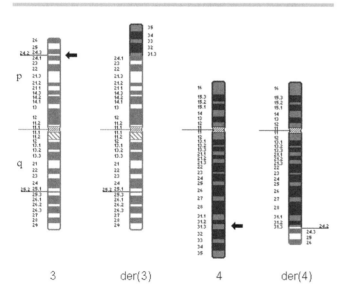

3   der(3)   4   der(4)

Figure 1.2   Balanced translocation between chromosomes 3 and 4.

to 10%, because of cryptic deletions/duplications at the break points or disruption of important genes.

b. *Robertsonian translocation*

Robertsonian chromosome translocations (RTs) involve only the acrocentric chromosomes: 13, 14, 15, 21 and 22. Acrocentric chromosomes have very small short (p) arm, coding DNA. The RT arises when two acrocentric chromosomes fuse at the centromere, each having lost their short (p) arm, to form a recombinant chromosome made up of the long arms of the chromosomes involved in the translocation (Fig. 1.3). The diploid number is therefore reduced by one chromosome and equals 45. As no coding DNA has been lost or gained, the carriers of RT do not exhibit any abnormalities. However, these translocations usually

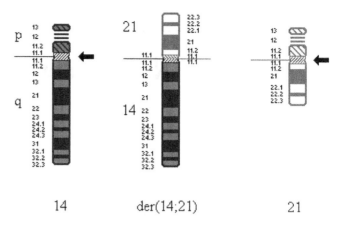

14   der(14;21)   21

Figure 1.3   Balanced Robertsonian translocation between chromosomes 14 and 21.

have reproductive implications. RTs often lead to chromosome imbalance in the offspring and predispose to early miscarriage. Males with RTs may have reduced fertility.

SINGLE GENE DISORDERS

The DNA sequence of a gene is a template for protein synthesis. A change in the DNA sequence (mutation) alters the template and interferes with protein synthesis. Depending on the nature of the mutation, protein synthesis may be completely abolished or a structurally or functionally abnormal protein may be produced.

Patterns of Inheritance

1. *Autosomal dominant* (AD) conditions are caused by an alteration in only one of the two copies of a particular gene. The offspring of an individual who carries a mutation in only one copy of a gene have a 50% chance of inheriting either the altered or the healthy gene. The inheritance of AD conditions is independent of the gender of either the parent or the offspring.

   AD genes have two important characteristics:
   a. *Variable expression*. This implies that the severity of phenotype between and within families may vary considerably. For example, the age at which individuals who carry mutations in the spastin gene, associated with AD spastic paraplegia, become symptomatic is highly variable, from childhood to well into adult life.
   b. *Variable penetrance* refers to the likelihood of any phenotypic features manifesting in those who carry a pathogenic mutation. For example, the Huntington disease gene is fully penetrant: all individuals who carry the mutation will develop the condition although the age of onset may vary. However, the breast/ovarian cancer predisposing genes (*BRCA1* and *BRCA2*) have reduced penetrance, as not all mutation carriers develop cancer in their lifetime.

A de novo gene mutation occurring in a gamete (sperm or egg) will affect all the cells of the embryo. Conditions like tuberous sclerosis and neurofibromatosis 1 and 2 have a high new mutation rate; therefore, a significant proportion of patients do not have a relevant family history. A new mutation may

Table 1.1 Risk Assessment in Autosomal Recessive Disorders

At conception		
Phenotype	Genotype	Risk
Affected	aa	1 in 4
Carrier	Aa	1 in 2
Not carrier	AA	1 in 4

Abbreviations: A, normal allele; a, allele carrying mutation.

also arise in an embryo as a post-zygotic event. When this occurs, the mutation will be present in some, but not all, cells. This is known as somatic mosaicism and usually gives rise to a milder form of the condition. The severity of phenotype depends on both the percentage and distribution of cells carrying the mutation. The level of mosaicism may vary in different tissues. A genetic test on blood lymphocytes does not necessarily identify or reflect the level of mosaicism in other tissues (e.g., skin or brain tissue) and may not be an accurate predictor of the phenotype.

2. *Autosomal recessive* (AR) conditions arise when both copies of a gene carry a pathogenic mutation. Both parents of individuals affected by AR conditions are almost always carriers. The presence of the same mutation on both copies of the gene is referred to as homozygosity and is more likely to be seen in consanguineous families. Two different mutations in the same gene imply double or compound heterozygosity.

    If both parents are carriers of a mutation in the same, AR gene, then, at conception, there is a 1 in 4 chance of both passing on faulty copies of the gene and having an affected child regardless of the child's sex. There is a 1 in 4 chance of the embryo inheriting two normal copies of the gene and a 50% chance of inheriting only one abnormal copy of the gene conferring a carrier status similar in both parents (Table 1.1).

    There is an increasing recognition of conditions caused by mutations in two different genes (digenic inheritance), which may, although not necessarily, be in the same pathway. For example, holoprosencephaly (a developmental abnormality associated with incomplete separation of the forebrain into two hemispheres) can be caused by simultaneous mutations in both the Sonic Hedgehog (*SHH*) gene (Sonic Hedgehog pathway) and *TGIF* gene (Nodal pathway) (see page 5).

3. *X-linked disorders* result from mutations in genes on the X chromosome. According to the traditional Mendelian teaching, they cause disease in males (X-linked recessive) because of their hemizygous state (having only one copy of X chromosome genes). Female carriers should remain symptom free because of the compensatory effect of the functional copy of the gene on their second X chromosome. X-linked dominant conditions, by contrast, present in females and males, and may be lethal for male embryos (Rett syndrome, Incontinentia pigmenti, Aicardi syndrome).

    However, it is well recognised that females may be manifesting carriers of X-linked recessive disorders and exhibit a wide variety of phenotypic features, from very mild to virtually the full clinical spectrum as seen in affected males (Duchenne/Becker muscular dystrophy). One of the explanations for this is non-random (skewed) X-inactivation. However, X-linked dominant conditions associated with lethality in male fetuses have been seen in male newborn babies, albeit rarely. Affected boys usually have severe phenotype and prolonged survival is rare. For example, Rett syndrome in boys is associated with severe neonatal encephalopathy, unlike in females who, following a period of relative normality in infancy, present with global developmental delay, microcephaly and characteristic behavioural phenotype.

    Therefore, the distinction between X-linked recessive and X-linked dominant disorders is not as strict, which is why the term X-linked disorders (genes) is more commonly used.

    Carrier females of X-linked conditions have a 1 in 2 chance of passing the gene onto their sons and 1 in 2 chance of having carrier girls. At conception, therefore, there is a 25% chance of having an affected offspring.

4. *Mitochondrial disorders* arise by mutations in the mitochondrial DNA (mtDNA) which is exclusively inherited from the mother. MtDNA is different from nuclear DNA and contains only about 30 genes. There are several copies of mtDNA in each mitochondrion and a number of mitochondria in each cell. A mutation may be present in some but not necessarily all mtDNA copies. The combination of normal and mitochondria carrying a mutation is known as heteroplasmy. The ratio between the altered and normal mtDNA determines the mutation load. The severity of phenotype correlates with the mutation load although it is likely that other, modifying genes in conjunction with the environment also contribute to the phenotypic diversity of the disorders caused by mutated mtDNA.

    A large number of nuclear genes regulate mitochondrial function and maintenance. These are transmitted in an AR or AD fashion. Consequently, the majority of mitochondrial disorders are caused by mutations in the nuclear genome, and may carry a 25% or 50% recurrence risk, respectively, in every pregnancy.

FAMILY HISTORY OF NEUROLOGICAL DISORDER
Epilepsy

Epilepsy is the most common neurological disorder requiring long-term and sometimes lifelong treatment. In one study, it was reported to affect 4/1000 people in the United Kingdom (1). The prevalence among women of childbearing age is estimated to be between 6.9 and 7.8 per 1000 (2). Aetiologically this is a very heterogeneous group; a proportion of cases are genetic.

The risk to any child of a mother with epilepsy is related to any potential genetic cause to maternal epilepsy and the effect of the intrauterine exposure to anti-epileptic drugs (AEDs).

Monogenic, AD epilepsy syndromes, for example, *SCN1A*-related Dravet syndrome, in either parent will incur a 50% risk of gene transmission; however, the degree of severity may be very variable. Epilepsy caused by mutations in an X-linked gene, for instance, *FLNA*-related periventricular nodular heterotopia (PNH)_ in the mother, will incur a 50% risk of transmission, with significantly reduced viability of male fetuses; hence the risk of epilepsy would apply largely to the daughters of a carrier mother. By contrast, *PDH19* gene is a gene on the X chromosome, mutations in which cause epilepsy in females; carrier males usually do not develop a seizure disorder, but are at increased risk of psychiatric illness.

It is recommendable that a potential genetic diagnosis is explored and the risk of epilepsy and teratogenic effects of AEDs or fetal anti-convulsant syndrome (FACS) are discussed prior to conception. If a disease-causing mutation is known, PND or pre-implantation genetic diagnosis may be available. Prospective parents should be given the opportunity to discuss these issues with a clinical geneticist to enable them to make an informed choice.

Fetal Anti-convulsant Syndrome

FACS refers to the teratogenic effects, including congenital malformations, dysmorphic facial features and developmental and behavioural difficulties, in children prenatally exposed to AEDs (3). This is also discussed in chapter 12.

Approximately 1 in 250 pregnancies is exposed to sodium valproate, carbamazepine, phenytoin, lamotrigine or a combination of AEDs. Studies have consistently shown a two- to three fold. Increase in the incidence of congenital anomalies (Table 1.2) in fetuses exposed to AEDs compared to a non-exposed group (Table 1.3). The highest incidence is associated with sodium valproate exposure and polytherapy, and the lowest with carbamazepine monotherapy (4,5). A dose-related effect has been seen with sodium valproate, with another study suggesting a dose-related effect with lamotrigine (chapter 12).

The highest prevalence of facial dysmorphic features (Table 1.4) is seen in the sodium valproate monotherapy group with a significant positive correlation between the severity of facial dysmorphic features and verbal IQ (4).

Table 1.2 Congenital Anomalies Associated with FACS

Major congenital malformations in FACS in order of frequency
Cardiovascular
Musculoskeletal
Cleft lip and/or palate
Neural tube defect
Structural brain malformations
Exomphalos
Reduction limb defects

Abbreviation: FACS, fetal anti-convulsant syndrome.

Table 1.3 Incidence of Major Congenital Anomalies in Pregnancies Exposed to AEDs in Selected Studies

	Kini et al., 2006 (4)	Meador et al., 2008 (5)
All births	6%	7.08%
Monotherapy, overall	–	5.30%
Carbamazepine	5%	5%
Sodium valproate	14%	17.64%
Polytherapy	5%	9.84%

Abbreviation: AEDs, anti-epileptic drugs.

Table 1.4 Dysmorphic Features in FACS

Facial features in FACS
• Bi-temporal narrowing
• Metopic ridge
• Upslanting palpebral fissures
• Hypertelorism
• Epicanthic folds
• Flat nasal bridge
• Infra-orbital creases
• Mid-facial flattening
• Long, poorly formed philtrum
• Thin upper lip

Abbreviation: FACS, fetal anti-convulsant syndrome.

The risk of long-term effect of antenatal exposure to AEDs on development, learning and behaviour has been controversial and difficult to establish due to ascertainment bias, inconsistent assessment strategies and length of follow-up. A 24% overall incidence of learning difficulties in the prenatally exposed children compared to 11% in non-exposed siblings was reported by Dean et al. (3); however, when only the children from families without history of learning difficulties were assessed, 19% of those exposed to AEDs presented with cognitive impairment compared to 3% of their non-exposed siblings (3). These figures are considerably higher than demonstrated in the more recent studies (4,5). After adjustment for maternal IQ, maternal age, AED dose, gestational age at birth and maternal preconception use of folate, at the age of 3 years the children exposed to valproate had an IQ score 9 points lower than the score of those exposed to lamotrigine, 7 points lower than the score of those exposed to phenytoin and 6 points lower than the score of the children exposed to carbamazepine (6) highlighting the highest risk of cognitive function impairment in children prenatally exposed to valproate in a dose-dependent fashion.

The prevalence of combined autistic spectrum and autistic disorder of 1.9% and 4.6%, respectively, in children exposed in utero to AEDs (7) is higher compared to 0.25% in a population-based survey in the United Kingdom using DSM-IV clinical criteria (8).

Confounding factors, including parental IQ, family history of learning and/or behavioural difficulties, autism or speech delay, may influence the neurodevelopmental pattern independently or concomitantly with the potential effects of prenatal AEDs exposure. In this context it is important to consider the possibility of a genetic aetiology of epilepsy in the mother who could present with variable phenotype including cognitive impairment.

The diagnosis of FACS is usually made by the clinical geneticists based on the maternal medical history, child's physical features and developmental pattern.

Preconception counselling should be offered to women of childbearing age to enable them to understand the risks of FACS and make an informed decision. Monotherapy and use of drugs with less teratogenic potential should be considered. However, the majority of epileptic mothers will give birth to a healthy child and the risk of FACS should be balanced against the risk associated with poor seizure control in pregnancy.

Tuberous Sclerosis Complex

Tuberous sclerosis complex (TSC) is an AD, multi-system disorder. The diagnosis is usually clinical and based on major and minor disease criteria (9). About 70% of affected individuals have seizures and a significant proportion have some degree of learning difficulties, behavioural problems and increased susceptibility to psychiatric illness. TSC causes a reduced life expectancy primarily because of CNS tumours and renal disease.

Nearly 60% of affected fetuses develop a cardiac rhabdomyoma. These are rarely seen before the third trimester and are therefore not helpful for early PND. They have a good prognosis and spontaneously resolve in the first few years of life. Active management is only required if they cause outflow obstruction, but if this is not the case at birth, it is highly unlikely that it will develop later.

Post-natally, the diagnosis is made on clinical grounds. As the features evolve over time the findings may not necessarily meet the diagnostic criteria early on and molecular

Table 1.5 Expansion Mutation in MD and Associated Phenotype

Allele size	Phenotype
5–34 (normal)	Healthy
35–49 (permutation)	Unaffected
50–100	Mild phenotype
100–1000 (expansion)	Classical MD
>2000 (expansion)	Congenital MD

Abbreviation: MD, myotonic dystrophy.

Table 1.6 Causes of Microcephaly

Cause	Inheritance/Comments
Genetic (Isolated)	AD, variable, mild/moderate delay to near normal for the family cognitive function
	AR, usually more severe and of prenatal onset
	X-linked, variable phenotype
Syndromic[a]	Chromosomal abnormalities (1p36 deletion)
	Microdeletion syndromes (Miller–Dieker syndrome)
	Single gene disorders (AD, AR and XL)
Environmental	Congenital infection (TORCH)
	Alcohol in pregnancy [Fetal alcohol syndrome (FAS)]
	Maternal phenylketonuria

[a]Microcephaly may be associated with
1. CNS abnormalities (agenesis of the corpus callosum, abnormal neuronal migration, cerebellar hypoplasia)
2. Extracranial abnormities (growth failure, congenital heart defect, structural eye abnormalities)
Abbreviations: AD, autosomal dominant; AR, autosomal recessive; XL, X-linked; TORCH, Toxoplasmosis, Rubella, Cytomegalovirus, Herpes simplex.

analysis may occasionally be undertaken to confirm the diagnosis.

The condition is caused by mutations in one of the two genes: *TSC1* and *TSC2*. Nearly two-thirds of cases represent a new mutation. The gene is considered fully penetrant, although the severity is highly variable within and between families. In some cases, a parent was diagnosed as having TSC only after a diagnosis was made in their child. The extent of clinical features is not a precise predictor of the disease severity, especially not in regard to the epilepsy and cognitive/behavioural phenotype.

The risk to a sibling of a singleton case is approximately 1%, assuming that the parents do not manifest any features of TSC on careful clinical examination by a trained professional, and that their ophthalmological examination and renal ultrasound scan are normal. The residual risk is due to germline mosaicism.

Molecular analysis of *TSC1* and *TSC2* genes identifies mutations in approximately 60% of clinically diagnosed cases. PND by gene testing is available if the disease-causing mutation in the proband has been confirmed. It is however not possible to predict the severity of the condition.

Myotonic Dystrophy

Myotonic dystrophy (MD) is an AD, multi-system disorder caused by a CTG triplet repeat expansion in the *DMPK* gene. The age of onset and disease severity correlate to some degree with the size of the expanded allele.

The expanded allele is unstable and tends to expand further when it is passed from one generation to the next (genomic anticipation) (Table 1.5). This phenomenon occurs more commonly in female meiosis. Congenital MD (caused by a large CTG repeat expansion) is rarely seen in the offspring of affected males.

Features of congenital MD include reduced fetal movements, contractures and polyhydramnios and may be detected prenatally. Affected neonates present with muscle weakness, hypotonia and respiratory difficulties. Congenital MD is associated with significant morbidity and mortality.

PND is available, but the disease severity is difficult to predict; large expansions of 500 or more CTG repeats are likely to cause congenital MD.

GENETIC IMPLICATIONS OF ABNORMAL ANTENATAL NEUROIMAGING

Antenatally identified brain abnormalities are always a considerable cause of concern for parents, and providing an aetiological diagnosis and prognosis is challenging for clinicians. CNS abnormality may be isolated or associated with cerebral or extracranial abnormalities. However, regardless of any associated abnormalities, the CNS malformation may be the major predictor of long-term outcome.

Microcephaly

Microcephaly is defined as head circumference of two or more standard deviations below the mean. It should be taken into the context of the other fetal growth parameters as well as the head circumference of both parents. Environmental and genetic causes, syndromic and non-syndromic, should be considered in the differential diagnosis. The prognosis for the pregnancy and long-term development depends on the underlying cause (Table 1.6).

Holoprosencephaly

Holoprosencephaly (HPE) is the most common neurodevelopmental disorder arising as a consequence of the failure of the forebrain to divide into two individual hemispheres and ventricles. HPE has a prevalence of 1 in 250 embryos and 1 in 10,000 births. The extent of the brain malformation is variable and mild cases are difficult to detect by antenatal ultrasound scan.

Associated brain abnormalities include absent corpus callosum, absent septum pellucidum, absent or hypoplastic olfactory bulbs and tracts (arrhinencephaly) and optic bulbs and tracts, microcephaly, hydrocephalus, Dandy–Walker malformation and neuronal migration anomalies. Craniofacial abnormalities are seen in about 80% of patients ranging from severe, such as cyclopia and arrhinencephaly, to ocular hypotelorism, choanal stenosis, cleft lip and palate and single central incisor.

HPE is an aetiologically heterogeneous (Table 1.7) and phenotypically very variable condition. Virtually all individuals with abnormal cranial imaging have developmental delay, the degree of which is comparable to the severity of HPE. HPE microforms refer to the presence of mild craniofacial features (hypotelorism, ptosis, cleft palate, choanal stenosis, single central incisor) and are less likely to be associated with significant developmental delay. The recurrence risk depends on the underlying cause.

SHH gene product is the key signalling molecule in patterning of the ventral neural tube (10), the anterior-posterior limb axis (11) and the ventral somites (12). Whole gene deletions (chromosome 7q36) and point mutations are

Table 1.7   Aetiology of Holoprosencephaly

Aetiology	Condition	Comments
Chromosomal 25–50%	Aneuploidies: Trisomy 13 Trisomy 18 Structural chromosomal abnormalities: 13q deletion 18p deletion 7q deletion 13p duplication 2p deletion	Sporadic unless parent carrier of balanced chromosome rearrangement
Monogenic (non-syndromic) 25–40%	Sonic hedgehog signalling: *SHH, PTCH, GLI2* Nodal/TGF signalling: *TDGF1, FAST1, TGIF SIX3* and *ZIC2*	Monogenic with reduced penetrance Concomitant heterozygous mutations in two different genes in same or different pathways
Syndromic 18–25%	Smith–Lemli–Opitz Meckel Palister–Hall Rubinstein–Taybi	AR AR AD AD
Environmental	Maternal diabetes Alcohol Retinoic acid Cholesterol-lowering drugs	

Abbreviations: AR, autosomal recessive; AD, autosomal dominant.

implicated in the AD HPE with variable expression and reduced penetrance. A heterozygous mutation in this gene in conjunction with a heterozygous mutation in one of the genes involved in the nodal/TGF signalling pathway may give rise to HPE in non-Mendelian, digenic constellation.

Agenesis of the Corpus Callosum

Agenesis of the corpus callosum (ACC) consists of complete or partial absence of the white matter fibres that cross the midline between the two hemispheres (13). This is one of the most frequent brain malformations with an incidence of 0.5 to 70 per 10,000 (14). The incidence of ACC in children with developmental delay is estimated at 2% to 3% (15).

ACC may present as isolated condition or in association with additional CNS abnormalities such as abnormalities of neuronal migration and cortical development, including polymicrogyria (PMG), pachygyria, lissencephaly and heterotopias, as well as HPE, Dandy–Walker malformation, Chiari malformation and schizencephaly (15).

ACC is aetiologically heterogeneous. It can be caused by extrinsic factors such as maternal alcohol use in pregnancy or maternal phenylketonuria. It may also be associated with, usually unbalanced, chromosome rearrangements or part of an AD (HPE), AR (acrocallosal syndrome – duplicated hallux, postaxial polydactyly, aganesis/hypoplasia of the CC, dysmorphic features) or X-linked (Aicardi syndrome – ACC with chorioretinal abnormality) syndrome.

Fetal MRI is recommended to look for any additional CNS abnormalities, the identification of which could facilitate an aetiological diagnosis in about 25% of cases (16,17). (see chapter 3).

The prognosis for neurodevelopmental outcome in children with isolated ACC appears to be good in approximately 50% of patients although some may have transient difficulties such as neonatal hypotonia and speech delay. Approximately 25% of cases of isolated ACC may have mild to moderate learning and behavioural difficulties. Severe disability is usually associated with additional brain abnormalities, although these may not always be identifiable antenatally (15).

These figures should be used with caution as the available studies have limitations because of ascertainment bias and lack of standardised assessment protocol and long-term follow-up.

Ventriculomegaly

Ventriculomegaly (VM) indicates the presence of excess fluid in the lateral ventricles of the developing brain. Hydrocephalus is associated with raised intracranial pressure (ICP) and given that it is not possible to measure it in utero, the term VM is used in reference to fetal ventricular enlargement (18).

VM is diagnosed prenatally by means of ultrasound scan when the atrium width is larger than 10 mm, measured on transverse view just above the thalami (which corresponds to 4SD above the mean), from 14 weeks gestation to term (19). It is considered severe if the atrium width is larger than 15 mm, moderate between 12 and 15 mm and mild/borderline between 10 and 12 mm.

The incidence of VM ranges from 0.5 to 2 per 1000 births; isolated VM is seen in 0.4 to 0.9 per 1000 births (18). Associated abnormalities are reported in 70% to 83% of cases, 60% of which are extracranial (19,20).

VM is aetiologically heterogeneous and its natural history is variable. Amongst the non-genetic causes, congenital infection (Cytomegalovirus, *Toxoplasma gondii*, herpes simplex, although the latter is very rare with only about 100 cases reported in the literature) is identified in approximately 10% to 20% of cases of isolated, severe VM (21,22). Intracranial/intraventricular haemorrhage with consequent obstruction of the cerebrospinal fluid flow should also be considered, especially if VM occurs in the context of alloimmune thrombocytopenia (23), but it is otherwise rare.

Genetic causes include chromosomal abnormalities, AR, AD and X-linked syndromic conditions. Unbalanced chromosome abnormalities may be found in about 15% of cases of isolated mild/severe VM in the presence of other, intra- or extracranial abnormalities (Tables 1.8–1.10) (20). More than 100 single gene disorders may present prenatally with VM.

Table 1.8 Structural Abnormalities Associated with VM in Order of Frequency

Structural abnormalities	Frequency (%)
Aqueductal stenosis	30–40
Chiari II malformation	25–30
Callosal dysgenesis	20–30
Dandy–Walker complex	7–10
Other	5–10

Abbreviation: VM, ventriculomegaly. *Source*: From Ref. 24.

Table 1.9 Frequency of Chromosomal Abnormalities Associated with VM

VM	Abnormal chromosomes	
	Nicolaides et al., 2007	Weichert et al., 2010 (25)
Isolated	3–6%	Not reported
VM + other congenital abnormalities	25–36%	4.6%

Abbreviation: VM, ventriculomegaly.

Table 1.10 Syndromes Associated with VM

Syndrome	Inheritance	Features
Miller–Dieker syndrome	Microdeletion	Severe lissencephaly, microcephaly
Walker–Warburg syndrome	AR	Encephalocele, lissencephaly, myopathy
Seckel syndrome	AR	Microcephaly, intrauterine growth restriction
Apert syndrome	AD	Craniosynostosis, syndactyly of fingers and toes
Smith–Lemli–Opitz syndrome	AR	Microcephaly, urogenital abnormalities
Aicardi syndrome	X-linked	Agenesis of the corpus callosum

Abbreviations: AR, autosomal recessive; AD, autosomal dominant.

Aqueduct stenosis is the most common structural brain abnormality leading to VM (24). It may be secondary to congenital infection or intracerebral/intraventricular haemorrhage associated with aqueduct narrowing by a blood clot/scar. About 5% of cases are caused by mutations in the *L1CAM* gene on the X chromosome and are therefore more likely to affect males.

Fetuses with severe VM have a 2.2-fold (isolated VM) and 3.6-fold (VM associated with other abnormalities) increased risk of progressive dilatation compared to mild VM (25). Fetuses with asymmetrical bilateral isolated VM are more likely to have severe ventricular enlargements (25).

The outcome for the pregnancy and for long-term development depends on the severity of VM, underlying aetiology and the presence of associated abnormalities. Isolated, mild VM with normal chromosome analysis is expected to have good outcome in nearly 90% of cases (22,25). The risk of abnormal neurodevelopmental outcome is highest in the presence of associated anomalies irrespective of the degree of dilatation (91%) and in cases with severe isolated VM (68%) (25).

Severe VM develops with progression of the pregnancy and is therefore often diagnosed in the late second or third trimester and it is more likely to be associated with additional abnormalities indicating a poor prognosis (20).

Table 1.11 Causes of Structural Brain Abnormalities

Aetiology	Frequency (%)
Chromosomal	6
Single gene disorders	7.5
Polygenic/multi-factorial	20
Environmental/Teratogens	5
Unknown	>60

Abnormalities of Neuronal Migration and Cortical Development

Neuronal migration disorders and cortical dysplasia are the cause of severe, refractory epilepsy and global developmental delay in about 25% of cases (26). Conceptuses are at high risk of intrauterine death (IUD). Forty percent of infant mortality is caused by consequences of abnormal development of the CNS and the long-term morbidity, including developmental delay and epilepsy, has significant impact on the affected individual, family and the society. The aetiology is heterogeneous and summarised in Table 1.11.

Lissencephaly spectrum

Lissencephaly entails a continuum of abnormalities, from complete absence of gyri (agyria) to the presence of larger and fewer gyri (pachygyria). It is always associated with thickening of the cortex which is identifiable by MRI imaging. There is an increased incidence of ACC and cerebellar hypoplasia. AR and X-linked genes have been implicated. Some genotype/phenotype correlation has been observed.

Miller–Dieker syndrome. Miller–Dieker syndrome (MDS) is associated with severe lissencephaly, affecting the whole hemispheres, microcephaly and dysmorphic features. It is caused by a contiguous gene deletion of the terminal short arm of chromosome 17 (del17p13.3). Majority of cases are sporadic implying a low recurrence risk of 1%. Occasionally, the deletion arises as a consequence of a balanced chromosome rearrangement in one of the parents. This confers an increased recurrence risk for future pregnancies, the magnitude of which depends on the nature of chromosome abnormality in the parent.

Subcortical band heterotopia/DCX-related lissencephaly in males. Subcortical band heterotopia (SBH) is an X-linked disorder caused by mutations in the *DCX* gene on the X chromosome. The disorder primarily affects heterozygous females. The clinical picture ranges from mild learning difficulties to severe seizure disorder and developmental delay, depending on the extent of brain abnormality. Affected males present with lissencephaly, usually with an anterior to posterior gradient, severe global delay and infantile spasms. There is a 10% risk of germline mosaicism in mothers who test negative for the mutation identified in their affected son. Carrier female have a 25% risk of having an affected offspring at conception; if the offspring is male there is a 50% chance it will be affected.

Periventricular Nodular Heterotopia

PNH is a rare form of neuronal migration disorder presenting in females with uncalcified nodules of neurons subependymal to the lateral ventricles. It is caused by inactivating mutations in the filamin A (*FLNA*) gene on the X chromosome. Affected male fetuses are usually not viable and die prenatally or in the neonatal period. The obstetric history of a carrier woman may reveal multiple miscarriages.

Eighty-eight percent of heterozygous females present with seizures (27) at an average age of 14 to 15 years, which in majority of cases have focal character. The severity may be variable, from rare seizure episodes not requiring medication to severe, difficult-to-treat epilepsy. Intelligence ranges from normal to borderline. The extent of radiological findings is variable and does not predict the severity of clinical phenotype.

The incidence of congenital heart disease (patent ductus arteriosus and bicuspid aortic valve) appears to be increased and stroke in young women has also been reported. The true frequency of the cardiovascular phenotype is not entirely clear and larger studies are required (28).

FLNA is currently the only known gene associated with PNH. Mutations are found in about 25% of singleton cases indicating that the condition is genetically heterogeneous. The mutation detection rate in clear X-linked pedigrees approaches 100%.

Mutations in *FLNA* are associated with four other phenotypes: oto-palato-digital syndrome type 1 and 2 (OPD1, OPD2), frontometaphyseal dysplasia (FMD) and Melnick–Needles syndrome (MNS). These conditions are characterised by skeletal dysplasia of variable severity in both affected males and females. PNH is usually not associated with these phenotypes.

Heterozygous women have a 50% chance of passing the gene in every pregnancy. Given the lethality in male fetuses, the risk of early miscarriage is close to 25%. PND, once the disease-causing mutation is known in the mother, is possible. The disease severity is not possible to predict, but it is important to emphasise that it can be variable. The unpredictability of disease severity may be a significant burden to prospective parents and families in making a decision about the pregnancy outcome.

Polymicrogyria

PMG is an abnormality of cortical development characterised by excessive number of gyri which are reduced in size. The distribution may be over the whole or only part of the brain surface thus defining the anatomically different forms of PMG. This is an aetiologically varied condition which may be isolated or part of a syndrome. Collectively, it is a relatively common abnormality of cortical development, although its true incidence is as yet not known.

The clinical manifestations range from mild neurological deficit to a severe encephalopathic picture, global developmental delay, visual impairment and refractory epilepsy, depending on the extent and distribution of cortical abnormality.

PMG may be caused by congenital infection (TORCH – Toxoplasmosis, Rubella, Cytomegalovirus, Herpes simplex) or impaired blood flow (twin-twin transfusion). The heritable forms of PMG are genetically heterogeneous, including syndromic and non-syndromic forms (Tables 1.12 and 1.13).

It is possible that rare AD and X-linked forms are clinically variable and may be inherited from an affected parent. Careful clinical examination of the parents for any mild neurological phenotype is therefore recommended and, if clinically indicated, followed by cranial MRI. Early PND is available if a genetic diagnosis is confirmed. The empiric risk

Table 1.12   Isolated (Non-Syndromic) PMG

Distribution	Inheritance	Gene
Bilateral frontal PMG	AR	Not known
Bilateral frontoparietal PMG	AR	GFR56
Bilateral perisylvian PMG	AD, AR, X-linked	Not known
Bilateral parasagittal parieto-occipital PMG	Sporadic	
Generalised PMG	AR	Not known

Abbreviations: PMG, polymicrogyria; AR, autosomal recessive; AD, autosomal dominant.

Table 1.13   Syndromic PMG

Syndrome	Inheritance
22q11 (Velocardiofacial syndrome)	AD
1p36 deletion	AD (rarely reproduce)
Aicardi syndrome	X-linked, only females
Fukuyama muscular dystrophy	AR
Muscle-eye-brain disease	AR
Walker–Warburg syndrome	AR
Joubert syndrome	AR
Zellweger syndrome	AR

Abbreviations: PMG, polymicrogyria; AD, autosomal dominant; AR, autosomal recessive.

Table 1.14   Outcome in ECM and DWC

	ECM		DWC	
Outcome	Isolated	Complex	Isolated	Complex
Favourable	97%	30–50%	12–40%	2%
Poor	3%	50–70%	60–88%	98%

Abbreviations: ECM, enlarged cisterna magna; DWC, Dandy–Walker complex. *Source*: From Ref. 32.

for siblings of a singleton, non-syndromic cases is 5% to 10% if congenital infection and environmental causes have been excluded.

Posterior Fossa Abnormalities

Posterior fossa abnormalities (PFAs) include enlarged cisterna magna (ECM), Dandy–Walker malformation (DWM) and Dandy–Walker variant (DWV). DWM and DWV share many features and may be indistinguishable on prenatal ultrasound scan; the term Dandy–Walker complex (DWC) encompasses both DWM and DWV (29–13).

Approximately two-thirds of pregnancies with PFAs result in IUD or termination. Although isolated ECM and DWC are more likely to have a favourable outcome if the chromosome analysis is normal, the prognosis should be guarded (Table 1.14). Postmortem analysis of apparently isolated DWC identifies additional abnormalities in about 50% of cases and a specific genetic diagnosis could be established in approximately 30% (32).

Anencephaly and Neural Tube Defect

Isolated neural tube defect (NTD) and anencephaly are multifactorial conditions, product of an interaction between genetic susceptibility and environment. Both conditions can be readily diagnosed on antenatal scan. The preconception and early pregnancy folic acid supplementation has reduced the recurrence risk following a singleton case to 1% for either

Table 1.15 Causes of FADS

Condition	Inheritance
Neurogenic disorders	
Neurodevelopmental abnormalities	Chromosomal, AD, AR, XL, sporadic
Spinal muscular atrophy (SMA)	AR
Penna–Shokeir syndrome	AR
Cerebro-oculo-facio-skeletal syndrome (COFS)	AR
Myopathic disorders	AD, sporadic
Arthrogryposis multiplex congenital (Amyoplasia)	AD, AR, XL
Congenital myopathies	AR
Popliteal pterygium syndrome	AD
Congenital myasthenia	AR
Congenital myotonic dystrophy	AD
Restrictive dermopathy	AR
Maternal myasthenia gravis	Environmental
Oligohydramnios	
Teratogens	

Abbreviations: FADS, fetal akinesia deformation sequence; AD, autosomal dominant; AR, autosomal recessive; XL, X-linked.

anencephaly or NTD. The risk to the offspring of an affected parent is approximately 3% to 4%. Rare X-linked pedigrees have been reported in the literature (33) as well as AR (Meckel–Gruber syndrome, Nail-patella syndrome) and AD (Currarino triad) syndromes.

Fetal Akinesia Deformation Sequence

Restriction of fetal movement can result in a pattern of abnormalities recognised as fetal akinesia deformation sequence (FADS) (Table 1.15). Aetiologically, this is an extremely complex group of disorders often clinically identifiable in the second trimester of pregnancy. Careful neurological assessment of the mother is recommended. Definite PND is very difficult. This is also discussed in chapter 26.

PRENATAL DIAGNOSIS

PND is undertaken during pregnancy to determine the clinical or genetic status of the fetus. PND can use non-invasive or invasive techniques:

1. *Non-invasive diagnostic techniques*
   a. Prenatal ultrasound scan, 3D imaging and fetal dysmorphology
   b. Diagnostic imaging (MRI and spectroscopy)
   c. Free fetal DNA in maternal circulation
2. *Invasive diagnostic techniques*
   a. Chorionic villus sampling (CVS)
   b. Amniocentesis
   c. Fetal blood sampling – cordocentesis
   d. Fetal tissue sampling for diagnosis of rare skin disorders

Genetic Investigations

1. *QF-PCR* (quantitative fluorescence polymerase chain reaction) – for rapid detection of common aneuploidies
2. *Standard chromosome analysis* – identifies abnormalities of chromosome number and structure (deletions, duplications, translocations)
   a. If anomalies are identified on the antenatal scan and are not due to common aneuploidies

   b. One of the parents is a carrier of chromosome rearrangement
   c. Sibling with chromosome abnormality
3. *FISH* (fluorescent in situ hybridisation) – a test using fluorescently labelled probe for identification of microdeletion syndromes (e.g., MDS)
4. *MLPA* (multiple-ligation-dependent probe amplification) – a DNA-based, very versatile technique that can be tailored for detection of small deletions and duplications and can be used as a screening tool unlike FISH
5. *Array CGH analysis (comparative genomic hybridisation array; aCGH)* – a new technique to scan the genome for gains or losses of genetic material (deletions and duplications) at a much higher resolution level than standard- or high-resolution chromosome analysis. This test cannot detect balanced chromosome rearrangements.

   aCGH is increasingly used as a first-line investigation instead of standard karyotype in individuals with suspected genetic conditions. It has been very helpful for patients with learning difficulties and multiple congenital anomalies. De novo rearrangements involving gene-rich areas are likely to be significant and therefore of diagnostic value. Some rearrangements are relatively frequent, for example, 16p11.2 deletion of approximately 500 kb associated with learning difficulties, susceptibility to autism spectrum disorder and seizures, although their true incidence, and phenotypic implications are, as yet, not known.

   Some rearrangements, also known as copy number variations (CNVs) are familial and may be seen in phenotypically normal people as well as in individuals with problems suggesting that CNVs may contribute to genetic variations as well as play a role in the aetiology of complex diseases in an, as yet, not fully understood fashion.

   aCGH is currently not routinely used for PND given the limitations in interpreting the results. However, PND for a pathogenic deletion/duplication identified in a sibling may be offered to look for the specific rearrangement. These are more likely to have arisen de novo, carrying a low recurrence risk.
6. *Mutation analysis* is a single gene testing used when
   a. The fetus is at risk of a genetic disorder and the mutation in the family is known
   b. A known single gene disorder is suspected on the basis of the prenatal scan finding

GENETIC COUNSELLING

Genetic counselling is the process by which patients or relatives at risk of an inherited disorder are advised of the consequences and nature of the disorder, the probability of developing or transmitting it, the management aspects and reproductive options (34). Genetic counselling aims to provide:

1. Diagnosis, prognosis and/or risk estimation (clinical geneticist)
2. Psychological support before, during and after pregnancy regardless of whether a diagnosis has been established (genetic counsellor, clinical geneticist)

The prenatal diagnostic process often requires input from a number of professionals including the fetal medicine obstetrician, neurologist, neuroradiologist, paediatrician, surgeon and geneticist to establish a diagnosis and provide as accurate as possible information about the outcome of pregnancy and long-term outcome for the child.

Given the fact that a significant proportion of neurodevelopmental disorders are genetic, it is important that the clinical genetics team is involved as early as possible as most genetic tests are time-consuming and often more than one test may be necessary.

Genetic counsellors are usually involved early on in the process to provide emotional and psychological support and facilitate the decision-making process when the outcome of pregnancy is considered. The counselling process may well extend to the next pregnancy.

REFERENCES

1. MacDonald BK, Cockerell OC, Sander JW, et al. The incidence and lifetime prevalence of neurological disorders in a prospective community-based study in the UK. Brain 2000; 123:665–676.
2. Purcell B, Gaitatzis A, Sander JW, et al. Epilepsy prevalence and prescribing patterns in England and Wales. Health Stat Q 2002; 15:23–31.
3. Dean CS, Hailey H, Moore SJ, et al. Long term health and neurodevelopment in children exposed to antiepileptic drugs before birth. J Med Genet 2002; 39:251–259.
4. Kini U, Adab N, Vinten J, et al. Dysmorphic features: an important clue to the diagnosis and severity of foetal anticonvulsant syndromes. Arch Dis Child Foetal Neonatal Ed 2006; 91:90–95.
5. Meador K, Reynolds MW, Creanb S, et al. Pregnancy outcomes in women with epilepsy: a systematic review and meta-analysis of published pregnancy registries and cohorts. Epilepsy Res 2008; 81:1–13.
6. Meador KJ, Baker GA, Browning N, et al. Cognitive function at 3 years of age after foetal exposure to antiepileptic drugs. N Engl J Med 2009; 360(16):1597–1605.
7. Rasalam AD, Hailey H, Williams JH, et al. Characteristics of foetal anticonvulsant syndrome associated autistic disorder. Dev Med Child Neurol 2005; 47:551–555.
8. Chakrabarti S, Fombonne E. Pervasive developmental disorders in preschool children. JAMA 2001; 285:3093–3099.
9. Roach ES, Sparagana SP. Diagnosis of tuberous sclerosis complex. J Child Neurol 2004; 19:643–649.
10. Roelink H, Augsburger A, Heemskerk J, et al. Floor plate and motor neuron induction by vhh-1, a vertebrate homolog of hedgehog expressed by the notochord. Cell 1994; 76(4):761–775.
11. Riddle RD, Johnson RL, Laufer E, et al. Sonic hedgehog mediates the polarizing activity of the ZPA. Cell 1993; 75(7):1401–1416.
12. Johnson RL, Laufer E, Riddle RD, et al. Ectopic expression of Sonic hedgehog alters dorsal-ventral patterning of somites. Cell 1994; 79(7):1165–1173.
13. Aicardi J, Chevrie JJ, Baraton J. Agenesis of the corpus callosum. In: Vinken PJ, Bruyn GW, Klawans HL, eds. Handbook of Clinical Neurology. Revised series, Vol 6. New York: Elsevier Science, 1987:149–173.
14. Schell-Apacik CC, Wagner K, Bihler M, et al. Agenesis and dysgenesis of the corpus callosum: clinical, genetic and neuroimaging findings in a series of 41 patients. Am J Med Genet A 2008; 146:2501–2511.
15. Chadie A, Radi S, Trestard L, et al. Neurodevelopmental outcome in prenatally diagnosed isolated agenesis of the corpus callosum. Acta Paediatr 2008; 97(4):420–424.
16. Gupta JK, Lilford RJ. Assessment and management of foetal agenesis of the corpus callosum. Prenat Diagn 1995; 15:301–312.
17. Glenn O, Goldstein R, Li K, et al. Foetal MRI in the evaluation of foetuses referred for sonographically suspected abnormalities of the corpus callosum. J Ultrasound Med 2005; 24:791–804.
18. Garel C, Luton D, Oury JF, et al. Ventricular dilatations. Childs Nerv Syst 2003; 19:517–523.
19. Nyberg DA, Mack LA, Hirsch J, et al. Foetal hydrocephalus: sonographic detection and clinical significance of associated anomalies. Radiology 1987; 163:187–191.
20. Nicolaides KH, Berry S, Snijders RJ. Foetal lateral cerebral ventriculomegaly: associated malformations and chromosomal defects. Foetal Diagn Ther 1990; 5:5–14.
21. Graham E, Duhl A, Ural S, et al. The degree of antenatal ventriculomegaly is related to pediatric neurological morbidity. J Matern Foetal Med 2001; 10(4):258–263.
22. Gaglioti P, Danelon D, Bontempo S, et al. Foetal cerebral ventriculomegaly: outcome in 176 cases. Ultrasound Obstet Gynecol 2005; 25(4):372–377.
23. Bussel JB, Primiani A. Foetal and neonatal alloimmune thrombocytopenia: progress and ongoing debates. Blood Rev 2008; 22 (1):33–52.
24. D'Addario V, Pinto V, Cagno L, et al. Sonographic diagnosis of foetal cerebral ventriculomegaly: an update. J Mat-Foetal Neonat Med 2007; 20:7–14.
25. Weichert J, Hartge D, Krapp M, et al. Prevalence, characteristics and perinatal outcome of foetal ventriculomegaly in 29,000 pregnancies followed at a single institution. Foetal Diagn Ther 2010; 27(3):142–148.
26. Reiss-Zimmermann M, Weber D, Sorge I, et al. Developmental malformations of the cerebral cortex. Rofo 2010; 182(6):472–478.
27. Guerrini R, Carrozzo R. Epileptogenic brain malformations: clinical presentation, malformative patterns and indications for genetic testing. Seizure 2001; 10:532–543.
28. Sheen VL, Jansen A, Chen MH, et al. Filamin A mutations cause periventricular heterotopia with Ehlers-Danlos syndrome. Neurology 2005; 64:254–262.
29. Barkovich AJ, Kjos BO, Normal D. Revised classification of the posterior fossa cysts and cystlike malformations based on the results of multiplanar MR imaging. Am J Neuroradiol 1989; 10:977–988.
30. Pilu G, Visentin A, Valeri B. The Dandy-Walker complex and foetal sonography. Ultrasound Obstet Gynecol 2000; 16(2): 115–117.
31. Glenn OA, Barkovich AJ. Magnetic resonance imaging of the foetal brain and spine: an increasingly important tool in prenatal diagnosis, Part 2. Am J Neuroradiol 2006; 27:1807–1814.
32. Forzano F, Mansour S, Ierullo A, et al. Posterior fossa malformation in foetuses: a report of 56 further cases and a review of the literature. Prenat Diagn 2007; 27:495–501.
33. Newton R, Stanier P, Loughna S, et al. Linkage analysis of 62 X-chromosomal loci excludes the X chromosome in an Icelandic family showing apparent X-linked recessive inheritance of neural tube defects. Clin Genet 1994; 45(5):241–249.
34. Harper P. General aspects of genetic counselling. In: Harper P, ed. Practical Genetic Counselling. 5th ed. Oxford: Butterworth-Heinemann, 1998:3–4.

2

Imaging during pregnancy

Francessa Wilson and Jozef Jarosz

PRACTICAL CONSIDERATIONS

Imaging the nervous system during pregnancy can be challenging as there are multiple factors for consideration to ensure safety of both the mother and the fetus. Radiological examinations should be kept to a minimum at all stages in pregnancy unless there is a clearly defined indication; however, maternal well-being and management should not be compromised because of concerns about fetal exposure to ionising radiation.

POSITIONING

In the later stages of pregnancy, the patient may be at risk of aortocaval compression from the second trimester when in the supine position for even short periods of time. The gravid uterus can compress the aorta and inferior vena cava causing problems from mild hypotension to reduced cardiac output and cardiovascular collapse. This in turn can cause fetal distress. All women should have a wedge inserted under their right hip whilst in the supine position from the middle of the second trimester (1). Alternatively, women may be imaged in the left lateral decubitus position which prevents compression of the vena cava. Scanning times should be kept as short as possible to reduce maternal fatigue and discomfort (2).

DOSE

Computerised tomography (CT) brain imaging can be performed if clinically indicated and should not be avoided because of concerns about radiation. The natural background radiation dose to the fetus during pregnancy is approximately 1 mGy (3) and the fetal absorbed doses from head CT are less than 0.1 mGy. The estimated radiation exposure is thus low for CT when the fetus is outside the field of view and CT of the brain can be safely performed during any trimester of pregnancy.

The 1977 report of the National Council on Radiation Protection and Measurements (US) stated: 'The risk [of abnormality] is considered to be negligible at 0.05 Gy or less when compared to the other risks of pregnancy, and the risk of malformations is significantly increased above control levels only at doses above 0.15 Gy. Therefore, the exposure of the fetus to radiation arising from diagnostic procedures would rarely be cause, by itself, for terminating a pregnancy'. The 'risks of pregnancy' referred to in this statement include the normal risks of pregnancy: 3% risk of spontaneous birth defects, 15% risk of spontaneous abortion, 4% risk of prematurity and growth retardation and 1% risk of mental retardation (4).

CT CONTRAST

Intravenous contrast crosses the placenta and into the fetus. There are no controlled studies on its effects and so a risk–benefit analysis should be conducted before use (5).

There have been concerns in the past about neonatal thyroid function after the administration of iodinated contrast media in pregnancy (12). Recent studies have shown that a single high-dose exposure is unlikely to have a clinically important effect on thyroid function at birth (13).

MAGNETIC RESONANCE IMAGING (MRI)

There is no scientific evidence to suggest that there is a significantly increased risk to the fetus in the first trimester when performing a routine MRI examination but because this is the period of active organogenesis, MRI should be avoided unless the potential benefits outweigh the theoretical risks (2). MRI has been used to evaluate obstetric and fetal conditions for over 20 years with no evidence of adverse effects (6). Some authorities do raise safety concerns due to the heating effects of radiofrequency pulses and the effects of acoustic noise on the fetus (7), and more research is needed.

Overall, the clinical need for imaging should be addressed and whether MRI is appropriate to answer the clinical question. Pregnant patients should be informed that there is no evidence that MRI imaging during pregnancy has resulted in deleterious effects to the developing fetus (11).

MRI CONTRAST

The safety of using intravenous contrast agents in pregnancy is not clear (7). Intravenous gadolinium-based contrast has been shown to cross the placenta and appear within the fetal bladder (8,9). It then enters the fetal bloodstream, is excreted into the amniotic fluid, swallowed by the fetus and reabsorbed from the gastrointestinal tract. The half-life of the drug in the fetal circulation and the effect of this drug on the developing human fetus are unknown (8,9). In animal studies, growth retardation and delay in ossification have been reported after administration of a high dose of the drug (10). The safety of intravenous administration of the drug in pregnant patients has not been widely tested and established (8,9). Therefore, use of the drug is generally not recommended in pregnant patients (8,9).

NEUROLOGICAL CONDITIONS
Headache

Headache is a common complaint and is prevalent in pregnancy. Neuroimaging (including CT and MRI) may reveal an underlying aetiology for headache in 27% of cases including cerebral venous sinus thrombosis, intracranial haemorrhage and posterior reversible leukoencephalopathy (14). The chances of having an intracranial pathology on neuroimaging have not been proven to be higher when there is positive neurology on clinical examination (14).

Pre-Eclampsia/Eclampsia (Fig. 2.1)

Indications for imaging. Neuroimaging may not be needed if the clinical picture is clearly defined. The diagnosis of eclampsia is made when pre-eclampsia is complicated by seizures in the absence of other causative conditions (15). However, if there is focal neurology or any deterioration in neurological status, imaging may be useful.

Modality and protocol. MRI is the superior imaging modality (20) with the most frequent abnormality seen on T2 and FLAIR sequences. Parieto-occipital hyperintense cortical/subcortical lesions are seen in 95% of patients (21). CT may be useful to rule out haemorrhage if MRI cannot be performed. Diffusion-weighted imaging can be useful in distinguishing reversible vasogenic oedema from infarction/cytotoxic oedema (16,18). This technique, if there is an early diagnosis of ischemia, may be helpful in predicting whether there will be an adverse outcome (18).

An MRI protocol should consist of T2, T1, FLAIR and DWI sequences. Gradient echo and contrast-enhanced sequences could also be performed but are not essential. The imaging should be repeated once the symptoms have resolved and the blood pressure has normalised.

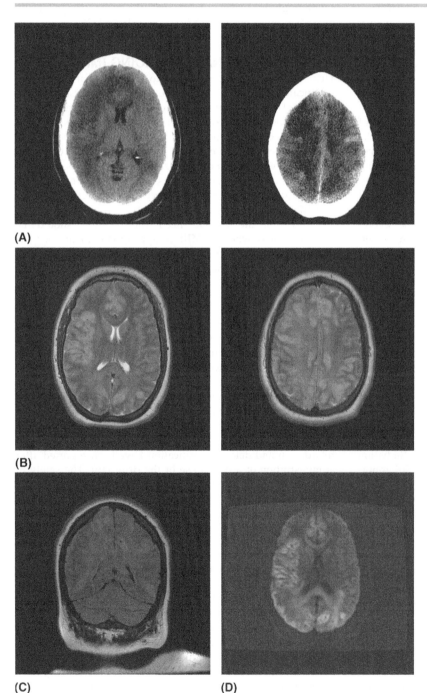

(A)

(B)

(C)   (D)

Figure 2.1 A 22-year-old pregnant woman with HELLP syndrome with a decreased Glasgow Coma Scale and dilated pupils. **(A)** CT brain (without contrast). Diffuse predominantly white matter low attenuation can be seen, more extensive on the right with mild mass effect. **(B)** Axial T2-weighted MRI. **(C)** Coronal FLAIR. **(D)** Axial diffusion. Cortical and subcortical T2 and FLAIR hyperintensity in parietal and occipital lobes and to a lesser extent the frontal lobes. Some of these lesions show restricted diffusion (low signal was seen on the corresponding ADC map). Appearances are consistent with eclampsia.

Findings. There is considerable clinical and radiological overlap between reversible posterior leukoencephalopathy syndrome, hypertensive encephalopathy and eclampsia (18).

CT Focal regions of asymmetric hemispheric oedema/hypodensity. There is a predilection for the posterior circulation with the parietal and occipital lobes most commonly affected, followed by frontal and inferior temporal lobes and cerebellum (16,18,20). The changes may be transitory (19). This resembles a watershed distribution with cortex and subcortical and deep white matter involved to varying degrees (16,18). The basal ganglia may be involved (19,20) but the brainstem is rarely of abnormal signal (20,21). Associated petechial haemorrhage can occur (19); haemorrhage is said to occur in 15% (16).

MR T1 hypointense, T2 and FLAIR hyperintense cortical/subcortical lesions. T2* punctuate low-signal lesions if haemorrhage is present (20). The DWI is usually normal with a high ADC value suggesting vasogenic oedema which usually completely reverses (16,20). Focal areas of restricted diffusion with high signal on the DWI with normal or decreased ADC are uncommon and may indicate irreversible infarction (16,20). If intravenous contrast is given there is variable enhancement (21). MR spectroscopy, although not routinely performed, may show widespread abnormality with increased choline and creatine and mildly decreased *N*-acetyl aspartate (NAA) that usually returns to normal within 2 months (20,21). MRA may show narrowing of the major intracranial vessels which can resolve with time (20).

Eclampsia may result in a posterior reversible encephalopathy syndrome. This is probably due to a multitude of factors including cytotoxic effects on the vascular endothelium and labile blood pressure which can lead to breakdown of the blood–brain barrier in the posterior circulation (17).

Cerebral Venous Thrombosis (Fig. 2.2)
Patients with cerebral venous thrombosis (CVT) in pregnancy tend to be younger and to present more acutely than patients

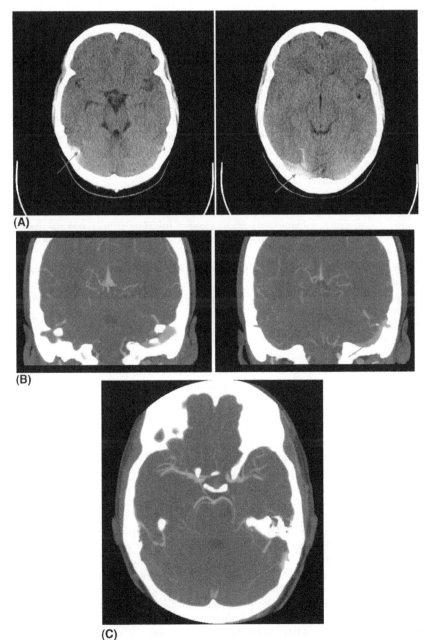

(A)

(B)

(C)

Figure 2.2 A 28-year-old woman who whilst 16 weeks pregnant developed sudden onset of headache and nausea. **(A)** CT brain scan showing hyperdense transverse and sigmoid sinuses. **(B)** coronal and **(C)** axial CT venograms demonstrating that there is no filling of the right lateral transverse sinus and sigmoid sinus due to venous sinus thrombosis.

with non-obstetric causes. Symptoms also tend to reach a plateau within 10 days of symptom onset compared to a longer course which could be progressive (23). There has been found to be no difference in the presenting neurological symptoms or radiological findings between the two groups but the outcome has been proven to be better in obstetric patients (23). Intracranial veno-occlusive disease is most common in the first 3 weeks following delivery (16).

Indications for imaging. Imaging should be performed when patients present with symptoms such as headache, confusion, decreased level of consciousness, and papilloedema when other potential causes have been excluded. Focal neurological deficit may reflect the venous sinus or cerebral vein involved (19) and if present it would be a strong indication for imaging. CVT can result in focal brain swelling and venous oedema or infarction due to raised venous pressure (25). There is poor correlation between extent of parenchymal changes and location and degree of clot (24) – probably due to collateral circulation.

Modality and protocol – CT versus MR venography. Brain imaging by itself is of little diagnostic value in CVT as it can be normal in 25% of cases especially in the acute stage. MRI is more sensitive than CT in early detection of thrombosis and more accurate in depicting the extent of the clot and any possible complications (25). Parenchymal changes are seen on MRI in 40% to 70% (22). Lack of enhancement of a sinus on CT/MRI is an early sign (21). MR venography (MRV) may not be able to differentiate between thrombosis and hypoplasia and is not sensitive in the diagnosis of cortical vein thrombosis (23). CT is quicker and therefore more tolerant of patient movement.

CT with CT venography (CTV), both with thin sections, is recommended as the initial screening examination. MRI (T1, T2, T2*, DWI) with phase-contrast MRV can be performed if the CT is negative. Intravenous gadolinium is relatively contraindicated in pregnancy.

Findings

CT   This may show hyperdensity in the dural venous sinuses, cortical veins ('cord sign') or deep cerebral veins, but there is low sensitivity due to slow flow (30,31). The dense vein sign is seen only in 20% to 55% of cases and is insensitive in chronic cases (25). In the parenchyma there may be signs of mass effect with sulcal effacement and/or venous infarcts, which do not conform to arterial vascular territories and may include areas of haemorrhage (24). However, these changes are not sensitive or specific (24). If the straight sinus or internal cerebral veins occlude, the thalami and basal ganglia may be hypodense (20,21). It may take 7 to 10 days after symptom onset for the empty delta sign (seen on post contrast imaging) to be detected on CT (20,30). Thick sections may miss both the hyperdense sinus or vessel and the 'empty delta sign' (24).

MR   T1: Acute thrombus is isointense. Subacute thrombus becomes hyperintense (21).

T2: The clot is initially hypointense then becomes hyperintense and isointense in the chronic stage (21). A venous infarct has mass effect with mixed hypo/hyperintense signal in the adjacent parenchyma (21).

FLAIR: The thrombus is hyperintense and venous infarcts are of high signal.

T2*: The thrombus is hypointense and 'blooms' (21). Parenchymal and/or petechial haemorrhage is of low signal (21).

DWI: In ADC/DWI parenchymal changes are variable and heterogeneous with a mixed picture of cytotoxic and vasogenic oedema (21). The parenchymal changes are more often reversible than in arterial occlusions (21).

MRV: absence of flow in occluded sinus. Collateral vessels may be seen (21). Phase-contrast MRV is not limited by hyperintense thrombus (21).

High signal in sinuses on T1, T2, FLAIR is a reliable sign (19). Filling defects following administration of gadolinium may develop within the first week (22). Imaging should be performed in axial and coronal planes so flow can be analysed perpendicular to the axis of the sinuses (24).

The sensitivity of T2* and T1 in the first 3 days is 90% and 71%, respectively. For cortical veins T2* has 97% detection compared with 78% on T1 (27). T2* provides the highest detection of cortical vein thrombosis followed by T1, FLAIR, and time-of-flight MR angiography (MRA), with sensitivities of CT and CT venography below 30% (27). Between days 1 and 5, isointense T1/hypointense T2 findings are due to deoxyhaemoglobin. Between days 5 and 15, hyperintense T1/T2 findings are due to extra cellular methaemoglobin, initially peripherally then centrally (27).

The main limitation is the similarity in signal of flow artefacts with acute thrombus (isointense T1, hypointense T2) (23). It is necessary to perform T1 and T2 in orthogonal planes to distinguish slow flow from thrombus (23). Other limitations are that absence or hypoplasia can simulate occlusion (30). Phase contrast is useful as it is dependent only on phase shifts engendered by moving blood (30).

Contrast MR venography can help but is contraindicated in pregnancy and not good in detection of chronic thrombosis (24,26).

Venous oedema/ischaemia is represented by high T2 signal which may persist up to 2 years and may eventually lead to infarction (24).

T2 high signal is usually subcortical but may involve cortex (28).

Haemorrhage is shown by low T2 signal early which extends from centre to periphery unlike arterial infarcts (29).

Haemorrhage in venous infarcts usually has extensive surrounding low attenuation in contrast to primary haemorrhage (29).

Peripheral gadolinium enhancement may look tumour-like (28).

Commonly, multiple sites are involved with more swelling than arterial infarcts (29).

Subarachnoid Haemorrhage

Indications for imaging. The risk of subarachnoid haemorrhage (SAH) is five times greater in pregnant than in non-pregnant women (15,19), and rupture of an intracranial aneurysm is the most common cause. Pregnancy-induced hypertension has also been linked to acute subarachnoid haemorrhage (19).

Modality and protocol. CT with CT angiography (CTA) is the gold standard for the initial investigation of subarachnoid haemorrhage due to its high sensitivity to acute SAH, short scan times and widespread availability; however, MR with MR angiography (MRA) allows assessment without the need for ionising radiation or intravenous contrast (15,32). The sensitivity of CT however drops rapidly with time with 95% positive within the first 24 hours dropping to less than 50% by 1 week (21) and approaching 0% at 3 weeks (32). Multi-slice CTA is 90% to 95% sensitive for detecting an aneurysm that measures 2 mm or greater (21). Lumbar puncture should be performed in all cases of suspected SAH if there is no clinical contraindication.

MR may be able to supplement CT in the subacute phase when the sensitivity falls or when the LP is inconclusive (32).

T2* is the most sensitive MRI sequence with a sensitivity of 94% in the acute phase and 100% in the subacute phase (32); however, this persists in 70% to 75% of patients with a prior history of subarachnoid haemorrhage (21). FLAIR has sensitivities of 81% and 87% (32); however, high signal in the subarachnoid space is not pathognomonic for SAH (32). Conventional T1- and T2-weighted images are relatively insensitive (32).

Imaging protocol: CT with CTA to be performed if acute SAH is seen.

Findings

CT Hyperdense CSF on non-contrast CT with a distribution of blood that may suggest the location of the aneurysm. Secondary hydrocephalus and arterial infarcts may develop secondary to vasospasm.

MR T1: isointense CSF

T2/FLAIR: hyperintense CSF

T2*: hypointense CSF

DWI: may show focal restricted diffusion secondary to vasospasm which is most common between days 3 and 8 (32).

MRA is 85% to 95% sensitive (32).

Conventional DSA is considered the gold standard for aneurysm detection although it is negative in 15% to 20% of acute SAH (32).

Headache with Visual Field Neurology

Pregnancy affects the pituitary gland significantly. The adenohypophysis increases in volume by approximately 30%, peaking at day 3 after delivery (Fig. 2.3) and the neurohypophysis loses its normal bright spot during the third trimester (36).

MRI is the preferred imaging modality in evaluating the pituitary gland. A standard protocol would include pre-contrast thin-section (<3mm) sagittal and coronal T1 and T2 sequences with a small field of view. Gadolinium is relatively contraindicated in pregnancy, so follow-up imaging may be necessary for complete interpretation of an abnormality.

Pituitary Adenoma

During pregnancy, prolactinomas are the most common pituitary tumours (19).

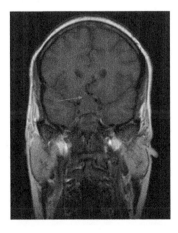

Figure 2.3 A 22-week pregnant lady presenting with a severe headache. Coronal T1 brain shows enlargement of the anterior pituitary (17 mm) extending into the suprasellar cistern and abutting the chiasm, consistent with physiological enlargement of the pituitary gland.

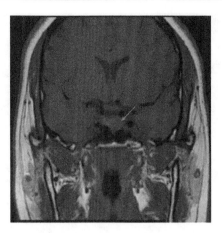

Figure 2.4 A 20-week pregnant lady presenting with a headache. Coronal T1: focal bulging and subtle low signal in the left side of the pituitary gland in keeping with a small adenoma.

Macroadenomas are greater than 10 mm in height (Fig. 2.4). They commonly have a 'snowman' configuration with the indentation caused by the diaphragma sellae (19).

Adenomas are commonly hypointense relative to the normal pituitary gland on T1 but are occasionally isointense and have a variable appearance on T2-weighted imaging (34). The adenoma may extend superiorly and compress the optic chiasm or infundibulum or extend laterally into the cavernous sinus (34). In the correct clinical context, a pituitary adenoma may be present if the pituitary height is greater than 12 mm (15).

The MR imaging protocol includes thin-section sagittal and coronal T1-weighted and T2-weighted scans without gadolinium.

CT. Uncomplicated adenomas are isodense to grey matter. Cyst formation and necrosis are common, creating focal low attenuation within the adenoma.

Large adenomas expand the sella and may erode the floor.

MR. T1: usually isointense with grey matter. Secondary subacute haemorrhage will have bright signal.

T2: usually isointense with grey matter. Cysts will be hyperintense, haemorrhage signal varies with age.

T2*: low signal if haemorrhage is present.

Pituitary Apoplexy

Pituitary apoplexy occurs when an existing pituitary adenoma (Fig. 2.5) or a physiologically enlarging pituitary gland is complicated by infarction or haemorrhagic infarction (19,33).

CT and MRI may show haemorrhage in a prominent pituitary gland; however, haemorrhage is not seen in all cases (19,33). Early MR depicts a heterogeneous mass which is predominantly hyperintense on T1 and hypointense on T2 (35). The sella may be enlarged if a macroadenoma is present (35). At a later stage, the sedimentation of any blood products present may create a fluid–debris level which is highly suggestive of haemorrhagic pituitary adenoma (35). Thickening of adjacent sphenoid sinus mucosa is seen in 80% of cases (35).

Follow-up imaging can show atrophy with the appearance of a partially empty sella (19). CT is useful in detecting haemorrhage within the pituitary in the acute phase (33).

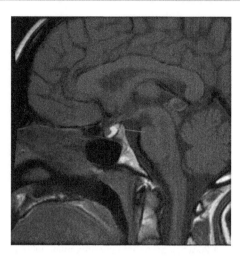

Figure 2.5 A 30-week pregnant lady with known pituitary adenoma and sudden onset of headache. Sagittal T1 shows a high T1 signal in the central and posterior aspect of the pituitary gland in keeping with haemorrhage.

The imaging protocol for suspected pituitary apoplexy should include standard MR pituitary sequences. DWI and T2* can also be useful (21).

CT. Sellar/suprasellar mass with patchy or confluent hyperdensity.

May be associated with subarachnoid blood (21).

Rim enhancement is suggestive but not diagnostic (21).

MR. T1: Early – enlarged gland, iso/hypointense with brain

Subacute – hyperintense

Chronic – empty sella

T2: Early – enlarged hypointense (haemorrhagic) or hyperintense (non haemorrhagic)

Subacute – hyperintense

Chronic – hyperintense (CSF) fills empty sella.

DWI: restricted diffusion within adenoma may be early sign (21).

T1 following contrast: rim enhancement is common.

Sheehan Syndrome
Sheehan syndrome occurs when there is pituitary infarction due to obstetric-related haemorrhage and subsequent hypotension (15,19).

In the acute phase, the pituitary gland is enlarged and of homogeneously low signal on T1 and high signal on T2 with a thin rim of irregular contrast enhancement (15). In the later stages, atrophy and a partial or completely empty sella may be seen (15,19).

Lymphocytic Adenohypophysitis
Lymphocytic adenohypophysitis (LA) is a rare inflammatory condition of the anterior lobe of the pituitary which is considered an autoimmune disease and occurs usually in the middle and third trimesters (15,19) and early post-partum (36). The hypothalamus and infundibulum may also be involved (36).

Imaging shows pituitary gland enlargement with suprasellar extension in the majority of cases which may displace the optic chiasm. There also may be cavernous sinus involvement (15,19). The gland may have a variable appearance with the majority of patients showing early and homogeneous enhancement (19). The mass is of relatively low signal on T1 and high signal on T2 (37). The enhancement may extend to involve the adjacent meninges with a 'dural tail' appearance (15). Thickening of the infundibulum and involvement of the neurohypophysis are reported in 15% of patients (19), and there may be local inflammatory reaction with thickening of the adjacent sphenoid sinus mucosa (35). It is difficult to distinguish this condition from a pituitary adenoma (19) although adenomas do tend to be asymmetric and more heterogeneous (36). A thickened stalk and loss of the normal posterior pituitary bright spot are reported in LA (36). Follow-up imaging shows regression of the pituitary gland to a normal or small size (19).

The MR imaging protocol should include standard pituitary imaging.

CT. Thick pituitary stalk with or without an enlarged pituitary gland.

Strong uniform enhancement.

MR. T1: Thick pituitary stalk (>2 mm) with or without an enlarged pituitary gland.

A large proportion show loss of the normal posterior pituitary 'bright spot'.

T2: Iso/hypointense

T1 with contrast: intense uniform enhancement

Meningioma (Fig. 2.6)
Pregnancy appears to enhance the growth of meningiomas (19). Meningiomas account for up to 20% of all intracranial tumours (34), and they commonly occur in a suprasellar or parasellar location. Suprasellar meningiomas commonly arise from the diaphragma sellae or tuberculum sellae and cause visual disturbance when they compress the optic chiasm (34). Large planum sphenoidale meningiomas can extend into the suprasellar cistern or parasellar regions (34).

Meningiomas are generally isointense relative to grey matter on T1- and T2-weighted images with some variation due to the presence of calcium (lower signal intensity), cystic or haemorrhagic changes (34).

Focal Neurology with or Without Headache
Stroke
The risk of ischaemic stroke is increased in the peripartum period but not during pregnancy itself (19).

Thrombotic infarcts can be due to the 'hypercoagulable state' of pregnancy and the puerperium on a background of pre-existing atherosclerotic plaque disease (15,19).

Embolic infarcts can result from carotid or vertebral dissections due to prolonged labour or cardiac valvular disease (16,19). Watershed infarcts can result from significant obstetric haemorrhage, sepsis or pulmonary embolus (16,19).

Multiple Sclerosis
The relapse rate of multiple sclerosis is said to be reduced during pregnancy and increases in the puerperium (23). The imaging findings are identical. This is discussed further in Chapter 21.

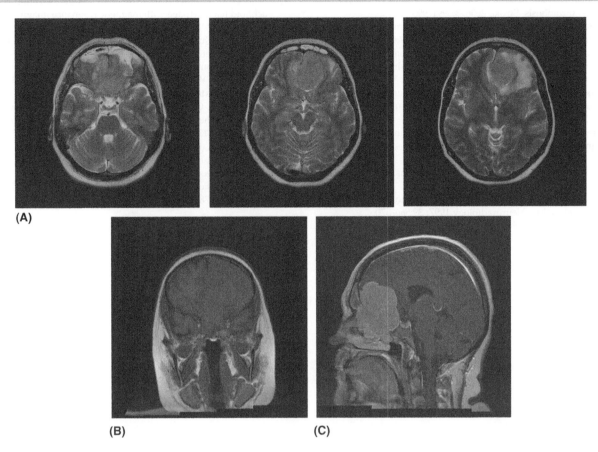

(A)

(B)   (C)

Figure 2.6 A 30-week pregnant lady with known meningioma complaining of headache and decreased visual acuity. **(A)** Axial T2 **(B)** Coronal T1 **(C)** Sagittal post contrast T1. Large extra-axial solid mass (meningioma) centred on the planum sphenoidale and involving the sella and extending into the ethmoid and sphenoid sinuses and encroaching on the medial walls of the orbits.

REFERENCES

1. Dineen R, Banks A, Lenthall, R. Imaging of acute neurological conditions in pregnancy and the puerperium. Clin Radiol 2005; 60:1156–1170.
2. Levendecker J, Gorengaut V, Brown JJ. MR imaging of maternal diseases of the abdomen and pelvis during pregnancy and the immediate postpartum period. Radiographics 2004; 24: 1301–1316.
3. Osei EK, Faulkner K. Fetal doses from radiological examinations. Br J Radiol 1999; 72:773–780.
4. Brent RL, Mettler FA. Pregnancy policy. AJR Am J Roentgenol 2004; 182:819–822.
5. Ultravist package insert. Montville, NJ: Berlex Laboratories, 2004.
6. Shellock FG, Crues JV. MR procedures: biologic effects, safety and patient care. Radiology 2004; 232:635–652.
7. Shellock FG, Kanal E. Magnetic resonance: bioeffects, safety and patient management. 2nd ed. Lippincott Williams and Wilkins Philadelphia PA USA.
8. Levine D, Barnes PD, Edelman RR. Obstetric MR imaging. Radiology 1999; 211:609–617.
9. Shellock FG, Kanal E. Safety of magnetic resonance imaging contrast agents. J Magn Reson Imaging 1999; 10:477–484.
10. Magnevist product information. Wayne, NJ: Berlex Laboratories, 2010.
11. Shellock FG. Reference manual for magnetic resonance safety, implants and devices: 2006 edition. Los Angeles, CA: Biomedical Research Group, 2006.
12. Atwell TD, Lteif AN, Brown DL, et al. Neonatal thyroid function after administration of IV contrast agent to 21 pregnant patients. AJR 2008; 191:268–271.
13. Bourjeily G, Chalhoub M, Phornphutkul C, et al. Neonatal thyroid function: effect of a single exposure to iodinated contrast medium in utero. Radiology 2010; 256(2) 744–750.
14. Ramchandren S, Cross BJ, Liebeskind DS. Emergent headaches during pregnancy. AJNR 2007; 28:1085–1087.
15. Dineen R, Banks A, Lenthall R. Imaging of acute neurologic conditions in pregnancy and puerperium. Clin Radiol 2005; 60:1156–1170.
16. Bartynski WS. Posterior reversible encephalopathy syndrome, Part 1. AJNR 2008; 29:1037–1042.
17. Schqartz RB, Feske SK, Polak JF, et al. Pre-eclampsia-eclampsia: clinical and neuroradiological correlates and insights into the pathogenesis of hypertensive encephalopathy. Radiology 2000; 217:371–376.
18. Koch S, Rabinstein A, Falcone S, et al. Diffusion-weighted imaging shows cytotoxic and vasogenic oedema in eclampsia. AJNR 2001; 22:1068–1070.
19. Zak IT, Dulai HS, Kisj KK. Imaging of neurologic disorders associated with pregnancy and the postpartum period. Radiographics 2007; 27:95–108.
20. Sengar AR, Gupta RK, Dhanuka RR, et al. MR imaging, MR angiography and MR spectroscopy of the brain in eclampsia. AJNR 1997; 18:1485–1490.
21. Diagnostic Imaging: Brain 2nd Ed 2010 Anne G. Osborn et al Amirsys Inc Salt Lake City, Utah USA.
22. Roncallo F, Turtulici I, Arena E, et al. Cerebral venous sinus thrombosis: prognostic and therapeutic significance of an early radiologic diagnosis. Riv Neuroradiol 1998; 11:479–505.
23. Cerebral venous thrombosis associated with pregnancy and puerperium.

24. Idbaih A, Boukobza M, Crassad I, et al. MRI of clot in cerebral venous thrombosis. Stroke 2006; 37:991–995.

25. Connor SEJ, Jarosz JM. Magnetic resonance imaging of cerebral venous sinus thrombosis. Clin Radiol 2002; 57:449–461.

26. Berguy M, Bradac GB, Daniele D. Brain lesions due to cerebral venous thrombosis do not correlate with sinus involvement. Neuroradiology 1999; 41:419–424.

27. Haroun, A. Utility of contrast enhanced 3D turbo flash MRA in evaluating the intracranial venous system. Neuroradiology 2005; 47:322–327.

28. Linn J, Michl S, Katja B, et al. Cortical vein thrombosis: the diagnostic value of different imaging modalities. Neuroradiology 2010; 52(10):899–911.

29. Chiras J, Dubs J, Bories J. Venous infarctions. Neuroradiology 1985; 27:593–600.

30. Bakac G, Wardlaw JM. Problems in the diagnosis of intracranial venous infarction. Neuroradiology 1997; 39:566–570.

31. Provenzale JM, Joseph GJ, Barboriak DP. Dural sinus thrombosis: findings on CT and MR imaging and diagnostic pitfalls. AJR 1998; 170(3):777–783.

32. Mitchell P, Wilkinson ID, Paley MNJ, et al. Detection of subarachnoid haemorrhage with magnetic resonance imaging. J Neurol Neurosurg Psychiatry 2001; 70(2):205–211.

33. Ostrov SG, Quencer RM, Hoffman JC, et al. Hemorrhage within pituitary adenomas: how often associated with pituitary apoplexy syndrome? AJNR 1989; 153:153–160.

34. Johnsen DE, Woodruff WW, Allen IS, et al. MR imaging of the sellar and juxtasellar regions. Radiographics 1991; 11(5):727–758.

35. Bonneville F, Cattin F, Marsot-Dupuch K, et al. T1 signal hyperintensity in the sellar region: spectrum of findings. Radiographics 2006; 26:93–113.

36. Gutenberg A, Larsen J, Lupi I, et al. A radiologic score to distinguish autoimmune hypophysistis from nonsecreting pituitary adenoma preoperatively. AJNR 2009; 30: 766–1772.

37. Lorenzi AR, Ford HL. Multiple sclerosis and pregnancy. Postgrad Med J 2002; 78:460–464.

3

Intrauterine imaging, diagnosis and intervention in neurological disease

William Dennes

INTRODUCTION

Ultrasound scans have for many years been the modality of choice for imaging the fetus in utero. More recently, the use of magnetic resonance imaging (MRI) has provided a novel imaging modality for suspected fetal anomalies in general and visualisation of fetal brain structures in particular. MRI has become increasingly important where ultrasound resolution is limited because of maternal obesity or the fetal position. Recent developments in MRI technology, and in particular shorter acquisition times, can now provide clinicians with good-quality, non-motion images. This chapter describes the principles and development of fetal imaging by ultrasound scan and MRI, their limitations, and the diagnosis and management of congenital neurological disease.

ULTRASOUND

Ultrasonography in obstetrics was first introduced in the late 1950s, and has since become commonplace for imaging the fetus. Whilst many groups were involved in the development of ultrasound, in the United Kingdom, Professor Ian Donald (Regius Chair of Midwifery at Glasgow University) has largely been credited with its early development in obstetric imaging. Whilst there are a number of different ultrasound methods, they rely on the same principle; that is, high-frequency ultrasound, generated from a piezoelectric transducer, results in an ultrasound wave. Ultrasound is partially reflected from layers within different tissues. Dense tissues such as bones have a high reflectivity and are therefore echo bright, whilst fluid (such as amniotic fluid) has low reflectivity and is echo lucent (dark). These differences in density and therefore reflectivity are referred to as acoustic impedance. The reflected sound wave (echo) is partially reflected back to the transducer and converted into electrical pulses which are processed to generate a digital image. The time taken for the reflected echo to be returned to the transducer can be measured, and used to determine tissue depth.

Initial work on medical ultrasound resulted in the generation of A-mode (*amplitude* mode) ultrasound. A-mode is the simplest form of ultrasound, where a single transducer scans a line through the tissue under examination, with echoes plotted on a screen as a function of depth. A-mode is still used in ophthalmology for imaging of the eye. Subsequent developments in technology resulted in B-mode (*brightness* mode) ultrasound where a linear array of transducers simultaneously scans a plane through the tissue, resulting in a two-dimensional (2D) image on a screen. Professor Donald's initial paper on the use of medical ultrasound, published in *Lancet* in 1958 (1), used B-mode ultrasound to image the pregnant uterus, ovarian cysts, fibroids and ascites on various normal and pathological conditions. Donald also used A-mode to measure the fetal biparietal diameter (BPD), and this work led to the

publication, by Professor Stuart Campbell in 1968, of a method of BPD measurement as a means of calculating gestational age (2). Subsequently, B-mode ultrasound was used in the first-trimester to determine gestational age by measurement of the crown-rump length (CRL) (3). With further developments in technology, fetal abnormalities such as anencephaly and spina bifida could be detected on ultrasound (4,5). The development of greyscale imaging and real-time scanning in the 1970s further improved visualisation of the moving fetus, with the development of high-frequency, transabdominal and transvaginal transducers. With improvements in resolution, prenatal diagnosis became increasingly possible in the late first and early second trimesters. Pulsed and colour Doppler allowed the detailed analysis of fetal perfusion/blood flow, and when this was combined with conventional B-mode scanning it improved the detection of fetal cardiac abnormalities. Further advances include the development of power Doppler, which displays the strength of Doppler signal rather than just the direction of flow. This development has become useful in assessing placental function (6).

Most recently, both 3D (three-dimensional) and 4D (four-dimensional – real-time 3D) scanning have become available (Fig. 3.1). These techniques rely on the acquisition of a tissue volume, enabling post-acquisition processing and image reconstruction. The use of 3D surface rendering has added a new dimension to fetal imaging. However, 3D ultrasound currently does not appear to have achieved its potential in improving diagnostic accuracy, and whilst in fetal scanning they generate images of great parental interest, it is currently a technology searching for a suitable clinical application.

ANTENATAL ULTRASOUND

The current minimum schedule of antenatal ultrasound scans in England, in line with current National Institute of Clinical Excellence (NICE) 2010 guidelines (7), is to offer a first-trimester ultrasound scan at 11 to 14 weeks, and a second-trimester scan at 20 to 24 weeks, often referred to as the 'anomaly scan'. The 20-24 week anomaly scan is offered in most developed countries.

The 11-14 Week Scan

This scan is usually performed transabdominally, although in some cases it may be necessary to do a transvaginal scan. The principal purpose of this scan is to confirm fetal viability by identifying normal fetal heart activity. In addition, measurement of the CRL is made to date the pregnancy accurately. This is particularly important for women who either are unable to recall the date of their last period or have an irregular menstrual cycle.

In addition, early ultrasound can be used to identify multiple pregnancies. Approximately 2% of natural conceptions

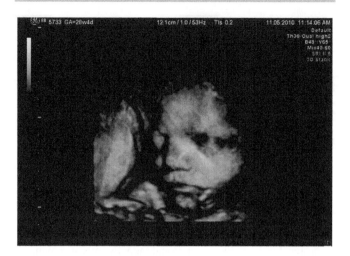

Figure 3.1   3D ultrasound image (surface rendering mode) showing a normal fetal face at 28 weeks of pregnancy.

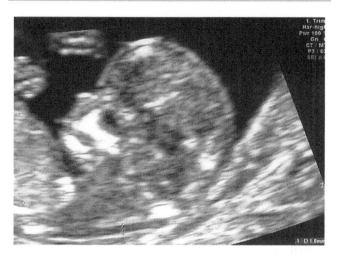

Figure 3.2   Fetal nuchal translucency measurement at 12 weeks of pregnancy (showing a normal nuchal translucency measurement – 1.0 mm).

and 10% of assisted conceptions result in multiple pregnancies. Early ultrasound scan can reliably distinguish dichorionic from monochorionic twin pregnancies (8) allowing for early development of an appropriate management plan, notably for monochorionic twin pregnancy where there is a risk of twin-twin transfusion syndrome. In general, the use of early ultrasound in pregnancy has been shown to improve neonatal outcomes (9).

In the United Kingdom, the 11-14 week scan can also be used to assess the risk of trisomy 21 (Down syndrome) and other chromosomal abnormalities. Widespread use of ultrasound scanning earlier in pregnancy led to the observation that an increased fetal neck fold thickness (nuchal translucency) was associated with poor pregnancy outcome in general and chromosomal abnormality (aneuploidy) in particular (10). This observation resulted in the development of the nuchal translucency test to assess the patient's adjusted risk of aneuploidy (11). This has been further refined by the measurement of additional, independent markers of trisomy, such as the presence or absence of the nasal bone, and blood flow through the tricuspid valve and ductus venosus. In combination with first-trimester biochemistry (beta human chorionic gonadotrophin and Pregnancy associated plasma protein-A) and these ultrasound markers, the combined test has a sensitivity of 97% in the detection of Down syndrome and is currently regarded as the 'gold standard' test for screening for Down syndrome in pregnancy. The sensitivity is 97%, for a fixed false positive rate of 5%.

With increasing improvements in ultrasound resolution (it is generally accepted that 40% to 70% of major abnormalities can be detected at this scan) major fetal abnormalities may be detected at 11-14 week scan, prior to a routine 20-week anomaly scan (Fig. 3.2). Increasingly, abnormalities such as neural tube defects (12) and holoprosencephaly (HPE) (13) can be identified on this early scan, allowing for the option of either prenatal diagnostic testing (Karyotype-chorionic villus sampling) or the offer of early termination of pregnancy.

Anomaly Scan

Table 3.1 details the periods when various organ systems are vulnerable to abnormal development.

The anomaly scan is a detailed transabdominal scan at 20 to 22 weeks of pregnancy. This scan involves an anatomical

Table 3.1   Times of Vulnerability to Congenital Abnormality in the Fetus (Weeks Past Last Menstrual Period)

	High vulnerability leading to major abnormality	Lower vulnerability leading to minor abnormality
CNS	4–22	22–delivery
Heart	4.5–6.5	6.5–10
Upper limbs	5–7	7–9
Eyes	5.5–9.5	9.5–delivery
Lower limbs	5.5–8.5	8.5–10
Teeth	8–10	10–delivery
Palate	8–10	10–11
External genitalia	8.5–11	11–delivery
Ear	5.5–10.5	10.5–18

survey of the fetus, imaging the brain, face, spine, heart, stomach, bowel, kidneys and limbs. In addition, the position of the placenta is determined, to exclude a low-lying placenta that may develop into placenta praevia, and an assessment is made of the amniotic fluid volume and fetal growth.

The ability of prenatal ultrasound scan to diagnose fetal malformations is principally dependent on both the equipment used and the experience of the operator. In experienced hands ultrasound can be expected to detect approximately 70% of all fetal malformations (14); its rate of detecting cleft palate can be about 75%, dependent on operator and equipment. The majority of spinal, renal and abdominal wall malformations are detected by screening on ultrasound; however, the detection rate for isolated abnormalities is considerably lower with, for example, only approximately 25% of isolated cardiac defects detected antenatally by ultrasound.

The ability of prenatal ultrasound to accurately determine fetal gestational age has resulted in a reduction in the number of women requiring induction of labour for post-term pregnancy, and in an improvement in the management of preterm delivery where the gestational age has previously been accurately determined (9).

For the majority of women no further ultrasound scans beyond 22 weeks are necessary; however, further assessments of fetal growth and well-being may be necessary in the third trimester. Fetal biometry (measurement of the fetal head, abdomen and femur length) enables an assessment of fetal growth and an estimate of fetal weight. In growth-restricted fetuses, measurement of the amniotic fluid volume and flow within the umbilical artery, middle cerebral artery and ductus venosus provides an assessment of fetal well-being, and may be used to determine the optimal timing of delivery.

Fetal echo scans (cardiac scans) are additional scans, usually at 20 to 24 weeks, that are indicated in patients who

- have had a previously affected fetus with cardiac abnormality;
- have family history of cardiac disease;
- have maternal conditions or drug treatment – diabetes, epilepsy, etc.;
- have increased first-trimester nuchal translucency;
- have other major fetal malformations.

Safety

The theoretical risks from medical ultrasound result from dissipation of energy from the ultrasound wave, resulting in the potential for both thermal and mechanical damage and subsequent tissue injury. The thermal effect is due to an increase in tissue temperature due to energy absorption from the ultrasound beam. The American College of Obstetricians and Gynaecologists (15) set an arbitrarily defined safe, cut-off level of 100 mW/cm^2 (returned energy). The majority of antenatal ultrasound examinations result in dissipated energy levels of 20 mW/cm^2, well below this cut-off level. Power Doppler, particularly in the first trimester, may be associated with significant energy transfer and the potential for thermal damage. Therefore, Doppler imaging in the first trimester should be limited, especially for imaging of the central nervous system.

The mechanical effects of ultrasound result from radiation force, streaming and cavitation. The risks of mechanical damage may be quantified in a *mechanical index*; however, available evidence suggests it is unlikely that obstetric ultrasound results in any significant adverse effect associated with mechanical effects.

Long-term randomised trials on the safety to ultrasound in pregnancy have demonstrated no significant differences in developmental, neurological and psychological outcomes at up to 12 years of follow-up (16). In addition, studies of elementary school performance and dyslexia in groups either exposed or not exposed to ultrasound in utero have found no differences in developmental 'milestones' or any objective measurements of development (17). There are some data to suggest an association between left-handedness and in utero exposure to ultrasound (18), although it is difficult to determine whether there is a causal relationship. Therefore, the current consensus is that routine ultrasound in pregnancy is not associated with any adverse outcome for the fetus.

FETAL NEUROIMAGING – ULTRASOUND

Traditionally, assessment of the fetal brain is determined from axial views of the fetal head, where the cerebral ventricles can be seen in a view that allows measurement of the BPD (Fig. 3.3). This transventricular plane is obtained by a transverse scan at the level of the cavum septum pellucidum, allowing investigations of the lateral border of the anterior (or frontal) horns, the medial and lateral borders of the posterior horns, the choroid plexus and the sylvian fissure. The transcerebellar view allows examination of the midbrain and posterior fossa and in particular the cerebellum and cisterna magna. Transabdominal scanning often results in limited views of the near-field cerebral hemisphere due to reverberations from the fetal cranium, requiring additional imaging in the sagittal and coronal planes.

Ultrasound is useful for screening for fetal neurological abnormalities particularly in early pregnancy, that is, less than 20 weeks. It is also useful at assessing cerebral blood flow (using power Doppler) and may be helpful in the assessment of ventriculomegaly, Holoprosencephaly, corpus callosal abnormalities, cerebellar abnormalities (Dandy–Walker malformations) and craniosynostosis. Its principal limitation is that it provides no information on neuronal migration disorders. Power or colour Doppler may be useful in delineating vascular lesions such as aneurysms of the vein of Galen or intracranial arteriovenous malformations (20,21).

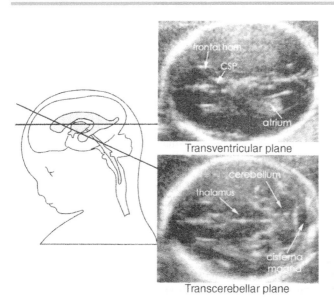

Transventricular plane

Transcerebellar plane

Figure 3.3 Standard views of the fetal head showing transventricular plane (frontal and lateral ventricles) and transcerebellar plane showing the posterior fossa. *Source*: From Ref. 19 with permission.

MAGNETIC RESONANCE IMAGING

MRI has become increasingly useful as a clinical application for fetal imaging in general and neuroimaging in particular. Whilst MRI has been available for many years, it has only recently been applied to prenatal diagnosis. The principal limitation on adequate imaging was the long acquisition times of standard images. Significant fetal movement during the scan affects image acquisition, resulting in image degradation. This is further compounded by noise generated within the MRI scanner, stimulating fetal movements.

The basis of MR imaging is that when an external magnetic field is applied across tissue, where individual magnetically resonant atomic nuclei are randomly aligned, the nuclei align themselves parallel to, or in opposition to the magnetic field. If a radio frequency (RF pulse) is applied the net magnetisation of vector is flipped by a certain angle, which has both longitudinal and transverse components. The transverse component induces a current in a receiver call, which can be translated into a signal. Developments in MRI acquisition, such as half-Fourier acquisition single-shot turbo spin-echo (*HASTE techniques*) – have allowed acquisition of a single T_2-weighted anatomic image in less than 500 milliseconds. These ultra-fast scanning techniques eliminate, or at least significantly reduce, the artefacts caused by movement (22). These adaptations to existing MR techniques have been applied to the fetal examinations with varying results. Whilst the consequences of fetal movements (secondary, for example, to maternal respiration) can be reduced by fast image acquisition times, an optimum solution would be to incorporate a motion correction or motion compensation technique (23). Techniques to reduce the consequences of fetal motion should further improve fetal MRI, such that investigations of brain growth and development in vivo might be achieved.

The most common indication for fetal MR imaging are suspected neurological abnormalities, previously identified on ultrasound [such as ventriculomegaly, suspected posterior fossa abnormalities and agenesis of the corpus callosum (ACC)]. Fetal MRI is preferred where ultrasound scans are limited due to oligohydramnios (reduced liquor volume) or maternal increased body mass index. MRI is generally superior to ultrasound (due to better resolution of intracranial structures, such as cortical tissue) for posterior fossa abnormalities, the detection of intracranial bleeding, tuberous sclerosis, schizencephaly, lissencephaly and severe microcephaly (24).

MRI is generally more informative the later it is performed in pregnancy (with a lower limit of gestation at around 23 weeks).

However, antenatal MR imaging does have its limitations. Limperopoulos et al. (25) reviewed details of fetuses referred for MRI with suspected posterior fossa abnormalities. They compared antenatal MRI findings with post-natal MRI findings in 39 of 42 live-born infants, showing agreement in fetal and post-natal MRI diagnosis in 59%. In 16 cases (41%), fetal and post-natal MRI diagnosis disagreed, with post-natal MRI excluding fetal MRI diagnosis in six cases and revealing additional anomalies in 10 cases. The authors concluded that in cases of suspected posterior fossa abnormalities, fetal MRI (particularly at early gestations) has limitations in accurately predicting post-natally detected MRI abnormalities. Currently, MRI is also limited in functional evaluation of the fetal brain, although developments in specialised techniques such as determination of fetal brain lactate by magnetic resonance spectroscopy and measurement of pO_2 by means of quantitative images of fluid oxygenation on standard single-shot turbo spin-echo sequences may have a clinical application in the future (26).

MRI Safety

There is no evidence of harmful effects of MR imaging in pregnancy, although potential safety issues have been raised in relation to the possible bioeffects of the static magnetic field of the MR system. In addition, concerns have been raised regarding possible risks associated with exposure to gradient magnetic fields, potential outburst effects of RF energy and the possible adverse effects related to the combination of these three electromagnetic fields. There are a relatively small number of studies investigating the outcome of fetuses exposed to MR imaging or the MR environment, with no reported adverse outcomes. Baker et al. (27) reported no demonstrable increase in disease, disability or hearing loss in children examined in utero using echo planar MRI for suspected fetal compromise. To date, there have been no recorded harmful effects in the developing fetus with the use of scanners at field strength of 1.5 T or less (28). Guidelines for patients' safety have been issued by the U.S. Safety Committee of the Society of Magnetic Resonance Imaging (1991) (29), who have recommended that

> *MR imaging may be used in pregnant women if other non-ionising forms of diagnostic imaging are inadequate or if the examination provides important information that would otherwise require exposure to ionising radiation (e.g. fluoroscopy, CT etc). Pregnant patients should be informed that to date, there has been no indication that the use of clinical MR imaging during pregnancy has produced deleterious effects.*

In the United Kingdom, the current advice from the Department of Health is that patients receiving MRI scans during their pregnancy should have details of the scan parameters recorded, and a copy kept for subsequent inclusion in the child's note.

FETAL ANATOMICAL DEVELOPMENT

Whilst the fetal brain undergoes major changes throughout pregnancy, from 7 weeks of gestation a sonolucent area can be seen in the cephalic pole on ultrasound scan. At 9 weeks, demonstration of the convoluted pattern of three vesicles is feasible, and from 11 weeks, large brightly echogenic choroid plexuses, filling the large lateral ventricles can be seen (the '*Butterfly sign*') (30). In the second trimester, the lateral ventricles and choroid plexus decrease in size relative to the brain mass.

CONGENITAL ABNORMALITIES
Neural Tube Defect

Neural tube defects reflect a spectrum of disease, from anencephaly to spina bifida. Anencephaly describes an absence of the cranial vault (acrania) with secondary degeneration of the brain as a result of exposure to amniotic fluid. Similarly, in spina bifida the neural arch, often in the lumbosacral region, is incomplete with secondary damage to the exposed nerves.

Incidence
The incidence of neural tube defects in the United Kingdom is approximately 5 per 1000 births, with anencephaly and spina bifida accounting for approximately 95% of cases (and encephaloceles for the remaining 5%).

Aetiology
Neural tube defects may be associated with chromosomal abnormalities, genetic syndromes (single mutant genes), maternal diabetes or secondary to maternal drug use such as

antiepileptic drug treatment. The precise aetiology for the majority of these defects remains unknown. The recurrence risk of neural tube defect following an affected pregnancy is 5% to 10%, and can be reduced by pre-conception supplementation with high-dose folic acid – at 5 mg daily.

Diagnosis

The majority of neural tube defects should be detected by ultrasound scan. Before the advent of detailed ultrasound, neural tube defects were diagnosed on the basis of increased maternal serum alpha-fetoprotein, which was the basis for maternal serum screening. Nowadays anencephaly can be diagnosed at 11 weeks of pregnancy by demonstration of an absent cranial vault and cerebral hemisphere (31). The facial bone, brainstem and occipital bones and midbrain are usually present.

Diagnosis of spina bifida is more frequently made initially on the basis of intracranial abnormalities rather than identification of the spinal lesion. Frontal bone scalloping (lemon sign) and obliteration of the cisterna magna with either an absent or abnormally shaped cerebellum (banana sign) are diagnostic of neural tube defects (32). These signs should prompt careful examination of the fetal spine to identify the level of neural tube defect. The spine should be systematically examined, both transversely and longitudinally. In the transverse plane, the normal neural arch appears as a closed circle with intact covering skin. In spina bifida, the arch is 'U-shaped' with an associated bulging meningocele (thin-walled) or myelomeningocele. A variable degree of ventricular enlargement is present in virtually all cases of spina bifida at birth, but in only about 70% of cases in the mid-trimester.

Prognosis

Anencephaly is universally fatal, at (or within hours of) birth. In patients who decline termination of pregnancy, for ethical or religious reasons, the pregnancy can further be complicated by polyhydramnios (secondary to reduced fetal swallowing) and this, in addition to an increased risk of malpresentation (face presentation due to an absent cranium), may further complicate the pregnancy and delivery. In spina bifida, surviving infants may be severely handicapped, with paralysis in the lower limbs and both urinary and bowel incontinence. Despite an often-associated hydrocephalus, intelligence is usually normal.

Fetal Therapy

Fetal therapy appears attractive in terms of reducing the risk of handicap due to exposure to amniotic fluid in the third trimester. However, in utero closure of spina bifida has been associated with a high risk of iatrogenic preterm delivery (due to hysterotomy) and has therefore previously been considered only in fetuses with life-threatening malformations. More recently, fetal surgery has been performed in selected patients (with a fetus with myelomeningocele), and is currently being investigated in a multi-centre, prospective, randomised study (*Management of Myelomeningocele Study* – MOMS). Preliminary (non-randomised) results suggest that fetal myelomeningocele closure may improve lower extremity function, neurodevelopmental outcome and reduce morbidity from hydrocephalus and hindbrain herniation (33).

Ventriculomegaly

Incidence

Hydrocephalus is a pathological increase in intracranial cerebrospinal fluid (CSF) volume. This may result from either fluid production that exceeds absorption or primary atrophy of the cerebral parenchyma. Hydrocephalus is found in approximately 2/1000 births.

Aetiology

Ventriculomegaly is a descriptive term of a pathological process with many causes. It may result from obstruction to CSF, or due to maldevelopment of the cerebral ventricles (such as ACC) or as a destructive process, secondary to cerebral atrophy. Ventriculomegaly (dilatation of the cerebral ventricles) is found in approximately 1% of all pregnancies at the 20- to 24-week scan. The majority of cases of ventriculomegaly do not therefore go on to develop hydrocephalus.

Diagnosis

A transverse scan of the fetal head at the level of the cavum septum pellucidum will demonstrate the lateral cerebral ventricles and the choroid plexus. The sonographic appearance of enlarged ventricles is often striking (Fig. 3.4). The fetal head biometry (BPD) may not be increased despite ventricular dilatation. The lateral ventricles can be visualised as early as 12 weeks, but ventriculomegaly is more often diagnosed at 20 to 24 weeks' gestation.

Ventriculomegaly is divided on the basis of atrial width into

— *Borderline* (9–10 mm)
— *Mild*   (11–12 mm)
— *Moderate* (13–15 mm)
— *Severe*   (>15 mm)

The prognosis is generally worse with increasing atrial measurement. Ventriculomegaly may be associated with aneuploidy (often trisomy 21), prompting the offer of prenatal diagnostic testing by amniocentesis. Although mild ventriculomegaly is generally associated with a good prognosis, affected fetuses from this group have the highest incidence of chromosomal abnormalities. The overall risk of karyotypic abnormality is between 12% and 25%. Associated intracranial anomalies, such as ACC or Dandy–Walker malformation, are present in at least one-third of cases.

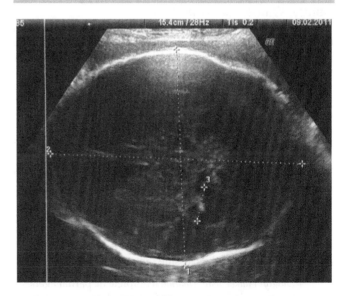

Figure 3.4 Ultrasound imaging of ventriculomegaly: 2D ultrasound image at 35 weeks of gestation, showing the lateral (posterior) cerebral ventricles, and unilateral, severe ventriculomegaly measuring 15.6 mm (Caliper 3).

Management

Management of ventriculomegaly should include detailed examination of fetal anatomy to exclude other defects, especially of the brain. Associated intracranial anomalies – such as ACC or Dandy–Walker malformation – are present in at least one-third of cases. A maternal infection screen [toxoplasmosis, syphilis and cytomegalovirus (CMV)] should be performed and patients offered fetal karyotyping. For patients who choose to continue the pregnancy, serial ultrasound scans every 2 to 3 weeks may be useful to define evolution of ventriculomegaly, which may be progressive in 2% to 5% of cases. In a number of cases of apparently isolated ventriculomegaly, there may be an underlying cerebral maldevelopment (such as lissencephaly) or destructive lesion (such as periventricular leukomalacia). It may therefore be appropriate to arrange fetal MR imaging at around 32 weeks to identify these lesions. In utero treatment (cephalocentesis) in an attempt to reduce progressive damage to the fetal brain by a chronic increase in CSF pressure has been attempted but is not currently recommended. The prognosis associated with isolated borderline ventriculomegaly (9–10 mm) is generally good and these findings may represent a normal variant (particularly if the fetus is male). The optimal management of these cases remains uncertain, although many units will arrange serial follow-up scans to exclude progressive ventricular dilatation.

Isolated mild ventriculomegaly (atrial width 10–12 mm) is generally associated with a good prognosis, and neurodevelopment may be similar to fetuses with no ventriculomegaly. Impaired neurodevelopment is observed in approximately 15% of cases with moderate ventriculomegaly (atrial width 13–15 mm) and in up to 50% of cases with severe ventriculomegaly. In these cases it may be appropriate to offer the option of termination of pregnancy. Infants who are delivered with a prenatal diagnosis of ventriculomegaly should have a detailed physical examination, and consultation with a geneticist and neurosurgeon. Infants who develop hydrocephalus may require placement of a ventriculoperitoneal shunt.

Dandy–Walker Malformation

The Dandy–Walker malformation is a non-specific congenital brain malformation resulting from a number of diverse causes. The two principal features of the Dandy–Walker malformation are as follows: aplasia or hypoplasia of the cerebellar vermis and posterior fossa cysts (representing cystic dilatation of the fourth ventricle). The features were originally described by Blackfan and Dandy in 1914, in a patient with a hindbrain abnormality, cystic dilatation of the fourth ventricle, hypoplasia of the cerebellar vermis and separation of the cerebellar hemispheres. The term Dandy–Walker was adopted in 1954, following publication of a case report by Blackfan and Dandy and a subsequent report from Taggart and Walker.

The Dandy–Walker malformation complex refers to a spectrum of abnormalities of the cerebellar vermis, cystic dilatation of the fourth ventricle and enlargement of the cisterna magna. It can be classified into

— *Dandy–Walker malformation* (complete or partial agenesis of the cerebellar vermis and enlarged posterior fossa).
— *Dandy–Walker variant* (partial agenesis of the cerebellar vermis without enlargement of the posterior fossa).
— *Mega-cisterna magna* (normal vermis and fourth ventricle).

Incidence

The incidence of true Dandy–Walker malformation is approximately 1 in 25,000 to 35,000 pregnancies. The Dandy–Walker variant (see below) may be more common. In a series of post-natally acquired Dandy–Walker malformations, it occurred in 12% of cases of congenital hydrocephalus and 2% to 4% of childhood-onset hydrocephalus.

Aetiology

The malformation occurs as a result of an uncharacterized insult to the developing cerebellar hemispheres and the fourth ventricle during embryogenesis. A number of theories exist to explain the underlying aetiology. It may be associated with aneuploidy (trisomy 13, 18 or triploidy) and genetic syndromes. Predisposing factors to Dandy–Walker syndrome include exposure to rubella, CMV, toxoplasmosis, maternal warfarin treatment, alcohol intake and isotretinoin during the first trimester of pregnancy.

Diagnosis

On ultrasound the posterior fossa is visualised on a transverse, suboccipito-bregmatic section of the fetal head (Fig. 3.5). In the Dandy–Walker malformation there is cystic dilatation of the fourth ventricle with partial or complete agenesis of the vermis; in more than 50% of cases there is associated hydrocephalus and other extracranial defects. An enlarged cisterna magna is diagnosed if the distance from the cerebellar vermis to the fetal cranium is ≥10 mm. A diagnosis of isolated partial agenesis of the cerebellar vermis may be difficult to make, as the appearances can be created (in a normal fetus) if the angle of insonation is too steep, or if there is a degree of abnormality in cerebellar vermis rotation. Fetal MRI may be particularly helpful in assessing rotation of the cerebellar vermis and identifying landmarks such as the fastigial point and primary cerebellar fissure.

Management

There is a high incidence of associated CNS and extra-CNS abnormalities associated with Dandy–Walker syndrome. The risk of associated intracranial abnormalities is 25% to 68%. Given the association with aneuploidy, prenatal diagnostic testing (amniocentesis) should be offered. There is a high risk of post-natal mortality, about 20%, and a >50% incidence

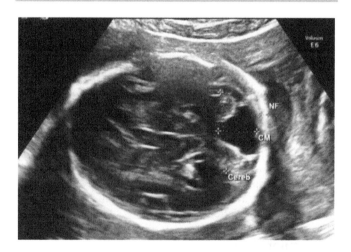

Figure 3.5 Ultrasound imaging of Dandy Walker Malformation: 2D ultrasound image at 25 weeks and 6 days gestation, showing the posterior fossa and a Dandy Walker malformation of the cerebellum. *Abbreviations*: Cereb, transcerebellar diameter; CM, cisterna magna; NF, Nuchal fold.

of impaired intellectual and neurological development. On this basis the option of termination of pregnancy should be discussed. Experience with Dandy–Walker variant (isolated partial agenesis of the vermis) is limited and the prognosis for this condition is uncertain. Isolated mega-cisterna is associated with a generally good prognosis.

Holoprosencephaly

HPE is a spectrum of cerebral (and facial) abnormalities resulting from incomplete cleavage of the forebrain. The abnormality occurs during the third week of gestation. HPE is sub-classified based on the extent of sagittal division of the cerebral cortex, thalamus and hypothalamus. The alobar type is the most severe, and is characterized by a single, monoventricular ventricle, with fusion of the thalami. In the semi-lobar type, there is partial segmentation of the anterior ventricles with incomplete fusion of the ventricles. In lobar HPE, there is normal separation of the ventricles and thalami but absent cavum septum pellucidum.

Incidence

HPE is a severe but relatively rare disorder that affects about 1 per 10,000 births.

Aetiology

In many cases the cause is chromosomal abnormality (more than 75% of cases of HPE are a result of trisomy 13). HPE can also result from genetic disorders. The risk of recurrence for non-chromosomal, sporadic HPE is approximately 6%. There is an excess of female fetuses in alobar (3:1) compared to lobar (1:1) HPE. Maternal diabetes increases the risk of HPE significantly compared to normal controls.

Diagnosis

Forebrain cleavage can be assessed in a standard transverse view of the fetal head, where in alobar HPE a single, dilated midline ventricle replaces the two lateral ventricles, or partial separation in semi-lobar HPE. Alobar and semi-lobar HPE may also be associated with microcephaly and facial abnormalities such as facial cleft, hypotelorism, cyclopia or proboscis.

Management

HPE is frequently lethal in fetal life. There is a high risk of extra-cerebral abnormalities associated with aneuploidy. Given the high risk of aneuploidy, prenatal diagnostic testing (amniocentesis) should be offered. Alobar and semi-lobar HPE are lethal. Lobar HPE is associated with mental retardation. The option of termination of pregnancy should be offered.

Agenesis of the Corpus Callosum

The corpus callosum is a major structure connecting the two cerebral hemispheres. Its development begins during the fifth week of fetal life. The mature corpus callosum is formed by the 17th week of fetal life. In ACC, the commissural fibres do not cross the midline, but pass posteriorly along the medial walls of the lateral ventricles.

Incidence

ACC is found in approximately 1 in every 200 births.

Aetiology

ACC may be an isolated finding but is frequently associated with other malformations and genetic syndromes. It is commonly associated with chromosomal abnormalities (trisomy 13, 18 and 8). It may be a result of maldevelopment or secondary to a destructive lesion.

Diagnosis

The corpus callosum is not visible in the standard transverse view of the fetal brain, but its absence may be suspected if the cavum septum pellucidum is not seen. The lateral ventricles may be dilated resulting in a 'teardrop' appearance of the ventricles with a 'dangling' choroid plexus. ACC can be demonstrated on a mid-sagittal view. Prenatal diagnosis of partial ACC has been reported; however, prenatal diagnosis may be difficult. Where there is a suspicion of ACC prenatal MRI may be needed to accurately confirm the diagnosis. In a series of antenatally suspected ACC, ultrasound confirmed the diagnosis in only four cases (of 14) while MRI confirmed the diagnosis in 13 cases (34).

Management

Where there is a suspicion of ACC, detailed ultrasound assessment should be made for both cranial and extracranial abnormalities. Because of the association with chromosomal abnormalities, prenatal diagnostic testing should be offered. If the diagnosis is in doubt fetal MR imaging should be arranged. If an isolated ACC is detected and the chromosomes are normal, standard obstetric management should be offered. In 50% of patients with apparently isolated ACC, development is normal. ACC with multiple major abnormalities is associated with a high risk of neurodevelopmental retardation and neonatal seizures. ACC with additional structural abnormalities should prompt a discussion regarding termination of pregnancy.

SUMMARY

Traditionally, ultrasound has been the principal method to assess fetal neurological development and to confirm normal brain development. With increasing developments in processor speeds and ultrasound resolution, diagnostic imaging has become possible in the first trimester allowing for both earlier diagnosis and management. Antenatal ultrasound has been used for many years and its safety profile has been well established.

Developments in MR imaging, and in particular shorter image acquisition times (HASTE techniques), have made MR imaging increasingly useful for prenatal diagnosis. MR imaging is particularly useful for fetal neuroimaging where ultrasound may not be diagnostic. Whilst there is little long-term data available regarding outcomes following in utero exposure to MRI, the available data suggest there is no increased risk to the fetus in terms of congenital abnormalities or subsequent neurodevelopment.

REFERENCES

1. Donald I, Macvicar J, Brown TG. Investigation of abdominal masses by pulsed ultrasound. Lancet 1958; 1(7032):1188–1195.
2. Campbell S. The prediction of fetal maturity by ultrasonic measurement of the biparietal diameter. J Obstet Gynaecol Br Commonw 1969; 76(7):603–609.
3. Robinson HP. Sonar measurement of fetal crown-rump length as means of assessing maturity in first trimester of pregnancy. Br Med J 1973; 4(5883):28–31.
4. Campbell S, Johnstone FD, Holt EM, et al. Anencephaly: early ultrasonic diagnosis and active management. Lancet 1972; 2(7789):1226–1227.
5. Campbell S, Pryse-Davies J, Coltart TM, et al. Ultrasound in the diagnosis of spina bifida. Lancet 1975; 1(7915):1065–1068.

6. Ogle RF, Rodeck CH. Novel fetal imaging techniques. Curr Opin Obstet Gynecol 1998; 10(2):109–115.

7. Antenatal care: routine care for the healthy pregnant woman. NICE clinical guidelines, No. 62. London: National Institute for Health and Clinical Excellence, 2010.

8. Shetty A, Smith AP. The sonographic diagnosis of chorionicity. Prenat Diagn 2005; 25(9):735–739.

9. LeFevre ML, Bain RP, Ewigman BG, et al. A randomized trial of prenatal ultrasonographic screening: impact on maternal management and outcome. RADIUS (Routine Antenatal Diagnostic Imaging with Ultrasound) Study Group. Am J Obstet Gynecol 1993; 169(3):483–489.

10. Nicolaides KH, Azar G, Snijders RJ, et al. Fetal nuchal oedema: associated malformations and chromosomal defects. Fetal Diagn Ther 1992; 7(2):123–131.

11. Nicolaides KH, Azar G, Byrne D, et al. Fetal nuchal translucency: ultrasound screening for chromosomal defects in first trimester of pregnancy. BMJ 1992; 304(6831):867–869.

12. Lachmann R, Picciarelli G, Moratalla J, et al. Frontomaxillary facial angle in fetuses with spina bifida at 11-13 weeks' gestation. Ultrasound Obstet Gynecol 2010; 36(3):268–271.

13. Faro C, Wegrzyn P, Benoit B, et al. Metopic suture in fetuses with holoprosencephaly at 11 + 0 to 13 + 6 weeks of gestation. Ultrasound Obstet Gynecol 2006; 27(2):162–166.

14. Boyd PA, Chamberlain P, Hicks NR. 6-year experience of prenatal diagnosis in an unselected population in Oxford, UK. Lancet 1998; 352(9140):1577–1581.

15. Ultrasonography in pregnancy. Technical Bulletin No. 187. Washington, DC: American College of Obstetricians and Gynecologists, 1993.

16. Stark CR, Orleans M, Haverkamp AD, et al. Short- and long-term risks after exposure to diagnostic ultrasound in utero. Obstet Gynecol 1984; 63(2):194–200.

17. Salvesen KA, Bakketeig LS, Eik-nes SH, et al. Routine ultrasonography in utero and school performance at age 8–9 years. Lancet 1992; 339(8785):85–89.

18. Salvesen KA, Vatten LJ, Eik-Nes SH, et al. Routine ultrasonography in utero and subsequent handedness and neurological development. BMJ 1993; 307(6897):159–164.

19. Pilu G, Nicolaides KH. Diagnosis of fetal abnormalities: the 18-23 week scan. New York and Carnforth: Parthenon Publishing, 1999.

20. Malinger G, Monteagudo A, Pilu G. Sonographic examination of the fetal central nervous system: guidelines for performing the 'basic examination' and the 'fetal neurosonogram'. Ultrasound Obstet Gynecol 2007; 29(1):109–116.

21. Hartung J, Heling KS, Rake A, et al. Detection of an aneurysm of the vein of Galen following signs of cardiac overload in a 22-week old fetus. Prenat Diagn 2003; 23(11):901–903.

22. Semelka RC, Kelekis NL, Thomasson D, et al. HASTE MR imaging: description of technique and preliminary results in the abdomen. J Magn Reson Imaging 1996; 6(4):698–699.

23. Jiang S, Xue H, Glover A, et al. MRI of moving subjects using multislice snapshot images with volume reconstruction (SVR): application to fetal, neonatal, and adult brain studies. IEEE Trans Med Imaging 2007; 26(7):967–980.

24. Pistorius LR, Hellmann PM, Visser GH, et al. Fetal neuroimaging: ultrasound, MRI, or both? Obstet Gynecol Surv 2008; 63(11):733–745.

25. Limperopoulos C, Robertson RL Jr., Khwaja OS, et al. How accurately does current fetal imaging identify posterior fossa anomalies? AJR Am J Roentgenol 2008; 190(6):1637–1643.

26. Zaharchuk G, Busse RF, Rosenthal G, et al. Noninvasive oxygen partial pressure measurement of human body fluids in vivo using magnetic resonance imaging. Acad Radiol 2006; 13(8):1016–1024.

27. Baker PN, Johnson IR, Harvey PR, et al. A three-year follow-up of children imaged in utero with echo-planar magnetic resonance. Am J Obstet Gynecol 1994; 170(1 pt 1):32–33.

28. Hubbard AM. Ultrafast fetal MRI and prenatal diagnosis. Semin Pediatr Surg 2003; 12(3):143–153.

29. Shellock FG, Kanal E. Policies, guidelines, and recommendations for MR imaging safety and patient management. SMRI Safety Committee. J Magn Reson Imaging 1991; 1(1):97–101.

30. Sepulveda W, Dezerega V, Be C. First-trimester sonographic diagnosis of holoprosencephaly: value of the "butterfly" sign. J Ultrasound Med 2004; 23(6):761–765; quiz 6–7.

31. Johnson SP, Sebire NJ, Snijders RJ, et al. Ultrasound screening for anencephaly at 10–14 weeks of gestation. Ultrasound Obstet Gynecol 1997; 9(1):14–16.

32. Sebire NJ, Noble PL, Thorpe-Beeston JG, et al. Presence of the 'lemon' sign in fetuses with spina bifida at the 10–14-week scan. Ultrasound Obstet Gynecol 1997; 10(6):403–405.

33. Danzer E, Gerdes M, Bebbington MW, et al. Preschool neurodevelopmental outcome of children following fetal myelomeningocele closure. Am J Obstet Gynecol 2010; 202(5):450 e1–e9.

34. d'Ercole C, Girard N, Cravello L, et al. Prenatal diagnosis of fetal corpus callosum agenesis by ultrasonography and magnetic resonance imaging. Prenat Diagn 1998; 18(3):247–253.

Disposition of drugs in pregnancy: anti-epileptic drugs

Dave Berry

INTRODUCTION

During pregnancy physiological changes occur which can alter drug absorption, distribution, metabolism and elimination (1,2). As a result, careful dose adjustments may be required throughout the pregnancy in order to improve the efficacy and safety of prescribed medication. Not only can gastrointestinal function be prolonged (particularly during the third trimester) but as gestation advances the quantity of total body water and fat increases which may lead to increased volume of distribution, and thus reduce drug plasma concentrations. Accompanying changes in cardiac output, ventilation and renal/hepatic blood flow also occur together with a decrease in plasma protein concentrations which increase the unbound (pharmacologically effective) fraction of a drug. Increased renal blood flow and glomerular filtration rate (GFR) may decrease serum concentrations of drugs predominantly eliminated unchanged by the kidneys. Furthermore, pregnancy can change the metabolising capacity of hepatic enzymes and increase the renal absorption of sodium; in addition, placental transport of drugs and their compartmentalisation in the embryo/placenta, along with metabolism by the placenta/fetus can play an important role in modifying the pharmacokinetics (PK) of a drug during gestation (3,4). Increased secretion of oestrogen and progesterone in pregnancy affects hepatic metabolism of drugs in different ways (5,6). Progesterone can increase the rate of metabolism of some drugs by induction of hepatic drug-metabolising enzymes; however, the contrary may occur such that hepatic metabolism may decrease because some drugs compete with progesterone and oestradiol for enzymatic hepatic metabolism, for example, theophylline and caffeine. Furthermore, the cholestatic effect of oestrogen may interfere with drug clearance, for example, rifampicin (7).

Lower serum concentrations of lithium occur in pregnancy which may be related to an increase in GFR; also, serum concentrations of ampicillin are reported to be 50% lower along with a faster clearance of penicillin V in pregnant women (7).

Pregnancy also affects the PK of some antiretroviral drugs, for example, the half-life of nevirapine is significantly prolonged. Furthermore, standard adult doses of nelfinavir and saquinavir produced lower drug concentrations in pregnant compared with non-pregnant women (3).

During gestation the thyroid is hyperstimulated which causes changes in thyroid hormone concentration; also, hypothyroidism is common and consistently lower serum concentrations of propylthiouracil have been observed in pregnant women compared with non-pregnant (8).

ANTI-EPILEPTIC DRUGS AND PREGNANCY

This topic is also discussed in chapter 12. About 0.5% to 1% of pregnant women have epilepsy (9,10) and they often discontinue or greatly reduce their prescribed medication without informing the managing clinician (11). Drug therapy in pregnant women usually focuses on safety for the fetus; however, PK of many drugs is altered during gestation and individual dose modifications may be required to account for pregnancy-related changes in disposition (7).

Pregnancy-related changes in maternal anti-epileptic drug (AED) concentrations may, to some extent, be predicted by the pharmacological properties of the drug, but many factors influence serum concentrations and there are large inter-individual differences in drug disposition which are impossible to predict. Co-medication with other drugs, which may themselves be subject to PK alterations, can be a further complicating factor and make it difficult to anticipate whether gestation-related changes in AED disposition will become clinically relevant.

For many AEDs, significant changes in both total and free drug concentrations occur throughout gestation and while the disposition of the first generation AEDs throughout pregnancy is reasonably well understood (12,13); the extent of the effect can vary widely between patients (13). At constant dosages, serum concentrations of most AEDs tend to decrease during gestation and return to pre-pregnancy concentrations usually by the third to the sixth week post-partum. While a decrease in adherence to the drug regimen and poorer bio-availability cannot be dismissed, these alterations are due mainly to decreased drug binding to serum proteins and increased metabolism and elimination (12,14,15).

Decreased protein binding will result in lower total (protein bound plus unbound) drug concentrations but may leave unchanged the unbound (pharmacologically active) concentration. Therapeutic drug monitoring (TDM) during gestation aims to facilitate individualised dosing by identifying pregnancy-induced pharmacokinetic changes, but for highly protein-bound drugs, for example, valproic acid and phenytoin, total serum concentrations during gestation may be misleading.

Significant changes in the clearance of some of the newer AEDs in pregnancy have now been reported with several studies demonstrating altered pharmacokinetics of lamotrigine, levetiracetam and the pharmacologically active metabolite of oxcarbazepine (MHD).

When pregnancy is planned and seizure control is optimal, it is advisable to obtain one or, preferably, two serum concentrations before conception, for future comparison (16). The timing and frequency of TDM during pregnancy should also be individualised, based on the AED prescribed and the patient's characteristics. Monitoring once each trimester is often recommended and probably sufficient in most women with adequate seizure control; however, more frequent sampling is advisable in patients with complicated epilepsy, those known to be sensitive to modest alterations in dose and serum concentrations and those treated with lamotrigine or oxcarbazepine, in whom monthly TDM would be justified. The need for monitoring in the post-partum period depends on the clinical situation and whether dose changes occurred during pregnancy.

There are few formal pharmacokinetic studies of AEDs throughout gestation, that is, determination of a sequence of plasma concentration profiles at various time points as a pregnancy progresses. Almost all the evidence for changes in pharmacokinetics of the various AEDs throughout gestation is derived from sequential drug monitoring and if doses are adjusted to maintain serum levels it is possible to determine apparent clearance (daily dose/steady-state plasma concentration mL/min).

PHARMACOKINETICS OF INDIVIDUAL DRUGS
Phenytoin

The plasma clearance of phenytoin was first studied during gestation in two prospective investigations (17,18) and in both studies changes in phenytoin plasma clearance were observed as the pregnancies progressed. Maximal clearance values were recorded at the time of delivery or in the preceding few weeks and clearance returned to pre-pregnancy levels 4 to 6 weeks after delivery. The plasma phenytoin concentration decrease starts shortly after conception and may fall by more than 60% in the third trimester, returning to pre-conception levels within a few weeks after delivery (19).

Enhanced metabolism of phenytoin to *p*-hydroxyphenytoin is the main reason for increased clearance (20). Increased secretion of oestrogen and progesterone in pregnancy affects hepatic metabolism of drugs in different ways. Progesterone can increase the rate of metabolism of phenytoin by induction of hepatic drug-metabolising enzymes and this is probably the main reason for increased clearance. However, another possible reason for decreased plasma phenytoin is described in a single case report of malabsorption during pregnancy, with 56% of the dose appearing in faeces (21).

Phenytoin is normally about 90% to 95% protein bound (mainly to albumin); however, in pregnancy there is a reduction in plasma albumin concentration and thus in the extent of protein binding (22). The overall effect is that while there is an increase in plasma clearance leading to a decrease in total phenytoin concentrations compared with pre-pregnancy levels (23), the decreased protein binding results in an increase in the free (pharmacologically active), unbound fraction. In one series, unbound plasma concentrations declined by only 18%, whereas total phenytoin declined by as much as 61% (14,15).

Phenobarbital

The plasma clearance of phenobarbital was also studied in the investigations cited above and both studies demonstrated that the plasma clearance of phenobarbital was increased, but this was much less marked than for phenytoin (17,18). Similar findings were reported more recently with total plasma concentrations declining by 55% and the sharpest decrease occurring in the first trimester (12), but considerable inter-individual variation has been demonstrated (24). Even more recently, a further study has reported that both total and free phenobarbital concentrations may decrease by 50% (23).

Primidone

Primidone is metabolised to phenobarbital, which slowly accumulates in plasma to account for some of the pharmacological effects, and phenylethylmalonamide (PEMA). Primidone is not protein bound and there have been only a few studies of its disposition during gestation with controversial results. In one

study of 14 patients, drug concentrations were lower after conception and in two patients the total clearance values increased after conception, persisted throughout pregnancy and then dropped after delivery (25). The authors concluded that both renal and hepatic clearance of primidone increased significantly during gestation. However, results from the prospective Helsinki study which contained 10 patients prescribed primidone indicated that there was no significant change in primidone clearance with gestation although there was marked intra- and inter-individual fluctuation (26). In this study sample collection times were not standardised with respect to dose. Primidone generally has a fairly short plasma elimination half-life ($t_{1/2}$) of around 5 hours, but it can be long in some patients (24 hours), so results from this study may be misleading. However, a later study concluded that primidone plasma concentrations did not significantly change during gestation (27), consistent with the findings of Bardy (28) and Battino et al. (29).

Carbamazepine

The plasma clearance of carbamazepine was also studied in three patients by Dam et al. (18), and this reached maximal values between 3 weeks before and 1 week after delivery, but it fluctuated considerably during the pregnancies (18).

The metabolism of carbamazepine is dose dependent in humans (30), and the drug is metabolised along several major pathways with the epoxide-diol pathway being quantitatively the most important (31). Carbamazepine epoxide is pharmacologically active being equipotent to the parent drug and the principal catalyst for the epoxidation reaction is CYP3A4; also the CYP2C8 isoenzyme is involved to a lesser extent (32). Further oxidation of epoxide to the pharmacologically inactive 10,11-trans-dihydroxy-10,11-dihydro-carbamazepine is catalysed by epoxide hydrolase (33). Both carbamazepine and the epoxide are protein bound, but to different extents, for example, carbamazepine is 70% to 80% and epoxide is 50% to 60%.

Data on the disposition of carbamazepine during pregnancy are conflicting with some studies finding no significant change in total plasma concentrations or intrinsic clearance (15,34). While there are differing reports regarding the disposition of carbamazepine during gestation, on balance it seems that clearance increases with a maximum in the third trimester. While plasma carbamazepine may decline by over 40% at constant dosage, non-protein bound drug is reported to be less affected (12). Another group found that compared with baseline, total carbamazepine concentrations were just 10% lower during the third trimester with the free concentrations only 4% lower (14,15). The ratio of epoxide metabolite to carbamazepine concentration usually increases during gestation, although not in a predictable manner. This has been attributed to reduced metabolism of epoxide through epoxide hydrolase inhibition (34), but equally epoxide formation might be enhanced. Overall, the evidence indicates that clinically significant changes in the clearance of carbamazepine and epoxide during gestation are uncommon.

Valproic Acid

Valproic acid (valproate) is extensively biotransformed with protein binding normally between 70% and 93% and is drug concentration dependent in the range <75 to 150 mg/L. Diminished protein binding of valproate has been observed in numerous pathophysiologic states associated with hypoalbuminaemia including pregnancy (35,36). The elimination kinetics are dose dependent and when maintenance doses are escalated in an individual, a non-linear relationship exists between plasma concentration and dose such that as dose is increased there is a less than proportional increase in steady-state plasma concentration. This convex, curvilinear relationship is caused by concentration-dependent protein binding such that the free fraction of valproate increases as total plasma concentration rises.

There are many reports of increased valproate clearance during gestation. In a single case review, the ratio of plasma valproate concentration to dose began to decline in the latter part of the second trimester and reached its lowest ratio 3 weeks before delivery. After parturition valproate concentrations in the mother regained pre-pregnancy values within 2 to 3 weeks (37). A similar experience was reported in five patients by Philbert and Dam (38). Other studies report a decline in *total* plasma valproate concentration by up to 50% during gestation with a return to pre-conception concentrations within 1 week of delivery (12).

Since valproate is extensively protein bound, it is susceptible to pregnancy-induced reduction in plasma albumin concentration and the non-protein bound fraction is inversely correlated with plasma albumin concentration. It is the free drug fraction that is pharmacologically active and to some extent the decrease in binding will compensate for the decline in total valproate as gestation proceeds; furthermore, one should not forget that the free fraction of valproate increases over-proportionally with increased total valproate plasma concentration. It was reported in nine pregnancies that total valproate concentrations decreased by 39%, while unbound concentrations increased by 25% (12).

Since, despite a decrease in total valproate concentration through gestation, the free concentration remains approximately constant; a need for dose adjustment would not be anticipated. The increased valproate clearance, particularly during late gestation, is the result of the previously recognised decrease in maternal plasma protein binding which arises because of elevated non-esterified fatty acids and hypoalbuminaemia (35). While it is still not known whether there is a change in intrinsic metabolic clearance of valproate during pregnancy, monitoring free rather than total valproate concentrations is probably more useful throughout the entire gestation and post-partum.

Ethosuximide

Ethosuximide is extensively biotransformed by oxidative and conjugation mechanisms with only about 20% of an administered dose being excreted unchanged in urine. It is a low-clearance drug with a plasma elimination half-life of 40 to 60 hours and is not protein bound. The relationship between daily dose and plasma concentration is somewhat controversial and while at low daily intake there is a linear relationship between plasma concentration and dose; it is reported that in some patients there is a disproportionate increase in plasma concentration with incremental doses and the drug is tending towards saturation kinetics in some patients within the plasma concentration target range.

There is some evidence that plasma ethosuximide concentrations decrease during gestation and return to baseline after delivery, but these are only small numbers of mothers that have been investigated (39–42).

Benzodiazepines

Benzodiazepines are used as anticonvulsants primarily to treat status epilepticus; however three of them, namely, clobazam, clonazepam and nitrazepam, are prescribed for maintenance treatment of various seizure disorders. Clobazam is the most widely prescribed benzodiazepines used in the treatment of epilepsy and differs from the others in that it has a 1,5- rather than 1,4-diazepine structure. Both clonazepam and nitrazepam are more widely used in children than adults and as such their disposition is not reported in gestation. Clobazam is less liable to the development of tolerance than other benzodiazepines and is more widely prescribed, however, there are no reports of clobazam disposition throughout pregnancy.

Clobazam is extensively biotransformed by N-demethylation at the 1-N-position of the benzodiazepine ring to produce N-desmethylclobazam. This metabolite accumulates to much higher concentrations than parent drug in plasma and is responsible for the majority of the pharmacological effect (43). Clobazam is 85% bound to serum proteins and elimination involves hydroxylation at the 4 position of the unsubstituted aromatic ring, resulting in formation of 4-hydroxyclobazam and 4-hydroxydesmethylclobazam, both of which are subsequently conjugated and excreted in urine. The plasma elimination half-life of clobazam is normally 10 to 30 hours, whilst the half-life of N-desmethylclobazam is 36 to 46 hours.

If clobazam is compared with the analogous drug, diazepam, where the pharmacokinetics have been evaluated in pregnancy, and which undergoes a similar metabolic sequence, then the normal $t_{1/2}$ for diazepam and nordiazepam are 21 to 37 hours and 50 to 99 hours, respectively, but gestation prolongs the $t_{1/2}$ of diazepam to 2 to 3 days, probably because of a change in the volume of distribution (44,45). Another study of desmethyldiazepam pharmacokinetics (administered as clorazepate) indicated that desmethyldiazepam $t_{1/2}$ was extended by three-fold during pregnancy (46). By analogy it is likely that the clearance of clobazam and its major plasma metabolite will be decreased significantly during gestation.

Lamotrigine

Lamotrigine is extensively metabolised primarily to the pharmacologically inactive 2-N-glucuronide, a reaction catalysed by UGT1A4. The plasma elimination half-life is 15 to 35 hours when given as monotherapy, and may be substantially shorter (8–20 hours) in patients taking enzyme-inducing AEDs; conversely, valproic acid inhibits lamotrigine metabolism and prolongs $t_{1/2}$ to about 60 hours (47,48). The drug is approximately 55% bound to plasma proteins and will not, therefore, be significantly affected by changes in serum albumin concentration.

At a constant lamotrigine dose, large decreases in plasma concentrations have been reported in pregnancy with apparent clearance increasing steadily as gestation progresses and peaking at around 32 weeks when plasma concentrations can be 40% to 60% below baseline (49,50). Another group studied 11 pregnant women that also demonstrated significant decreases in the ratio of plasma lamotrigine concentration to dose compared with pre-pregnancy values (51). Five patients in another study experienced seizure deterioration during gestation and there was significant inter-patient variability in the pharmacokinetics of lamotrigine (52).

There are several other reports that lamotrigine clearance may be increased by up to 300% during pregnancy (53–55) and this is probably a consequence of an increased rate of lamotrigine glucuronidation in pregnancy caused by up-regulation of UGT1A4 by 17β-estradiol (56). The decrease in lamotrigine plasma concentration occurs shortly after conception, continues throughout gestation (first trimester 197%, second trimester 236% and third trimester 248%) and may result in increased seizures (55). However, large inter-individual variability in the degree of enhanced clearance is reported thus making it important to personalise any dose increases. Furthermore, while lamotrigine clearance may be increased by up to 300% during pregnancy this increase is attenuated in women that are co-medicated with enzyme-inducing or -inhibiting medications (54,57) which also suggests an enhanced rate of glucuronidation as the underlying mechanism. This effect was recently confirmed by demonstrating an increased lamotrigine 2-N-glucuronide/lamotrigine ratio in serum during pregnancy (58).

Since large inter-individual differences in the inductive effect occur even with monotherapy, which results in the extent of lamotrigine clearance changes being quite unpredictable; and since frequent dose adjustments may be required to maintain stable plasma concentrations, it is recommended that these are best guided by TDM. Lamotrigine pharmacokinetics appears to revert to pre-pregnancy conditions within a few days of delivery, hence monitoring plasma concentrations second daily for 1 week after delivery could also be justified in order to guide the mother's post-partum treatment (see chapter 12).

Levetiracetam

Oral absorption of levetiracetam is efficient and there is an individual linear plasma concentration/dose response. The major route of elimination is renal, with approximately 66% of a dose being cleared unchanged and 27% as the pharmacologically inactive acid metabolite, LO59 (59). This metabolite is formed by hydrolysis of levetiracetam with a cytosolic amidase which oxidises the acetamide side chain; however, some additional minor metabolic oxidative pathways exist which are catalysed by hepatic isoenzymes and are therefore inducible (60). The drug is not bound to plasma proteins and renal function is the main determinant of its rate of elimination with the plasma $t_{1/2}$ being 6 to 8 hours in healthy adults (61,62). However, despite the fact that hepatic biotransformation is reported to account for only about 3% of metabolism via two hydroxylated metabolites, this pathway is inducible and enzyme-inducing AEDs can moderately decrease serum levetiracetam concentrations (63–65).

During pregnancy, the apparent clearance of levetiracetam increases significantly and case series have demonstrated reduced serum concentration/dose ratios as low as 50% of baseline (66,67). The underlying mechanism for this effect has not been identified and both increased hydrolysis in the peripheral compartment and/or increased renal blood flow with consequent higher renal clearance are considered possible.

Oxcarbazepine

Following oral ingestion, oxcarbazepine is rapidly biotransformed via pre-systemic 10-keto reduction, which is catalysed by a cytosolic arylketone reductase (68–70), to the two enantiomers of the monohydroxy derivative (MHD), 10,11-dihydro-10-hydroxy-carbamazepine. The enantiomers have similar pharmacological activity and accumulate in plasma to much higher concentration (about 10-fold) than the parent drug (71,72). MHD is 40% protein bound, shows linear pharmacokinetics and, since the conversion of oxcarbazepine to MHD is stereoselective, the plasma concentrations of the S-enantiomer are considerably higher than those of the R-enantiomer (69,73). The plasma elimination half-life of both enantiomers is 7 to 12 hours, and they are metabolised primarily by glucuronidation prior to renal clearance.

Pharmacokinetic data on oxcarbazepine in human pregnancy are limited with Bülau et al. (74) reporting concentrations from one mother and neonate, and Pienimäki et al. (75) reporting drug concentrations of three mothers. These cases indicate significant fetal exposure to oxcarbazepine/MHD with the maternal and fetal concentrations being similar. There have also been two studies that report a decrease of MHD plasma concentration of at least 36% during pregnancy compared with pre- and post-pregnancy values (76,77) and an increase in the rate of glucuronide metabolism is suggested to be the mechanism responsible for the increased MHD clearance.

The information above will also apply to the recently introduced eslicarbazepine acetate which is also metabolised to produce mainly S-MHD and will accumulate in plasma in the same way described previously.

Topiramate

Following oral ingestion, topiramate is efficiently absorbed with a linear relationship between dose and serum concentration. When administered alone a high proportion of the drug is cleared renally unchanged, but topiramate also undergoes oxidative biotransformation which is significantly enhanced when it is prescribed together with enzyme-inducing drugs. The plasma elimination half-life is 20 to 30 hours in monotherapy, but this can decrease to about 12 hours with enzyme induction (78,79).

Topiramate is only 15% bound to serum proteins, but it does have a high-affinity/low-capacity binding site on erythrocytes (80). There is limited pharmacokinetic data on topiramate in human pregnancy, and first reports only looked at transfer of the drug into the neonate and breast milk rather than disposition during gestation (81). A recent study of 10 pregnancies, where samples were available from all three trimesters, compared the drug clearance with the pre-pregnancy values and found it was significantly increased during the second and third trimesters but not during the first; however, there was a pronounced intra-individual variability in topiramate clearance between subjects (82). Another recent study of 15 pregnancies found a similar result, and it is postulated that a pregnancy-related increase in renal blood flow might lead to an increase in renal clearance and a consequent decline in topiramate serum concentrations if the drug dose is not adjusted (83).

Zonisamide

Following oral ingestion, zonisamide is efficiently absorbed and subsequently eliminated by mixed hepatic (70%) and renal (30%) routes of elimination. In humans, metabolism is primarily via opening of the benzisoxazole ring to produce 2-sulfamoylacetylphenol (SMAP) which is subsequently glucuronide linked and also by N-acetylation of the sulfonamide side chain to produce N-acetyl zonisamide. Zonisamide is 40% to 60% bound to plasma proteins and the mean elimination half-life of the drug from plasma is 50 to 60 hours, although hepatic enzyme-inducing drugs increase zonisamide clearance.

There are no systematic studies of the pharmacokinetic of zonisamide during gestation, but decreased serum albumin concentrations and increased glomerular filtration would not be expected to produce large changes in pharmacokinetics. However, other pregnancy-related changes, for example, increased volume of distribution might affect zonisamide plasma concentrations and one case reports a slight increase 9 days after delivery (84). More recently, another case report indicates that the change in zonisamide serum concentrations in a pregnant woman could be due to an increase in clearance at the end of the second trimester (85).

Gabapentin and Pregabalin

Both drugs are absorbed and transported by the L-amino acid transporter system and neither is metabolised. There have been no systematic investigations into the disposition of either gabapentin or pregabalin throughout pregnancy, but theoretically the increase in glomerular filtration may result in decreased drug concentrations. One study of six pregnancies in women prescribed gabapentin investigated the pharmacokinetics of gabapentin during delivery, lactation and into the neonatal period, but did not follow plasma concentrations throughout the whole period of gestation and compare them with pre-conception data (86).

Other Newer Drugs

There are no systematic studies of disposition throughout gestation of the remaining drugs that are available at the present time, namely vigabatrin, felbamate, tiagabine, brivaracetam, rufinamide, stiripentol, lacosamide and retigabine. Because of their specific indications, some of these drugs, for example, stiripentol and rufinamide, are unlikely to be prescribed to women of childbearing age, while others, for example, felbamate and tiagabine, are rarely prescribed at the present time. With the latest AEDs such as lacosamide and retigabine it will be a question of studying their disposition during gestation as the opportunity arises.

Transfer of AEDs into Breast Milk

All of the AEDs transfer into the mother's milk to some degree (Table 4.1). However, the importance of this phenomenon may be overemphasised, since all of the drugs used to treat epilepsy cross the placenta to some extent and therefore the child is born fully loaded with the mother's drug if she has continued maintenance treatment throughout the pregnancy. Some AEDs may cause neonatal difficulty with withdrawal symptoms if exposure is stopped abruptly. The neonatal withdrawal syndrome was described by Desmond et al. (87) and there has

Table 4.1 Transfer of AEDs into Breast Milk.

AED	Milk/Plasma ratio
Carbamazepine	0.17–0.69
Carbamazepine epoxide	0.3–0.5
Ethosuximide	0.77–1.0
Felbamate	Not known
Gabapentin	0.73
Lamotrigine	0.47–0.77
Levetiracetam	0.76–1.33
Oxcarbazepine + MHD	0.5
Primidone	0.4–0.96
Phenytoin	0.06–0.69
Tiagabine	Not known
Topiramate	0.88–1.2
Valproate	0.01–0.1
Vigabatrin	0.04–0.22
Zonisamide	0.93
Pregabalin	Not known[a]
Clobazam + desmethylclobazam	0.13–0.36
Brivaracetam	Not known[b]
Rufinamide	Not known, but likely to be excreted in milk
Lacosamide	Not known[c]
Retigabine	Not known[c]

[a]Passes into breast milk in animals. Probably similar to gabapentin.
[b]Probably similar to levetiracetam.
[c]Passes into breast milk in animals.
Abbreviations: AED, anti-epileptic drug; MHD, monohydroxy derivative.

been subsequent studies of the phenomena in neonates passively exposed to phenobarbital and primidone (88,89); furthermore, the elimination of phenobarbital in neonates is significantly slower than in other patient groups which can cause the withdrawal period to be prolonged. The withdrawal syndrome has also been observed with other AEDs, notably benzodiazepines (90); however, the phenomenon has not been associated with any of the second- or third-generation AEDs to date. Since most of the AEDs pass into breast milk, normal feeding will continue the neonate's exposure and a weaning regimen can then be initiated (see chapters 5 and 12).

DISCUSSION

Maternal serum AED concentration in pregnancy not only reflects the therapeutic and adverse effects in the mother, but also the extent of drug exposure to the fetus. The pharmacokinetics of many AEDs undergo significant changes during pregnancy because of modifications in body weight, altered serum composition, haemodynamic changes, hormonal influences and contribution of the foetoplacental unit to drug distribution and disposition (91). Pregnancy may also affect AED absorption, binding to serum proteins and distribution, metabolism and renal elimination (13).

TDM is of particular value in pregnancy because the pharmacokinetic alterations noted above represent average changes, but the extent of these changes varies extensively between individuals with the decline in plasma drug concentration being insignificant in some pregnant patients and pronounced in others. If the aim is to maintain the mother's AED concentration constant throughout gestation (and preferably similar to successful pre-conception values), regular monitoring as outlined in best practice guidelines should be undertaken in order to guide dose adjustments (16). Other guidelines and recommendations are discussed in more detail in chapter 12. In particular with drugs that are extensively protein bound, monitoring the non-protein bound (free) drug concentration is recommended since decreased protein binding may result in a lower *total* (protein bound plus unbound) drug concentrations but may leave unchanged the unbound (pharmacologically active) concentration. TDM during pregnancy aims to facilitate individualised dosing by identifying pregnancy-induced pharmacokinetic changes, but for highly protein-bound drugs, for example, valproic acid and phenytoin, total serum concentrations during pregnancy may be *misleading*. Furthermore, since less information is available regarding disposition of the second- and third-generation AEDs throughout pregnancy, TDM of these drugs during pregnancy would help to guide any dose adjustments required to ensure stability of serum levels.

REFERENCES

1. Anderson GD. Pregnancy-related changes in pharmacokinetics: a mechanistic-based approach. Clin Pharmacokinet 2005; 44:989–1008.
2. Krauer B, Krauer F. Drug kinetics in pregnancy. Clin Pharmacokin 1979; 2:167–181.
3. Rakhmanina N, van den Anker, Soldin SJ. Safety and pharmacokinetics of antiretroviral therapy during pregnancy. Ther Drug Monit 2004; 26:110–115.
4. Rane A, Von Bahr Chr, Orrenius S, et al. Drug metabolism in human fetus. In: Boreus A, ed. Fetal Pharmacology. New York: Raven Press, 1973:287–301.
5. Davis M, Simmons CJ, Dordoni B, et al. Induction of hepatic enzymes during normal pregnancy. J Obstet Gynaecol Br Commonw 1973; 80:690–694.

6. Tephly TR, Mannering GJ. Inhibition of drug metabolism by steroids. Mol Pharmacol 1968; 4:10–14.

7. Loebstein R, Koren G. Clinical relevance of therapeutic drug monitoring during pregnancy. Ther Drug Monit 2002; 24:15–22.

8. Koren G, Soldin O. Therapeutic drug monitoring of antithyroid drugs during pregnancy. Ther Drug Monit 2006; 28:8–11.

9. Nulman I, Laslo D, Koren G. Treatment of epilepsy in pregnancy. Drugs 1999; 57:535–544.

10. Morrell MJ. Antiepileptic drug use in women. In: Levy R, et al. eds. Antiepileptic Drugs. 5th ed. Philadelphia: Lippincott Williams & Wilkins, 2002:132–148.

11. Williams J, Myson V, Steward S, et al. Self-discontinuation of antiepileptic medication in pregnancy: detection by hair analysis. Epilepsia 2002; 43:824–831.

12. Yerby MS, Friel PN, McCormick K. Antiepileptic drug disposition during pregnancy. Neurology 1992; 42:12–16.

13. Pennell PB. Antiepileptic drug pharmacokinetics during pregnancy and lactation. Neurology 2003; 61(suppl 2):S35–S42.

14. Tomson T, Lindborn U, Ekqvist B, et al. Epilepsy and pregnancy: a prospective study of seizure control in relation of free and total plasma concentrations of carbamazepine and phenytoin. Epilepsia 1994; 35:122–130.

15. Tomson T, Lindborn U, Ekqvist B, et al. Disposition of carbamazepine and phenytoin in pregnancy. Epilepsia 1994; 35: 131–135.

16. Patsalos PN, Berry DJ, Bourgeous BFD, et al. Antiepileptic drugs—best practice guidelines for therapeutic drug monitoring. Epilepsia 2008; 49(7):1239–1276.

17. Bossi L, Assael BM, Avanzini G, et al. Plasma levels and clinical effects of antiepileptic drugs in pregnant epileptic patients and their newborns. In: Johannessen SI, Morselli PL, Pippenger CE, et al. eds. Antiepileptic Therapy: Advances in Drug Monitoring. New York: Raven Press, 1980:9–14.

18. Dam M, Christiansen J, Munck O, et al. Antiepileptic drugs: metabolism in pregnancy. Clin Pharmacokinet 1979; 4:53–62.

19. Bardy AH, Hiilesmaa VK, Teramo KA. Serum phenytoin during pregnancy, labour and puerperium. Acta Neurol Scand 1987; 75:374–375.

20. Bernus I, Hooper WD, Dickinson RG, et al. Effects of pregnancy on various pathways of human antiepileptic drug metabolism. Clin Neuropharmacol 1997; 20:13–21.

21. Ramsay RE, Strauss RG, Wilder BJ, et al. Status epilepticus in pregnancy: effect of phenytoin malabsorption on seizure control. Neurology 1978; 28:85–89.

22. Yerby MS, Friel PN, McCormick K. Pharmacokinetics of anticonvulsants in pregnancy: alterations in plasma protein binding. Epilepsy Res 1990; 5:223–228.

23. Tomson T. Gender aspects of pharmacokinetics of new and old AEDs: pregnancy and breast feeding. Ther Drug Monit 2005; 27:718–721.

24. Luoma PV, Heikkinen JE, Ylostalo PR. Phenobarbitone pharmacokinetics and salivary and serum concentrations in pregnancy. Ther Drug Monit 1982; 4:65–68.

25. Nau H, Schmidt D, Beck-Mannagetta G, et al. Pharmacokinetics of primidone and metabolites during human pregnancy. In: Janz D, et al. eds. Epilepsy, Pregnancy and the Child. New York: Raven Press, 1982:121–129.

26. Bardy AH, Teramo KA, Hiilesmaa VK. Apparent plasma clearance of phenytoin, phenobarbitone, primidone and carbamazepine during pregnancy: results of the prospective Helsinki study. In: Janz D, et al. eds. Epilepsy, Pregnancy and the Child. New York: Raven Press, 1982:141–145.

27. Kaneko S, Otani K, Fujita S, et al. The pharmacokinetics of primidone during pregnancy. In: Porter RJ, et al. eds. Advances in Epileptology: XVth Epilepsy International Symposium. New York: Raven Press, 1984:259–263.

28. Bardy AH. Epilepsy and pregnancy. A Prospective Study of 154 Pregnancies of Epileptic Women [dissertation]. Helsinki: University of Helsinki, 1982.

29. Battino D, Avanzini G, Bossi L, et al. Monitoring of antiepileptic drugs plasma levels during pregnancy and puerperium. In: Janz D, et al. eds. Epilepsy, Pregnancy and the Child. New York: Raven Press, 1982:147–154.

30. Bernus I, Dickinson RG, Hooper WD, et al. Dose-dependent metabolism of carbamazepine in humans. Epilepsy Res 1996; 24:163–172.

31. Spina E. Carbamazepine: chemistry, biotransformation, and pharmacokinetics. In: Levy R, et al. ed. Antiepileptic Drugs. 5th ed. Philadelphia: Lippincott Williams & Wilkins, 2002:236–246.

32. Kerr BM, Thummel KE, Wurden CJ, et al. Human liver carbamazepine metabolism. Role of CYP3A4 and CYP2C8 in 10,11-epoxide formation. Biochem Pharmacol 1994; 47:1969–1979.

33. Faigle JW, Feldmann KF. Carbamazepine: chemistry and biotransformation. In: Levy R, et al. eds. Antiepileptic Drugs. 4th ed. New York: Raven Press, 1995:499–513.

34. Yerby MS, Friel PN, Miller DQ. Carbamazepine protein binding and disposition in pregnancy. Ther Drug Monit 1985; 7:269–273.

35. Nau H, Krauer B. Serum protein binding of valproic acid in fetus-mothers pairs throughout pregnancy: correlation with oxytocin administration and albumin and free fatty acid concentrations. J Clin Pharmacol 1986; 26:215–221.

36. Perucca E. Free level monitoring of antiepileptic drugs: clinical usefulness and case studies. Clin Pharmacokinet 1984; 9(suppl 1): 71–78.

37. Plasse J-C, Revol M, Chabert G. Neonatal pharmacokinetics of valproic acid. In: Schaaf D, Van de Kleijn E, eds. Progress in Clinical Pharmacy, Amsterdam: Elsevier, North-Holland Biomedical Press, 1979:247–252.

38. Philbert A, Dam M. The epileptic mother and her child. Epilepsia 1982; 23:85–99.

39. Koup JR, Rose JQ, Cohen ME. Ethosuximide pharmacokinetics in a pregnant patient and her newborn. Epilepsia 1978; 19:535–539.

40. Kuhnz W, Koch S, Jacob S, et al. Epileptic women during pregnancy and lactation: placental transfer, serum concentration in nursed infants and clinical status. Br J Clin Pharmacol 1984; 18:671–677.

41. Rane A, Tunell R. Ethosuximide in human milk and in plasma of a mother and her nursed infant. Br J Clin Pharmacol 1981; 12:855–858.

42. Eadie MJ, Lander CM, Tyrer JH. Plasma drug level monitoring in pregnancy. Clin Pharmacokinet 1977; 2:427–436.

43. Aucamp AK. Aspects of the pharmacokinetics and pharmacodynamics of benzodiazepines with particular reference to clobazam. Drug Dev Res 1982; (suppl 1):117–126.

44. Mandeli M, Morselli PL, Nordio S, et al. Placental transfer of diazepam in the newborn. Clin Pharmacol Ther 1975; 17:564–572.

45. Anderson GD, Miller JW. Benzodiazepines. Chemistry, biotransformation and pharmacokinetics. In: Levy RH, Mattson R, Meldrum BS, et al. eds., Antiepileptic Drugs. 5th ed. Philadelphia: Lippincott Williams & Wilkins, 2002:187–205.

46. Rey E, d'Arthis Ph, Giraux P, et al. Pharmacokinetics of clorazepate in pregnant and non-pregnant women. Eur J Clin Pharmacol 1979; 15(3):175–180.

47. Rambeck B, Wolf P. Lamotrigine clinical pharmacokinetics. Clin Pharmacokinet 1993; 25:433–443.

48. Biton V. Pharmacokinetics, toxicology and safety of lamotrigine in epilepsy. Expert Opin Drug Metab Toxicol 2006; 2:1009–1018.

49. Pennell PB, Newport DJ, Stowe ZN, et al. The impact of pregnancy and childbirth on the metabolism of lamotrigine. Neurology 2004; 62:292–295.

50. Tomson T, Ohman I, Vitols S. Lamotrigine in pregnancy and lactation: a case report. Epilepsia 1997; 38:1039–1041.

51. Franco V, Mazzucchelli I, Gatti G, et al. Changes in lamotrigine pharmacokinetics during pregnancy and the puerperium. Ther Dug Monit 2008; 30(4):533–537.

52. Petrenaite V, Sabers A, Hansen-Schwartz J. Individual changes in lamotrigine plasma concentration during pregnancy. Epilepsia 2005; 65:185–188.

53. Ohman I, Vitols S, Tomson T. Lamotrigine in pregnancy: pharmacokinetics during delivery, in the neonate, and during lactation. Epilepsia 2000; 41:709–713.

54. Tran TA, Leppik IE, Blesi K, et al. Lamotrigine clearance during pregnancy. Neurology 2002; 59:251–255.

55. Pennell PB, Peng L, Newport DJ, et al. Lamotrigine in pregnancy: clearance, therapeutic drug monitoring, and seizure frequency. Neurology 2008; 70:2130–2136.

56. Chen H, Yang K, Choi S, et al. Up-regulation of UDP-glucuronosyltransferase (UGT) 1A4 by 17β-estradiol: a potential mechanism of increased lamotrigine elimination in pregnancy. Drug Metab Dispos 2009; 37:1841–1847.

57. Tomson T, Luef G, Sabers A, et al. Valproate effects on kinetics of lamotrigine in pregnancy and treatment with oral contraceptives. Neurology 2006; 67:1297–1299.

58. Ohman I, Beck O, Vitols S, et al. Plasma concentrations of lamotrigine and its 2-N-glucuronide metabolite during pregnancy in women with epilepsy. Epilepsia 2008; 49:1075–1080.

59. Patsalos PN. Clinical pharmacokinetics of levetiracetam. Clin Pharmacokinet 2004; 43:707–724.

60. Patsalos PN, Ghattaura S, Ratnaraj N, et al. In situ metabolism of levetiracetam in blood of patients with epilepsy. Epilepsia 2006; 47:1818–1821.

61. Patsalos PN. Levetiracetam: pharmacology and therapeutics in the treatment of epilepsy and other neurological conditions. Rev Contemp Pharmacother 2004; 13:1–168.

62. Johannessen SI, Battino D, Berry DJ, et al. Therapeutic drug monitoring of the newer antiepileptic drugs. Ther Drug Monit 2003; 25:347–363.

63. Perucca E, Gidal BE, Baltes E. Effects of antiepileptic comedication on levetiracetam pharmacokinetics: a pooled analysis of data from randomized adjunctive therapy trials. Epilepsy Res 2003; 53:47–56.

64. Contin M, Albani F, Riva R, et al. Levetiracetam therapeutic monitoring in patients with epilepsy: effect of concomitant antiepileptic drugs. Ther Drug Monit 2004; 26:375–379.

65. Hirsch LJ, Arif H, Buchsbaum R, et al. Effect of age and comedication on levetiracetam pharmacokinetics and tolerability. Epilepsia 2007; 48:1351–1359.

66. Tomson T, Palm R, Kallen K, et al. Pharmacokinetics of levetiracetam during pregnancy, delivery, in the neonatal period and lactation. Epilepsia 2007; 48(6):111–116.

67. Westin AA, Reimers A, Helde G, et al. Serum concentration/dose ratio of levetiracetam before, during and after pregnancy. Seizure 2008; 17:192–198.

68. Tecoma ES. Oxcarbazepine. Epilepsia 1999; 40:S37–S46.

69. Wellington K, Goa KL. Oxcarbazepine: an update of its efficacy in the management of epilepsy. CNS Drugs 2001; 15:137–163.

70. Kalis MM, Huff NA. Oxcarbazepine, an antiepileptic agent. Clin Ther 2001; 23(5):680–700.

71. Schultz H, Feldman K, Faigle JW, et al. The metabolism of 14C-oxcarbazepine in man. Xenobiotica 1986; 16:769–778.

72. Lloyd P, Flesch G, Dieterle W. Clinical pharmacology and pharmacokinetics of oxcarbazepine. Epilepsia 1994; 35(suppl 3):10–13.

73. Volosov A, Xiaodong S, Perucca E, et al. Enantioselective pharmacokinetics of 10-hydroxycarbazepine after oral administration of oxcarbazepine to healthy Chinese subjects. Clin Pharmacol Ther 1999; 66:547–553.

74. Bülau P, Paar WD, von Unruh GE. Pharmacokinetics of oxcarbazepine and 10-hydroxy-carbazepine in the newborn child of an oxcarbazepine-treated mother. Eur J Clin Pharmacol 1988; 34:311–313.

75. Pienimäki P, Lampela E, Hakkola J, et al. Pharmacokinetics of oxcarbazepine and carbamazepine in human placenta. Epilepsia 1997; 38(3):309–316.

76. Christensen J, Sabers A, Sidenius P. Oxcarbazepine concentrations during pregnancy: a retrospective study in patients with epilepsy. Neurology 2006; 67:1497–1499.

77. Mazzucchelli I, Onat FY, Ozkara C, et al. Changes in the disposition of oxcarbazepine and its metabolites during pregnancy and the puerperium. Epilepsia 2006; 47:504–509.

78. Sachdeo RC, Sachdeo SK, Walker SA, et al. Steady-state pharmacokinetics of topiramate and carbamazepine in patients with epilepsy during monotherapy and concomitant therapy. Epilepsia 1996; 37:774–780.

79. Britzi M, Perucca E, Soback S, et al. Pharmacokinetic and metabolic investigation of topiramate disposition in healthy subjects in the absence and in the presence of enzyme induction by carbamazepine. Epilepsia 2005; 46:378–384.

80. Doose DR, Streeter AJ. Topiramate: chemistry, biotransformation, and pharmacokinetics. In: Levy R, et al. eds. Antiepileptic Drugs. 5th ed. Philadelphia: Lippincott Williams & Wilkins, 2002:727–734.

81. Ohman I, Vitols S, Luef G, et al. Topiramate kinetics during delivery, lactation, and in the neonate: preliminary observation. Epilepsia 2002; 43(10):1157–1160.

82. Ohman I, Sabers A, de Flon P, et al. Pharmacokinetics of topiramate during pregnancy. Epilepsy Res 2009; 87(2–3):124–129.

83. Westin AA, Nakken KO, Johannessen SI, et al. Serum concentration/dose ratio of topiramate during pregnancy. Epilepsia 2009; 50(3):480–485.

84. Kawada K, Itoh S, Kusaka T, et al. Pharmacokinetics of zonisamide in perinatal period. Brain Dev 2002; 24:95–97.

85. Oles KS, Bell WL. Zonisamide concentrations during pregnancy. Ann Pharmacother 2008; 42(7):1139–1141.

86. Ohman I, Vitols S, Tomson T. Pharmacokinetics of gabapentin during delivery, in the neonatal period, and lactation: does a fetal accumulation occur during pregnancy? Epilepsia 2005; 46(10): 1621–1624.

87. Desmond MM, Schwanecke RP, Wilson G, et al. Maternal barbiturate utilisation and neonatal withdrawal symptomatology. J Pediatr 1972; 80:190–197.

88. Bleyer WA, Marshall RE. Barbiturate withdrawal syndrome in a passively addicted infant. JAMA 1972; 221:185–186.

89. Kuhnz W, Kock H, Helge H, et al. Primidone and phenobarbitone during lactation period in epileptic women: total and free drug serum levels in the nursed infant and their effects on neonatal behaviour. Dev Pharmacol Ther 1988; 11:147–154.

90. Weber LWD. Benzodiazepines in pregnancy: academic debate or teratogenic risk? Biol Res Preg 1985; 6:151–167.

91. Perucca E. Drug metabolism in pregnancy, infancy and childhood. Pharmacol Ther 1987; 34:129–143.

Therapeutics and breastfeeding

Thomas W. Hale

INTRODUCTION

The rate of breastfeeding worldwide has continued to increase over the last few decades. In many countries the rate exceeds 90% of mothers opting to breastfeed. It has become increasing clear to women that this provides their infant with the best and cleanest source of nutrition. Benefits for the infant also include enhanced neurocognitive development; stronger immune function; reduced rates of sudden infant death syndrome (SIDS) and significant reductions in infectious diseases such as upper respiratory infections, otitis media and necrotising enterocolitis (1–6).

Although the number of women opting to breastfeed is increasing, the number that prematurely discontinue breastfeeding remains high. While this is often for personal reasons, it may also be because of the use of maternal medications. Virtually all women will consume a medication at some time while breastfeeding and usually do not stop breastfeeding. Stopping breastfeeding is common in women who must use medications for chronic syndromes.

Because so many women ingest medications during the early neonatal period, it is not surprising that one of the most common questions encountered by paediatricians and obstetricians is concerning the use of specific drugs during lactation. While in the past two decades an extensive literature on the transfer of drugs into human milk has developed, little of this data seems to have transferred to the practicing clinician. Too often clinicians simply read the package insert, which always suggests discontinuing breastfeeding. Discontinuing breastfeeding is often the wrong decision and most mothers could easily continue to take the medication and continue to breastfeed their infants without risk to the infant.

The following review covers a basic model for understanding how drugs enter milk, and numerous recommendations for drugs of choice for breastfeeding mothers.

THE ALVEOLAR SUBUNIT

The parenchyma of the breast consists of approximately 10 to 15 quadrants or ductal regions that ultimately drain towards the nipple. The alveolus is lined with a specialised epithelial cell, formerly called the alveolar epithelial cell, but now called the lactocyte. During lactation, the breast is heavily perfused with capillaries and lymphatics. Closely juxtaposed to the basal membrane of the alveolus are numerous capillaries that serve as the primary source of nutrients, fatty acids and many other components needed for the production of human milk. Surrounding the alveolus like a basket is a specialised smooth muscle cell called the myoepithelial cell. This cell contains receptor sites for oxytocin. On attachment of the infant to the breast and release of oxytocin from the pituitary, the myoepithelial cells contract around the alveolus thus propelling the milk down towards the nipple via the ductal system.

Plasma cells (also called plasma B cells or plasmocytes) surround the entire alveolar unit and provide most of the immunoglobulins present in milk. Each day an infant receives between 800 and 1200 mg of secretory IgA and smaller amounts of IgM and IgG. Millions of living cells also enter milk, including lymphocytes, T cells and macrophages, particularly during the early stages of lactation (days 1–7). The presence of large numbers of immune cells in milk protects the infant's gut from exposure to microbes.

DRUG TRANSFER INTO HUMAN MILK

The ability of a medication to transfer into the milk compartment is largely determined by their physicochemical properties, such as molecular weight, pKa, lipophilicity and plasma protein binding, as discussed below. Maternal factors include the concentration of medication in the plasma compartment, with higher transfer at higher plasma levels (particularly Cmax). The only source of medications to the breast milk compartment is the plasma.

The transfer of drugs into human milk is usually accomplished by passive diffusion down a concentration gradient. At this time, we only know of a few transport systems for drugs.

Fewer than six drugs are known to transfer against the concentration gradient. The vast majority of drugs transfer from areas of high concentration (plasma) to areas of low concentration (milk) by passive diffusion between compartments.

During the first few days post-partum, drugs may transfer into milk at slightly higher concentrations due to a relatively open alveolar system. The retrograde diffusion of drugs from the milk back into the plasma is well documented and is probably controlled by the same kinetic factors as entry (molecular size, pKa and lipophilicity). As the maternal plasma level of medication increases, so does the transfer into milk. As the maternal plasma level of medication drops, most drugs diffuse out of the milk compartment and back into the maternal plasma for elimination. Few drugs are actually trapped in milk but these include iodine, cimetidine, ranitidine, nitrofurantoin and others.

The most important factors that determine milk levels are as follows:

- *Molecular weight*: Drugs with lower molecular weights (<250 Da) generally enter the milk compartment resulting in higher milk drug levels. Drugs >800 Da are virtually excluded from milk. Thus, large molecular weight proteins (etanercept, heparin) are virtually excluded from the milk compartment.
- *pKa*: Drugs are either weak acids (which can disassociate hydrogen ions or protons) or bases (which can associate the same). The measure of the ease of proton disassociation in a compound, the disassociation or ionisation

constant, is referred to as pKa. It is defined by pKa = pH + log (protonated/unprotonated). The balance of the equilibrium of a sample can be shifted by varying the acidity. If pH is higher than the pKa, the drug site is mostly deprotonated; and if the pH is lower than the pKa, the site is mostly protonated. Drugs with a basic pKa may become highly ionised at the pH of milk (7.2) and thus become trapped in the milk compartment (barbiturates).

- *Protein binding*: As with any drug in any compartment, the more protein binding in the maternal plasma compartment, the less drug available for transfer into the milk compartment. Warfarin is virtually excluded from milk due to its massive binding to plasma albumin.
- *Maternal Cmax*: Drugs that produce low levels in the plasma compartment produce even lower levels in the milk compartment. Thus topical or inhaled medications are largely excluded from the milk compartment.
- *CNS activity*: These medications invariably enter the milk compartment to some degree due to their ability to pass tight endothelial barriers. Therefore, expect milk levels from CNS-active drugs (anticonvulsants, antidepressants and neuroleptics) to be somewhat higher.
- *Oral bioavailability*: Bioavailability is used to describe the fraction of an administered dose that bypasses hepatic uptake and catabolism and reaches the systemic circulation. Medications taken by the mother that are poorly bioavailable produce lower maternal plasma levels and hence lower milk levels. Medications that are poorly bioavailable in the mother are often poorly bioavailable in the infant, thus producing lower plasma levels in the infant.

Medications present in milk can and do in rare instances produce gastrointestinal (GI) symptoms in the infant such as diarrhoea or constipation. Diarrhoea has been reported in some infants exposed to antibiotics or 5-aminosalcylic acid products, but most medications must be systemically absorbed in the infant's plasma compartment to produce untoward systemic effects. Thus, in breastfeeding mothers, poorly bioavailable drugs are often preferred as it ultimately reduces the infants' oral absorption and produces fewer systemic side effects. Table 5.1 lists a number of medications that are poorly bioavailable and are ideal for breastfeeding mothers simply because they are poorly absorbed even in infants.

Table 5.1 Oral Bioavailability of Various Medications

Drug	Oral absorption
Omeprazole	Minimal
Morphine	25%
Infliximab	0%
Gentamycin	<1%
Enoxaparin	Minimal
Lansoprazole	Minimal
Ceftriaxone	Minimal
Gadopentetate	0.8%
Radiocontrast agents	Nil
Sumatriptan	10–15%
Heparin	Nil
Glatirimer	Nil
Natalizumab	Nil
Interferon beta	Nil

Lower maternal oral absorption generally leads to lower maternal plasma levels and reduced milk levels. Drugs with poor oral bioavailability are preferred because they are probably minimally absorbed orally in infants as well.

DETERMINING INFANT EXPOSURE

One of the most accurate determinations of infant exposure is to calculate the daily dose the infant is receiving via milk (Dose.infant). Infants ingest milk at the rate of 150 mL/kg/day for the first 6 months of life, although this is highly variable. If the actual concentration of drug in milk has been published then the absolute infant dose is calculated using the formula below:
(Dose$_{inf}$) = Drug concentration in milk (mg/L) × 0.15 L/kg/day

The relative infant dose (RID) provides an estimate of the weight-normalised dose relative to the mother's dose. This is far more meaningful for the clinician as it gives an estimate of the infant's dose compared to the mother's dose. It is simply calculated by using the formula below:

$$\frac{\text{Dose.infant} \left(\frac{mg/kg}{day} \right)}{\text{Dose.mother} \left(\frac{mg/kg}{day} \right)}$$

This value provides a percent of the mother's dose that reaches the infant via milk.

The vast majority of medications fall below 4% of the maternal dose. In full-term infants, Bennett suggests that an RID of less than 10% is probably safe (7). In premature infants, a safe percentage estimate may be lower. Preterm infants may be more sensitive to even these levels in milk. A clinical evaluation is required in each individual premature infant's case. While RID values greater than 10% should be evaluated cautiously, many drugs can exceed this limit (metronidazole, fluconazole) and can still be used safely. Therefore, the overall risk of the individual medication must be closely correlated with the RID to determine the absolute risk to the infant. As infants age past 6 months, they consume less human milk (and more solid foods) and their ability to metabolise drugs increases incrementally to that of an adult by 9 to 12 months. Milk volumes produced by the mother vary enormously, but in general the volume of milk drops to 100 to 200 cc/day after the first year. Thus, the clinical dose of medication transferred in this volume is reduced as well. For this reason, it is always important to ask the infant's age before evaluating the risk of the drug.

SELECTED DRUG CLASSES
Sedatives and Hypnotics

The benzodiazepine family has been thoroughly studied in breastfeeding mothers. Milk levels of diazepam, lorazepam, midazolam and others have been published and are not excessive. Rarely, sedation has been reported in breastfed infants.

In a study of nine mothers receiving diazepam post-partum, milk levels varied from approximately 0.01 to 0.08 mg/L (8). Other reports suggest slightly higher values. Taken together, most results suggest that the RID of diazepam and its metabolite, desmethyldiazepam, will be on average 0.78% to 9.1% of the weight-adjusted maternal dose (9). Some reports of lethargy, sedation and poor suckling have been found, although these were with prolonged use. Acute use such as in surgical procedures is not likely to lead to clinical effects in breastfed infants.

If a sedative is required, the shorter half-life analogues such as lorazepam and midazolam are preferred (10). The RID

Table 5.2 Relative Infant Dose of Various Anticonvulsants

Drug	Relative infant dose (%)	Compatibility with breastfeeding	References
Carbamazepine	4.35	Compatible. No adverse effects reported.	14,15,16
Ethosuximide	31.4	Levels high in milk and infants. Caution: Poor suckling, sedation and hyperexcitability reported.	17
Gabapentin	3.7–6.6	Compatible. Plasma levels in infants low. No adverse effects reported.	18,19
Lamotrigine	22.8	Compatible with caution. Infant levels fall with time but average about 40–50% of maternal levels.	20,21,22,23
Levetiracetam	3.3–7.8	Compatible. No complications reported in infants. Infant plasma levels reported to be 13% of maternal level.	24,25
Phenobarbital	23.9	Compatible with caution. Expect infant plasma levels of one-third of maternal levels.	26,27
Phenytoin	7.74	Compatible. Infant plasma levels low to undetectable.	14,28,29
Topiramate	24.5	Compatible with caution. Levels in infants 10–20% of maternal levels.	30
Valproic acid	0.68	Compatible. Liver Function tests (LFTs) for infant may be required.	31,32,33
Zonisamide	<33	Caution: Levels in milk high (10.5 mg/L).	34

Source: Adapted from Ref. 136.

of lorazepam (2.5%) and midazolam (0.6%) are quite low and sedation in breastfeeding infants is unlikely. Chronic use of alprazolam has been reported to induce minimal withdrawal in some infants (11).

The use of phenothiazine analogues should be avoided. Chlorpromazine (Thorazine) and promethazine (Phenergan) may increase sleep apnoea (12) and the risk of SIDS (13), and should probably be avoided in breastfeeding mothers. Ondansetron or analogues are preferred for treating nausea and vomiting. Levels of ondansetron in milk are unknown, but this agent is very safe and is commonly used in pregnant patients and young infants.

Anti-Epileptic Medications

Table 5.2 provides the RID of most anti-epileptic drugs.

Valproic Acid

Valproic acid levels in milk are quite low with an RID of approximately 0.68%. In a study of 16 patients receiving 300 to 2400 mg/day, valproic acid concentrations in breast milk ranged from 0.4 to 3.9 mg/L (mean = 1.9 mg/L) (31). In another group of six women, receiving 9.5 to 31 mg/kg/day valproic acid, milk levels averaged 1.4 mg/L while serum levels averaged 45.1 mg/L (35). The average milk/serum ratio was 0.027. It is generally agreed that the amount of valproic acid transferring to the infant via milk is low.

Phenytoin

Phenytoin has been extensively studied in breastfeeding mothers. Levels tend to peak in milk at about 3.5 hours post-dose.

In one study of six women receiving 200 to 400 mg/day, plasma concentrations varied from 12.8 to 78.5 µmol/L, while their milk levels ranged from 1.61 to 2.95 mg/L (28).

In only two of these infants were plasma concentrations of phenytoin detectible (0.46 and 0.72 µmol/L). No untoward effects were noted in any of these infants.

Others have reported milk levels of 6 µg/mL (29) or 0.8 µg/mL (14). Breast milk concentrations ranged from 0.26 to 1.5 mg/L depending on the maternal dose.

The neonatal half-life of phenytoin is highly variable for the first week of life. Monitoring of the infants' plasma may be useful although it is not definitely required. All of the current studies indicate rather low levels of phenytoin in breast milk and minimal plasma levels in breastfeeding infants.

Lamotrigine

Lamotrigine has been extensively studied in breastfeeding mothers and their infants.

In a study of a 24-year-old female receiving 300 mg/day lamotrigine during pregnancy, maternal serum levels and cord levels of lamotrigine at birth were 3.88 µg/mL and 3.26 µg/mL, respectively (20). By day 22, the maternal serum levels were 9.61 µg/mL, the milk concentration was 6.51 mg/L and the infant's serum level was 2.25 µg/mL. The RID was estimated at 22%. Despite this RID, the infant plasma levels continued to drop over time. The infant was asymptomatic during the period of feeding.

The manufacturer reported that in a group of five women (no dose listed), breast milk concentrations of lamotrigine ranged from 0.07 to 5.03 mg/L (21). Breast milk levels averaged 40% to 45% of maternal plasma levels. No untoward effects were noted in the infants.

In a study by Ohman of nine breastfeeding women at 3 weeks post-partum, the median milk/plasma ratio was 0.61, and the breastfed infants maintained lamotrigine concentrations of approximately 30% of the mothers' plasma levels (36). The authors estimated the mean dose to the infant at 0.2 to 1 mg/kg/day. No adverse effects were noted in the infants.

The use of lamotrigine in breastfeeding mothers produces clinically relevant plasma levels in some breastfed infants, although they are apparently not high enough to produce side effects. It is probably advisable to monitor the infant's plasma levels if the infant is symptomatic to insure safety.

Exposure levels in utero are much higher than those via milk. Premature infants exposed to maternal milk containing lamotrigine should be closely monitored for apnoea, sedation and weakness. However, plasma levels reported thus far in full-term breastfeeding infants suggest that their levels fall rapidly during the first month post-partum. The maternal use of lamotrigine is probably compatible with in premature and full-term breastfeeding infants as long as the infant is closely observed for symptoms above.

Topiramate

In two women who received 150 to 200 mg/day, the concentration of topiramate in milk averaged 7.9 µM (range: 1.6–13.7) (30). The weight-normalised RID, assuming a milk intake of 150 mL/kg/day, ranged from 3% to 23% of the maternal dose/day. The absolute infant dose was 0.1 to 0.7 mg/kg/day. The plasma concentrations of topiramate in two infants were 1.4 and 1.6 µM, respectively. The plasma level in a third infant was undetectable. The plasma concentrations in the two infants were 10% to 20% of the maternal plasma level. At 4 weeks, the mean milk/plasma ratio had dropped to 0.69 and plasma levels in the infants were <0.9 µM and 2.1 µM.

Due to the fact that the plasma levels found in breast-feeding infants were significantly lower than in maternal plasma, the risk of using this product in breastfeeding mothers is probably acceptable. Close observation, including plasma levels in symptomatic infants is advised.

Carbamazepine
Carbamazepine (CBZ) use in breastfeeding mothers has been thoroughly studied.

In a study of three patients who received from 5.8 to 7.3 mg/kg/day, milk levels of CBZ were reported to vary from 1.3 to 1.8 mg/L, while the epoxide (ECBZ) metabolite varied from 0.5 to 1.1 mg/L (15). No adverse effects were noted in any of the infants.

In another study by Niebyl, breast milk levels were 1.4 mg/L in the lipid fraction and 2.3 mg/L in the skim fraction in a mother receiving 1000 mg CBZ daily (16). This author estimated that the infant's daily intake is 2 mg CBZ (0.5 mg/kg) in an infant ingesting 1 L of milk per day.

In a study of 16 mothers who received an average dose of 13.8 mg/kg/day, the average maternal serum levels of CBZ and ECBZ were 7.1 and 2.6 µg/mL, respectively (37). The average milk levels of CBZ and ECBZ were 2.5 and 1.5 mg/L, respectively. The relative percent of CBZ and ECBZ in milk were 36.4% and 53% of the maternal serum levels. A total of 50 milk samples from 16 patients were analysed. Of these, the lowest CBZ concentration in milk was 1.0 mg/L and the highest was 4.8 mg/L. All infants had CBZ levels below 1.5 µg/mL.

In a study of seven women receiving 250 to 800 mg/day, the CBZ level ranged from 2.8 to 4.5 mg/L in milk and from 3.2 to 15.0 mg/L in plasma (38). The levels of ECBZ ranged from 0.5 to 1.7 mg/L in milk and from 0.8 to 4.8 mg/L in plasma.

The amount of CBZ transferred to the infant is apparently quite low. Although the half-life of CBZ in infants appears shorter than in adults, infants should still be monitored for sedative effects.

Antidepressants

Tricyclic Antidepressants
Almost all of the current antidepressants have been studied in breastfeeding mothers. More than 40 studies of the tricyclic antidepressants are available and suggest that levels of these agents in milk are low and that they are compatible with breastfeeding. But patient compliance is poor with the tricyclics due to anticholinergic symptoms, such as xerostomia, blurred vision and sedation, and as a result they are less often used than other antidepressant drugs. The RID of amitriptyline is less than 1.5% of the maternal dose (39).

Studies thus far have been unable to detect it in the infant's plasma. Doxepin should be avoided due to reported hypotonia, poor suckling, vomiting and jaundice (40). Desipramine levels in breast milk are minimal. One study of desipramine suggests an RID of about 1% following a dose of 30 mg/day (41).

SSRIs
The selective serotonin reuptake inhibitors (SSRIs) are presently the mainstay of antidepressive therapy, primarily because of their efficacy and minimal toxicity in overdose. Table 5.3 provides the RID of most antidepressants. Interestingly, the most often studied drug family in breastfeeding mothers in the last decade has been the SSRI antidepressants.

Clinical studies of breastfeeding patients taking sertraline, fluvoxamine and paroxetine clearly indicate that the transfer of these medications into human milk is low and uptake by the infant is even lower. Thus far, no untoward effects have been reported following the use of these three agents in breastfeeding mothers. Sertraline appears to be the overwhelming favourite of most mothers and clinicians, as more than 50 infants have been evaluated in numerous studies and milk and infant plasma levels are quite low to undetectable.

Fluoxetine has been studied in at least 50 breastfeeding infants. Fluoxetine transfers into human milk in relatively higher concentrations, ranging to as high as 9% of the maternal dose (50). Because of its long half-life, clinically relevant plasma levels in infants have been reported. Because of a higher RID, fluoxetine is somewhat less preferred unless lower doses are used during pregnancy and early post-partum. However, in reality, the incidence of untoward effects is probably remote, and mothers who cannot tolerate other SSRIs should be maintained on fluoxetine while breastfeeding.

Citalopram and its new congener, escitalopram, transfer into milk moderately. In a study of seven women receiving an average of 0.41 mg/kg/day citalopram, the average milk level was 97 µg/L for citalopram and 36 µg/L for its metabolite (RID = 3.7%) (60). Low concentrations of citalopram were noted in the infants' plasma (2 and 2.3 µg/L in two infants). While no untoward effects have been noted in the published studies, two cases of somnolence have been reported to the manufacturer and at least four other anecdotal cases have been reported to this author. In a recent study of eight breastfeeding women taking an average of 10 mg/day of escitalopram, the total RID of escitalopram and its metabolite was reported to be 5.3% (44). The drug and its metabolite were undetectable in

Table 5.3 Relative Infant Dose of Various Antidepressant Levels in Human Milk

Drug	Relative infant dose (%)	Comments	References
Amitriptyline	1.5	Compatible; observe for sedation in infant.	39
Bupropion	0.7–2	Compatible; do not use in patients subject to seizures. Observe for possible milk suppression.	42,43
Citalopram, escitalopram	0.4–3.7	Caution; somnolence reported in some newborns.	44,45
Desipramine	1	Compatible; observe for sedation in infant.	41
Desvenlafaxine	6.8–9.3	Probably safe; no side effects noted in one study; however, RID is somewhat high.	46,47
Doxepin	1.2–2.8	Unsafe; respiratory arrest and sedation reported.	48,49
Fluoxetine	2.6–6.81	Compatible	50,51,52,53
Paroxetine	<2.9	Compatible for infant; avoid use in adolescent mothers.	54,55
Sertraline	0.4–2.2	Compatible; preferred SSRI	56,57,58
St. John's Wort	—	Compatible; recent data suggest transfer to milk is minimal. No untoward effects noted.	59
Venlafaxine	6.4	Probably safe; no side effects noted in one study; however, RID is somewhat high.	46

most of the infants tested. No adverse events in the infants were reported. Escitalopram is probably preferred in breast-feeding mothers over citalopram.

Neonatal withdrawal symptoms have been commonly reported in infants (30%) exposed to SSRIs in utero. These symptoms, which occur early post-natally, consist of poor adaptation, irritability, jitteriness and poor gaze control in neonates exposed to fluoxetine (61,62) and paroxetine (63). Most clinicians do not treat neonatal withdrawal symptoms unless they are severe. Continued breastfeeding is certainly advised. Because levels of the antidepressants in milk are so low, they are ineffective in reducing withdrawal symptoms.

Immune Modulating Agents
The use of immunosuppressants and immune modulating agents in breastfeeding mothers is poorly understood. We unfortunately have limited studies on most of these agents. This, however, does not preclude the use of these agents in breastfeeding mothers.

Methotrexate
Methotrexate is a potent and potentially dangerous folic acid antimetabolite used in arthritic and other immunologic syndromes. It is also used as an abortifacient in tubal pregnancies. Methotrexate is secreted into breast milk in small amounts.

Two hours after a dose of 22.5 mg to one patient, the methotrexate concentration in breast milk was 2.6 µg/L with a milk/plasma ratio of 0.08 (64).

The cumulative excretion of methotrexate in the first 12 hours after oral administration was only 0.32 µg in milk. These authors concluded that methotrexate therapy in breastfeeding mothers would not be a contraindication to breastfeeding. However, methotrexate is believed to be retained in human tissues (particularly neonatal GI cells and ovarian cells) for long periods (months) (65).

One study has indicated a higher risk of fetal malformation in mothers who received methotrexate months prior to becoming pregnant (66). Therefore, pregnancy should be delayed if either partner is receiving methotrexate for at least 3 months following therapy. Elimination of methotrexate is by a two-compartment model with a terminal elimination half-life of 8 to 15 hours (67).

It is apparent that the concentration of methotrexate in human milk is minimal, although due to the toxicity of this agent, it is probably wise to pump and discard the mother's milk for a minimum of 4 days.

Azathioprine
Azathioprine is a powerful immunosuppressive agent that is metabolised to 6-mercaptopurine (6-MP). In numerous studies of more than 25 infants whose mothers consumed azathioprine, levels were exceedingly low in milk (68–70). The RID ranged from 0.06% to 0.26% of the maternal dose. None of the infants in these studies had detectable plasma levels of 6-MP or any symptoms of immunosuppression.

Methylprednisolone
Pulsed-dose methylprednisolone is one of the mainstays of therapy in multiple sclerosis (MS). Fortunately, the transfer of corticosteroids into human milk is poor at best. Studies of radiolabelled prednisolone have found that the total dose after 48 hours was only 0.14% of the maternal dose (71). In another study of prednisolone, where women consumed 10 to 80 mg/day prednisolone, the milk levels ranged from 1.6 to 2.67 µg/L

(72). However, in the case of MS massive intravenous doses such as 1 to 2 gm have been used. We do not have published levels in milk following such doses. However, following pharmacokinetic modelling, levels of methylprednisolone in maternal plasma fall rapidly within 8 to 12 hours to levels less than 1 µg/mL in plasma (73). Levels in milk would be at least 50- to 100-fold less. Thus, breastfeeding mothers should be advised to pump and discard their milk for approximately 12 hours following intravenous methylprednisolone.

Beta Interferons
Information on the transfer of beta interferons into human milk has not been published. Beta interferon is a large molecular weight peptide of 22,500 Da. As such, it is virtually excluded from the milk compartment. Unpublished data from six mothers in my laboratories now suggest beta interferon transfer into human milk is virtually nil. In five patients receiving 30 µg/wk, levels in milk ranged from 2 to 200 pg/mL. Thus levels of beta interferon in human milk are negligible.

Glatiramer Acetate
Glatiramer acetate is a random polymer ranging from 4700 to 13,000 Da and is composed of four amino acids found in myelin basic protein. At present, we do not have data on its transfer into human milk, but it will be low to nil due solely to its large molecular weight. Any present in milk would likely not be orally bioavailable in the infant. It is not a contraindication to breastfeeding.

Natalizumab
Natalizumab is a humanised IgG4k monoclonal antibody. While we do not have data on its transfer into human milk, levels are likely to be low to nil. IgG levels in milk are extraordinarily low as IgG is not actively transported into human milk. When small amounts of natalizumab is admixed with the patient's plasma IgG intravenously, only minuscule levels of this drug would expected to be found in milk.

Mitoxantrone
Mitoxantrone is an antineoplastic agent used in the treatment of relapsing MS. It is a DNA-reactive agent that intercalates into DNA via hydrogen bonding, causing cross-links. It inhibits B cell, T cell and macrophage proliferation. In a study of a patient who received three treatments of mitoxantrone (6 mg/m^2) on days 1 to 5, mitoxantrone levels in milk measured 120 ng/mL just after treatment (on the third day of treatment), and dropped to a stable level of 18 ng/mL for the next 28 days (74). This agent has an enormous volume of distribution and is sequestered in at least seven organs including the liver and bone marrow. In another study, 15% of the dose remained 35 days after exposure. Were a mother to breastfeed, these levels would provide about 18 µg of mitoxantrone per litre of milk after the first few days following exposure to the drug. As this is a DNA-reactive agent, and it has a huge volume of distribution leading to prolonged tissue, plasma and milk levels, mothers should be strongly advised to not breastfeed following its use.

SUMMARY
The transfer of medications into milk is often quite low. There are thousands of studies presently available which suggest that most medications can be safely used in breastfeeding mothers. For this reason, the mother requiring treatment should almost always be advised to continue breastfeeding. While the vast

majority of medications transfer into milk in subclinical levels and pose almost no problem to a breastfed infant, the physician must always weigh the risk of the medication against the enormous benefit of breastfeeding.

Health care professionals should not jump to conclusions that all medications are unsafe for breastfeeding mothers. Indeed, interrupting breastfeeding carries risks for the infant, which include higher rates of GI syndromes, allergies and upper respiratory tract infection, which are well documented in formula-fed infants.

In most cases the amount of medication delivered to the infant via milk is far less than 1% of the maternal dose, and the amount the infant actually absorbs orally is often less than this. In healthy infants this amount is often easily tolerated without untoward effects. However, as the RID rises above 7% to 10%, and the toxicity of the medication increases, clinicians should be more cautious in recommending breastfeeding.

Medications that may require discontinuation of breastfeeding include anticancer, antimetabolite and radioactive drugs. Radioactive iodine-131 is particularly dangerous and infants should completely discontinue breastfeeding until radiation counts in milk are baseline.

The evaluation of the risk of the medication must always include the infant. Premature and neonatal infants are always at slightly higher risk to any medication and the clinician must always include the age of the infant in the overall evaluation of risk. Older infants are metabolically more capable of metabolising drugs and are generally at less risk to drugs in breast milk. Most older infants (>6 months) generally consume less human milk, thus the clinical dose transferred is reduced. Infants older than 1 year are at very little risk to drugs in breast milk, with some exceptions.

In infants exposed to drugs in utero, neonatal withdrawal has been commonly reported, though it often goes untreated. Neonatal withdrawal is common following gestational exposure to opiates, and antidepressants. Infants exposed to opiates in utero often require exogenous supplementation to prevent severe withdrawal symptoms. We know definitively that there is insufficient opiate (or antidepressant) in milk to prevent withdrawal in breastfed infants.

In almost all situations there are numerous medications that can be safely used for specific syndromes and should be carefully chosen with the breastfeeding mother in mind (75,76). Numerous texts now document hundreds of studies concerning medications and their use in breastfeeding mothers.

Most importantly, we all know that human milk is the finest and safest nutrition a mother can give her infant. The benefits to the infant are now overwhelmingly documented in the literature. Interrupting breastfeeding for unsound reasons may actually increase the risk to the infant and should be avoided if possible.

REFERENCES

1. Cochi SL, Fleming DW, Hightower AW, et al. Primary invasive Haemophilus influenzae type b disease: a population-based assessment of risk factors. J Pediatr 1986; 108(6):887–896.
2. Ford RP, Taylor BJ, Mitchell EA, et al. Breastfeeding and the risk of sudden infant death syndrome. Int J Epidemiol 1993; 22(5):885–890.
3. Goldman AS. The immune system of human milk: antimicrobial, anti-inflammatory and immunomodulating properties. Pediatr Infect Dis J 1993; 12(8):664–671.
4. Goldman AS, Chheda S, Keeney SE, et al. Immunologic protection of the premature newborn by human milk. Semin Perinatol 1994; 18(6):495–501.
5. Goldman AS, Hopkinson JM, Rassin DK. Benefits and risks of breastfeeding. Adv Pediatr 2007; 54:275–304.
6. Pisacane A, Graziano L, Mazzarella G, et al. Breast-feeding and urinary tract infection. J Pediatr 1992; 120(1):87–89.
7. Bennett PN. Use of the monographs on drugs. In: Bennett PN, ed. *Drugs and Human Lactation.* Vol 2. Amsterdam: Elsevier, 1996:67–74.
8. Cole AP, Hailey DM. Diazepam and active metabolite in breast milk and their transfer to the neonate. Arch Dis Child 1975; 50(9):741–742.
9. Spigset O. Anaesthetic agents and excretion in breast milk. Acta Anaesthesiol Scand 1994; 38(2):94–103.
10. Kanto JH. Use of benzodiazepines during pregnancy, labour and lactation, with particular reference to pharmacokinetic considerations. Drugs 1982; 23(5):354–380.
11. Anderson PO, McGuire GG. Neonatal alprazolam withdrawal—possible effects of breast feeding. DICP 1989; 23(7–8):614.
12. Kahn A, Hasaerts D, Blum D. Phenothiazine-induced sleep apneas in normal infants. Pediatrics 1985; 75(5):844–847.
13. Cantu TG. Phenothiazines and sudden infant death syndrome. DICP 1989; 23(10):795–796.
14. Kaneko S, Sato T, Suzuki K. The levels of anticonvulsants in breast milk. Brit J Clin Pharmaco 1979; 7(6):624–627.
15. Pynnonen S, Kanto J, Sillanpaa M, et al. Carbamazepine: placental transport, tissue concentrations in foetus and newborn, and level in milk. Acta Pharmacol Toxicol (Copenh) 1977; 41(3):244–253.
16. Niebyl JR, Blake DA, Freeman JM, et al. Carbamazepine levels in pregnancy and lactation. Obst Gynecol 1979; 53(1):139–140.
17. Kuhnz W, Koch S, Jakob S, et al. Ethosuximide in epileptic women during pregnancy and lactation period. Placental transfer, serum concentrations in nursed infants and clinical status. Br J Clin Pharmacol 1984; 18(5):671–677.
18. Kristensen JH, Ilett KF, Hackett LP, et al. Gabapentin and breastfeeding: a case report. J Hum Lact 2006; 22(4):426–428.
19. Ohman I, Vitols S, Tomson T. Pharmacokinetics of gabapentin during delivery, in the neonatal period, and lactation: does a fetal accumulation occur during pregnancy? Epilepsia 2005; 46(10):1621–1624.
20. Rambeck B, Kurlemann G, Stodieck SR, et al. Concentrations of lamotrigine in a mother on lamotrigine treatment and her newborn child. Eur J Clin Pharmacol 1997; 51(6):481–484.
21. Biddlecombe RA. Analysis of breast milk samples for lamotrigine. Internal document BDCR/93/0011. GlaxoWellcome, 2004.
22. Page-Sharp M, Kristensen JH, Hackett LP, et al. Transfer of lamotrigine into breast milk. Ann Pharmacother 2006; 40(7–8):1470–1471.
23. Tomson T, Ohman I, Vitols S. Lamotrigine in pregnancy and lactation: a case report. Epilepsia 1997; 38(9):1039–1041.
24. Johannessen SI, Helde G, Brodtkorb E. Levetiracetam concentrations in serum and in breast milk at birth and during lactation. Epilepsia 2005; 46(5):775–777.
25. Tomson T, Palm R, Kallen K, et al. Pharmacokinetics of levetiracetam during pregnancy, delivery, in the neonatal period, and lactation. Epilepsia 2007; 48(6):1111–1116.
26. Horning MG. Identification and quantification of drugs and drug metabolites in human milk using GC-MS-COM methods. Mod Probl Pediatr 1975; 15:73–79.
27. Pote M, Kulkarni R, Agarwal M. Phenobarbital toxic levels in a nursing neonate. Indian Pediatr 2004; 41(9):963–964.
28. Steen B, Rane A, Lonnerholm G, et al. Phenytoin excretion in human breast milk and plasma levels in nursed infants. Ther Drug Monit 1982; 4(4):331–334.
29. Svensmark O, Schiller PJ, Buchthal F. 5, 5-Diphenylhydantoin (dilantin) blood levels after oral or intravenous dosage in man. Acta Pharmacol Toxicol (Copenh) 1960; 16:331–346.
30. Ohman I, Vitols S, Luef G, et al. Topiramate kinetics during delivery, lactation, and in the neonate: preliminary observations. Epilepsia 2002; 43(10):1157–1160.
31. von Unruh GE, Froescher W, Hoffmann F, et al.. Valproic acid in breast milk: how much is really there? Ther Drug Monit 1984; 6(3):272–276.

32. Alexander FW. Sodium valproate and pregnancy. Arch Dis Child 1979; 54(3):240.

33. Dickinson RG, Harland RC, Lynn RK, et al. Transmission of valproic acid (Depakene) across the placenta: half-life of the drug in mother and baby. J Pediatr 1979; 94(5):832–835.

34. Shimoyama R, Ohkubo T, Sugawara K. Monitoring of zonisamide in human breast milk and maternal plasma by solid-phase extraction HPLC method. Biomed Chromatogr 1999; 13(5):370–372.

35. Nau H, Rating D, Koch S, et al. Valproic acid and its metabolites: placental transfer, neonatal pharmacokinetics, transfer via mother's milk and clinical status in neonates of epileptic mothers. J Pharmacol Exp Ther 1981; 219(3):768–777.

36. Ohman I, Vitols S, Tomson T. Lamotrigine in pregnancy: pharmacokinetics during delivery, in the neonate, and during lactation. Epilepsia 2000; 41(6):709–713.

37. Froescher W, Eichelbaum M, Niesen M, et al. Carbamazepine levels in breast milk. Ther Drug Monit 1984; 6(3):266–271.

38. Shimoyama R, Ohkubo T, Sugawara K. Monitoring of carbamazepine and carbamazepine 10,11-epoxide in breast milk and plasma by high-performance liquid chromatography. Ann Clin Biochem 2000; 37(pt 2):210–215.

39. Bader TF, Newman K. Amitriptyline in human breast milk and the nursing infant's serum. Am J Psychiatry 1980; 137(7): 855–856.

40. Frey OR, Scheidt P, von Brenndorff AI. Adverse effects in a newborn infant breast-fed by a mother treated with doxepin. Ann Pharmacother 1999; 33(6):690–693.

41. Stancer HC, Reed KL. Desipramine and 2-hydroxydesipramine in human breast milk and the nursing infant's serum. Am J Psychiatry 1986; 143(12):1597–1600.

42. Baab SW, Peindl KS, Piontek CM, et al. Serum bupropion levels in 2 breastfeeding mother-infant pairs. J Clin Psychiatry 2002; 63(10):910–911.

43. Haas JS, Kaplan CP, Barenboim D, et al. Bupropion in breast milk: an exposure assessment for potential treatment to prevent post-partum tobacco use. Tob Control 2004; 13(1):52–56.

44. Rampono J, Hackett LP, Kristensen JH, et al. Transfer of escitalopram and its metabolite demethylescitalopram into breastmilk. Brit J Clin Pharmaco 2006; 62(3):316–322.

45. Jensen PN, Olesen OV, Bertelsen A, et al. Citalopram and desmethylcitalopram concentrations in breast milk and in serum of mother and infant. Ther Drug Monit 1997; 19(2):236–239.

46. Ilett KF, Hackett LP, Dusci LJ, et al. Distribution and excretion of venlafaxine and O-desmethylvenlafaxine in human milk. Br J Clin Pharmacol 1998; 45(5):459–462.

47. Newport DJ, Ritchie JC, Knight BT, et al. Venlafaxine in human breast milk and nursing infant plasma: determination of exposure. J Clin Psychiatry 2009; 70(9):1304–1310.

48. Matheson I, Pande H, Alertsen AR. Respiratory depression caused by N-desmethyldoxepin in breast milk. Lancet 1985; 2(8464):1124.

49. Kemp J, Ilett KF, Booth J, et al. Excretion of doxepin and N-desmethyldoxepin in human milk. Br J Clin Pharmacol 1985; 20(5):497–499.

50. Kristensen JH, Ilett KF, Hackett LP, et al. Distribution and excretion of fluoxetine and norfluoxetine in human milk. Brit J Clin Pharmaco 1999; 48(4):521–527.

51. Burch KJ, Wells BG. Fluoxetine/norfluoxetine concentrations in human milk. Pediatrics 1992; 89(4 pt 1):676–677.

52. Isenberg KE. Excretion of fluoxetine in human breast milk. J Clin Psychiatry 1990; 51(4):169.

53. Kim J, Riggs KW, Misri S, et al. Stereoselective disposition of fluoxetine and norfluoxetine during pregnancy and breast-feeding. Br J Clin Pharmacol 2006; 61(2):155–163.

54. Ohman R, Hagg S, Carleborg L, et al. Excretion of paroxetine into breast milk. J Clin Psychiatry 1999; 60(8):519–523.

55. Stowe ZN, Cohen LS, Hostetter A, et al. Paroxetine in human breast milk and nursing infants. Am J Psychiatry 2000; 157(2):185–189.

56. Altshuler LL, Burt VK, McMullen M, et al. Breastfeeding and sertraline: a 24-hour analysis. J Clin Psychiatry 1995; 56(6): 243–245.

57. Kristensen JH, Ilett KF, Dusci LJ, et al. Distribution and excretion of sertraline and N-desmethylsertraline in human milk. Br J Clin Pharmacol 1998; 45(5):453–457.

58. Stowe ZN, Owens MJ, Landry JC, et al. Sertraline and desmethylsertraline in human breast milk and nursing infants. Am J Psychiatry 1997; 154(9):1255–1260.

59. Lee A, Minhas R, Matsuda N, et al. The safety of St. John's wort (Hypericum perforatum) during breastfeeding. J Clin Psychiatry 2003; 64(8):966–968.

60. Rampono J, Kristensen JH, Hackett LP, et al. Citalopram and demethylcitalopram in human milk: distribution, excretion and effects in breast fed infants. Brit J Clin Pharmaco 2000; 50(10):263–268.

61. Chambers CD, Johnson KA, Dick LM, et al. Birth outcomes in pregnant women taking fluoxetine [see comments]. New Engl J Med 1996; 335(14):1010–1015.

62. Spencer MJ, Escondido CA. Fluoxetine hydrochloride (Prozac) toxicity in a neonate. Pediatrics 1993; 92(5):721–722.

63. Stiskal JA, Kulin N, Koren G, et al. Neonatal paroxetine withdrawal syndrome. Arch Dis Child Fetal Neonatal Ed 2001; 84(2): F134–F135.

64. Johns DG, Rutherford LD, Leighton PC, et al. Secretion of methotrexate into human milk. Am J Obstet Gynecol 1972; 112 (7):978–980.

65. Fountain JR, Hutchison DJ, Waring GB, et al. Persistence of amethopterin in normal mouse tissues. Proc Soc Exp Biol Med 1953; 83(2):369–373.

66. Walden PA, Bagshawe KD. Pregnancies after chemotherapy for gestational trophoblastic tumours. Lancet 1979; 2(8154):1241.

67. Grochow LB, Ames MM. A clinician's guide to chemotherapy pharmacokinetics and pharmacodynamics. Baltimore, MD: Williams & Wilkins, 1998.

68. Coulam CB, Moyer TP, Jiang NS, et al. Breast-feeding after renal transplantation. Transplant Proc 1982; 14(3):605–609.

69. Moretti ME, Verjee Z, Ito S, et al. Breast-feeding during maternal use of azathioprine. Ann Pharmacother 2006; 40(12):2269–2272.

70. Sau A, Clarke S, Bass J, et al. Azathioprine and breastfeeding: is it safe? BJOG 2007; 114(4):498–501.

71. McKenzie SA, Selley JA, Agnew JE. Secretion of prednisolone into breast milk. Arch Dis Child 1975; 50(11):894–896.

72. Ost L, Wettrell G, Bjorkhem I, et al. Prednisolone excretion in human milk. J Pediatr 1985; 106(6):1008–1011.

73. Morrow SA, Stoian CA, Dmitrovic J, et al. The bioavailability of IV methylprednisolone and oral prednisone in multiple sclerosis. Neurology 2004; 63(6):1079–1080.

74. Azuno Y, Kaku K, Fujita N, et al. Mitoxantrone and etoposide in breast milk. Am J Hematol 1995; 48(2):131–132.

75. Hale TW. Medications and mothers' milk. Amarillo, TX: Hale Publishing LP, 2008.

76. Hale TW, Berens PD. Clinical therapy in breastfeeding patients. Amarillo, TX: Pharmasoft Publishing LP, 2003.

Neuroanaesthesia in pregnancy

James Arden

INTRODUCTION

It is estimated that 1% to 2% of pregnant women will have non-obstetric surgery. Most of these procedures will be to treat conditions common in this age group, such as appendectomy or operations related to trauma. Pregnant patients requiring neurosurgery are a small subset of the 1% to 2% of this surgical population. Data on which to base specific management guidelines for these patients are sparse, consisting of case reports or small group studies and reviews of pregnant neurosurgical patients (1,2).

A rational management plan for neuroanaesthesia for the pregnant patient must balance the physiology of pregnancy (e.g., increased plasma volume) with the pathophysiology of the neurosurgical disease [e.g., elevated intracranial pressure (ICP)]. This chapter focuses specifically on incorporating the physiology of pregnancy (e.g., avoidance of caval compression) into the intraoperative requirements of specific neurosurgical procedures (e.g., prone position for laminectomy) to develop a coordinated approach to the pregnant neurosurgical patient.

The anaesthetic management of the pregnant woman who has previously had neurosurgery presents several problems which may be unfamiliar to the obstetric anaesthetist. For these patients, reports are again scant, but available information will be reviewed here to suggest reasoned management choices in these uncommon cases.

NEUROANAESTHESIA AND PHYSIOLOGY OF PREGNANCY

Alterations in maternal physiology are described in textbooks and reviews. The physiological changes of pregnancy suggest modifications of the standard anaesthetic management of neurosurgical patients:

- Cardiac output and plasma volume increase by 30% to 50% in pregnancy, reaching their peak at 24 to 28 weeks of gestation. The placental circulation, in contrast to the cerebral circulation, is not autoregulated and receives 10% of the maternal cardiac output. Thus, the status of the maternal circulating blood volume and mean blood pressure directly affect the fetus. Standard interventions in neuroanaesthesia, such as fluid restriction or diuresis for the management of intracranial masses, volume replacement during meningioma resection or treatment of vasospasm with hypervolaemia, hypertension and haemodilution ('triple H therapy') must be adjusted relative to this maternal baseline.

- Oxygen consumption and minute ventilation increase during pregnancy. With chronic increased ventilation, the resting P_{CO_2} decreases to 4.3 kP (32 mmHg) producing a respiratory alkalosis. During neurosurgery, hypocapneia may be instituted temporarily to lower cerebral blood flow (CBF) in the management of raised ICP. Since the maternal cerebral vasculature adjusts to the decreased P_{CO_2}, the target P_{CO_2} to achieve reduction in CBF must incorporate the maternal baseline respiratory alkalosis and should be just below 4 kP. Hyperventilation must be instituted cautiously since a reduction much greater than the baseline in pregnancy may result in marked cerebral vasoconstriction and cerebral ischaemia in non-pregnant patients. Following traumatic brain injury marked hypocapneia is associated with a poor outcome (3), and hyperventilation to P_{CO_2} = 3.3 to 4 kPa (25–30 mmHg) is no longer recommended.

- Hypothermia has neurological benefit following cardiac arrest, and longer periods of hypothermia appear to be of value in neurocritical care (4). However, hypothermia decreases uteroplacental blood flow and may result in fetal stress and fetal bradycardia (5). Recent data also indicate that acute hypothermia is of no proven value in cerebral aneurysm surgery (6) or in head injury (7). Thus maternal physiology and current information suggest that normothermia is frequently the preferred management goal.

Balancing the gestational age with the urgency of neurosurgery can be a challenge to the surgeon and the anaesthetist. At term, a combined neurosurgical procedure and delivery can provide a solution (8). At the opposite extreme, surgical intervention and anaesthetic exposure in early pregnancy present both known risks, such as spontaneous abortion (9) and neonatal death (10), and uncertain risks, such as cognitive dysfunction in the child (11–13). Perioperative or intraoperative fetal heart rate (FHR) monitoring is often suggested to follow the effects of surgery on the fetus (14,15). However, the value of intraoperative FHR monitoring in non-obstetric surgery is unclear, and neither U.K. nor U.S. national guidelines consider intraoperative FHR monitoring (16–18). The FHR shows reduced beat-to-beat variability during maternal general anaesthesia and with the administration of opioids (15,19,20). Reduced beat-to-beat variability is a sign of fetal sleep if short term (40–60 minutes) and of fetal hypoxia if prolonged. In the absence of any other CTG abnormality, a reduced beat-to-beat variability can be considered as normal for women who are undergoing general anaesthesia. Misinterpretation of the FHR tracing has been reported to have prompted an unnecessary Caesarian section (21); thus, a skilled interpreter, such as an obstetrician, a midwife or trained obstetrical nurse, familiar with drug effects on the FHR, is essential. Providing the FHR pattern is interpreted correctly, fetal monitoring may provide evidence of fetal hypoxia (e.g., decelerations or a change of baseline rate) which may alter management. However, the value of intraoperative FHR monitoring currently remains controversial and some have advocated not monitoring the FHR during neurosurgery (22).

The complex topic of the effects of anaesthetic agents on the fetus and the newborn has been a focus of recent research.

Generic assurances simply to minimise fetal exposure to anaesthetics are frequently given to the patient, but the rationale for this is not well defined. The choice of anaesthetics in pregnancy is often unsystematically based on the absence of reported problems for commonly used agents in the general population. Data acquired during drug evaluation on anaesthetic teratogenicity can be considered, but the range of doses and the absence of specific human data make the information difficult to apply to clinical situations. It is known that certain drugs, such as the opioids, propofol and midazolam, are passively transferred to the newborn from the mother (see chapter 6b, 'Neurocritical Care'), and the short-term depressant effects of opioids are known to every neonatal resuscitation team. Recently, it has been suggested that a child's neurodevelopment during the post-natal period may show subtle, late effects of early exposure to anaesthetics (11). Conversely, recent animal studies suggest a protective role for anaesthetics in preconditioning against neonatal brain injury (12). The late effects of anaesthetic agents in the newborn remain to be defined.

NEUROSURGICAL PROCEDURES
Intracranial Surgery
Subarachnoid haemorrhage (SAH) results from bleeding from an intracranial aneurysm or an arteriovenous malformation. SAH is uncommon; only 5% of strokes result from SAH. Rebleeding from aneurysmal SAH, however, carries an 80% mortality, so early treatment either by endovascular coiling or surgical clipping is essential in all but the worst grades of SAH. The incidence of SAH is 6 to 8 per 100,000 in the United Kingdom (23), which is similar to the rate in pregnancy, which is 10 to 20 per 100,000 pregnancies (24). Despite the rarity of SAH, it accounted for 5% of maternal deaths in the United Kingdom (25) and there are multiple case studies of SAH during pregnancy.

Given the risk, a ruptured SAH is one of the few situations during pregnancy requiring urgent neurosurgical or interventional radiology treatment, and a general anaesthetic is necessary (see chapter 6c, 'Neurovascular Intervention During Pregnancy: Cerebral Aneurysms and Vascular Malformations'). Near-term, combined delivery and aneurysm treatment may be completed with a single anaesthetic (26–28). But treating SAH earlier in pregnancy presents several difficult anaesthetic choices because of the physiological changes in pregnancy. For example, the anaesthetic management for a pregnant woman includes left lateral tilt after 20 weeks to prevent caval compression, but aneurysm clipping demands optimal positioning for surgical access. In pregnancy, the 'full-stomach' status after midterm dictates rapid airway control at anaesthetic induction, and laryngeal engorgement in pregnancy can result in difficult laryngoscopy and increased ICP. In contrast, elevated ICP dictates a slow, smooth neuroanaesthesia induction and intubation. Maintaining increased maternal plasma volume and fetal perfusion can conflict with the restrictive fluid management and intraoperative diuresis used for ICP control. Finally, endovascular coiling requires exposure to potentially harmful radiation and anticoagulation of a hypercoagulable pregnant patient (29).

Some of these management dilemmas are simplified by recent clinical advances. On the basis of outcome studies, the preferred first choice for aneurysm therapy in the United Kingdom currently is endovascular coiling (30–32). Coiling is quicker and may be less haemodynamically stressful than surgical clipping, and therefore offers added benefit to the pregnant patient. Diagnostic MRI/MRA is readily available, and guidelines have been developed for exposure to radiation during pregnancy (33; see chapter 3, 'Intrauterine Imaging, Diagnosis and Intervention in Neurological Disease'). Several advances in airway management, such as the video laryngoscope, have facilitated a less stressful, rapid sequence intubation, essential to the pregnant neurosurgical patient. Anaesthetic agents now employed in neuroanaesthesia, including remifentanil, propofol and sevoflurane, are rapidly eliminated and provide the haemodynamic stability to maintain uterine perfusion. Nitrous oxide, once implicated in a variety of toxic effects, has been shown in large studies to have no demonstrable association with congenital abnormalities (34) or with adverse outcome in aneurysm surgery (35).

A craniotomy may be performed during pregnancy for other indication besides aneurysm clipping including brain tumour resection, haematoma evacuation or in traumatic brain injury (see chapter 7, 'Analgesia and Anaesthesia in Neurological Disease and Pregnancy'). The decision to operate will depend on the urgency of surgery, the stage of pregnancy and treatment alternatives. The anaesthetic considerations described above for aneurysm surgery apply equally to the anaesthetic management of any craniotomy. In certain, more limited, intracranial procedures, such as burr hole drainage of a haematoma, neurosurgery may be performed with infiltration of local anaesthetic alone, and this option should be considered, depending on the patient's cooperation.

Spinal Surgery
Urgent surgery for discectomy, decompression or stabilisation at any level of the spinal cord may be indicated during pregnancy. Indications for emergency spine surgery include cauda equina syndrome, spinal instability, spinal cord compression, trauma or intractable pain. Lower back pain, which is frequent in pregnancy (36,37) generally does not require surgical intervention. Back pain without signs of a progressive deficit is generally managed conservatively with a range of therapeutic modalities.

Nevertheless, procedures at any level from the base of the skull to the sacrum may be indicated during pregnancy. Clearly, the point in the pregnancy (>20 weeks for caval compression) and any observed haemodynamic effects will modify the choice of positioning. The prone position is usually avoided after the beginning of the second trimester and a lateral (38) or kneeling (tuck) position are alternatives for spine surgery. Some operations on the cervical spine may be performed under local anaesthesia and both epidural and spinal anaesthetics have been employed effectively for lumbar spine surgery (39,40). In cervical spine procedures, limited neck mobility due to exacerbation of symptoms, muscle spasm or instability may complicate the well-described progression of upper airway engorgement and oedema during pregnancy. A cautious approach to the airway is imperative, and intubation with local anaesthetic ('awake') or with minimal sedation may be advisable.

Neurotrauma
Trauma is a leading cause of death in women of childbearing age, and maternal death is an important cause of fetal demise. Road traffic accidents, falls, assault and burn injuries are the leading causes of trauma in this age group. Neurotrauma is anatomically and pathologically divided into head injury and spinal cord injury, but brain and spine injuries are not distinct in several ways. Primary injury of both the brain and spinal

cord is defined as the instantaneous damage caused by the traumatic event and is irreversible. Secondary injury in both head and spine is the focus of treatment in neurotrauma, and it may be reversible to differing degrees. Secondary injury results from the action of multiple factors at and near the site of injury, including inflammatory mediators, amino acids, altered perfusion, ischaemia, oedema, axonal and structural disruption and cell death. Head injuries occur in up to 50% of spinal cord injuries, and spinal injury is found in 2% to 5% of severe head injuries (41). For this reason, head injury patients are transferred with spine stabilisation precautions and head injury should be suspected in spinal cord trauma. Finally, it must be remembered that 20% to 50% of spine and head injury patients have associated injuries to other organ systems which may also require emergency intervention.

Altered consciousness is a component of many of these injuries and pregnancy must be assumed in any female trauma victim of childbearing age with diminished responsiveness and a pregnancy screen should be part of initial testing. Pregnancy is assumed in all women of child-bearing age until proven otherwise. Pregnancy tests are generally routine for trauma patients and surgical patients in this age group. Pregnancy brings additional complexity to the anaesthetic management of neurotrauma, but little information is available about anaesthetic strategies (42). In the initial assessment and management of the pregnant woman's 'ABC' (airway, breathing and circulation), the pulmonary, cardiovascular and airway changes described earlier must be remembered. When intubation is required in major trauma patients, a smaller-diameter endotracheal tube is placed and cervical spine stabilisation is maintained until diagnostic tests are completed. The challenges of intubating during stabilisation are compounded by the airway changes and full-stomach status of pregnancy. In this context, if emergency intubation is required (GCS < 8, loss of airway), the option of a percutaneous or surgical cricothyroidotomy should be readily available.

The chronic respiratory alkalosis of pregnancy and the resultant compensatory metabolic acidosis may limit buffering capacity and maternal resistance to hypotension, so acidosis must be diagnosed early. Uteroplacental perfusion is directly related to systemic pressure, and plasma volume is expanded in the pregnant woman, so resuscitation must be appropriately vigorous. In this complicated scenario, many management decisions must be simplified by the recognition that fetal survival is closely coupled to maternal survival, and diagnostic procedures and emergency surgery must be directed simply towards limiting secondary injury in the mother.

PREGNANCY FOLLOWING NEUROSURGERY

Previous spinal surgery can have significant implications for anaesthesia during labour and delivery. Cervical spine disease can limit neck flexion and extension and surgical decompression or discectomy may leave some degree of limitation in neck mobility. The range of neck motion must be carefully evaluated in any patient with cervical spine disease. Cervical spine fusion (fixation) procedures can significantly diminish mobility of the spine, causing direct visualisation of the glottis to be extremely difficult. Further difficulty with laryngoscopy from airway changes during pregnancy, plus the risk of aspiration during pregnancy can render rapid intubation at emergency Caesarean section virtually impossible. A thorough pre-assessment of the airway of these patients and a clear management plan, incorporating the airway management algorithm (43), are essential. The support of experienced airway trained personnel, a video

laryngoscope or bronchoscope, laryngeal mask airways (LMA), and emergency cricothyroidotomy and tracheostomy supplies must be readily available.

Epidural analgesia during labour, and spinal or epidural anaesthesia for delivery, can be technically challenging following lumbar surgery. Removal of the spinous processes at laminectomy eliminates palpable surface landmarks for epidural or spinal needle placement. Identification of a particular lumbar level by surface palpation, which has been reported to be only 30% accurate normally (44,45), is made even more difficult after laminectomy. Adhesions and scarring following discectomy or laminectomy can alter the feel of the needle in the tissues (46) and may affect the localisation of the epidural and subarachnoid spaces, which can result in an inadvertent subarachnoid block (47). Adhesions may also make epidural catheter placement difficult and may affect the spread of injected local anaesthetic. These changes can result in repeated attempts to place the block, traumatic needle placement or failure to place a block in patients who have had spine surgery (48). The availability of higher-resolution ultrasound equipment for needle placement has facilitated block placement in these patients (45,49).

Reports of the anaesthetic management of pregnant patients with shunts are limited (50). Bradley et al. (51) reviewed 77 pregnancies in 37 women in whom shunts had been placed prior to their pregnancies. The shunts had been placed in the years between 1940 and 1993, to treat hydrocephalus of various aetiologies. During this period, improvements in shunt technology have been made and this study probably included a range of devices. In 44 pregnancies, the patients had epidural anaesthesia, in two, spinal, and in nine, general anaesthesia. No complications directly related to anaesthesia were described. On the basis of this review, any of these anaesthetic techniques is suitable in the shunt-dependent pregnant woman. Though not reported, the theoretical concerns raised about spinal or epidural anaesthesia in these patients have been the following: risk of infection of the CSF and the shunt, sudden reduction of ICP with uncal herniation following dural puncture and shunt malfunction of unclear cause. Appropriate aseptic technique should prevent infection. The standard small-bore, pencil-point spinal needle should minimise CSF leak and a functioning valved shunt should keep ICP controlled in the event of CSF loss. If an inadvertent dural puncture during epidural placement occurs, a functioning shunt should limit CSF loss if ICP drops, and the recommendation is to institute the standard conservative treatments (hydration, head flat) (52). A small, transient increase in ICP occurs with epidural injection, which should also be attenuated by the shunt, if required. Headache in the parturient following spinal or epidural anaesthesia does create a diagnostic problem, since shunt malfunction must be distinguished from post-dural puncture headache or meningitis (infectious or aseptic). An MRI scan, compared to the baseline scan with a functioning shunt, and any clinical signs or laboratory evidence of infection help clarify the diagnosis. Any deterioration in neurological function warrants urgent consultation with a neurosurgeon. If intrapartum shunt revision is required, a general anaesthetic will be needed, and an adequate level of anaesthetic to enable rapid intubation and limit the further elevation of ICP should be administered.

Elevation of ICP in patients with Arnold-Chiari malformation (ACM) presents a theoretical risk that a patent's neurological condition will deteriorate, if the pressure gradient between cranial and spinal subarachnoid spaces is increased by removal of CSF during intended or inadvertent lumbar dural pucture. Multiple case reports (53–57) and small case reviews (58,59) of both corrected and uncorrected ACM in pregnancy have documented that uncomplicated spinal, epidural and general anaesthetics have been administered. However, two earlier reports (60,61) of the onset of neurological signs or intractable headache following spinal anaesthesia in undiagnosed ACM have alerted anaesthetists to include ACM in the differential diagnosis of post spinal anaesthetic complications. While general anaesthesia has been suggested with the presence of elevated ICP in ACM on theoretical grounds, a trial of neck extension to define any limitation and to test for neurological symptoms is recommended prior to airway manipulation for intubation.

SUMMARY

The physiological changes in pregnancy, especially those affecting the airway, vascular volume and maternal blood pH, plus the importance of maintaining fetal perfusion, modify neuroanaesthesia management during pregnancy. Although the need for neurosurgery during pregnancy is uncommon, the point in pregnancy, the urgency of surgery and the treatment alternatives, including a more limited or modified surgical approach, must all be considered. In the reverse situation, where a post-neurosurgery patient becomes pregnant, the functional implications of the surgery, such as limitation of cervical spine mobility, must be carefully factored into the anaesthetic management during labour and delivery.

REFERENCES

1. Ng J, Kitchen N. Neurosurgery and pregnancy. J Neurol Neurosurg Psychiatry 2008; 79:745–752.
2. Wang LP, Peach MJ. Neuroanaesthesia for the pregnant woman. Anesth Analg 2008; 107:193–200.
3. Warner K, Cuschieri J, Copass M. The impact of prehospital ventilation on outcome after severe traumatic brain injury. J Trauma 2007; 62:1330–1338.
4. Poulderman K. Application of therapeutic hypothermia in the ICU: opportunities and pitfalls of a promising treatment modality. Intensive Care Med 2004; 30:555–575.
5. Usman S, Menon V. Avoiding caesarean section in maternal hypothermia associated with marked fetal distress. Emerg Med J 2007; 25:177.
6. Todd M, Hindman B, Clarke W. Mild intraoperative hypothermia during surgery for intracranial aneurysm. N Engl J Med 2005; 352:135–145.
7. Alderson P, Gadkary C, Signorini D. Therapeutic hypothermia for head injury. Cochrane Database Syst Rev 2004; 4: CD0011048.
8. Alareibi A, Coveny L, Sing S, et al. Case report: anesthetic management for sequential Caesarian delivery and laminectomy. Can J Anaesth 2007; 54:471–474.
9. Duncan P, Pope W, Cohen M, et al. Fetal risk of anesthesia and surgery during pregnancy. Anesthesiology 1986; 64:790–794.
10. Mazze R, Kallen B. Reproductive outcome after anesthesia and operation during pregnancy: a registry study of 5404 cases. Obstet Gynecol 1989; 161:1178–1185.
11. Davidson AJ, McCann M, Morton N, et al. Anesthesia and outcome after neonatal surgery. Anesthesiology 2008; 109:941–944.
12. Sun L, Li G, DiMaggio C, et al. Anesthesia and neurodevelopment in children. Anesthesiology 2008; 109:757–761.
13. Luo Y, Ma D, Ieong E, et al. Xenon and sevoflurane protect against brain injury in a neonatal asphyxia model. Anesthesiology 2008; 109:782–789.
14. Caforio L, Draisci G, Ciampelli M, et al. Rectal cancer in pregnancy: a new management based on blended anesthesia and monitoring of fetal well being. Eur J Obstet Gynecol Reprod Biol 2000; 88:71–74.
15. van Buul BJ, Nijhuis JG, Slappendel R, et al. General anesthesia for surgical repair of intracranial aneurysm in pregnancy: effects on fetal heart rate. Am J Perinatol 1993; 10:183–186.
16. Intrapartum fetal heart rate monitoring: nomenclature, interpretation, and general management principles. ACOG Practice Bulletin No. 106. American College of Obstetricians and Gynecologists. Obstet Gynecol 2009; 114:192–202.
17. Intrapartum care: care of healthy women and their babies during childbirth, NICE Clinical Guidelines No. 55. London: RCOG Press, 2007.
18. Macarthur A. Editorial: craniotomy for suprasellar meningioma during pregnancy: role of monitoring. Can J Anesth 2004; 51:535–538.
19. Katz JD, Hook R, Barash PG. Fetal heart rate monitoring in pregnant patients undergoing surgery. Am J Obstet Gynecol 1976; 125:267–269.
20. Fedorkow DM, Stewart TJ, Parboosingh J. Fetal heart rate changes associated with general anesthesia. Am J Perinatol 1989; 6:287–288.
21. Immer-Bansi A, Immer FF, Henle S, et al. Unnecessary emergency caesarean section due to silent CTG during anaesthesia? Br J Anaesth 2001; 87(5):791–793.
22. Balki M, Manninen PH. Craniotomy for suprasellar meningioma in a 28-week pregnant woman without fetal heart rate monitoring. Can J Anaesth 2004; 51(6):573–576.
23. Linn F, Rinkle G, Algra A, et al. Incidence of subarachnoid haemorrhage: role of region, year and rate of computed tomography: a meta-analysis. Stroke 1996; 27:625–629.
24. Dias M, Sekhar L. Intracranial haemorrhage from aneurysms and arteriovenous malformations during pregnancy. Neurosurgery 1990; 27:855–865.
25. Why Mothers Die, 1997-98. The fifth report from the confidential enquiries into maternal death in the United Kingdom. London: RCOG Press, 2001.
26. Whitburn RH, Laishley R, Jewkes D. Anaesthesia for simultaneous caesarean section and clipping of an intracerebral aneurysm. Br J Anaesth 1990; 64:642–645.
27. Jaeger K, Ruschulte H, Muhlhaus K, et al. Combined emergency caesarean section and intracerebral aneurysm clipping. Anaesthesia 2000; 55:1138–1140.
28. Selo-Ojeme DO, Marshman LA, Ikomi A, et al. Aneurysmal subarachnoid haemorrhage in pregnancy. Eur J Obstet Gynecol Reprod Biol 2004; 116:131–143.
29. James AH, Pregnancy and thromboembolic risk, Critical Care Medicine 2010; 38:S57–S63.
30. Molyneux AJ, Kerr RS, Yu YM, et al. International Subarachnoid Aneurysm Trial (ISAT) Collaborative Group, International subarachnoid aneurysm trial (ISAT) of neurosurgical clipping versus endovascular coiling in 2143 patients with ruptured intracranial aneurysms: a randomised comparison of effects on survival, dependency, seizures, rebleeding, subgroups, and aneurysm occlusion. Lancet 2005; 366:809–817.
31. Marshman LA, Rai MS, Aspoas AR. Comment to 'endovascular treatment of ruptured intracranial aneurysms during pregnancy: report of three cases'. Arch Gynecol Obstet 2005; 272:93.
32. Piotin M, DeSouza Filho C, Kothimbakam R, et al. Endovascular treatment of acutely ruptured intracranial aneurysm in pregnancy. Am J Obstet Gynecol 2001; 185:1261–1262.
33. Fielding JR, Washburn D. Imaging the pregnant patient. J Wom Imag 2005; 7:16–21.
34. Mazze RI, Kallen B. Reproductive outcome after anesthesia during pregnancy: a registry study of 5405 cases. Am J Obstet Gynecol 1986; 161:1178–1185.
35. McGregor DG, Lanier WL, et al. Effects of nitrous oxide on neurologic and neuropsychological function after intracranial aneurysm surgery. Anesthesiology 2008; 108:568–579.
36. Fast A, Shapiro D, Ducommun EJ, et al. Low back pain in pregnancy. Spine 1987; 12:368–371.
37. Berg G, Hammar M, Moller-Nielsen J, et al. Low back pain during pregnancy. Obstet Gynecol 1988; 71:71–75.
38. Dubey P, Kumar A. Case report: anesthesia for resection of spinal meningioma during pregnancy. J Neurosurg Anesthesiol 2005; 17:120.

39. Brown M, Levi A. Surgery for lumbar disc herniation during pregnancy. Spine 2001; 26:440–443.

40. McLain R, Bell G, Kalfas I, et al. Complications associated with lumbar laminectomy. Spine 2004; 29:2542–2547.

41. Gupta A, Gelb A, eds. Essentials of Neurotrauma and Neuro-intensive Care. Philadelphia: Saunders Elsevier, 2008:153 and 213.

42. Kuczkowski K. Trauma in the pregnant patient. Curr Opin Anaesthesiol 2004; 17:145–150.

43. American Society of Anesthesiologists Task Force on the Difficult Airway. Practice guidelines for management of the difficult airway. Anesthesiolgy 2003; 98:1269–1277.

44. Broadbent CR, Maxwell WB, Ferrie R, et al. Ability of anaesthetists to identify a marked lumbar interspace. Anaesthesia 2000; 55:1122–1126.

45. Furnesss G, Reilly MP, Kuchi S. An evaluation of ultrasound imaging for identification of lumbar intervertebral level. Anaesthesia 2002; 57:277–280.

46. Chin KL, Macfarlane AJ, Chan V, et al. The use of ultrasound to facilitate spinal anaesthesia in a patient with previous lumbar laminectomy and fusion: a case report. J Clin Ultrasound 2009; 3:482–485.

47. Lee YS, Bundschu RH, Moffat EC. Unintentional subdural block during labor epidural in a parturient with prior Harrington rod insertion for scoliosis. Reg Anesth 1995; 20:159–162.

48. Kuczkowski KM. Labor analgesia for the parturient with prior spinal surgery: what does an obstetrician need to know? Arch Gynecol Obstet 2006; 274:373–375.

49. Yamuchi M, Honma E, Mimura M, et al. Identification of the intervertebral level using ultrasound imaging in a post-laminectomy patient. J Anesth 2006; 20:231–233.

50. Littleford JA, Brockhurst NJ, Bernstein EP. Georgoussis, obstetrical anesthesia for a parturient with a ventriculuoperitoneal shunt and a third ventriculostomy. Can J Anaesth 1999; 46:1057–1063.

51. Bradley NK, Liakos AM, McAllister JP, et al. Maternal shunt dependency: implications for obstetric care, neurosurgical management, and pregnancy outcomes and a review of selected literature. Neurosurgery 1998; 43:448–460.

52. Preston R. Comment on 'obstetrical anesthesia for a parturient with ventriculostomy'. Can J Anaesth 1999; 46:1061–1062.

53. Semple DA, McClure JH, Wallace EM, Arnold-Chiari malformation in pregnancy. Anaesthesia 1996; 51:580–582.

54. Nel MR, Robson V, Robinson PN, Extradural anaesthesia for Caesarean section in a patient with Syringomyelia and Chiari type I anomaly. British Journal of Anaesthesia 1998; 80:512–515.

55. Parker JD, Broberg JC, Napolitano PG, Maternal Arnold-Chiari Type I Malformation and Syringomyelia: A Labor Management Dilemma. American Journal of Perinatology 2002; 19:445–50

56. Landau R, Giraud M, Delrue V, Kern C, Spinal Anesthesia for Cesarean Delivery in a Woman with Surgically Corrected Type I Arnold Chiari Malformation, Anesth Analg 2003;97:253–5.

57. Newhouse BJ, Kuczkowski KM, Uneventful epidural labor analgesia and vaginal delivery in a parturient with Arnold-Chiari malformation type and sickle cell disease Arch Gynecol Obstet 2007; 275:311–313.

58. Chartigian RC, Koehn MA, Ramin KD, Warner MA, Chiari I malformation in partuients. J Clin Anesth 2002; 14:201–205.

59. Mueller DM, Oro JJ, Chiari I Malformation with or without Syringomyelia and Pregnancy: Case Studies and Review of the Literature. American Journal of Perinatology 2005; 22:67–70.

60. Hullander MR, Bogard TD, Leivers D, et al. Malformation presenting as recurrent spinal headache. Anesth Analg 1992; 75:1025–1026.

61. Barton JJ, Sharpe JA. Oscillopsia and horizontal nystagmus with accelerating slow phases following lumbar puncture in the Arnold-Chiari malformation. Ann Neurol 1993; 33:418–421.

Neurocritical care for the pregnant woman

Clemens Pahl

INTRODUCTION

Obstetric patients admitted to an intensive care unit (ICU) fall into one of two categories: those with an obstetric cause of their critical illness (50–80%) and those with a non-obstetric aetiology.

Obstetric causes of pregnant patients admitted to ICU are most frequently pre-eclampsia/eclampsia, and non-obstetric causes are most often sepsis from community-acquired pneumonia or urinary tract infection.

More generally, neurological syndromes caused either by primary disorders of the nervous system or by systemic illness with secondary neurological manifestation are common reasons for referral to intensive care, and these cases will include pregnant women.

This chapter gives an overview of neurocritical care for the pregnant patient. The section 'Neurological Syndromes in Critically Ill Pregnant Patients' describes the neurological syndromes that critically ill pregnant patients commonly present with, their causes and emergency management. The section 'Intensive Care Therapy for TBI and Non-Traumatic SAH in the Pregnant Woman' outlines the principles of intensive care therapy in pregnancy, followed by summaries of the specific management of traumatic brain injury (TBI) and aneurysmal subarachnoid haemorrhage (SAH), common diagnoses on neurocritical care units. The chapter concludes with a section on maternal brain stem death and issues that arise in relation to support for the fetus in this case.

NEUROLOGICAL SYNDROMES IN CRITICALLY ILL PREGNANT PATIENTS
Altered Mental Status and Coma

The commonest neurological syndrome in obstetric patients needing intensive care consultation is reduced levels of consciousness, or coma, defined by a Glasgow Coma Scale (GCS) ≤ 8 (Table 6b.1).

The immediate management of a patient with a low level of consciousness follows the A (airway), B (breathing), C (circulation), D (disability of the nervous system) approach. An anaesthetist or intensivist must be called. All pregnant women who are 20 or more weeks pregnant should be nursed in the left lateral rescue position. Oxygen should be supplied at 15 L/min via a non-rebreathing (reservoir bag) mask. Venous access needs to be secured and the capillary blood glucose measured urgently. Immediate testing of a small sample of blood in a modern blood gas analyser provides essential information about the metabolic and respiratory state, and about haemoglobin and electrolyte levels.

The pregnant patient is particularly vulnerable to aspiration of saliva and regurgitated gastric contents, as a result of the normal physiological changes in pregnancy leading to reduced oesophageal sphincter tone, delayed gastric emptying and increased gastric pressure (1). In addition, falling levels of consciousness reduce pharyngeal sensations and pharyngeal muscle tone as well as upper and lower oesophageal sphincter tone, progressively increasing the risk of aspiration. For this reason, intubation of the trachea must be considered early when GCS is falling, and it is strongly indicated for patients with a GCS ≤8. Intubation provides a patent upper airway, protects the lower airways from aspiration and enables mechanical ventilation as necessary.

Prior to induction of general anaesthesia and intubation, it is prudent to document the results of a neurological assessment with a view to further diagnostic and therapeutic planning. This should include assessment of GCS, looking for signs of meningeal irritation, noting pupillary size and reaction, tone (including clonus) and muscle strength and reflexes (including the plantar response).

Common disorders that produce focal neurological deficits, for example, an asymmetric response to pain, are cerebral infarction, intra-cerebral haemorrhage, cerebral venous sinus thrombosis and brain abscess. Signs of meningeal irritation may be present in meningitis and in SAH. The absence of meningeal irritation or focal deficits suggests metabolic or toxic causes or cerebral involvement in systemic sepsis.

The next steps in making a diagnosis are brain imaging (see chapter 12) and examination of cerebrospinal fluid (CSF).

Seizures

In general, all conditions with reduced levels of consciousness and coma in pregnancy (Table 6b.1) may elicit seizures. The commonest cause of seizures in pregnancy is pre-existing epilepsy (see chapter 12).

Maternal seizures lead to a redistribution of blood to brain and muscle with reduction in uterine and visceral blood flow (2). Status epilepticus is associated with high maternal and fetal mortality and needs to be treated aggressively (3). The immediate management again follows the ABCD approach.

Benzodiazepines, for example, lorazepam 2 mg i.v., repeated every 5 minutes, are the first-line drugs for non-eclamptic convulsive seizures lasting more than 5 minutes. An intravenous loading dose of phenytoin is started simultaneously if the patient is not already receiving oral phenytoin. The dose recommended in the general population is 18 to 20 mg/kg, with a maximum rate of 50 mg/min.

It is uncertain if pregnant patients require a higher loading dose of phenytoin per kilogram weight per se, or if any calculated dose should be based on current pregnancy weight or on pre-pregnancy weight. The volume of distribution (Vd) and the degree of plasma protein binding determine the required total loading dose. In non-pregnant patients, phenytoin is 90% bound to plasma proteins, mostly albumin, and the Vd lies between 0.5 to 1.2 L/kg. This moderately high Vd does not suggest excessive drug accumulation in tissues. Pregnancy is associated with a larger Vd for this drug resulting in a higher calculated loading dose. In vivo, however, the effect

Table 6b.1 Causes of Reduced Levels of Consciousness in Pregnancy

Vascular
    Cerebral ischaemic and haemorrhagic infarction
    Cerebral venous sinus thrombosis
    Subarachnoid haemorrhage
Hypertensive encephalopathy/Posterior reversible encephalopathy
    syndrome (PRES)
Infections
    Meningoencephalitis
    Cerebral abscess
    Sepsis from extracranial sources
Intracranial space-occupying lesions
    Primary intracranial tumours
    Metastasis
Trauma
Metabolic disorders
    Hypoglycaemia
    Electrolyte disturbances
Hepatic encephalopathy, for example, acute fatty liver of pregnancy
    and HELLP syndrome (haemolysis, elevated liver enzymes, low
    platelets)
Porphyria
Drugs and toxins
    Magnesium
    Sedatives
    Ethanol
    Illicit drug abuse
    Poisoning
Miscellaneous
    Epilepsy
    Eclampsia
    Sheehan syndrome

of a higher Vd might be offset, to an unknown degree, by a higher free and hence active drug fraction in pregnant patients, so that the required loading dose may only slightly differ from that in non-pregnant patients (4,5). A reasonable approach, given the current evidence, is to use a phenytoin loading dose of 20 mg/kg of ideal, pre-pregnancy body weight. In patients currently on phenytoin with a known plasma level below the therapeutic range, a reduced reloading dose adjusted to the plasma level should be given. This dose may be calculated as: Loading dose = Vd × (desired plasma concentration − actual plasma concentration). Actual plasma concentration in general patients should be corrected for low plasma albumin concentration. In pregnant patients with mild pregnancy-induced hypoalbuminaemia it seems appropriate from the considerations made above to use for this equation a Vd as in general patients, and to use the actual plasma concentration, not corrected for low albumin.

For eclampsia, intravenous magnesium (loading dose of 5 g, then infusion of 2–3 g/hr) should be used instead of phenytoin (6). Phenytoin is not effective for the treatment of eclamptic seizures. If seizures continue, or there is continued unconsciousness, an anaesthetist or intensive care specialist must be called as general anaesthesia with thiopentone, propofol or benzodiazepines as hypnotic agents is the next step in stopping the seizures and protecting the airway. Cessation of seizures must then be confirmed by electroencephalography (EEG). Artificial coma is continued until sufficient non-sedative anti-epileptic therapy has been established.

Respiratory Muscle Weakness (See Chapters 25 and 26)

Respiratory muscle weakness may result from disorders of the neuromuscular junction (e.g., myasthenia gravis, which may

worsen during pregnancy), from peripheral neuropathies (e.g., Guillain–Barre syndrome) or from spinal cord disorders (e.g., from trauma or demyelination). Muscle weakness may be so severe as to require mechanical ventilation.

PRINCIPLES OF INTENSIVE CARE MEDICINE FOR PREGNANT PATIENTS

There are two general aspects of patient management on an ICU:

- *support of organs that have become dysfunctional as a consequence of the disease process*, and
- *specific therapy of the underlying cause(s) of critical illness.*

For example, seizures in status epilepticus can be stopped temporarily by ventilating the patient in a barbiturate coma (organ support) until non-hypnotic anti-epileptic therapy has been established (specific therapy) and the patient can be woken up.

The following paragraph gives an introduction to organ support in neurocritical care with particular regard to the impact of physiological changes in pregnancy.

Airway

Difficult or failed intubation and aspiration of stomach contents on induction of anaesthesia are more common in pregnant women than in the general population (7).

Physiological swelling of nasal, oral, pharyngeal and/or laryngeal mucosa may hinder visualisation of the larynx at laryngoscopy and insertion of an endotracheal tube. Increased breast size can interfere with introduction of a laryngoscope into the mouth. Anaesthesia should ideally be induced in the operating theatre or on the ICU where advanced equipment for dealing with difficult airways and trained assistance are available.

Respiratory System and Mechanical Ventilation Support

Upward displacement of the enlarging uterus in pregnancy (diaphragmatic splinting) causes mechanical compression of basal alveoli (atelectasis) when the woman lies supine. General anaesthesia causes additional alveolar collapse (8). Alveolar gas volume (specifically functional residual capacity) and oxygen content diminish, which render the woman prone to hypoxaemia on induction of anaesthesia.

Mechanical *v*entilation with *i*ntermittent *p*ositive *p*ressure (IPPV) is radically different from the mechanisms of normal physiology in spontaneous respiration. IPPV is likely to sustain or exacerbate atelectasis in dependent lung areas (9). Pulmonary blood flowing through atelectic areas no longer takes part in gas exchange (shunt flow), and arterial partial pressure of oxygen (PaO_2) decreases as a result. PaO_2 is stabilised during IPPV by choosing inspired fractions of oxygen (FiO_2) above 30% in the gas mixture, and by using *p*ositive *e*nd-*e*xpiratory *p*ressure (PEEP). PEEP reduces pulmonary shunt flow by reopening and splinting alveoli. It should be titrated to achieve a normal PaO_2 (≥ 11 kPa) initially with an $FiO_2 < 60\%$. Prolonged use of $FiO_2 > 60\%$ causes pulmonary oxygen toxicity (10).

IPPV may also increase lung water because lymphatic drainage is hindered, and capillary leak may develop because of ventilation-induced inflammation (8).

Diaphragmatic splinting can be minimised by positioning the patient with the upper body raised at 15° to 40°. This position has the additional advantage of reducing the incidence of ventilator-associated pneumonia, and represents a standard of care for all ventilated patients (11). Patients after the 20th week of gestation should, in addition, be turned on to their left side (see below).

Normal pregnancy induces hyperventilation during spontaneous breathing. Partial pressure of carbon dioxide in arterial blood ($PaCO_2$) falls to between 3.7 and 4.1 kPa (4.8–6.4 kPa in healthy non-pregnant subjects). Arterial pH is incompletely compensated by renal mechanisms, with a slight rise to around 7.44. Standard bicarbonate falls from 22 to 26 mmol/L in healthy, spontaneously breathing, non-pregnant subjects to 19 to 20 mmol/L during normal pregnancy. This has important implications for setting mechanical ventilation. Setting the ventilator to achieve normal non-pregnancy $PaCO_2$ values will cause an immediate respiratory acidosis, because renal compensation for increased $PaCO_2$ lags behind in time. Acidosis threatens normal organ function in both mother and fetus. Maintenance of the diffusion gradient for transfer of CO_2 from fetal to maternal circulation dictates keeping the maternal $PaCO_2$ below 4.5 kPa.

$PaCO_2$ is also a major regulator of cerebral vessel tone, as discussed below.

Sedation and Analgesia

Mechanically ventilated patients require sedation and analgesia to tolerate endotracheal intubation and artificial ventilation, and to control pain. Propofol, midazolam and opioids are used most commonly in various combinations.

All sedative and analgesic agents used in intensive care cause a variable degree of peripheral vasodilatation and a fall in cardiac output and systemic blood pressure. Oversedation causes cardiovascular instability and delays recovery from critical illness. Daily interruptions of sedative infusions in general intensive care patients reduce the duration of mechanical ventilation and the length of stay on ICU (12). Respiratory depression and low APGAR scores occur in the newborn of mothers who receive these drugs prepartum.

Propofol, a hypnotic agent, crosses the placenta and reaches blood levels in the cord of about 70% of those in maternal blood. Animal studies and limited human data on propofol as a bolus for induction of general anaesthesia suggest a low risk of lasting fetal harm (13). There are no studies investigating fetal sequelae of propofol infusions on ICU, although its short-term use seems to be safe (14). Long-term propofol sedation in high doses (>4 mg/kg/hr for >48 hr) should be avoided as this may cause a shock-like syndrome (propofol infusion syndrome) with multi-organ failure (15). However, propofol is non-cumulative, even with significant liver and renal dysfunction, and allows rapid recovery from sedation.

The benzodiazepine midazolam is an alternative sedative agent, often chosen if long-term sedation is required. Midazolam can effectively control seizures in ventilated patients. It may be preferable in patients with hypotension and/or low cardiac output because of its favourable cardiovascular profile over propofol. Midazolam crosses the placenta and reaches 60% of the maternal blood concentration in the cord. Human data suggest a low risk of adverse effects to the fetus when midazolam is given as a single dose at term. However, teratogenicity with neurological and facial abnormalities is associated with maternal abuse of benzodiazepines (diazepam/oxazepam) during pregnancy (13). The risk of fetal harm caused by midazolam infusions for maternal sedation on ICU is unknown. A major drawback of using prolonged, continuous infusions of midazolam is its tendency to accumulate and delay recovery from sedation. Withdrawal symptoms in the newborn or 'floppy baby syndrome' can occur when midazolam is infused prepartum.

The barbiturate thiopentone has a long safety record as a general anaesthesia induction agent for caesarean section. Thiopentone is an effective drug for intractable intracranial hypertension after TBI, and for treatment-resistant status epilepticus. It is, however, not routinely used as a sedative infusion on ICU because its hypnotic effect perseveres after discontinuation of the drug because of its low clearance and accumulation of the active metabolite pentobarbitone. It can cause severe hypokalaemia because of a shift of potassium into the intracellular space, and hyperkalaemia after stopping the infusion.

Analgesia in intensive care patients is often provided by infusions of opioids. There are no reports of long-lasting adverse effects of short-term use of morphine, fentanyl, alfentanil and remifentanil in offspring (16), although withdrawal symptoms in the newborn should be anticipated.

Impact of Mechanical Ventilation on the Systemic Circulation

Cardiac Output

Oxygen demand in pregnancy is increased by 30% to 60%, met by an increase in oxygen delivery, which is achieved by a rise in cardiac output (maximally by 50% at the end of the second trimester). On the ICU, maintenance of high cardiac output is threatened by both aortocaval compression and mechanical ventilation.

Compression of the inferior vena cava by the gravid uterus in the supine position reduces venous return to the heart and cardiac output. The effect develops at around 13 weeks' gestation and becomes maximal at 36 to 38 weeks. From the 20th week of gestation at the latest, critically ill pregnant patients must be nursed on the left lateral side to displace the uterus away from the inferior vena cava and restore venous return.

Positive intrathoracic pressure and raised pulmonary vascular resistance during mechanical ventilation further reduce venous return and cardiac output by causing resistance to right ventricular in- and outflow (17). The fall in cardiac output can be reversed by expanding intravascular volume with intravenous fluids. For this reason, ventilated patients often require positive daily fluid balances, at least over the initial days on ICU.

Organ Perfusion in Ventilated and Sedated Patients

Renal blood flow (RBF) and glomerular filtration rate (GFR) rise by 30% to 50% in pregnancy. Plasma concentrations of urea and creatinine decrease progressively during pregnancy. Any rise in the normal values of urea and creatinine for each trimester needs to be addressed promptly to prevent progression to acute ischaemic renal failure. The upper limit of normal of serum creatinine in pregnancy is around 80 µmol/L and that of urea is 4.5 mmol/L and values above these need clinical evaluation. Estimation of creatinine clearance using the Cockroft–Gault or the modification of diet in renal disease study (MDRD) equations is not validated in pregnancy (18).

It is important to understand that both IPPV with PEEP and the infusion of sedative agents as well as aortocaval compression in pregnancy tend to reduce GFR and urine output. The fall in cardiac output is a major, but not the sole, reason for renal impairment caused by IPPV, because an expansion in intravascular blood volume fails to completely correct urine output to normal (19). Other mechanisms such as an increase in renal vein pressure may have relevance. The renal arteries in normal subjects maintain constant RBF between mean arterial pressures (MAPs) of 80 mmHg and 150 mmHg through autoregulation, but RBF falls directly with MAPs below 80 mmHg. Drugs used for sedation impair RBF through their vasodilating and blood pressure–lowering effect. An infusion of a vasopressor (such as noradrenaline) is often required to balance the vasodilator effects and ensure adequate RBF.

Liver and utero-placental blood flows are not autoregulated and tend to fall in ventilated and sedated patients because of reductions in cardiac output and blood pressure, and because of IPPV-related elevations in hepatic and uterine venous pressure. Blood flow to these organs can often be restored by intravascular volume expansion, but normalisation of blood pressure with a vasopressor may also be necessary (20).

Haemoglobin

In general intensive care patients, the haemoglobin concentration (Hb) commonly falls below 10 g/dL for a variety of reasons, including blood loss with incomplete replacement, reduced bone marrow red cell formation and iatrogenic plasma volume expansion. Threshold haemoglobin levels for transfusing red blood cells to general intensive care patients lie between 7.0 and 8.0 g/dL. This somewhat restricted transfusion policy is supported by a randomised controlled trial suggesting that a more liberal use of blood transfusions may result in higher hospital mortality rates (21).

There is no established transfusion trigger for neurocritical care patients. In healthy volunteers it has been shown that cerebral function remains normal until haemoglobin levels fall to 5 to 7 g/dL (22). Observational data in patients with TBI, ischaemic stroke or aneurysmal SAH suggest that both severe anaemia and red blood cell transfusion (RBCT) are associated with poor outcomes. It remains unclear whether anaemia or RBCT per se influences outcome or just indicates poor prognosis determined by other factors (23).

Packed red blood cells stored for more than 20 days have reduced oxygen delivery capacity and their transfusion may compromise microvascular blood flow. Such red cells are less deformable (reducing rheology) and leak haemoglobin into plasma, where free haemoglobin binds to endothelial nitric oxide and may result in deleterious cerebral and uterine vasoconstriction (24).

It remains a matter of debate which transfusion trigger should be used for the pregnant patient. Haemoglobin concentration during normal pregnancy commonly falls to about 10 g/dL. It is common practice to maintain an Hb of about 10 g/dL in critically ill pregnant patients, that is, higher than in non-pregnant patients as discussed above, although there is no evidence to support the use of different transfusion criteria in pregnant patients with neurological/neurosurgical disease than in other critically ill obstetric patients.

Central Nervous System

Subarachnoid Space

CSF pressure is increased by uterine-caval compression. The important consequence for obstetric patients with intracranial pathologies associated with brain oedema formation is an escalated risk of developing raised intracranial pressure (ICP). The pivotal significance of nursing obstetric patients in the left lateral position is again emphasised.

Cerebral Haemodynamics

Maternal cerebral blood vessels are adapted to low $PaCO_2$ values (3.7–4.1 kPa), so that the diameter of large cerebral arteries is unchanged despite hypocapnia (25). Studies using transcranial Doppler indicate that both autoregulation of cerebral blood flow (CBF) in response to changes in MAP and cerebrovascular reactivity to $PaCO_2$ remain intact in normal pregnancy (26). This is an important consideration when treating pregnant patients with or at risk of raised ICP (as discussed further below).

Nutritional Support

It is widely accepted practice to provide early nutritional support for all critically ill patients. The enteral route is preferred over the parenteral route as it may be associated with fewer complications of feeding.

Maternal malnutrition has lasting effects on the fetus. Furthermore, malnutrition exacerbates critical illness–related muscle catabolism and hence weakness related to neuromuscular disease. A useful initial approach is to provide pregnant patients on ICU with protein at the upper limit of the recommended intake for general ICU patients of 1 to 1.25 g/kg/day (6). Caloric requirements are calculated with standard equations, such as the Schofield equation, and adjusted for critical illness–related stress. Vitamins and trace elements, especially selenium, may need to be supplemented in addition to feeding with standard formulae, as in general critical care management.

Prevention of Teratogenicity

Causes of teratogenicity are diverse but include physiological derangements in association with the ICU admission; for example, infection, hypoxia, systemic hypotension, acidosis, dehydration, in addition to the hazards of drugs. The goal of critical care in any patient, including pregnant women, is to correct these abnormalities early in the course of critical illness.

INTENSIVE CARE THERAPY FOR TBI AND NON-TRAUMATIC SAH IN THE PREGNANT WOMAN

TBI

Trauma including TBI is one of the leading causes of death in women of childbearing age and one of the leading causes of coincidental death during pregnancy. The aetiology of maternal trauma is most often road traffic accidents. With life-threatening polytrauma, a 50% fetal loss rate is described (27). In the general population, the 1-year mortality after severe TBI is around 30% to 40% and a favourable outcome (moderate disability or good recovery) in up to 60% of patients may be achieved in neurosurgical centres (28). Close collaboration between critical care specialists, surgeons and obstetricians ensures optimal care for both mother and fetus.

Detailed discussion of the neurocritical care management of TBI is beyond the scope of this chapter. A brief outline of the approach to treating TBI is given in this section. The approach to the pregnant patient does not differ to that in other patients.

Patients with TBI and GCS ≤ 8 (which defines severe TBI) require intubation, ventilation and admission to ICU. Emergency and neurocritical care aim to prevent the development of secondary brain damage that readily follows the primary injury. The predominant pathophysiological mechanism of secondary brain injury is ischaemia, closely linked with inflammation and oedema formation.

Intensive care focuses on prevention and correction of brain ischaemia. Ischaemia has a variety of causes. An important mechanism is the build-up of resistance to CBF in the wake of raised ICP. ICP rises in the presence of space-occupying intracranial haematomas and secondary to cytotoxic and/or vasogenic brain oedema.

Surgical interventions to reduce ICP include evacuation of haematomas, drainage of CSF and removal of skull to allow more room for swelling without increases in pressure (decompressive craniectomy).

Medical therapy for intracranial hypertension aims both to remove brain water and to regulate cerebral blood volume (CBV), a major determinant of ICP. Brain water can be reduced by intravenous osmotherapy with hypertonic saline (HS) or mannitol. HS often appears superior for several reasons. It expands plasma volume without a secondary diuretic effect. The latter is typical for mannitol and may result in detrimental reductions of cerebral and utero-placental blood flow. HS also seems to have favourable rheological effects in the microcirculation (29). HS and mannitol can be administered repeatedly as long as plasma sodium concentration remains below 155 mmol/L and osmolality below 320 mosmol/kg plasma water to prevent hypertonic acute renal failure. CBV is regulated by sedative medications, by titration of $PaCO_2$ and by manipulation of cerebral perfusion pressure (CPP). Sedative agents (propofol, midazolam or thiopentone) reduce global cerebral metabolic rate, coupled with similar reductions in CBF and CBV. $PaCO_2$ is a major regulator of cerebral vessel tone. Rising $PaCO_2$ causes cerebral vasodilatation, whereas falling $PaCO_2$ induces vasoconstriction in a linear relationship. Hence, CBF is directly proportional to $PaCO_2$ over a wide range of values. International guidelines recommend a $PaCO_2$ target of 4.5 to 5.0 kPa for ventilated patients with or at risk of raised ICP (30). This $PaCO_2$ achieves a balance between over-vasoconstriction risking cerebral ischaemia, and vasodilatation resulting in increased CBV and hence raised ICP. However, maternal blood vessels are adapted to lower $PaCO_2$ values. A $PaCO_2$ of 4.5 to 5.0 kPa in a pregnant woman with TBI may cause cerebral vasodilatation and rise in ICP, and may also jeopardise CO_2 transfer from the fetal to maternal circulation. A $PaCO_2$ target nearer to 4.0 kPa is therefore recommended in pregnancy.

CPP is calculated as MAP minus ICP. In normal brain, CBF is kept constant in the face of changes in CPP between 50 and 150 mmHg by altering cerebral arteriolar diameter (autoregulation). CBF falls sharply when CPP falls below 50 mmHg, risking brain ischaemia. If brain autoregulation remains intact in TBI, then increasing CPP will cause progressive vasoconstriction, reduction in CBV and fall in ICP with constant CBF. However, in many patients with severe TBI, autoregulation is abolished. In this situation, first, CPP may be critically reduced even at 50 mmHg and needs to be increased pharmacologically. Second, when CPP increases, cerebral arterioles passively dilate. The effect is an increase in CBV and ICP. In clinical practice, a balance needs to be found between providing a sufficient CPP, and preventing intracranial hypertension secondary to elevations in CBV. A general CPP target of 60 mmHg in patients with severe TBI is currently advocated (30). The maintenance of an adequate CPP requires infusion of a vasopressor agent such as noradrenaline in most patients.

Hypoxaemia is another cause of brain ischaemia. A normal PaO_2 (>11 kPa) should be targeted with the lowest FiO_2 possible. Care must be taken to avoid a PaO_2 < 8.0 kPa because CBF, hence CBV and ICP, will increase sharply below this value (31).

Hyperglycaemia and hyperthermia both increase cerebral oxygen consumption and CBF (hence CBV) through flow-metabolism coupling. Blood glucose and temperature must be controlled promptly to prevent effects on ICP and avoid oxygen deficits in brain cells (30).

The timing of introduction of heparin for prophylaxis of venous thromboembolism depends on the severity and nature of the brain injury. The risk of causing intracranial bleeding must be weighed against the increased risk of thromboembolic events in pregnancy. Non-pharmacological measures, namely compression stockings, pneumatic calf compression and physiotherapy, should be employed vigorously in all intensive care patients.

Non-Traumatic SAH

The majority of cases of non-traumatic SAH are caused by ruptured aneurysms (85%). Patients presenting with reduced levels of consciousness need prompt admission to intensive care. Intubation and ventilation are necessary when GCS is ≤8. Even with a higher GCS, after SAH, patients may develop later deterioration from a variety of intracranial and extracranial complications, hence observations to detect change are important. Admission to high-dependency and/or intensive care facility is often necessary later.

Intracranial Complications of SAH

There are three major intracranial complications of SAH: re-bleeding, acute hydrocephalus and cerebral vasospasm.

Re-bleeding. Re-bleeding usually results in a drop in conscious level. Urgent intubation and resuscitation may be necessary, followed by CT scanning of the brain. If re-bleeding occurs, 80% die or are severely disabled but not all re-bleeds are unsurvivable and such deterioration should be treated (32).

Acute hydrocephalus. This may occur within the first 24 hours after SAH or later. It typically results in a drop in GCS (often by 1 point), exacerbation of headache, a sluggish pupillary response and downward deviation of the eyes ('sunset eyes'). CT scanning will confirm the diagnosis. Patients with acute hydrocephalus should be moved to a high-dependency/critical care facility for close observation. Ventricular or lumbar CSF drainage may be required.

Cerebral vasospasm. Vasospasm following SAH may cause delayed cerebral ischaemia. Although vasospasm can be observed angiographically in 60% to 70% of patients with SAH, only 30% develop a delayed ischaemic neurological deficit (DIND), the incidence of which peaks between days 5 and 14 post-SAH. Amongst those with DIND, 64% develop cerebral infarction (33). In the awake patient, repeated clinical examination is the gold standard for detecting neurological deterioration. However, neurological examination in ventilated patients on ICU is not a suitable tool for detection of brain ischaemia, and cerebral angiography and transcranial Doppler ultrasonography (TCD) are used to aid diagnosis of cerebral vasospasm. Angiography is the gold standard, but both angiography and TCD lack specificity in diagnosing relevant reductions in CBF. On ICU, the trend in blood flow velocities measured by daily TCD examinations informs decisions around further diagnostic procedures and specific therapy.

The only proven intervention to prevent or reduce the severity of DINDs secondary to cerebral vasospasm is the administration of oral nimodipine, a dihydropyridine calcium channel blocker, at 60 mg 4 hourly for 21 days (34). In ventilated patients, this is given via a nasogastric tube. In the first trimester, nimodipine may potentially cause fetal harm as indicated by experimental studies that suggest that early embryonic differentiation can be disturbed by calcium channel blockers (13). Potential risks and benefits of nimodipine must be considered in individual cases, and a decision for or against its use be made together with the patient if possible. Nimodipine has been used safely in the second and third trimester to control blood pressure in pre-eclampsia (35), although it is not recommended as a first-line drug for this indication (36).

Adequate hydration is of paramount importance to prevent low CBF and ischaemia. Three litres of crystalloid (0.9% saline or Hartman's) per day are commonly given to patients with all grades of SAH, with close monitoring of fluid balance. Haemodilution and increased urine output achieved with this regime often lead to a fall in plasma concentrations of potassium, magnesium and phosphate. Electrolytes must be replaced promptly to avoid further morbidity. Significant systemic arterial hypotension despite adequate hydration is not infrequently encountered in the general population of patients with SAH. Causes include peripheral vasodilatation by nimodipine and myocardial dysfunction induced by SAH. The hypotensive effect of nimodipine can be mitigated by splitting the daily drug dose further up, for example, to 30 mg 2 hourly. The use of a vasopressor such as noradrenaline and/or of an inotropic drug such as dobutamine must be considered early to prevent low cerebral and low utero-placental blood flow.

Magnesium and the statin class of drugs show promise for the prevention of vasospasm and DIND. International multi-centre studies to determine the effect of these agents on outcome after SAH are currently being conducted (the MASH and STASH trials) (37,38).

Patients who develop symptomatic vasospasm should be managed in a critical care area. The aim is to restore CBF through the narrowed arteries to prevent reversible cerebral ischaemia from progressing to established cerebral infarction. This may be achieved by hypertensive hypervolaemic haemodilution, the so-called triple H therapy, and by intra-arterial administration of a vasodilator such as nimodipine via an intravascular catheter. Systemic hypertension is induced by intravenous infusion of a vasopressor, commonly noradrenaline, while intravenous fluid loading is being continued. Triple H therapy is a plausible and acutely effective intervention, although no level 1/2 evidence exists for its use. There are no generally agreed blood pressure targets for induced hypertension. In patients with a secured aneurysm, an MAP of 130 mmHg is targeted in our institution, and in patients with an unsecured aneurysm, it is an MAP of 100 to 110 mmHg. Triple H therapy requires intensive monitoring, including invasive arterial and central venous pressure, in addition to neurological monitoring. It must be taken into account that raising MAP significantly above normal by vasopressor administration may cause critical degrees of vasoconstriction in uterine arteries, leading to underperfusion of the placenta. In cases where induced hypertension may be indicated, early delivery of the fetus must be considered, or close monitoring, for example, by cardiotocography (CTG) and Doppler velocimetry of uterine arteries, with delivery where possible if there is suggestion of fetal compromise. Noradrenaline passing the placental membrane may have undue vasopressor effects in the fetus.

Extracranial Complications of SAH
Extracranial complications are common and encroach significantly on outcome in patients with SAH (Table 6b.2). Extracranial organ dysfunction may render the patient too unstable to undergo operative clipping or radiological coiling of the aneurysm in the acute phase.

Table 6b.2 Extracranial Complications of SAH

Pneumonia
Neurogenic pulmonary oedema
Adult respiratory distress syndrome
Heart failure
Arrhythmias
Liver dysfunction
Renal dysfunction
Hyponatremia

It is essential to identify these complications early by close clinical observation, repeated clinical examination, regular blood tests, including inflammatory markers, and chest radiography. Patients should be considered early for critical care unit admission.

BRAIN DEATH IN THE PREGNANT PATIENT ON ICU

Brain death may result from severe TBI, catastrophic SAH and other cerebrovascular accidents, and from other critical illnesses.

The medical Royal Colleges in the United Kingdom define brain death as a complete, irreversible loss of brainstem function that is equivalent to death of the individual (39). Brain death will result in cardiac asystole within days or weeks, despite continuation of mechanical ventilation and full life-support, as documented in over 1000 cases in the literature. Therefore, once brainstem death has been confirmed, death is declared, medical interventions are stopped and the body is discontinued from mechanical ventilation. In cases in which it has been agreed to proceed to organ transplantation, full somatic support continues until explantation of organs is completed in the operating theatre.

In the case of pregnant patients, this is the only situation in which continued mechanical ventilation and full additional somatic support for a prolonged period are considered when there is brain death. The goal is to extend the pregnancy to improve fetal outcome. Powner and Bernstein reviewed 10 wcases published before 2003 where somatic support was provided after maternal brain death (40). In all cases the fetuses survived with good outcomes. The longest reported duration of successful somatic support after maternal brain death is 107 days. This case was also the earliest gestational age (15 weeks) when such support began and was continued until delivery at 32 weeks (34). In this scenario, particular support for the patient's family may be needed (see also discussion below).

Diagnosis of Brain Death (39)

Diagnosis of brainstem death in the United Kingdom must be made by two doctors who have been fully registered with the General Medical Council for at least 5 years. One of these should be a consultant. This is usually an intensivist.

The diagnosis of brainstem death is in three parts.

First, the patient must fulfil two preconditions: He/she is in an unresponsive coma (GCS 3/15), and the patient's condition is secondary to irreversible brain damage of known aetiology.

Second, reversible causes of coma must be excluded. Potentially reversible causes are as follows: drugs; hypothermia; and circulatory, metabolic and endocrine disturbances. For example, sedative medications should have been stopped at least 24 hours before brainstem testing. Longer washout periods may be required after use of thiopentone or prolonged use of midazolam.

Third, a series of neurological tests is applied to the patient. The test battery has two parts: the brainstem reflexes and the apnoea test. The following must be confirmed: no pupillary response to light, absent corneal reflex, absent vestibulo-ocular reflex, no motor response to central stimulation, absent gag reflex, absent cough reflex; and in the apnoea test, the absence of respiratory movements with hypercarbia when the patient is disconnected from the ventilator, while oxygenation is maintained. Two sets of tests must be carried out, but there is no prescribed time interval between tests.

The diagnosis of brain death in the United States and Europe is based on similar clinical tests to in the United Kingdom. The United States and European countries also embrace the concept of brain death being equal to death of the individual. Differences to the approach in the United Kingdom exist in the duration of the recommended clinical observation period that should have elapsed between the time of the brain injury events and the time brainstem testing is conducted, and in the use of confirmatory investigations. EEG is frequently used as a confirmatory test in many countries. EEG is a mandatory component in the diagnosis of brain death in some countries, for example, in Austria, or in Germany when the lesion is primarily infratentorial. In the United Kingdom, EEG is not considered to be a valuable tool in the diagnosis of brain death.

The predictable pathophysiological changes after brainstem death must be managed if pregnancy is to be extended in a brain-dead patient. These changes are discussed below together with some recommendations for somatic support.

Pathophysiological Changes After Brainstem Death

Cardiovascular Changes

Brain death is followed by massive sympathetic discharge causing severe hypertension, tachycardia, rise in systemic vascular resistance, myocardial ischaemic damage and neurogenic pulmonary oedema. Subsequently, sympathetic output is lost leading to hypotension. Inotropic and vasopressor support, in addition to intravenous fluids, is often necessary to maintain cardiac output, systemic blood pressure and uterine blood flow.

Respiratory System

Pulmonary dysfunction may be secondary to ventilator-associated pneumonia (requiring antibiotics), neurogenic pulmonary oedema (requiring careful titration of PEEP) or pulmonary trauma.

Endocrine System

Panhypopituitarism causes significant reductions in the circulating levels of tri-iodothyronine (T3) and thyroxine (T4), antidiuretic hormone (ADH) and cortisol. ADH deficiency causes diabetes insipidus, which must be treated aggressively with intravenous fluids and ADH analogues to avoid intravascular volume depletion. Replacement of thyroid hormones and cortisol is guided by measurements of adrenal and thyroid function.

Temperature Regulation

Poikilothermia, where body temperature is dependent on that of the environment, is frequently described after brain death as a result of the loss of hypothalamic function. Labile temperatures and hyperthermia can occur, but hypothermia is more common after brain death. This can be managed with warm air blankets.

Throughout the period of somatic support, assessments of fetal growth and maturation include fetal heart rate monitoring and serial ultrasound scanning. Administration of drugs to reduce uterine contractions, such as nifedipine, may be necessary, and their successful use under these circumstances is described in the literature (40).

Ethical Issues

The issue of somatically supporting a brain-dead woman until delivery of the fetus raises ethical questions. The situation may be no different from the somatic support for a time of a brain-dead organ donor, with support for the benefit of another person (the organ recipient). The question then arises if it could be justified for doctors to use the woman's body as an 'incubator' for the growing fetus, if the woman had previously indicated her wishes in favour of being an organ donor.

Unfortunately, the exact wishes of the woman on how to proceed in such a situation are rarely, if ever, known. In practice, consent from the next of kin, particularly the father and other family members, is sought, and psychological support should be provided.

In making any decision it is important to inform the family of the risks of delivery of a severely premature fetus with the associated emotional, physical and economic costs.

In addition, there is currently no agreed gestational age below which somatic support of the mother should not be attempted.

CONCLUSIONS

Many issues arising in the neurocritical care management of the pregnant patient can be managed in similar ways to the non-pregnant patient. However, it is important that the physiology of pregnancy is understood and related to pathophysiological changes expected in critical care caused by neurological and neurosurgical disease. In addition, the clinician should be particularly aware of the effects of management on the fetus and its development. Particular issues arise when the pregnant patient is brain-dead and support is prolonged to help fetal development. Close cooperation between different specialists during a neurocritical illness will result in the best outcomes for the woman and the fetus.

REFERENCES

1. Munnur U, de Boisblanc B, Suresh MS. Airway problems in pregnancy. Crit Care Med 2005; 33(suppl):S259–S268.
2. Karnad DR, Guntupalli KK. Neurologic disorders in pregnancy. Crit Care Med 2005; 33(suppl):S362–S371.
3. Pennel PB. Pregnancy in the woman with epilepsy: maternal and fetal outcomes. Semin Neurol 2002; 22:299–307.
4. Freed CR, Gal J, Manchester DK. Dosage of phenytoin in pregnancy. JAMA 1985; 253(19):2833–2840.
5. Chen SS, Perucca E, Lee JN, et al. Serum protein binding and free concentration of phenytoin and phenobarbitone in pregnancy. Br J Clin Pharmacol 1982; 13(4):547–552.
6. Warwick D, Ngan WD, Gin T. Pre-eclampsia and eclampsia. In: Bersten AD, Soni N, eds. Oh's Intensive Care Manual. 6th ed. London: Butterworth-Heinemann, 2009:665–671.
7. McDonnell NJ, Paech MJ, Clavisi OM, et al. Difficult and failed intubation in obstetric anaesthesia: an observational study of airway management and complications with general anaesthesia for caesarean section. Int J Obstet Anaesth 2008; 17(4):292–297.

8. Hedenstierna G, Edmark L. The effects of anaesthesia and muscle paralysis on the respiratory system. Intensive Care Med 2005; 31:1327–1335.

9. Soni N, Williams P. Positive pressure ventilation: what is the real cost? Br J Anaesth 2008; 101:446–457.

10. Deneke SM, Fanburg BL. Normobaric oxygen toxicity in the lung. N Engl J Med 1980; 303(2):76–86.

11. Collard HR, Saint S, Matthay M. Prevention of ventilator-associated pneumonia: an evidence-based systemic review. Ann Intern Med 2003; 138:494–501.

12. Kress JP, Pohlman AS, O'Connor MF, et al. Daily interruption of sedative infusions in critically ill patients undergoing mechanical ventilation. N Engl J Med 2000; 342:1471–1477.

13. Briggs GG, Freeman RK, Yaffe SJ, eds. Drugs in Pregnancy and Lactation. 8th ed. Philadelphia: Lippincott Williams & Wilkins, 2008:1542–1544, 1218–1220, 200–203.

14. Bacon RC, Razis PA. The effect of propofol sedation in pregnancy on neonatal condition. Anaesthesia 1994; 49(12):1058–1060.

15. Kam PC, Cardone D. Propofol infusion syndrome. Anaesthesia 2007; 62(7):690–701.

16. Reuvers M, Schaefer C. Analgesics and anti-inflammatory drugs. In: Schaefer C, Peters P, Miller RK, eds. Drugs During Pregnancy and Lactation. 2nd ed. London: Elsevier, 2007:33–36.

17. Morgan BC, Martin WE, Hornbein TF, et al. Hemodynamic effects of intermittent positive pressure ventilation. Anesthesiology 1966; 27:584–590.

18. Levey AS, Bosch JP, Breyer Lewis J, et al. A more accurate method to estimate glomerular filtration rate from serum creatinine: a new prediction equation. Ann Intern Med 1999; 130:461–470.

19. Qvist J, Pontoppidan H, Wilson RS, et al. Hemodynamic responses to mechanical ventilation with PEEP: the effect of hypervolaemia. Anesthesiology 1975; 42:45–55.

20. Matuschak GM, Pinsky MR, Rogers RM. Effect of positive end-expiratory pressure on hepatic blood flow and performance. J Appl Physiol 1987; 62:1377–1383.

21. Hebert PC, Wells G, Blajchman MA, et al. A multicenter, randomized, controlled clinical trial of transfusion requirements in critical care. N Engl J Med 1999; 340:409–417.

22. Weisskopf RB, Kramer JH, Neumann M, et al. Acute severe isovolemic anemia impairs cognitive function memory in humans. Anesthesiology 2000; 92:1646–1652.

23. Leal-Noval SR, Munoz-Gomez M, Murillo-Cabezas F. Optimal hemoglobin concentration in patients with subarachnoid hemorrhage, acute ischemic stroke and traumatic brain injury. Curr Opin Crit Care 2008; 14:156–162.

24. Tinmouth A, Fergusson D, Yee IC, et al; The ABLE investigators and Canadian Critical Care Trial Group. Transfusion 2006; 46:2014–2027.

25. Zeeman GG, Hatab M, Twickler DM. Maternal cerebral blood flow changes in pregnancy. Am J Obstet Gynecol 2003; 189:968–972.

26. Sherman RW, Bowie RA, Henfrey MME, et al. Cerebral haemodynamics in pregnancy and pre-eclampsia as assessed by transcranial Doppler ultrasonography. Br J Anaesth 2002; 89:687–692.

27. Mattox KL, Goetzl L. Trauma in pregnancy. Crit Care Med 2005; 33(suppl):S385–S389.

28. Patel HC, Menon DK, Tebbs S, et al. Specialist neurocritical care and outcome from head injury. Intensive Care Med 2002; 28(5):547–553.

29. Strandvik GF. Hypertonic saline in critical care: a review of the literature and guidelines for use in hypotonic states and raised intracranial pressure. Anaesthesia 2009; 64(9):990–1003.

30. The Brain Trauma Foundation. Guidelines for the management of severe traumatic brain injury. J Neurotrauma 2007; 24(suppl 1): S32–S36.

31. Gupta AK, Menon DK, Czosnyka M, et al. Threshold for hypoxic cerebral vasoconstriction in volunteers. Anaesth Analg 1997; 85:817–820.

32. Van Gijn J, Kerr RS, Rinkel GJ. Subarachnoid haemorrhage. Lancet 2007; 27(9558):306–318.

33. Vajkoczy P, Horn P, Thome C, et al. Regional cerebral blood flow monitoring in the diagnosis of delayed ischemia following aneurysmal subarachnoid hemorrhage. J Neurosurg 2003; 98:1227–1234.

34. Allen GS, Ahn HS, Preziosi TJ, et al. Cerebral arterial spasm – a controlled trial of nimodipine in patients with subarachnoid hemorrhage. N Engl J Med 1983; 308(11):619–624.

35. Belfort MA, Saade GR, Moise KJ, et al. Nimodipine in the management of preeclampsia: maternal and fetal effects. Am J Obstet Gynecol 1994; 171(2):417–424.

36. Duley L, Henderson-Smart DJ, Meher S. Drugs for the treatment of very high blood pressure during pregnancy. Cochrane Database Syst Rev 2006; 3:CD001449.

37. Van den Bergh WM, Algra A, Van Kooten F, et al; MASH study group. Magnesium sulfate in aneurysmal subarachnoid hemorrhage: a randomized controlled trial. Stroke 2005; 36(5):1011–1015.

38. Tseng MY, Hutchinson PJA, Czosnyka M, et al. Effects of acute pravastatin on intensity of rescue therapy, length of inpatient stay and 6-months outcome in patients after subarachnoid haemorrhage. Stroke 2007; 38:1545–1550.

39. Academy of Medical Royal Colleges. A code of practice for the diagnosis and confirmation of death. London: PPG Design and Print Ltd, 2008.

40. Powner DJ, Bernstein IM. Extended somatic support for pregnant women after brain death. Crit Care Med 2003; 31:1241–1249.

Neurovascular intervention during pregnancy: cerebral aneurysms and vascular malformations

Daniel Walsh

INTRODUCTION

Intracranial haemorrhage is a condition which may mandate emergency treatment during a pregnancy. There may be no warning that the mother is at risk of this complication in the course of her antenatal care excepting cases of pre-eclampsia which may require medical management to minimise risk. Although intracranial haemorrhage is uncommon in women with pre-eclampsia, when hypertension is managed suboptimally intracranial haemorrhage remains an important complication of pre-eclampsia (1). This chapter focuses on instances where there is a structural cause accounting for the haemorrhage and considers the practical management of acutely raised intracranial pressure as well as intervention to secure a bleeding vascular abnormality or aneurysm during pregnancy. It is now best practice to make these decisions as part of a neurovascular multidisciplinary team which should include specialist neurovascular surgeons and interventional neuroradiologists. The reader may wish to refer to chapters 2, 6, 16 and 17 for related topics.

CONDITIONS THAT MAY REQUIRE INTERVENTION DURING PREGNANCY
Aneurysmal Subarachnoid Haemorrhage

Aneurysmal subarachnoid haemorrhage (aSAH) is uncommon during pregnancy but, as in the non-pregnant patient, its consequences can be devastating. Approximately one-third of all affected patients lose their lives to this condition and another third live on with disability both physical and psychological. It is estimated to affect 0.01% to 0.05% (2–4) of all pregnancies and is one of the commoner causes of maternal death. It has been cited as the third most common cause of non-obstetric death and the eighth greatest cause of maternal death overall (5,6). The rates of maternal death vary widely in the literature from 30% to 83%. Fetal mortality has been quoted between 7% and 42% and is obviously affected by the stage to which the pregnancy has progressed (1,2,5–8).

Discovery of an Unruptured Cerebral Aneurysm

Pregnancy itself has been considered a risk factor for aneurysmal rupture, although this remains controversial. The Rochester study recorded no cases of subarachnoid haemorrhage in 26,099 live births over a 25-year period (9). This is important as high-quality neuroimaging has proliferated and clinically silent, unruptured aneurysms are discovered more frequently. The International Study of Unruptured Intracranial Aneurysms (10,11) suggested that the risk from small aneurysms of the anterior circulation was rather less than had been believed previously. When one considered the complications of treatment that were recorded in the same study, this has led to a

more conservative approach to incidental lesions by most authorities. Given the lack of high-quality evidence that pregnancy increases rupture rates, there seems no reason at present to treat incidental aneurysms presenting during pregnancy any differently to those in the rest of the population.

The Symptomatic Aneurysm

Cerebral aneurysms become symptomatic when they

1. rupture producing subarachnoid haemorrhage
2. cause symptoms by compression or irritation of adjacent structures.

Decision-making is simplified considerably when an aneurysm ruptures. Re-bleeding from a ruptured aneurysm is frequently fatal and securing the aneurysm is, in most cases, a neurosurgical emergency. Mortality from a second haemorrhage ranges from 50% to 70% and the greatest risk is in the first 24 hours after the initial rupture (12).

The management of symptoms by compression or irritation of adjacent structures is more variable and depends on the site. An oculomotor palsy may be caused by a posterior communicating aneurysm or superior cerebellar artery aneurysm because of their close anatomical relationship to the third cranial nerve. This sign may be considered a prelude to rupture of the aneurysm and should be managed as such. A patient presenting in this way should have the aneurysm secured as soon as practicable. Cavernous sinus syndromes resulting from intracavernous aneurysms are often not at high risk of rupture (9,10) and can be managed symptomatically except when very large aneurysms protrude into the subarachnoid space. Giant aneurysms, for example, of the basilar trunk, presenting with slowly progressive brainstem symptoms represent a difficult management problem even outside of pregnancy. Treatment needs to be individualised to the patient's circumstances but will often be appropriately deferred until completion of the pregnancy. The axiom 'keep it simple' is a useful touchstone and a management algorithm for any complex aneurysm is suggested in Figure 6c.1.

Timing of Repair

Securing a ruptured aneurysm as soon as possible significantly reduces mortality and morbidity from bleeding (12–16). There are proponents for *ultra early* repair as an emergency 'out-of-hours' procedure (13). The standard we adhere to is to secure the aneurysm as early as possible and within 48 hours of ictus. Delaying repair may result in fewer ischaemic events associated directly with surgery by selecting survivors to be treated when brain swelling has subsided and dysautoregulation has recovered, but does not serve the overall outcome and salvageable patients are lost to re-bleeding (13–17). Consequently,

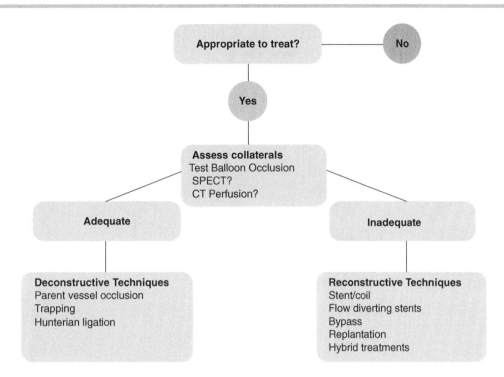

Figure 6c.1 An algorithm for the general management of complex aneurysms.

we delay only when faced with a complex aneurysm requiring more sophisticated reconstructive repairs.

Obstetric Considerations
If the mother presents in a state of depressed consciousness because of a life-threatening aneurysmal haematoma, this should be addressed as for any other patient. This will usually include securing the aneurysm during surgery. It is probably advisable to deliver a viable pregnancy as soon as possible so that the mother can be afforded the full range of critical care treatment without additional risk to the fetus. Similarly, if the mother presents with consciousness intact, already in labour with a viable pregnancy, then a caesarean section is usually recommended followed by definitive treatment of the aneurysm. If caesarean section is declined or were haemorrhage to occur during a spontaneous vaginal delivery, then epidural anaesthesia could be used to minimise the duration of the second stage and the haemodynamic or intracranial pressure effects of delivery. An algorithm for managing mother and viable pregnancy is offered in Figure 6c.2.

Mode of Repair
There has been a paradigm shift in the treatment of ruptured cerebral aneurysm since the International Subarachnoid Aneurysm Trial (ISAT) (18) and the majority of aneurysms are now secured endovascularly (Figure 6c.2). Endovascular repair has proven robust and safe (19) with suggested benefits on cognitive outcomes and epilepsy risk emerging (20,21). Not every aneurysm is best secured endovascularly however, so decisions are best made within an experienced multidisciplinary team that can offer surgical repair also (21,22). The development of stent-assisted coiling has increased the range of aneurysms which can be secured endovascularly but does require the patient to remain on anti-platelet and/or anti-thrombotic medication. Furthermore, it adds to the morbidity

of the treatment (23–25). However, comparable outcomes can be obtained with balloon-assisted techniques where any recurrence or residuum may be dealt with electively at a later date. This may be a preferable strategy for a critically ill patient as the need for anticoagulation is avoided or reduced.

Delayed Ischaemic Neurological Deficit and Vasospasm
Cerebral ischaemia will complicate the recovery of a significant number of patients with subarachnoid haemorrhage. In a U.K. audit of all neurosurgical units treating subarachnoid haemorrhage, 22% suffered a deterioration attributed to cerebral ischaemia (25). A significant proportion of these ischaemic episodes are contributed to by angiographic vasospasm defined as a transient narrowing of the intradural vasculature occurring after aSAH. Typically, the vessels begin to narrow around day 3 after haemorrhage and they are most severely affected by day 6 to 8. Vasospasm will resolve in the majority by day 14. Angiographic vasospasm may be observed in 30% to 43% of all subarachnoid haemorrhages during this interval (26–28).

The circulation is dysautoregulated during the vasospasm period and a more linear relationship between the arterial blood pressure and the cerebral perfusion pressure prevails than when autoregulation is functioning (27). The patient should be managed in an environment where the extracellular fluid volume may be carefully monitored and maintained in the normal range and thus support as constant a cerebral arterial perfusion pressure as possible. Prophylactic hypervolaemia is not beneficial and can contribute to morbidity and it should be remembered the pregnant patient will have a hyperdynamic circulation.

Presently, pharmacological prophylaxis of delayed ischaemic neurological deficit (DIND) relies on the administration of calcium channel blockers. The use of nimodipine 60 mg orally 4 hourly is supported by prospective, randomised,

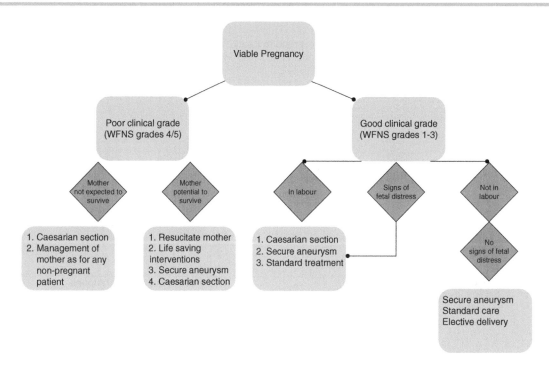

Figure 6c.2 Management of SAH where the pregnancy is viable.

Table 6c.1 World Federation of Neurological Surgeons SAH Grading System

WFNS grade	Glasgow Coma Scale	Motor deficit
0	15	Unruptured aneurysm
1	15	Absent
2	13–14	Absent
3	13–14	Present
4	7–12	Present or absent
5	3–6	Present or absent

controlled trials (28,29). It has been shown to reduce morbidity from ischaemia but does not abolish angiographic vasospasm. Nimodipine may be safely used during pregnancy and has been subject to clinical trial as a potential preventative treatment for eclampsia although without significant benefit (30). Although animal studies have suggested a potential teratogenic effect of calcium channel blockers, the magnitude of this effect is probably very small (31).

The recognition that magnesium sulphate was effective in reversing placental vasoconstriction prompted its examination as an agent to treat vasospasm and DIND after subarachnoid haemorrhage. Furthermore, hypomagnesaemia is associated with a poor outcome after subarachnoid haemorrhage (32,33). A clinical trial demonstrated a protective effect of magnesium therapy broadly comparable to the effect of nimodipine and with improved functional outcomes over placebo. Another trial failed to replicate the finding and larger

trials are ongoing to establish the place of magnesium replacement in the prevention and treatment of DIND as well as to determine what the appropriate dose should be (34,35).

Many other pharmacological treatments have been advanced to prevent or treat vasospasm and associated ischaemia. Clinical trials to date of endothelin receptor antagonists have not thus far proven safe or effective in human clinical trials (36). Statin therapy remains controversial and awaits the results of ongoing trials; as such these cannot be recommended therapy in a pregnant patient (37–42).

Vascular Malformations

Vascular malformations are classified according to their architecture and flow characteristics. Their risk of haemorrhage seems to vary accordingly. One such classification is as follows:

A. Arteriovenous shunts: Blood flows directly into the venous system from the arteries without passing through a capillary bed and/or supplying tissue with oxygen and nutrients.
   - *Arteriovenous malformations (AVM)* – characterised by the presence of a nidus of vessels at the centre.
   - *Cerebral arteriovenous fistulae*
   - *Dural arteriovenous fistulae*

B. No arteriovenous shunting:
   - *Capillary malformations (Telangiectasia)*
   - *Cavernous malformations*
   - *Mixed malformations*

Haemorrhage occurring in the context of an arteriovenous shunt poses the greater risk for early re-bleeding and consequent morbidity. Usually AVMs are thought to account for about 5% of all subarachnoid haemorrhage but in pregnancy they are associated with 21% to 48% of bleeds (45,46). Malformations are thought to bleed most commonly during the second or third trimesters, possibly affected by the maternal hyperdynamic circulation. Although early re-bleeding rates have been estimated as high as 27% during pregnancy, it is by no means clear that mother or baby always benefits from definitive treatment at this stage (47). AVMs are a heterogeneous collection of lesions with individual architectures. The ease by which they may be obliterated is affected by these characteristics making the generalisation of risk to a small population problematic.

Haemorrhage can occur from the nidus itself and aneurysms within it. There may be flow aneurysms on vessels associated with or remote from the nidus. When these aneurysms can be related to the radiological pattern of haemorrhage then it is reasonable to secure them in the same way that other cerebral aneurysms might in order to render the AVM 'safe'.

Ultimately, the only way to remove all risk of further haemorrhage is to abolish the arteriovenous shunt completely whether by division or embolisation of a fistula or by surgical excision of a nidus.

It is our practice where possible to attend to the immediately life-threatening consequences of an arteriovenous malformation first and leave definitive treatment until pregnancy has completed or terminated. This may mean endovascular or surgical treatment of aneurysms soon after rupture. Surgically significant haematomas may be removed and bleeding controlled without necessarily attempting complete extirpation of the nidus. This can be addressed later by further microsurgical, endovascular, stereotactic radiosurgical or multimodality means.

Stereotactic Radiosurgery
Stereotactic radiosurgery has become a mainstay of treatment of AVMs of the brain over the past 30 years. For the best results the target lesion needs to be carefully selected. Obliteration rates are affected by the volume of the malformation of the dose of radiations which can be safely delivered to the nidus. The treatment itself is very palatable to patients and it can be delivered on an outpatient basis. Various tools to deliver radiosurgery are available. Robotically guided delivery systems such as Cyberknife or Novalis do not even require placement of a stereotactic frame. Where a frame-based system such as Gamma Knife is preferred the frame can be applied under local anaesthetic with a minimum of discomfort. The details of the various platforms for delivery of stereotactic radiosurgery is beyond the scope of this chapter and the tool used for treatment will be in part be determined by local availability, clinician experience and the proposed target.

As stated above, it is our present practice to defer radiosurgical treatment of an arteriovenous malformation until a pregnancy had completed. The obliteration of the malformation takes place slowly and the time to obliteration is determined by

– the volume treated
– radiation dose

Three-dimensional stereotactic angiography and MRI allow the exact shape of the nidus to be described and planning of the treatment takes place on a computer workstation. It is planned so that the collimated beams of radiations result in delivery of the treatment dose only within the nidus of the lesion with a margin surrounding it of rapid drop-off in radiation dose sparing the adjacent nervous tissue in so far as is possible. The total volume of tissue which receives 12 Gy or more significantly affects the risk of side effects and so the volume that may be successfully treated is limited. The obliteration rate increases towards a dose of 25 Gy before radiation-related side effects reach unacceptable levels (48–50). It is tempting to believe the reduction in the volume of the nidus by partial endovascular embolisation would enable the safer treatment of larger-volume AVMs and success has been reported in otherwise untreatable lesions (51,52). However, partial embolisations are also well recognised to make accurate targeting of remaining nidus more difficult. It is presently our practice to confine endovascular treatment of AVMs to components of the lesions believed to pose an imminent threat of haemorrhage, for example, associated aneurysms (29,30). Fractionation of AVM treatment has also been used to treat larger lesions by targeting separate compartments within a lesion at intervals in hopes of mitigating the dose delivered to adjacent brain while ensuring a sufficiently high total dose to the nidus to obliterate it. This strategy does have a lower overall obliteration rate for these lesions and the exact dosing strategies are still developing (53,54).

The smallest lesions can disappear well within 2 years from the time of treatment. Larger lesions will take longer and gradual competed obliteration is observed up to 5 years after treatment. The definition of cure is abolition of arteriovenous shunting on a catheter angiogram. As this definition relies on a haemodynamic examination of the malformation it cannot be established by static imaging such as CT or MR. Patients planning a family and who have previously received treatment of any sort for a vascular malformation would ideally have a normal control angiogram prior to becoming pregnant.

Cavernomas during Pregnancy
Cavernomas are often reported to enlarge and haemorrhage more frequently during pregnancy, (55–57) although this does not appear to be under direct hormonal influence (58). Cavernomas present a different management conundrum. The risk of bleeding from a cavernoma is less than from a lesion with an arteriovenous shunt. Furthermore, large-volume catastrophic haemorrhage is unusual and good functional recovery from small-volume haemorrhages in the short term is the norm. Therefore we tend to prefer conservative management from these lesions and expect good outcomes.

Anaesthetic Considerations
These are also discussed in chapters 6a and 6b. Intervention following any intracerebral haemorrhage is either immediate to prevent death or disability, or urgent to prevent further bleeding. Life-saving interventions such as the insertion of a ventricular drainage catheter for acute hydrocephalus can be carried out under local anaesthesia or a brief general anaesthetic. In reality, patients whose consciousness is so impaired

as to require these treatments are already in need of ventilatory support. When more complex interventions are required, such as repair of an aneurysm, general anaesthesia is mandatory. Tight control of the patients' ventilation and cardiovascular system is maintained to minimise brain swelling and ensure adequate brain perfusion. Absolute stillness is a requirement of good microsurgical technique. This is also true of endovascular repair. Coiling of aneurysms has been carried out under local anaesthesia but most practitioners prefer the controlled conditions afforded by general anaesthesia (59).

Ventilation

Hyperventilation is generally avoided. Maternal resting $PaCO_2$ may be reduced over the non-pregnant baseline and the functional residual capacity (FRC) reduced by up to 20%. Resultant respiratory alkalosis will shift the oxygen dissociation curve to the left and could impair the release of oxygen to the fetus. Alkalosis may also produce vasoconstriction of the vessels in the placental circulation (60).

Arterial Hypotension

There is a temptation to manage intraoperative rupture of an aneurism by lowering the blood pressure while control of the bleeding is established. In reality it is not usually necessary in experienced hands and the risk of ischaemia occurring as a result of reduced blood flow outweighs the risk from blood loss. Turgor in the aneurysm can be reduced by the judicious use of temporary clipping of the parent vessels and without additional risk to the maternal-fetal circulation (32), although successful use of electively induced hypotension has been reported (33). Measures have been used to temporarily arrest the circulation so as to facilitate repair of particularly complex aneurysms. These include deep hypothermic cardiac arrest, adenosine induced arrest and high-flow vascular bypass. Such measures are only necessary with the most complex, high-risk lesions and the risk-benefit ratio will favour carrying them out once a pregnancy has completed or has been terminated.

Arterial hypotension may be a useful surgical adjunct when treating certain AVMs but as the definitive treatment of these lesions may be best as an elective procedure it is rarely necessary to expose the mother to the risk of arterial hypotension and the baby to the risk of fetal asphyxiation.

Positioning During Treatment

Positioning of neurosurgical patients for long, complex procedures is a challenge always and a lot of care is required in the set-up to protect cutaneous pressure areas, peripheral nerves and eyes. Aortocaval compression becomes an issue after approximately 20 weeks of pregnancy. The positioning of the patient is to a large extent determined by the pathology one is operating on. The majority of anterior and posterior circulation aneurysms can be operated on in the supine position. The effect of aortocaval compression may be minimised by judicious placement of pillows, gel padding and/or a left uterine displacement device (63–65). Table tilting will help further. Even with these precautions the maternal cardiac output can be reduced significantly, however, in the supine compared to the lateral position and so it is wise to consider the lateral position. It does not add to the difficulties of surgical dissection for most anterior circulation pathology. It is the position of choice for posterior circulation aneurysms and posterior fossa craniotomies. The prone position for cranial procedures can and should be avoided with a gravid uterus.

For endovascular repair of an aneurysm left lateral positioning may be more problematical and a supine position, with the modifications described above, is generally preferred for all aneurysms.

RADIATION SAFETY

The advent of effective endovascular therapies for cerebral aneurysms has inevitably resulted in an increase in exposure of the patient to ionising radiation. The bulk of a patients' exposure during their hospitalisation will be due to biplanar fluoroscopy while securing the aneurysm or diagnostic angiography (66).

The dose during repair of the aneurysm may range from <6 Gy to 12.8 Gy and morbidity relating to radiation exposure has been observed following aneurysm treatment, epilation (67–69) and skin erythema being the best known. There is little information yet on the long-term consequences of this exposure and it is far from certain it would outweigh the survival and disability benefits of endovascular repair of a ruptured aneurysm. From fertilisation to implantation (approximately day 15), the most likely result of any radiation exposure is embryonic death. The greatest concern about teratogenic effects arises during the organogenesis period from day 15 to day 50. After this, the most likely consequence is growth retardation of the fetus. It would seem prudent to counsel the patient about these risks as part of the consent process. There are many techniques to minimise intraprocedural exposure. Staff awareness and education are an important part. Lead shielding can be applied to protect the pelvis. Modern well-maintained equipment and software with effective shielding are mandatory. Magnification and exposure times can be minimised and collimators used to avoid scatter.

CONCLUSION

Vascular diseases pose a rare but significant risk of maternal and fetal mortality. aSAH in the case of a mother in salvageable condition and with a viable pregnancy may require the aneurysm be secured by endovascular or surgical means. This should usually be done as soon as possible to minimise mortality from re-bleeding. The urgency of delivery of the baby will also help determine the sequence of events. AVMs which have bled will often be definitively treated once the pregnancy is complete. Blood clots and hydrocephalus from either condition are managed according to their effects and similarly to any other clinical context.

REFERENCES

1. Cantwell R, Clutton-Brock T, Cooper G, et al. Saving mothers' lives: reviewing maternal deaths to make motherhood safer: 2006-2008. The Eighth Report of the Confidential Enquiries into Maternal Deaths in the United Kingdom. BJOG 2011; 118 (suppl 1):1–203.
2. Dias MS, Sekhar LN. Intracranial haemorrhage from aneurysms and arteriovenous malformations during pregnancy and the puerperium. Neurosurgery 1990; 27:855–865.
3. Cannell DE, Bottrell EH. Subarachnoid haemorrhage and pregnancy. Am J Obstet Gynecol 1956; 72:844–855.

4. Copeland EL, Mahon RF. Spontaneous intacranial bleeding in pregnancy. Obstet Gynecol 1967; 20:373–378.

5. Crawford S, Varner MW, Digre KB, et al. Cranial magnetic resonance imaging in eclampsia. Obstet Gynecol 1987; 70:474–477.

6. Drife J, Lewis G, eds. Why Mothers Die, 1997–1998. The Fifth Report from the Confidential Enquiries into Maternal Death in the United Kingdom. London: RCOG Press, 2001.

7. Barno A, Freeman DW. Maternal deaths due to spontaneous subarachnoid haemorrhage. Am J Obstet Gynecol 1967; 125: 384–392.

8. Robinson JL, Hall CJ, Sedzimir CB. Subarachnoid haemorrhage in pregnancy. J Neurosurg 1972; 36:27–33.

9. Wiebers DO, Whisnant JP. The incidence of stroke amongst amongst pregnant women in Rochester, Minn, 1955 through 1979. JAMA 1985; 254:3055–3057.

10. Investigators. The International Study of Unruptured Intracranial Aneurysms. Unruptured intracranial aneurysms—risk of rupture and risks of surgical intervention. N Engl J Med 1998; 339: 1725–1733.

11. Wiebers DO, Whisnant JP, Huston III J, et al. Unruptured intracranial aneurysms: natural history, clinical outcome and risks of surgical and endovascular treatment. Lancet 2003; 362:103–119.

12. Kassell NF, Torner JC. Aneurysmal rebleeding: a preliminary report from the co-operative aneurysm study. Neurosurgery 1983; 13:479–481.

13. Laidlaw JD, Siu KH. Ultra-early surgery for aneurysmal subarachnoid hemorrhage: outcomes for a consecutive series of 391 patients not selected by grade or age. J Neurosurg 2002; 97(2):250–258; discussion 247–249.

14. Sundt TM, Kobayashi S, Fode NC, et al. Results and complications of surgical management of 809 intracranial aneurysms in 722 cases. Related and unrelated to grade of patient, type of aneurysm, and timing of surgery. J Neurosurg 1982; 56(6):753–765.

15. Miyaoka M, Sato K, Ishii S. A clinical study of the relationship of timing to outcome of surgery for ruptured cerebral aneurysms. A retrospective analysis of 1622 cases. J Neurosurg 1993; 79(3):373–378.

16. Whitfield PC, Kirkpatrick PJ. Timing of surgery for aneurysmal subarachnoid haemorrhage. Cochrane Database Syst Rev 2001; 62(2):CD001697.

17. Ross N, Hutchinson P, Seeley H, et al. Timing of surgery for supratentorial aneurysmal subarachnoid haemorrhage: report of a prospective study. J Neurol Neurosurg Psychiatry 2002; 72(4):480–484.

18. Molyneux AJ, Kerr RSC, Yu L-M, et al. International subarachnoid aneurysm trial (ISAT) of neurosurgical clipping versus endovascular coiling in 2143 patients with ruptured intracranial aneurysms: a randomised comparison of effects on survival, dependency, seizures, rebleeding, subgroups, and aneurysm occlusion. Lancet 2002; 366:809–817.

19. Molyneux AJ, Kerr RS, Birks J, et al. Risk of recurrent subarachnoid haemorrhage, death, or dependence and standardised mortality ratios after clipping or coiling of an intracranial aneurysm in the International Subarachnoid Aneurysm Trial (ISAT): long-term follow-up. Lancet 2009; 8(5):427–433.

20. Scott RB, Eccles F, Molyneux AJ, et al. Improved cognitive outcomes with endovascular coiling of ruptured intracranial aneurysms: neuropsychological outcomes from the International Subarachnoid Aneurysm Trial (ISAT). Stroke 1743–1747; [Epub 8 Jul 2010].

21. Raper DMS, Allan R. International subarachnoid trial in the long run: critical evaluation of the long-term follow-up data from the ISAT trial of clipping vs coiling for ruptured intracranial aneurysms. Neurosurgery 2010; 66(6):1166–1169.

22. Society of British Neurological Surgeons and British Society of Neuroradiology. Consensus Conference on Neurovascular Services, 2004.

23. Piotin M, Blanc R, Spelle L, et al. Stent-assisted coiling of intracranial aneurysms: clinical and angiographic results in 216 consecutive aneurysms. Stroke 2010; 41(1):110–115.

24. Van Rooij WJ, Sluzewski M, Beute GN, et al. Procedural complications of coiling of ruptured intracranial aneurysms: incidence and risk factors in a consecutive series of 681 patients. AJNR Am J Neuroradiol 2006; 27(7):1498–1501.

25. Lubicz B, Lefranc F, Bruneau M, et al. Balloon-assisted coiling of intracranial aneurysms is not associated with a higher complication rate. Neuroradiology 2008; 50(9):769–776.

26. Society of British Neurological Surgeons, The British Society of Neuroradiologists Clinical Effectiveness Unit, The Royal College of Surgeons of England. National Study of Subarachnoid Haemorrhage: Final Report of an Audit carried out in 34 Neurosurgical Units in the UK and Ireland between 14 September 2001 to 13 September 2002.

27. Weir B, Grace M, Hansen J, et al. Time course of vasospasm in man. J Neurosurg 1978; 48:173.

28. Petruk KC, West M, Mohr G, et al. Nimodipine treatment in poor grade aneurysm patients. Results of a multicentre double blind placebo controlled Trial. J Neurosurg 1988; 68:505.

29. Pickard JD, Murray GD, Illingworth R, et al. Effect of oral nimdipine on cerebral infarction and outcome after subarachnoid haemorrhage: British Aneurysm Nimodipine Trial. BMJ 1989; 298:636.

30. Belfort MA, Anthony J, Saade GR, et al. Nimodipine Study Group. A comparison of magnesium sulfate and nimodipine for the prevention of eclampsia. N Engl J Med 2003; 348(4):304–311.

31. Magee LA, Schick B, Donnenfeld AE, et al. The safety of calcium channel blockers in human pregnancy: a prospective, multicenter cohort study. Am J Obstet Gynecol 1996; 174(3):823–828.

32. Van den Bergh WM, Algra A, Van Der Sprenkel JW, et al. Hypomagnesemia after aneurysmal subarachnoid haemorrhage. Neurosurgery 2003; 52:276–281.

33. Marinov MB, Harbaugh KS, Hoopes PJ, et al. Neuroprotective effects of pre-ischaemia intra-arterial magnesium sulphate in reversible focal cerebral ischaemia. J Neurosurg 1996; 85:117–124.

34. van den Bergh WM, Algra A, van Kooten F, et al. Magnesium sulfate in aneurysmal subarachnoid hemorrhage: a randomized controlled trial. Stroke 2005; 36:1011–1015.

35. Wong GK, Chan MT, Boet R, et al. Intravenous magnesium sulfate after aneurysmal subarachnoid hemorrhage: a prospective randomized pilot study. J Neurosurg Anesthesiol 2006; 18: 142–148.

36. Macdonald RL, Higashida RT, Keller E, et al. Clazosentan, an endothelin receptor antagonist, in patients with aneurysmal subarachnoid haemorrhage undergoing surgical clipping: a randomised, double-blind, placebo-controlled phase 3 trial (CONSCIOUS-2). Lancet Neurol 2011; 10(7):618–625; [Epub 2 Jun 2011].

37. Tseng MY, Hutchinson PJ, Czosnyka M, et al. Effects of acute pravastatin treatment on intensity of rescue therapy, length of inpatient stay, and 6-month outcome in patients after aneurysmal subarachnoid hemorrhage. Stroke 2007; 38:1545–1550.

38. Chou SH, Smith EE, Badjatia N, et al. A randomized, double-blind, placebo-controlled pilot study of simvastatin in aneurysmal subarachnoid hemorrhage. Stroke 2008; 39:2891–2893.

39. Vergouwen MD, Meijers JC, Geskus RB, et al. Biologic effects of simvastatin in patients with aneurysmal subarachnoid hemorrhage: a double-blind, placebo-controlled randomized trial. J Cereb Blood Flow Metab 2009; 29:1444–1453.

40. Vergouwen MD, de Haan RJ, Vermeulen M, et al. Effect of statin treatment on vasospasm, delayed cerebral ischemia, and functional outcome in patients with aneurysmal subarachnoid hemorrhage: a systematic review and meta-analysis update. Stroke 2010; 41:e47–e52.

41. Kern M, Lam MM, Knuckey NW, et al. Statins may not protect against vasospasm in subarachnoid haemorrhage. J Clin Neurosci 2009; 16:527–530.

42. Bleck TP. Statin use was not associated with less vasospasm or improved outcome after subarachnoid hemorrhage. Neurosurgery 2008; 62:422–427.

43. Dorsch NWC, King MT. A review of cerebral vasospasm in aneurysmal subarachnoid haemorrhage. J Clin Neurosci 1994; 1:19.

44. Kassell N, Torner J, Haley E, et al. The International Cooperative Study on the Timing of Aneurysm Surgery. Part 1: Overall management results. J Neurosurg 1990; 73:18–36.

45. Robinson JL, Hall CJ, Sedzimir CB. Arteriovenous malformations, aneurysms and pregnancy. J Neurosurg 1974; 41:63–70.

46. Lanzino G, Jensen ME, Cappelletto B, et al. Arteriovenous malformations that rupture during pregnancy: a management dilemma. Acta Neurochir 1994; 126(2–4):102–106.

47. Horton J, Chambers W, Lyons S, et al. Pregnancy and the risk of haemorrhage from cerebral arteriovenous malformations. Neurosurgery 1990; 27:867–872.

48. Flickinger JC, Kondziolka D, Maitz AH, et al. Analysis of neurological sequelae from radiosurgery of arteriovenous malformations: how location affects outcome. Int J Radiat Oncol Biol Phys 1998; 40(2)273–278.

49. Karlsson B, Lindquist C, Steiner L. Prediction of obliteration after gamma knife surgery for arteriovenous malformations. Neurosurgery 1997; 40(3):425–430.

50. Zipfel GJ, Bradshaw P, Bova FJ, et al. Do the morphological characteristics of arteriovenous malformations affect the results of radiosurgery? J Neurosurg 2004; 101(3):393–401.

51. Duffner F, Freudenstein D, Becker G, et al. Combined treatment effects after embolisation and radiosurgery in high-grade arteriovenous malformations. Case report and review of the literature. Stereotact Funct Neurosurg 2000; 75(1):27–34.

52. Gobin YP, Laurent A, Merienne L, et al. Treatment of brain arteriovenous malformations by embolisation and radiosurgery. J Neurosurg 1996; 85(1):19–28.

53. Kubo HD, Wilder RB, Pappas CT, et al. Two-staged radiosurgical treatment of large arteriovenous malformations. J Radiosurg 2000; 3(3):105–111.

54. Pendl G, Unger F, Papaefthymiou G, et al. Staged radiosurgical treatment for large benign cerebral lesions. J Neurosurg 2000; 93 (suppl 3):107–112.

55. Sawin PD. Spontaneous subarachnoid haemorrhage in pregnancy. In: Loftus CM, ed. Neurosurgical Aspects of Pregnancy. 1st ed. Park Ridge: American Association of Neurological Surgeons, 1996:85–100.

56. Pozzati E, Acciarri N, Tognetti F, et al. Growth, subsequent bleeding, and de novo appearance of cerebral cavernous angiomas. Neurosurgery 1996; 38(4):662–669.

57. Safavi-Abbasi S, Feiz-Erfan I, Spetzler RF, et al. Hemorrhage of cavernous malformations during pregnancy and in the peripartum period: causal or coincidence? Case report and review of the literature. Neurosurg Focus 2006; 21:1 e12.

58. Kaya AH, Ulus A, Bayri Y, et al. There are no estrogen and progesterone receptors in cerebral cavernomas: a preliminary immunohistochemical study. Surg Neurol 2009; 72(3):263–265.

59. Ogilvy CS, Yang X, Jamil OA, et al. Neurointerventional procedures for unruptured intracranial aneurysms under procedural sedation and local anesthesia: a large-volume, single-center experience. J Neurosurg 2011; 114(1):120–128.

60. Levinson G, Shrider SM, de Lorimer NA, et al. Effect of maternal hyperventilation on uterine blood flow and fetal oxygenation and acid base status. Anaesthesiology 1974; 40:340–347.

61. Giannotta SL, Oppenheimer JH, Levy ML, et al. Management of intraoperative rupture of aneurysm without hypotension. Neurosurgery 1991; 28(4):531–535; discussion 535–536.

62. Maissin F, Mesz M, Roualdès G, et al. Hypotension induced by isoflurane for the treatment of intracranial aneurysm in late pregnancy. Ann Fr Anesth Reanim 1987; 6(5):453–456.

63. Bieniarz J, Yoshida T, Romero-Salinas G, et al. Aortocaval compression by the uterus in late human pregnancy. IV. Circulatory homeostasis by preferential perfusion of the placenta. Am J Obstet Gynecol 1969; 103(1):19–31.

64. Goodwin AP, Pearce AJ. The human wedge. A manoeuvre to relieve aortocaval compression during resuscitation in late pregnancy. Anaesthesia 1992; 47(5):433–434.

65. Milsom I, Forssman L. Factors influencing aortocaval compression in late pregnancy. Am J Obstet Gynecol 1984; 148(6):764–771.

66. Moskowitz SI, Davros WJ, Kelly ME, et al. Cumulative radiation dose during hospitalization for aneurysmal subarachnoid hemorrhage. AJNR Am J Neuroradiol 2010; 31(8):1377–1382.

67. Huda W, Peters KR. Radiation-induced temporary epilation after a neuroradiologically guided embolization procedure. Radiology 1994; 193(3):642–644.

68. D'incan M, Roger H, Gabrillargues J, et al. Radiation-induced temporary hair loss after endovascular embolization of the cerebral arteries: six cases. Annales de dermatologie et de venereologie, 2002; 129(5 pt 1):703–706.

69. Tosti A, Piraccini BM, Alagna G. Temporary hair loss simulating alopecia areata after endovascular surgery of cerebral arteriovenous malformations: a report of 3 cases. Arch Dermatol 1999; 135(12):1555–1556.

Analgesia and anaesthesia in neurological disease and pregnancy

Jayaram K. Dasan

INTRODUCTION

The choice of analgesia methods for pregnant women with neurological disease must be based on a wide knowledge of pathophysiology and the state of the disease in question. Historically, the use of regional techniques in patients with pre-existing neurological diseases has been considered relatively contraindicated. The fear of worsening neurological outcome secondary to mechanical trauma, local anaesthetic toxicity or neural ischaemia are all common concerns. A retrospective review from Mayo Clinic (1) investigated 139 patients during a period of 12 years with a history of neurological disease who subsequently received neuraxial anaesthesia or analgesia. A satisfactory block was reported in 98% of patients. No new or worsening post-operative neurological deficit occurred when compared to pre-operative findings. The conclusion was the risk commonly associated with neuraxial anaesthesia or analgesia in patients with pre-existing neurological disease may not be as frequent as once was thought. However, post-partum published data on this area are limited. A few disorders contraindicate the use of regional anaesthesia. Early anaesthesia consultation should allow accurate assessment of the extent and pattern of the disease and formulation of the analgesia plan. Neurological disease complicating pregnancies require highly individualised care to balance complex medical conditions and their specific presentations during pregnancy. Consultation with obstetricians and anaesthetists is important to optimise the management of these patients.

MYOTONIC DISORDERS

These are autosomal-dominant degenerative diseases, including myotonia congenita, myotonic dystrophy and a rare paramyotonia congenita. Skeletal muscles are generally involved characterised by weakness and wasting. Smooth muscles can also be affected. Delayed muscle relaxation following contraction is characteristic of myotonia; a defect in membrane chloride permeability may be the responsible mechanism. Myotonic dystrophy is most common and most severe of these syndromes.

Anaesthetic management should include initial estimation of pulmonary function and electrocardiogram (ECG) to determine the potential for restrictive lung disease and cardiac arrhythmias. Holter monitoring and baseline blood gas may prove useful in some cases. For analgesia in labour, opioids and sedatives should be used with caution. All central nervous system (CNS) depressants including inhalational induction agents and diazepam have been associated with apnoea in these women with this condition (2). Regional analgesia and anaesthesia including epidural, spinal and pudendal block avoid the risk of respiratory depression. Keeping the patient warm reduces the risk of a myotonic crisis (3). If general anaesthesia is required, it should be given with great caution as patients may be extremely sensitive to induction agents. Use of depolarising muscle relaxants in a patient with myotonic dystrophy is extremely dangerous and should be avoided. Marked generalised skeletal muscle contracture, proportional to the dose of these muscle relaxants, can develop and may lead to great difficulty in ventilating the patient (4). The chance and extent of this adverse response are unpredictable. The response of these pregnant women with myotonia to non-depolarising muscle relaxants appears normal. Generalised contractures may result from mechanical and electrical stimulation. Neither regional anaesthesia nor non-depolarising relaxants prevent myotonic spasms. However, muscle in myotonic spasm will relax when injected with a local anaesthetic.

In summary, patients with myotonic syndromes often present with significant multi-system diseases having variable effects on pregnancy. For labour and delivery, regional anaesthesia may avoid many of the risks of general anaesthesia (5). Neuromuscular monitoring should be used to assess degree of muscle recovery.

NEUROFIBROMATOSIS

The disease is autosomal dominant and occurs 1 in 3000 births. The associated tumours may involve nerve roots or blood vessels and arise in or around most organs and body cavities. Occasionally, they produce serious problems, such as intracranial tumours or a compromised airway, the latter developing particularly if they are within the mediastinum or neck and cervical region (6). Initial evaluation including a careful history is paramount. A history of labile hypertension might be indicative of endocrine disorders such as pheochromocytoma which is associated with neurofibromatosis. Cardiac lesions such as pulmonary stenosis and coarctation of aorta also have been reported in these patients, as have spontaneous haemothorax and rupture of renal artery aneurysms. There are several reports of abnormal responses to muscle relaxants, including prolonged response to non-depolarising muscle relaxants and resistance to suxamethonium, in patients with neurofibromatosis (7–9). Given the diversity of clinical response, administering the minimal effective dose of muscle relaxants and monitoring neuromuscular blockade are recommended. The anaesthetist must also examine the airway for evidence of laryngeal or neck involvement, which would make intubation difficult. Regional anaesthesia is perfectly acceptable, but before performing an epidural block, all efforts should be made to exclude the presence of paraspinal tumours. Epidural analgesia in labour has been successful, but careful selection of cases has been suggested to avoid epidural in those women with spinal cord tumours.

LANDRY–GUILLAIN–BARRE SYNDROME

The overall incidence rate of Guillain–Barre syndrome (GBS) is less frequent during pregnancy, but the risk of GBS increases for the mother during the post-partum period (10). GBS in pregnant woman may worsen after delivery even if no epidural is administered for labour pain. There are no established guidelines for the analgesic management of the GBS parturient. GBS occurring in pregnancy is associated with an increased need for ventilatory support and an increase in maternal mortality.

The syndrome is an acute inflammatory, demyelinating disease with axonal degeneration of the peripheral nerves. Anaesthetic management for patients with GBS is controversial. If general anaesthesia is required, these patients are similar to any patients with generalised weakness and disability. Succinylcholine should not be used because of excessive release of potassium, which can cause cardiac systole. These patients may also be sensitive to non-depolarising muscle relaxants. In some cases, the need to support ventilation post-operatively should be anticipated. If intravenous analgesia is considered opioids should be used with care for patients with bulbar involvement. Autonomic nerve system dysfunction may occur with wide fluctuations in heart rate and blood pressure. Serial measurement of pulmonary dysfunction may be necessary during labour and delivery. The use of regional anaesthesia is controversial. A regional anaesthetic may be beneficial because an exaggerated haemodynamic response to labour pain can occur. Successful use of an epidural has been reported for labour analgesia and caesarean delivery with no complications (11,12). No established case of GBS relapse related to the regional anaesthesia has been reported. If caesarean delivery is indicated for patients with severe bulbar involvement, a general anaesthesia is more appropriate than regional analgesia as there is a fair potential for respiratory compromise.

SPINAL CORD INJURY

Patient disability and residual function depend on the anatomic location of the injury (13). Patients with lesion above T6 spinal segment have varying degree of respiratory compromise and are at risk of autonomic hyperreflexia. Autonomic hyperreflexia is a life-threatening complication that results from the absence of central inhibition on the sympathetic neurons in the cord below the injury. Administration of regional anaesthesia is the most common method for the prevention or treatment of autonomic hyperreflexia during labour and delivery. Spinal anaesthesia has been shown to effectively control blood pressure in paraplegic patients undergoing general surgical procedures (14–16).

MULTIPLE SCLEROSIS

Multiple sclerosis is a major cause of neurological disability in young adults. The anaesthetist should assess patient's degree of compromise, document the pattern of deficits and pay special attention to respiratory involvement. Historically there has been a great controversy regarding the administration of anaesthesia in patients with multiple sclerosis. Most anaesthetists have considered general anaesthesia to be safe, although published data are limited (17,18). Many anaesthetists have been reluctant to administer spinal or epidural anaesthesia because the effect of local anaesthetic drugs on the course of the disease is unclear. Some worried that spinal or epidural anaesthesia may expose demyelinated areas of the spinal cord to the potential neurotoxic effect of local anaesthetic agents. There are few published data regarding the use of epidural anaesthesia in patients with multiple sclerosis. Crawford et al. reported only one post-operative relapse in 50 non-obstetric and 7 obstetric patients who received epidural anaesthesia. Confavreux et al. (19) reported a study of 269 pregnancies in 254 women with multiple sclerosis, of whom 42 received epidural analgesia. They noted that epidural anaesthesia did not have an adverse effect on the rate of relapse or on the progression of the disability in these patients. Another retrospective study (20) of 32 pregnancies in women with multiple sclerosis found that women who received epidural analgesia during vaginal delivery did not have a higher incidence of relapse than those who received only local infiltration. Among the five patients who underwent caesarean delivery, one had a post-partum relapse. The authors suggested that the concentration of local anaesthetic used for epidural anaesthesia may influence the relapse rate because all patients in the relapse group had received higher concentration of bupivacaine or lignocaine (38).

The concentration of local anaesthetic in the cerebrospinal fluid (CSF) progressively increases during prolonged administration of epidural anaesthesia. The increased concentration may overwhelm the protective effect of dilution within the CSF. These observations suggest that anaesthetists should use dilute solutions of local anaesthetic for epidural analgesia during labour. Administration of anaesthesia during caesarean section is more problematic. However, given the limited duration of surgery, multiple doses of local anaesthetics are not needed, and CSF concentration should not increase over time. In summary, either spinal or epidural anaesthesia may be administered for caesarean delivery in patients with multiple sclerosis and published data suggest that regional anaesthesia may be safely used for labour and delivery. The patient should be aware that there is a high incidence of relapse during post-partum period, regardless of the type of anaesthesia used.

MYASTHENIA GRAVIS

Myasthenia gravis is an autoimmune disorder characterised by episodes of muscle weakness that are made worse by activity. Patients with myasthenia gravis should undergo consultation with an anaesthetist in early pregnancy. This assessment should include an estimation of the degree of bulbar and respiratory involvement. Pulmonary function tests should be performed should there any significant respiratory involvement. These patients may be susceptible to respiratory depression associated with opioids. Regional anaesthesia allows prevention of respiratory depression associated with opioids, and is the preferred method of analgesia during labour (21,22). Plasma cholinesterase activity is decreased in patients taking an anticholinesterase drugs. Ester local anaesthetic drugs like procaine may have a prolonged half-life, and patients may be at risk of local anaesthetic toxicity. Therefore, an amide local anaesthetic agent like bupivacaine should be given for epidural anaesthesia. D'Angelo and Gerancher (22) reported the administration of combined spinal-epidural (CSE) analgesia for labour and spontaneous vaginal delivery in a patient with severe myasthenia gravis. The CSE technique offers the advantage of effective analgesia with minimal motor block, but intrathecal opioid component is associated with some risk of respiratory depression. For caesarean section regional anaesthesia is the preferred method of anaesthesia unless complicated by severe bulbar involvement. Muscle relaxants have an unpredictable effect in these patients. It is worth including a list of drugs and supplements that are contraindicated in the hand-held notes of a pregnant woman with myasthenia gravis.

EPILEPSY

Epilepsy in pregnant women, usually starting in childhood or early life, is the commonest cause of seizures in pregnancy, affecting 1 in 200 women. Diagnostic confusion can occur with eclampsia, which is the most common cause of seizure during the peripartum period. Both can be confused with other conditions such as syncope, migraine, metabolic and cerebral disorders. Epilepsy was responsible for 10% to 15% of the indirect cause of maternal death in the U.K. Confidential Enquiry in Maternal Deaths reports during the period 1997 to 2006 (23). Interaction among anaesthetic drugs and anti-epileptic drugs takes many forms. Phenytoin and other hepatic microsomal enzymes inducing AEDs will enhance the breakdown of opioids, neuromuscular blocking drugs and volatile anaesthetic agents. In turn, this affects drug dosing and production of toxic metabolites. Some anaesthetic agents are epileptogenic particularly in presence of hypocapnia. Pethidine and its metabolite norpethidine with its long half-life can cause CNS excitability. Propofol has been implicated in epileptogenesis, with myoclonic activity and opisthotonus. However, propofol effectively stops seizures in humans and animals (24) and seizure time is shortened when compared to methohexital for electroconvulsive therapy. Low serum concentrations of amide local anaesthetics are anticonvulsant, but at high serum concentrations they cause convulsions. The action of non-depolarising neuromuscular blockers may be enhanced by concomitant use of anticonvulsants. Anaesthetists must also be aware of the side effects of anti-epileptic drugs. Communication between anaesthetist, obstetrician and neurologist is important. Provision of effective labour analgesia to reduce anxiety and hyperventilation are the goals anaesthetic care. Anaesthetic evaluation should include an assessment of seizure control, side effects of therapy, the patient's mental and physical status and proposed obstetric management. Parenteral opioid analgesia can be used with a dose modification to prevent worsening CNS depression in the parturient using anticonvulsants. However, epidural analgesia provides superior pain relief and does not depress the CNS. Patients with evidence of bleeding diathesis require coagulation assessment prior to regional analgesia. Low-dose epidural analgesia for labour pain and slow incremental to up for caesarean section would avoid high plasma concentrations of local anaesthetic, which are epileptogenic. Choice of general or regional anaesthesia for operative delivery is determined by a combination of maternal, fetal and obstetric factors. Post-ictal and drug-induced somnolence and status epilepticus mandate general anaesthesia. Regional anaesthesia is appropriate for elective caesarean section. Potential local anaesthetic toxicity should be kept in mind. There is no contraindication to the administration of regional anaesthesia in patients with epilepsy. In a review of 100 epileptic parturients, 19 received general anaesthesia, 48 received spinal anaesthesia, 21 received epidural or caudal anaesthesia and 12 received pudendal block (25). Of the five patients who had a post-partum seizure, four had received spinal anaesthesia and one had received general anaesthesia. No seizure occurred in patients who received epidural or caudal anaesthesia. Transcutaneous electrical nerve stimulation (TENS) is not contraindicated in women with epilepsy.

BRAIN NEOPLASMS

The anaesthetic management is guided by the presence or absence of symptoms and signs of elevated blood pressure and intracranial pressure (ICP). Pain during labour and pushing can increase ICP, while good pain control by regional analgesia helps to minimise any fluctuations. This analgesic effect has to be balanced against the risk of brainstem herniation following an inadvertent dural puncture. Epidural injection of local anaesthetics increases epidural space pressure, possibly causing a worsening of symptoms. Vadhera (26) described exacerbation of CNS symptoms, dizziness, paraesthesia in both hands, and transient rigid immobility, after an epidural in a parturient with an unknown large cerebello-pontine angle tumour and obstructive hydrocephalus. For caesarean section in a parturient with raised ICP, pre-induction measurement and control of ICP and blood pressure is mandatory. An arterial line and ventriculostomy with an ICP pressure transducer assist in controlling the response to tracheal intubation, as therapy can be titrated to maintain homoeostasis. Neurosurgical intervention at the time of caesarean section may be considered in some cases.

The choice of anaesthesia for labour and vaginal delivery is controversial in patients with brain neoplasm. Epidural analgesia prevents increase in ICP that can result with pushing during second stage of labour (27). However, there is concern that unintentional dural puncture might result in herniation in women with increased ICP. There are several published reports of successful use of epidural analgesia in labour and vaginal delivery in women with intracranial neoplasms (27–29).

SUBARACHNOID HAEMORRHAGE

If the parturient has undergone surgical repair of either an aneurysm or an arteriovenous malformation, analgesic and anaesthetic management need not differ from that of other obstetric patients. Those with untreated lesions should be managed to maintain haemodynamic stability and avoid hypertension. Regional anaesthesia is generally preferred (30,31). If vaginal delivery is planned, epidural or CSE anaesthesia should be considered. For caesarean delivery, either epidural or spinal can be used. Some anaesthetists consider that epidural anaesthesia provides greater haemodynamic stability and is thus preferred for operative delivery (31).

BENIGN INTRACRANIAL HYPERTENSION

Benign intracranial hypertension is defined as an increase in ICP without a demonstrable aetiology. Symptoms of benign intracranial hypertension worsen during pregnancy in 50% of cases (32). Surgical management with shunt placement has resulted in clinical improvement and normal pregnancy outcome in women with severe symptoms (33). Deliberate lumbar puncture represents a common form of treatment for this disorder. Cerebellar tonsillar herniation does not occur because of the uniform, global increase in ICP. Paruchuri et al. (34) noted that there are only two reported cases of cerebellar tonsillar herniation after diagnostic lumbar puncture in patients with this disorder. Both patients had presented with severe headache, neck pain exacerbated with movement. In the absence of these signs and symptoms, anaesthetists can safely give regional anaesthesia for labour and delivery (35). Some anaesthetists recommend the administration of general anaesthesia for caesarean section for patients with lumboperitoneal shunt (35). They postulate that local anaesthetic agent that reaches the subarachnoid space may escape in to the peritoneum, and that therefore it will be difficult to achieve adequate anaesthesia. Moreover, the performance of regional anaesthesia may result in trauma to the shunt catheter. However, Bedard et al. (36) reported the successful administration of epidural anaesthesia in a pre-eclamptic patient with a lumboperitoneal shunt for the treatment of benign intracranial hypertension. Epidural anaesthesia also has been used successfully in patients with ventriculoperitoneal and ventriculoatrial shunts (37,38).

ARNOLD–CHIARI MALFORMATION

Many women diagnosed with Chiari malformation are concerned about whether they can safely have children. Increased CSF pressure during labour and delivery is a concern. Research is limited but several case studies have been published demonstrating that labour and delivery can be successful for women with Chiari malformation. In a case series of seven women with Chiari during pregnancy (39), labour and delivery, there were only minor symptom changes during pregnancy. There was no significant worsening of symptoms either during or after labour. There were no complications due to epidural anaesthesia.

CONCLUSION

Lack of uniform anaesthetic guidelines for pregnant patients with neurological disease such as multiple sclerosis, myasthenia gravis, epilepsy, spinal cord injury and subarachnoid haemorrhage means that the decision whether or not to administer regional anaesthesia should be based on an individual case-by-case basis. However, few of these neurological diseases contraindicate the use of neuraxial anaesthesia. The successful management of the pregnant patient with neurological disorder depends on the cooperative efforts of the obstetrician, the neurologist and the anaesthetist involved in peripartum care. A comprehensive understanding of physiology of pregnancy and pathophysiology of underlying neurological disease is of primary importance in the analgesic and anaesthetic management of these women.

REFERENCES

1. Hebl HR, Horlocker TT. Neuraxial blockade. Anesth Analg 2010; 111(6):1511–1519.
2. Ravin M, Newmark Z. Myotonia dystrophia. Anesth Analg 1975; 54:261–268.
3. Camann WR, Johnson MD. Anesthetic management of a parturient with myotonia dystrophica. Reg Anesth 1990; 15:41–43.
4. Paterson IS. Generalised myotonia following suxamethonium. Br J Anaesth 1962; 34:340–342.
5. Campbell AN, Thompson N. Anaesthesia for caesarean section in a patient with myotonic dystrophy. Can J Anaesth 1995; 42:409–414.
6. Holt GR. ENT manifestations of Von Reclinghausen's disease. Laryngoscope 1978; 88:1617–1632.
7. Baraka A. Myasthenia response to muscle relaxants in Von Reclinghausen's disease. Br J Anaesth 1974; 46:701–703.
8. Mittershciffthaler G, Maurhard U. Prolonged action of vecuronium in neurofibromatosis. Anaesthesiol Reanim 1989; 14:175–178.
9. Naguib M, Al-Rajeh SM. The response of a patient with Von Reclinghausen's disease to succinylcholine and atracurium. Middle East J Anesthesiol 1988; 9:429–434.
10. Rockel A, Wissel J, Rolfs A. Guillain-Barre' syndrome in pregnancy. J Perinat Med 1994; 122:393–399.
11. Crawford JS, James FM, Nolte H. Regional analgesia for patients with chronic neurologic disease. Anaesthesia 1981; 36:821.
12. McGrady EM. Management of labour in patient with Guillain-Barre'syndrome. Anaesthesia 1987; 42:899.
13. Donaldson JO. Neurology of Pregnancy. 2nd ed. London: WB Saunders, 1989:11.
14. Lambert DH, Deane RS, Mazuzan JE. Anaesthesia and the control of blood pressure in patients with spinal cord injury. Anesth Analg 1982; 61:344–348.
15. Ciliberti PJ, Goldfein J, Rovenstine EA. Hypertension during anaesthesia in patients with spinal cord injuries. Anesthesiology 1954; 15:273–279.
16. Thorn-Alquist AM. Prevention of hypertensive crisis in patients with high spinal lesions during cystoscopy and lithotripsy. Acta Anaethesiol Scan (suppl) 1975; 57:79–82.
17. Baskett PJ, Armstrong, R. Anaesthetic problems in multiple sclerosis. Anaesthesia 1970; 25:397–401.
18. Bamford C, Sibley W, Laguna J. Anaesthesia in multiple sclerosis. Can J Neurol Sci 1978; 5:41–44.
19. Confavreux C, Hutchinson M, Hours MM, et al. Rate of pregnancy-related relapse in multiple sclerosis. N Engl J Med1998; 339:285–291.
20. Bader AM. Obstetric Anesthesia: Principles and Practice. 2nd ed. 1999:963–965.
21. Rolbin WH, Levinson G, Shnider SM, et al. Anesthetic considerations for myasthenia gravis and pregnancy. Anesth Analg 1978; 57:441–447.
22. D'Angelo R, Gerancher JC. Combined spinal and epidural analgesia in a parturient with severe myasthenia gravis. Reg Anesth Pain Med 1998; 23:201–203.
23. Cantwell R, Clutton-Brock T, Cooper G. Saving mothers' lives: reviewing maternal deaths to make motherhood safer: 2006–2008. BJOG 2011; 118:1–203.
24. Smith M, Smith SJ, Scott CA, et al. Activation of the electrocorticogram by propofol during surgery for epilepsy. Br J Anaesth 1996; 76:499–502.
25. Aravapalli R, Abouleish E, Aldrete JA. Anesthetic implications in the parturient epileptic patients. Anesth Analg 1988; 67:S266.
26. Martinez-Tica J, Vadhera RB. Section 3: Disorders of the Central Nervous System in Pregnancy; Obstetric Anaesthesia and Uncommon Disorders. 2nd ed. 1998:167–190.
27. Kepes ER, Andrews IC, Radnay PA, et al. Conduct of anaesthesia for delivery with grossly raised cerebrospinal fluid pressure. N Y State J Med 1972; 72:1155–1156.
28. Goroszeniuk T, Howard RS, Wright JT. The management of labour using continuous lumbar epidural analgesia in a patient with malignant cerebral tumour. Anaesthesia 1986; 41:1128–1129.
29. Boyd AH, Pigston PE. Postpartum headache and cerebral tumour. Anaesthesia 1992; 47:450–451.
30. Hudspith NJ, Popham PA. Anaesthetic management of intracranial haemorrhage from arteriovenous malformation during pregnancy. Int J Obstet Anesth 1996; 5:189–193.
31. Viscomi CM, Wilson J, Bernstein I. Anaesthetic management of a parturient with an incompletely resected cerebral arteriovenous malformation. Reg Anesth 1997; 22:192–197.
32. Koontz WL, Herbert WNP, Cefalo RC. Pseudotumor cerebri in pregnancy. Obstet Gynecol 1983; 62:324–327.
33. Shapiro S, Yee R, Brown H. Surgical management of pseudotumor cerebri in pregnancy. Neurosurgery 1995; 37:829–831.
34. Paruchuri SRA, Lawlor M, Kleinhomer K, et al. Risk of cerebellar tonsillar herniation after diagnostic lumbar puncture in pseudotumor cerebri. Reg Anesth 1993; 18(suppl):99.
35. Abouleish E, Ali V, Tang RA. Benign intracranial hypertension and anesthesia for caesarean section. Anesthesiology 1985; 63:705–707.
36. Bedard JM, Richardson MG, Wissler RN. Epidural anaesthesia in a parturient with lumboperitoneal shunt. Anesthesiology 1999; 90:621–623.
37. Yu J. Pregnancy and extracranial shunts. J Fam Pract 1994; 38:622–626.
38. Gast MJ, Grubb RL, Strickler RC. Maternal hydrocephalus and pregnancy. Obstet Gynecol 1983; 62:29S–31S.
39. Mueller DM, Oro'J. Chiari1 malformation. Am J Perinatol 2005; 22(2):67–70.

8

Psychiatric and neuropsychiatric disorders in pregnancy and the post-partum period

John Moriarty and Trudi Seneviratne

INTRODUCTION

Childbearing should be a happy time for women and their families. However, research has shown us that psychological and psychiatric abnormalities during pregnancy and the post-natal period are common and that episodes of mood disorder occurring at this time are of significant clinical and public health importance, with suicide a leading cause of maternal death in the developed world (1,2). Provision of services to support the mental health needs of women during pregnancy and the post-partum varies enormously across the world, with countries such as the United Kingdom and Australia, for example, investing more towards service provision in recent decades. Pregnancy and childbirth are major life events when women are susceptible to both physiological and psychological stress. This 'stress', whatever the aetiology, may cause new-onset psychopathology and morbidity as well as causing difficulties for women who have chronic psychological or mental health problems. Most vulnerable women have multiple stressors, such as sexual, reproduction or social problems. Women are at risk of related life events such as relationship, employment or financial difficulties. The psychological response to a new baby, no matter how planned the pregnancy is, may vary from joy to despair. The response may depend on factors such as the woman's own perspective on the pregnancy, and social circumstances such as adequate support, expectations of motherhood and cultural beliefs. Women's mental health may be at risk secondary to physical health problems or a personal or family predisposition to mental illness.

The stress that women experience could in turn have an influence on fetal development during pregnancy. There is a growing body of evidence suggesting that the maternal stress axis and psychological state during pregnancy and post-partum have a direct impact on the fetus with potential longer term consequences for the developing child (1–3). Maintaining maternal mental health and well-being during pregnancy, childbirth and the post-natal period is crucial not only for the mother but also for the developing child and the wider family.

In recent years, the importance of perinatal mental health problems has been recognised nationally in the United Kingdom with the highly publicised Confidential Enquiry into Maternal Deaths. The report, 'Why Mothers Die' (1) showed that suicide was the leading cause of maternal death in the United Kingdom. Saving Mothers' Lives 2003–2005, the subsequent report (2) continued to recognise these concerns. Factors contributing to death from suicide included lack of recognition of high-risk factors for mental health and/or lack of suitable care plans even when risk was identified. Another finding was misattribution of physical illness as psychological in origin causing delayed diagnosis and inappropriate management. The reports (1,2) have recommended that all women should be asked at a booking clinic about their previous psychiatric history in a sensitive and systematic way, that women with a history of serious psychiatric disorder should be seen by a psychiatrist during pregnancy and a written management plan, shared with the woman, her family and maternity services, should be in place prior to the delivery. It also recommended that women who have suffered from a severe episode of illness, following birth or at other times, discuss with their psychiatrist and obstetrician their plans for future childbearing and the risk of recurrence following childbirth. These reports have also highlighted the important contribution that substance misuse makes to perinatal mortality (1,2). The recently published National Institute for Health and Clinical Excellence (NICE) guidelines 'Antenatal and Postnatal Mental Health' in the United Kingdom (4) and the Scottish Intercollegiate Guidelines Network (SIGN) guidelines for 'Post Natal Depression and Puerperal Psychosis' (5) give evidence-based guidelines for clinical practice and service development and highlight the need for recognition of mental health problems during the perinatal period.

The main diagnostic manuals for mental illness include the International Classification for Mental and Behavioural Disorders (ICD 10, World Health Organisation, Geneva, 1992, used more in Europe) (6) and the Diagnostic and Statistical Manual of Mental Disorders (DSM), used more in the United States (7). Unfortunately, within these manuals the classification of mental illness during pregnancy, childbirth and post-natal period is unclear and inconsistent. The section of ICD-10 specifically dealing with mental and behavioural disorders in the puerperium (F53) is mainly concerned with post-partum depression and post-partum psychosis, if this cannot be diagnosed elsewhere in the diagnostic schedule. Post-partum depression and psychosis, as defined in the ICD-10, commence during the first 6 weeks post-delivery. The diagnoses are given on the basis of proximity to the delivery of a baby rather than any distinct symptom clustering. There is some controversy about their classification and whether they should even be considered in a separate category, or whether they should be classified with the specific disorders, for example, depression, psychosis, with a specifier which described the onset of the episode as during pregnancy or the post-partum period. Future editions of both classifications will hopefully address these difficulties.

This chapter considers the common psychiatric and neuropsychiatric sequelae of pregnancy and childbirth. Thus we have brought together the more common disorders which are likely to pose clinical dilemmas. We have divided the chapter into two broad sections: the first part examining common psychiatric disorders seen during pregnancy and the post-partum, and the second looking more specifically at neuropsychiatric conditions which could pose a clinical conundrum. We examine the major disorders likely to be encountered by health professionals during this period and outline general considerations when dealing with mental disorder at this time. There are, however, several other disorders, for example, substance misuse, obsessive-compulsive disorders, personality disorders and eating disorders, which can have a profound effect upon the perinatal period. Minor psychiatric or psychological problems in pregnancy are also common, such as milder forms of depression, adjustment reactions and anxiety disorders. For the subjects not covered in this chapter, the reader is referred to our suggestions for further reading.

PSYCHIATRIC DISORDERS DURING PREGNANCY

While some women develop mental disorders during pregnancy, others have a pre-existing psychiatric illness which needs to be carefully managed during pregnancy because it may increase the risk of a poor maternal and fetal outcome. Women with a pre-existing mental illness (especially severe mental illness) should be identified at routine screening when they book for antenatal care and referred to mental health or specialist perinatal psychiatry services. Also, women who have suffered from mental illness following the births of previous children should be monitored throughout pregnancy and the post-partum period as their risk of illness will be higher than in the general population (for further reading concerning screening for disorders, see Ref. 8).

Depression

Depression during pregnancy is a common condition, affecting 7% to 15% of women during pregnancy in the developed world (9) and probably more women in developing countries. For women with a history of depression, rates of relapse during pregnancy are about 50% (10). Depressive symptoms have been found to be higher during pregnancy than in the post-partum period in some studies (9). Antenatal depression may continue into the post-partum, depression in pregnancy being a predictor of post-partum depression (11). The risk of developing depression in pregnancy is highest in women with pre-existing bipolar disorder. Affective illness may increase the risk of obstetric complications such as preterm delivery (12,13) and intrauterine growth restriction (13).

Risk factors for depression in pregnancy include the following: past history of mood disorder, younger age, being single during pregnancy, unplanned pregnancy, lower education, discontinuation of antidepressants, poverty, sexual inequality and exposure to domestic violence. Maternal depression is associated with poor self-care, poor attendance for obstetric care, increased substance intake and increased smoking, which are all risk factors for poor obstetric outcomes, with potential harm to the fetus.

The association between antenatal maternal stress and preterm delivery or low birth weight or both, especially for socially deprived groups is thought to be mediated by the hypothalamic-pituitary-adrenal (HPA) axis, the main human stress axis. HPA axis function is upregulated in response to stress leading to increased cortisol levels. Cortisol is one of the major determinants of the timing of labour, therefore high cortisol levels can lead to preterm labour (14). It is also thought that high levels of maternal cortisol can cause levels of fetal cortisol to be raised, increasing the risk of abnormal infant stress responses and the development of depression in later life (3).

Management

Psychological management. The severity of the depressive illness should guide the mode of treatment. Mild depression may be managed with support and psychological interventions (4,15) with women encouraged to make an informed choice. Treatment options include the following: self-help strategies [guided self-help, computerised cognitive behavioural therapy (CBT) or exercise]; non-directive counselling delivered at home (listening visits); brief CBT or interpersonal psychotherapy. Women should be seen for psychological treatment normally within 1 month of initial assessment, and no longer than 3 months afterwards as timely access to such psychological treatment is important but there is often delay due to lack of such services (4).

Pharmacological management. A pharmacological approach should be considered for women with moderate to severe depression and/or a history of recurrent depression which has responded to antidepressant medication in the past. A multimodal approach may be appropriate for some women, using a combination of psychological and pharmacological therapies. When prescribing medication for maternal mental illnesses during pregnancy and breastfeeding, the principles of balancing risks of medication versus benefits to mother should apply (4,16,17).

When choosing an antidepressant for pregnant or breastfeeding women, prescribers should consider that while these drugs are usually indicated in women with a severe episode or a history of recurrent depression, their safety is not well established (3). Tricyclic antidepressants have been widely used throughout pregnancy and have not been shown to cause harm to the fetus, but can cause a neonatal withdrawal syndrome if used in the third trimester, although this is uncommon. Most tricyclic antidepressants have a higher fatal toxicity index than selective serotonin reuptake inhibitors (SSRIs) in terms of overdose and maternal morbidity. Most SSRIs have not been found to be teratogenic, with most data available for fluoxetine, sertraline and citalopram. Paroxetine taken in the first trimester may be associated with fetal heart defects (18) but data are conflicting (19). SSRIs taken after 20 weeks' gestation are associated with an increased risk of persistent pulmonary hypertension in the neonate (20). Information concerning neurodevelopmental outcome of fetal exposure to SSRIs suggests that these drugs are broadly safe, although this has not been conclusively demonstrated and concerns remain (21). Depression itself may have more obvious adverse effects on development (22). Venlafaxine may be associated with increased risk of high blood pressure at high doses, higher toxicity in overdose than SSRIs and some tricyclic antidepressants, and increased difficulty in withdrawal. Monoamine Oxidase Inhibitors (MAOIs) should be avoided in pregnancy because of a risk of fetal malformation and hypertensive crisis (16).

All antidepressants carry the risk of withdrawal or toxicity in neonates (23,24). In most cases the effects are mild and self-limiting. The risk may be particularly high with drugs which have a short half-life such as paroxetine and venlafaxine. Imipramine, nortriptyline and sertraline are present in breast milk at relatively low levels, while citalopram and fluoxetine are present at relatively high levels. Conflicting results from current data mean it is important to be mindful of any new safety data as they become available.

Benzodiazepines should not be routinely prescribed as psychotropic medication for pregnant women, unless clinically needed such as for the short-term treatment of extreme anxiety and agitation. This is because of the risks to the fetus (e.g., cleft palate) and the neonate (e.g., floppy baby syndrome). Gradually stopping benzodiazepines in pregnant women who are already taking these should be considered (16).

Although it remains a controversial treatment, electroconvulsive therapy (ECT) has not been shown to cause harm to the mother or fetus during pregnancy (4).

Bipolar Disorder

Women with a history of bipolar disorder are at risk of a relapse during pregnancy, although the risk of relapse is highest during the post-partum period, when the risk is around 50%, ranging between 30% and 70%, depending on familial factors. A relapse of bipolar disorder during pregnancy, especially a manic relapse, can cause considerable risk to the mother and baby through disturbed behaviour, poor self-care and increased alcohol and substance use. Women with bipolar disorder are at higher risk of post-partum psychosis. For episodes of severe affective psychosis, and for bipolar episodes in particular, there is very clear evidence of a specific relationship to childbirth (25). In a large study employing the Danish admission and birth registries that examined over 600,000 pregnancies and post-partum periods, women were over 23 times more likely to be admitted with an episode of bipolar disorder in the first post-partum month compared with any other month (26). A previous history of admission with bipolar disorder was associated with an even larger increased risk of admission following pregnancy (27). Women with bipolar disorder have at least a 1-in-4 risk of suffering a severe recurrence following delivery (25) and such women with a previous history of a severe post-partum episode (post-partum/puerperal psychosis) and those with a family history of post-partum psychosis are at particularly high risk, with greater than 1 in 2 deliveries affected (28). For post-partum psychotic episodes, there is a characteristic and close temporal relationship to childbirth. In a study of 111 episodes of post-partum psychosis, 97% of women retrospectively reported the onset of symptoms within the first two post-partum weeks with the majority on days 1 to 3. Familial factors have been implicated in the vulnerability to post-partum triggering of bipolar episodes (28) with evidence from linkage studies indicating the possible location of susceptibility genes (29).

Management

This should begin prior to conception if possible, and the woman should be followed up regularly during and after pregnancy, by mental health and ideally a specialist perinatal psychiatric service (4). If there is a high risk of relapse, or a previous episode of post-partum psychosis, a prophylactic admission to a mother and baby unit in the late stages of pregnancy may be considered, if this is available as many countries do not have such facilities. The obstetric team should be kept well informed about risks and management. Women should be advised about the importance of maintaining regular sleep patterns to reduce the risk of relapse (30) both before and after delivery.

Pharmacological management. This is tailored to the individual and should ideally be discussed with the patient prior to conception. Women planning a pregnancy should be fully aware of the risks and benefits of taking mood-stabilising medication during pregnancy and breastfeeding. It is very important to give good family planning advice to women of childbearing age being treated for bipolar disorder as, for example, carbamazepine interacts with the oral contraceptive

pill, making it less effective. Oral contraceptives decrease the serum concentration of lamotrigine by 50%.

Lithium

When given during pregnancy, lithium reduces the risk of relapse of bipolar disorder, and can also be prescribed in the second or third trimester for women at high risk of post-partum psychosis. When used during the period of fetal development lithium increases the rate of fetal heart defects to around 60 in 1000, compared with the risk of 8 in 1000 in the general population. It is estimated that lithium increases the risk of Ebstein anomaly (a major cardiac malformation) from 1 in 20,000 to 10 in 20,000. The risk is highest in the first trimester. Recent studies suggest that risk is not as high as was previously considered (16). Lithium should not be routinely prescribed for women, particularly in the first trimester of pregnancy, and should not be prescribed during breastfeeding because of the high levels in breast milk (4), unless serum lithium levels are checked in the neonate. Measuring lithium levels in the baby is understandably not a management strategy that many women choose. Discontinuing lithium should be weighed against risk to mother and fetus of severe relapse of illness. Factors to take into account are as follows: frequency and severity of previous relapses, stability in the past when untreated, previous pregnancies, compliance and engagement with services in the past when unwell and family/social support. Abrupt discontinuation of lithium can increase risk of relapse; therefore, the drug should be tapered off slowly over several weeks.

If a woman who is taking lithium becomes pregnant and if the pregnancy is confirmed in the first trimester, and the woman is well and not at high risk of relapse, lithium should be stopped gradually over 4 weeks. It should be explained that this may not remove the risk of cardiac defects in the fetus. If a woman continues taking lithium during pregnancy, serum lithium levels should be checked every 4 weeks, then weekly from the 36th week, and less than 24 hours after childbirth. The dose should be adjusted to keep serum levels towards the lower end of the therapeutic range (about 04–0.8 mmol/L), and the woman should maintain adequate fluid intake. The obstetric team should be notified and advised to check the lithium level, within the first 24 hours following delivery (4) and adjusted accordingly as levels can rise dramatically and cause toxicity. Women taking lithium should deliver in hospital, and be monitored during labour by the obstetric team. Monitoring should include fluid balance, because of the risk of dehydration and lithium toxicity. In prolonged labour it may be appropriate to check serum lithium levels. Thyroid function, urea and electrolytes, calcium and creatinine should be checked routinely during pregnancy and post-partum.

If a woman is at high risk of relapse, the following strategies can be considered: switching gradually to an antipsychotic; stopping lithium and restarting it in the second trimester if the woman is not planning to breastfeed and her symptoms have responded better to lithium than to other drugs in the past; continuing with lithium if she is at high risk of relapse. If lithium is to be continued, drug levels should be monitored frequently, especially during the third trimester, as physiological changes during pregnancy tend to reduce serum levels. There should be detailed ultrasound scanning and echocardiography looking for fetal malformations, and the baby should be monitored after birth for evidence of hypothyroidism, and cardiac arrhythmias. Women should be advised during pregnancy that breastfeeding while taking lithium is contraindicated unless they are prepared to have lithium levels checked frequently in their baby.

Sodium Valproate

Sodium valproate increases the risk of neural tube defects (mainly spina bifida and anencephaly) from around 6 in 10,000 pregnancies in the general population to around 100 to 200 in 10,000 (4,31). Valproate is often prescribed for epilepsy and results of a systematic literature review (32) suggest that the overall incidence of congenital malformations in children born to women with epilepsy is approximately threefold that of healthy women. The risk is elevated further for antiepileptic drug (AED) monotherapy and even more elevated for AED polytherapy. The risk is significantly higher for children exposed to valproate monotherapy and to polytherapy of two or more drugs when the polytherapy combination included phenobarbital, phenytoin or valproate. The risk associated with valproate is dose related and is greater than the risk associated with lamotrigine or carbamazepine (33). Further research is needed to delineate the specific risk for each individual AED and to determine underlying mechanisms including genetic risk factors. At present, it seems reasonable to extrapolate these figures to the population of women with bipolar disorder on valproate.

Valproate also has effects on the child's intellectual development (see chapter 12). Since many pregnancies are unintended and/or not confirmed until after the 28th day (when the neural tube closes), care is needed whenever it is prescribed for women of childbearing age, and women must be informed regarding the risks (34). If possible, valproate should be discontinued prior to conception (4) and if a pregnant woman presents early in the first trimester on sodium valproate, it is advisable to stop it and commence an alternative mood stabiliser. The fetus should have detailed ultrasonography (USS) at 12 and around 20 weeks to detect malformations, in particular neural tube defects. For women who need to remain on sodium valproate, as with other mood-stabilising medication, they should be given folic acid prior to conception and during the first trimester and have detailed scanning. Teratogenic effects are dose dependent, therefore slow-release formulations and dosages as low as possible should be used, for example, a valproate dosage of <900 mg/day with serum concentrations <80 mg/L (32). It is also recommended that doses are split to avoid high peak levels.

Carbamazepine and Lamotrigine

Carbamazepine is estimated to increase the risk of neural tube defects from 6 in 10,000 to around 20 to 50 in 10,000, and carries a risk of other major fetal malformations including gastrointestinal tract problems and cardiac abnormalities. Lamotrigine carries the risk of oral cleft (estimated at nearly 9 in 1000 exposed fetuses) according to one study (32), although this was not observed in the U.K. pregnancy register (34). A dose-related effect has been observed with lamotrigine (35). If a woman who is taking carbamazepine or lamotrigine is planning a pregnancy or has an unplanned pregnancy, and if this is appropriate in the individual case, health care professionals should advise her to stop taking these drugs because of the risk of malformations in the fetus. If appropriate, an alternative drug (such as an antipsychotic, haloperidol or olanzapine) should be considered. Carbamazepine or lamotrigine should not be routinely prescribed for women who are pregnant because of the lack of evidence of efficacy and the risk of neural tube defects in the fetus. Lamotrigine should not

be routinely prescribed as a new treatment for women who are breastfeeding because of the risk of dermatological problems in the infant, such as Stevens–Johnson syndrome. However, it may be used in breastfeeding when the women have already taken during pregnancy, as long as the infant is well and monitored.

Other Mood-Stabilising Drugs

Like all drugs, it is difficult to assess the safety and efficacy of newer mood stabilisers due the ethical difficulties of conducting trials on pregnant women and most data available are from case reports or short case series.

Clinicians now tend to use the second-generation atypical antipsychotics, which also have mood-stabilising properties, such as olanzapine (16). Unwanted consequences of olanzapine are a higher rate of metabolic complications in pregnancy, particularly diabetes. Data concerning quetiapine and risperidone are inconclusive (36). There is no clear evidence that olanzapine has teratogenic potential, and it is increasingly being used for treatment of psychotic and manic episodes by perinatal psychiatry services in the United Kingdom. Screening for gestational diabetes around 28 weeks in women taking atypical antipsychotics is commonly advocated.

Other Psychotic Disorders

Prior to the advent of atypical antipsychotics, women of childbearing age with schizophrenia were less likely to conceive than the general population because of the dopamine blockade caused by their medication as well as the reduced background level of fertility seen in schizophrenia. It is important to advise women of childbearing age taking atypical antipsychotics about the use of appropriate contraception. In addition, women who are taking typical antipsychotics and trying to conceive should consider switching to an antipsychotic that does not raise prolactin levels, for example, olanzapine or quetiapine (16).

For women with pre-existing psychotic disorders, unplanned pregnancy is more common than in the general population. Women may be reluctant to disclose their pregnancy for fear of intervention or even removal of the baby by local authorities or social services, and may present late to obstetric services. Psychosis during pregnancy increases the risk of stillbirth, fetal malformation (even in unmedicated women), other obstetric complications (37), cot death and accidental death of the baby. Interestingly, in contrast to bipolar disorder, there is no clear association between schizophrenia onset or relapse and the post-natal period.

Management

As with bipolar disorder, the risks and benefits of remaining on antipsychotic medication during pregnancy should be weighed carefully and discussed with the mother, ideally before conception. The potential risks to mother and fetus of an untreated psychosis should not be underestimated.

It may be necessary to admit the mother to a psychiatric unit for treatment of a psychotic episode in order to maintain a safe environment for her and the fetus.

Antipsychotic Medication

Conventional (first generation) antipsychotics, such as haloperidol and chlorpromazine, have not been found to be teratogenic and have been found to be safe for use in pregnancy. There are no reports of increased malformation rates after intrauterine exposure with atypical antipsychotics;

however, antipsychotic discontinuation symptoms can occur in the neonate, for example, crying, agitation and suckling difficulties (16). Mothers may continue to breastfeed with these known concerns, if the neonate is alert and well. Some centres use mixed feeding between breast and bottle to avoid this, although such mixed feeding reduces the chances of successful long-term breastfeeding. A few authorities also recommend discontinuation of antipsychotic medication 5 to 10 days before delivery to minimise withdrawal effects on the neonate. Gestational diabetes mellitus (GDM) may be a problem with the second-generation antipsychotics such as olanzapine and clozapine (16) and women taking these medications should have screening for GDM.

POST-PARTUM PSYCHIATRIC DISORDERS

Post-partum psychiatric disorders are associated with increased maternal mortality. Twenty-eight percent of maternal deaths are suicides (38). Infant mortality is also increased, and there can be long-term consequences for the child's emotional, cognitive and behavioural development. These disorders range in severity from the mild and self-limiting 'baby blues' to severe post-partum psychosis. Pre-existing disorders, for example, anxiety disorders or obsessive-compulsive disorder may be exacerbated by the presence of the new baby.

Post-Partum Blues – 'Baby Blues'

This is not a psychiatric disorder per se but the symptoms may mimic the early stages of a psychotic relapse. It is characterised by transient symptoms of irritability, lability of mood and tearfulness following delivery (39). It affects 50% to 75% of women post-partum. The symptoms peak on day 3 or 4 post-partum and rarely last more than 10 days. It is more common after a first baby. A proposed aetiological mechanism is the rapid fall in levels of oestrogen and progesterone following delivery, but there is no robust evidence for this. There is a positive association between poor family relationships and post-partum blues, and also an association between mood disturbances before or during pregnancy and development of the blues. Symptoms resolve spontaneously without treatment. Although usually a benign condition, emotional lability post-partum may herald the development of a post-partum psychosis and concern should be raised if this does not settle quickly.

Post-Partum Depression

This is the most frequent psychiatric disorder seen after childbirth, affecting 10% of women. Studies have found little difference between rates of depression just after childbirth and rates of depression in women at other times (40). Fifty percent of post-partum depressive episodes commence during pregnancy. It is associated with the following: previous depressive episodes, family history of depression, life events and relationship disturbance. Risk factors include previous psychiatric illness (especially bipolar disorder), high parity, prepartum distress and social isolation (41). Untreated depression which continues from the antepartum to post-partum period may also affect the well-being of the infant due to impaired attachment, impaired cognition and behavioural disturbance (42). Maternal depression may lead to neglect of the infant and in rare severe cases infanticide (43), so it may necessitate the separation of mother and baby. Although maternal infanticide is a rare event, a high proportion of cases occur in the context of post-partum mental illness, such as depression or psychosis.

In the United States, according to available death certificate records, one infant under age 1 year is killed every day, yet the national rate may be double that number; the complexity of the response to infanticide is demonstrated by the judicial system's reaction to such cases. Whereas England's Infanticide Law provides probation and mandates psychiatric treatment for mothers with mental illness who commit infanticide, mothers may face the death penalty in the United States (43).

Diagnosis
Primary care staff are usually the first to detect the condition. A careful assessment by the general practitioner should follow if the screening test is positive, identifying both risk and protective factors. This may result in a psychiatric referral. There will be the usual symptoms of low mood, anhedonia, but the so-called biological symptoms of depressions, such as disturbed sleep, appetite and concentration, may be masked by the feeding demands of the baby which may mask early morning wakening or diurnal mood variation. It is crucial to enquire about suicidal or indeed infanticidal thoughts as women may not offer these spontaneously. Cognitive features of the depression may include guilt, low esteem and thoughts of parental inadequacy.

Management
This should take a multimodal approach, including biological, psychological and social interventions working with a woman's choice of treatment, and choosing medication which allows breastfeeding. As with depressive disorders in other settings, medical causes of depression, for example, hypothyroidism, need to be excluded. Women experiencing severe post-partum depression should be considered for admission to a mother and baby unit for further assessment and management.

When using antidepressants, treatment of maternal illness should usually take priority over breastfeeding (3). The lowest effective dose of a single agent should be used. For significant anxiety lorazepam can be used and zolpidem considered for sleep (16). Antidepressants are excreted into breast milk, but infant serum levels are generally low and adverse effects have been reported very rarely. Some clinicians advise the patient to time feeds in order to avoid peak drug levels, that is, take the antidepressant after a feed or last thing at night, but this may be impractical advice for small infants feeding every 1 to 3 hours. The SSRIs paroxetine and sertraline are often recommended (16).

Non-Biological Interventions
Various psychological interventions have been used for treatment of post-partum depression (15) including interpersonal psychotherapy, CBT, peer and partner support, non-directive counselling, relaxation/massage therapy, infant sleep interventions, infant-mother relationship therapy and maternal exercise. Recent research from Canada has demonstrated that telephone-based peer support can be effective in preventing post-natal depression among women at high risk (44).

Post-Partum Psychosis

This is a psychiatric emergency, which if left untreated can have severe adverse consequences for the mother, infant and family (45). It should be managed promptly and in a safe environment for both mother and baby. This may involve admission to an inpatient unit, ideally to a specialised mother and baby unit.

This disorder is distinct from post-partum or post-natal depression and should not be referred to as such. It occurs in 1 to 2 in 1000 childbearing women within the first 2 to 4 weeks after delivery. It most commonly presents as a manic psychosis but also as severe psychotic depression or an acute polymorphic psychosis (40) and a history of bipolar affective disorder is a major risk factor (25,26,28,46). It is characterised by a rapid onset; paranoid, grandiose or bizarre delusions; mood swings; confused thinking; and disorganized behaviour that represents a dramatic change from previous functioning (47). Symptom clusters that precede onset of psychosis include feeling excited, elated or high, not needing to sleep or not able to sleep and feeling very active or energetic. There is a high and specific heritability (25,28) and a recurrence rate is 1 of every 4 subsequent pregnancies (48).

Management
Pharmacological management involves antipsychotic and mood-stabilising medication with the possible addition of sedating medications, for example, benzodiazepines in the acute phase. Olanzapine is commonly used because of its sedative and mood-stabilising properties in combination with lithium or sodium valproate. (See above section on bipolar disorder for information about the safety of breastfeeding whilst taking mood-stabilising medications and chapter 5.) ECT is less commonly used for the treatment of post-partum psychosis (4).

These women will need a great deal of support in order to parent their children during the psychotic illness, and because of the sleep cycle implications, they may be advised not to breastfeed at night. Bottle-feeding may be more appropriate for some women. If the psychosis is severe and there is a possible risk of harm to the baby (see point about rare event of infanticide above), a separation should be considered during the acute phase. In this case, social services may need to be involved in decision-making alongside the multidisciplinary team.

During the resolution phase of the illness, women may be very distressed at what has happened to them, especially if they have never experienced a mental illness before. Supportive psychotherapy, information giving and ongoing contact with appropriate services may be necessary. Women should be advised about the potential for a recurrence in future pregnancies, the association with bipolar affective disorder and the need for careful preparation.

SPECIFIC NEUROPSYCHIATRIC CONDITIONS
Neuropsychiatry generally refers to the psychiatric complications of neurological disease, the neurological complications of psychiatric disease and some specific syndromes which occur at the interface between the two disciplines. In general, the psychiatric management of the psychiatric complications of neurological illnesses should be according to the same principles of management already described. Thus, a woman with, for example, a demyelinating illness who becomes depressed will broadly be helped in the same way as any other depressed woman. Close liaison between a treating psychiatrist and the neurologist is important. Good liaison between the obstetrician and midwives, the perinatal psychiatrist and the neurologist is likely to be the key to effective management.

It is inevitable that most diseases of the CNS can and will have psychiatric manifestations. We will consider some of the most relevant.

Epilepsy
The commonest psychiatric problems of women with epilepsy are depression and anxiety (49). The causes of depression and anxiety in epilepsy are multifactorial but can include psychosocial factors (50), factors related to the seizures themselves, factors relating to the cause of the epilepsy (e.g., cerebrovascular disease, head injury and learning disability) and antiepileptic medication (51). The management of depression or anxiety in epilepsy should not differ greatly from that of depression generally described already. However, some specific aspects will need to be considered.

Antidepressant medications carry a risk of lowering the seizure threshold. In reality, this risk may not be as great as some prescribers fear. The incidence has been thought to be between 0.1% and 1.5%. The risk at therapeutic doses is considerably less than at higher doses or in overdose (52). It has been claimed that SSRI antidepressant medication at therapeutic dose may even be anticonvulsant (53). Although the reversible monoamine oxidase inhibitor moclobemide is generally thought to be a good choice in epilepsy, safety of use in pregnancy has not been established as it has been little used. Therefore, moclobemide is not recommended in women who may be pregnant unless the expected benefits to the patient markedly outweigh the possible risk to the fetus. The limited safety data available for alternative antidepressants suggest they may be a better choice. Tricyclic antidepressants, which have a fairly good evidence base for their relative safety in pregnancy, should generally be avoided in pregnant women with epilepsy as they clearly lower the seizure threshold in the non-pregnant patient. In summary, current data suggest that if antidepressant medication is indicated in the pregnant woman with epilepsy SSRIs would seem to be the drugs of first choice (see section 'Depression' above).

Psychological management of depression in epilepsy will share many of the features of management of depression in any context. However, there are likely to be specific concerns faced by pregnant women with epilepsy about risks to their health and that of the fetus, and the challenges posed by having seizures while caring for an infant. Sensitive and knowledgeable discussion of these issues is likely to be of benefit.

Psychosis in epilepsy is less common than mood disorder. The most useful distinction in clinical practice is between inter-ictal psychosis (unrelated to seizure activity) and post-ictal psychosis (having its onset following a seizure or cluster of seizures). In addition, complex partial status may present as a psychotic illness. In the investigation of patients with psychosis and suspected seizures, caution needs to be exercised in the interpretation of the EEG, as many psychotropics are associated with quite marked EEG abnormalities which if overinterpreted can lead to diagnostic confusion. (see also chapters 11 and 12)

Post-ictal psychosis, on one hand, usually follows a severe seizure or cluster of seizures. The onset of the psychotic illness may be delayed by one or several days. A degree of impaired consciousness with reduced attention is not unusual and the effect may be one of intense fear, agitation or rage (54). The duration of such episodes is usually of the order of days with one study giving a mean of 3.5 days and a range of 16 hours to 18 days (55). The prognosis even without treatment may be relatively good, although symptomatic treatment is usually required because of the degree of distress and the associated risks to self and others. The primary prevention of post-ictal psychosis will be any reduction in frequency and severity of the epileptic seizures themselves.

Table 8.1 Clinical Features Which May Help Distinguish Epileptic from Non-Epileptic Seizures

	Epilepsy	Dissociative seizures
Onset and duration	Highly stereotyped, relatively short (few minutes)	Variable, prolonged
Eyes	Open	Closed or deviated to ground (non-physiological)
Convulsive movements	Tonic followed by clonic with decreasing frequency and amplitude	Asymmetrical, asynchronous, fluctuating or episodic
Awareness	Absent	Usually absent but partial not uncommon
Recovery	Gradual reorientation	Abrupt reorientation but prolonged fatigue or distress
Injury	From falls, lateral tongue biting	Carpet burn type, tip of tongue biting

Inter-ictal psychosis, on the other hand, typically complicates chronic epilepsy (56). It presents rather like schizophrenia. Although psychotic symptoms may be exacerbated post-ictally, there is no simple relationship to seizures. The management is essentially that of any chronic psychosis.

In the investigation of patients with psychosis and suspected seizures, caution needs to be exercised in the interpretation of the EEG, as many psychotropics are associated with quite marked EEG abnormalities which if overinterpreted can lead to diagnostic confusion.

Dissociative Seizures

Non-epileptic or dissociative seizures are seizures of essentially psychological origin which can be mistaken for epilepsy and which indeed mimic that disorder. Patients with dissociative seizures are overrepresented in specialist epilepsy clinics and among patients with treatment resistant epilepsy. Twenty percent of patients who undergo video EEG telemetry are diagnosed with non-epileptic seizures (57), and pseudo-status epilepticus is the most common explanation for pharmacoresistant status epilepticus (58). Although there is often a considerable time delay between presentation and diagnosis of dissociative seizures of many years (59), there are numerous features which suggest the diagnosis (Table 8.1). There are, however, numerous pitfalls in the distinction between epileptic and non-epileptic attacks, including the bizarre manifestations of frontal lobe epilepsies. Although there is no literature on the incidence or prevalence of dissociative seizures in pregnancy, some clinicians feel it is not uncommon (Prof Dr Bettina Schmitz Chefärztin der Klinik für Neurologie, Stroke Unit und Zentrum für Epilepsie, Vivantes Humboldt-Klinikum, Am Nordgraben 2, 13509 Berlin, personal communication). A single case report (60) in which a woman underwent iatrogenic premature delivery at 31 weeks because of what were at the time was thought to be status epilepticus, but which subsequently proved to be dissociative seizures, emphasises the important of accurate diagnosis. The baby in this case died 3 hours after birth.

The management of dissociative seizures is a complex area, but initial communication of the diagnosis in an authoritative but non-judgemental manner may of itself be therapeutic (61). AEDs should be avoided or withdrawn if they have already been prescribed. Formal psychological therapies such as CBT may be useful (62,63). Psychological treatment strategies include psychoeducation, distraction techniques, anxiety management and exposure. The patients may be difficult to engage initially as they may need to change the attribution of their seizure episodes as being due to epilepsy or at least to revise their beliefs about whether they can learn to control the episodes and their beliefs about the risks from the seizures. They may then through a process of guided diary keeping, self-assessment and behavioural experiments learn to identify the early warnings of a seizure and to avert it using distraction and relaxation techniques. Fears they may have of the catastrophic consequences of having seizures can be challenged by graded exposure and by minimising avoidance. During pregnancy it is important to explain to women who have a clear diagnosis of dissociative seizures that the baby should not be affected by the seizures per se, and that early delivery or instrumental delivery is not indicated. Measured reassurance that the fetus is safe and explanation of the potentially adverse neonatal effects of early delivery to women with dissociative seizures may be followed by a reduction in dissociative seizure frequency. It may be that the effect of pregnancy on dissociative seizures is linked in part to whether the pregnancy is wanted or a source of stress or distress. Pre-existing dissociative seizures can improve with a wanted pregnancy or seizures may be the presenting symptom of the distress experienced by some pregnant women. Of course the interplay of psychological factors in patients with dissociative seizures is complex and may reflect difficulties in interpersonal relationships as well as the mixture of positive and negative emotional reactions which may accompany pregnancy (MM, personal communication).

Other Non-Organic or Medically Unexplained Disorders

Somatoform disorders are among the most problematic conditions to assess, manage and treat for all medical practitioners. Each medical discipline has its own particular disorder or group of disorders and clinicians may vary considerably as to how much they are comfortable with a psychogenic as opposed to an organic attribution. The assessment of these conditions is particularly complex because the way of classifying these disorders in medicine and psychiatry may differ. Thus, psychiatrists may speak of conversion/dissociation disorders, somatisation, somatoform disorders and physicians may speak of non-organic, psychogenic, functional or specific syndromes such as fibromyalgia and chronic fatigue.

Up to one-third of neurology outpatients in specialist settings are thought to have primarily non-organic or functional disorders. These patients are more distressed, disabled and more difficult to help than those with more clearly organic disorders (64). Patients with functional illness have been thought to be more likely to be female (65), so one might expect this to be a significant problem during pregnancy. Surprisingly there is very little literature on this subject.

Smith and Farkas (66) describe a case of a sudden-onset tetraparesis in a 28-year-old primagravida at 36 weeks' gestation. The case has some of the typical features of functional disorder (67), with neurologically inconsistent signs and symptoms and a plausible psychogenic hypothesis. The case, fortunately, resolved rapidly with multidisciplinary input. Other features typical of this and other cases is a history of somatisation and employment in paramedical professions.

Multiple Sclerosis

Multiple sclerosis (MS) (see chapter 21) is the commonest neurological cause of disability in young adults. The disease has a prevalence which seems to relate in part to latitude with rates of 1 per 100,000 at the equator rising to over 50 per 100,000 in Northern Europe. Women are affected two to three times more than men and it has its onset typically during childbearing years, with two-thirds of cases presenting first between the ages of 20 and 40. Relapse of MS appears to be less common in pregnancy but raised in the post-partum period (68).

Psychiatric aspects of the disorder are important and common. The two important types of disorder are cognitive impairment and mood disorders.

Cognitive impairment affects perhaps 50% of patients although this will be very dependent on what stage of disease is studied with patients with progressive MS typically more impaired than those with a relapsing-remitting course (69). The pattern of cognitive impairment probably reflects the subcortical nature of the disease with deficits of attention, speed of processing and executive function being particularly common. Screening tests which focus on cortical functions (such as the widely used Mini Mental State Examination (MMSE)) may therefore miss early or less florid, though significant impairments. Cognitive performance may respond to disease-modifying treatments. Specific treatments for cognitive dysfunction, such as anticholinesterase medications have shown some possible beneficial effects (70), but the evidence remains limited and the lack of good safety information with respect to their prescription in pregnancy means they are unlikely to be used.

Depression is also common in MS and the relative contribution of disability, loss and more biological factors due to direct brain involvement can be difficult to disentangle. Perhaps 50% of patients with MS suffer from significant mood problems. In addition to depression, bipolar disorder appears to be about twice as common in MS as in the general population (71). Treatment of depression in MS is generally based on extrapolation from the general psychiatry literature with SSRIs and tricyclics being considered. Moclobemide is an alternative. Mirtazepine may be useful if sexual side effects are common. For treatment resistance lithium or ECT may be considered but ECT may provoke a relapse of the MS itself (72). (In the context of pregnancy, however, the general guidelines for the use of these agents in pregnancy described above should be observed.)

A striking feature of some patients with MS is that they have a rather euphoric mood with inappropriate cheerfulness or denial of illness. It is thought to be more common in more disabled and impaired patients and cognitive impairment is invariable (73). For a thorough review of neuropsychiatric aspects of MS see Feinstein, 2004 (74).

Parkinson's Disease

Parkinson's disease (PD) and other akinetic-rigid syndromes are primarily diseases of later life. Only a small percentage of patients present with the condition before age 50, so the condition is extremely uncommon in pregnancy (see chapter 20). The psychiatric manifestations, and more generally the non-motor manifestations of PD are increasingly recognised, which may reflect increased survival and wider treatment options for the disease. They are of particular clinical importance as they are linked to quality of life, carer burden and distress, and because they are perhaps particularly difficult to treat (75). The commonest psychiatric disorder is depression, occurring in up to 8% of community samples (76) and as much as 40% to 50% of neurology clinics (77). The diagnosis of depression in PD is however problematic because there is considerable overlap of the symptoms of depression and the primary symptoms of PD such as psychomotor slowing, reduced facial expression, reduced volume and inflexion of speech, fatigue, disturbed sleep and apathy. While the evidence base for the treatment of depression in PD is in reality very thin, treatment is likely to include the following: optimising the dopaminergic medication and SSRI antidepressants.

An important area, increasingly recognised in patients with PD is the development of impulse control disorders (ICDs) in patients with PD on dopaminergic treatment. These disorders include pathological gambling, hypersexuality, compulsive shopping and the dopamine dysregulation syndrome (DDS) (78,79).

Huntington's Disease

Huntington's disease (HD), though rare [prevalence of 6 per 100,000 in most European populations (80)] is likely to be most frequently encountered by the obstetrician in the context of clinical genetics, genetic counselling and prenatal or pre-implantation diagnosis. The disorder can present with primarily psychiatric features. The commonest is probably personality change with the patient becoming insensitive and argumentative or apathetic and showing self-neglect. Mood symptoms such as depression and anxiety may be present as may paranoia or frank psychosis. Progression to manifest chorea and a frontal-type dementia is inevitable. Later complications include swallowing difficulties, rigidity and epilepsy. Pregnancy in the symptomatic HD patient is rare. However, a case described by Hoskins et al. (81) details significant morbidity due to dysphagia, compromised nutrition and complications of a preterm labour.

Tic Disorders

Tourette syndrome or Gilles de la Tourette syndrome is a chronic disorder of motor and vocal tics. It is commoner in men, with a ratio of 4:1. Most cases are relatively mild and it is relatively uncommon to see the full-blown syndrome of echolalia, coprolalia, echophenomena and coprophenomena for which the disorder is widely recognised (82). Some patients with tics will be taking neuroleptic medications such as haloperidol, pimozide, sulpiride, risperidone or aripiprazole. The use of these drugs to control tics is essentially symptomatic and not thought to have any effect on the underlying disorder. Careful consideration should therefore be given to withdrawing medications if tolerable prior to conception or during pregnancy. There is no literature on the effect of pregnancy on the syndrome nor on the effect of the syndrome on pregnancy.

Attention Deficit and Hyperactivity Disorder

Attention deficit and hyperactivity disorder (ADHD) has traditionally been thought of as a disorder of children. However, longitudinal studies suggest that deficits in attention persist into adult life and may still be helped by stimulant medication such as methylphenidate and atomoxetine (83,84). There is very limited evidence on the safety of methylphenidate or atomoxetine in human pregnancy, although available evidence suggests no increased risk of malformations with therapeutic doses. Adult women who are taking stimulant medication and who wish to conceive or who become pregnant while on medication should therefore discuss the risks and benefits of continued medication with their obstetricians and treating psychiatrist or family physician (85). They may also benefit from targeted educational or psychological input in the post-partum period, as the ADHD may result in parenting difficulties.

PERINATAL PSYCHIATRY SERVICES

Countries such as the England and Scotland in the United Kingdom have developed perinatal mental health services (4)]. The Confidential Inquiry into Maternal Deaths in the United Kingdom (1,2) has recommended that a perinatal mental health team should be available to every woman at risk of or suffering from a serious post-partum mental illness and protocols for the management of women at risk of mental illness following delivery should be in place for every trust providing maternity services. Mental health problems should be screened for at the first antenatal appointment as part of the booking routine with access to specialist services to care for women at high-risk mental illness. Perinatal psychiatry services need to consist of community teams, perinatal liaison psychiatry teams within the general hospital and inpatient mother and baby units. Perinatal services are highly multidisciplinary, including psychiatry, psychology, developmental psychology specialist nursing, social work, nursery nursing, occupational therapy and pharmacy with links to specialist alcohol and substance misuse teams as well as midwives, specialist midwives and obstetricians.

CONCLUSIONS

Women facing pregnancy and childbirth face a range of biological and psychological challenges which put them at increased risk of psychiatric disorder. Good principles and clinical guidelines exist for the management of these disorders in terms of service provision, pharmacological and psychosocial interventions. Women with neurological disease are also at increased risk of psychiatric disorder and the neurological disorder may have implications for the management of the mental illness. Pregnant women with neurological disorder will pose a management challenge to the obstetrician, neurologist and psychiatrist as well as primary care. Good collaboration and liaison between these disciplines is likely to benefit the patients and their clinicians alike.

REFERENCES

1. The Confidential Enquiry into Maternal and Child Health (CEMACH). Why Mothers Die 2000–2002. The Sixth Report on Confidential Enquiries into Maternal Deaths in the United Kingdom. London: DOH, 2004.
2. The Confidential Enquiry into Maternal and Child Health (CEMACH). Saving Mothers' Lives 2003–2005. The Seventh Report on Confidential Enquiries into Maternal Deaths in the United Kingdom. London: CEMACH, 2007.
3. O'Keane V. Mood disorder during pregnancy: aetiology and management. In: O'Keane V, Marsh M, Seneviratne G, eds. Psychiatric Disorders and Pregnancy. London: Taylor and Francis Group, 2006:69–107.
4. National Collaborating Centre for Mental Health, National Institute for Health and Clinical Excellence. Antenatal and Postnatal Mental Health. The NICE Guideline on Clinical Management and Service Guidance. London: The British Psychological Society and the Royal College of Physicians, 2007. Available at: http://guidance.nice.org.uk/CG45.
5. Scottish Intercollegiate Guidelines Network [SIGN]: Postnatal Depression and Puerperal Psychosis. SIGN Publication No. 60. ISBN 1899893 18 0. 2002.
6. International Classification for Mental and Behavioural Disorders (ICD 10), World Health Organisation, Geneva, 1992.
7. American Psychiatric Association. Diagnostic and Statistical Manual of Mental Disorders. 4th ed. Washington, DC: American Psychiatric Association, 1994.
8. Cantwell R, Oats M. Screening in pregnancy for risk of serious postnatal illness. In: O'Keane V, Marsh M, Seneviratne G, eds. Psychiatric Disorders and Pregnancy. London: Taylor & Francis, 2006:5–21.
9. Evans J, Heron J, Francomb H, et al. Cohort study of depressed mood during pregnancy and after childbirth. BMJ 2001; 323(7307): 257–260.
10. O'Keane V, Marsh MS. Depression during pregnancy. BMJ 2007; 334(7601):1003–1005.
11. O'Hara MW, Schlechte JA, Lewis DA, et al. Controlled prospective study of postpartum mood disorders: psychological, environmental, and hormonal variables. J Abnorm Psychol 1991; 100 (1):63–73.
12. MacCabe JH, Martinsson L, Lichtenstein P, et al. Adverse pregnancy outcomes in mothers with affective psychosis. Bipolar Disord 2007; 9:305–309.
13. Copper RL, Goldenberg RL, Das A, et al. The preterm prediction study: maternal stress is associated with spontaneous preterm birth at less than thirty-five weeks' gestation. Am J Obstet Gynecol 1996; 175(5):1286–1292.
14. Diego MA, Field T, Hernandez-Reif M, et al. Prenatal depression restricts fetal growth. Early Hum Dev 2009; 85(1):65–70.
15. Ward A. The place of psychological therapies in the perinatal period. In: O'Keane V, Marsh M, Seneviratne G, eds. Psychiatric Disorders and Pregnancy. London: Taylor and Francis Group, 2006:261–277.
16. Taylor D, Paton C, Kapur S, eds. The Maudsley Prescribing Guidelines. 10th ed. London: Informa Healthcare, 2009.
17. McElhatton PR. General principles of drug use in pregnancy. Pharmacol J 2003; 270:232–234.
18. Berard A, Ramos E, Rey E, et al. First trimester exposure to paroxetine and risk of cardiac malformations in infants: the importance of dosage. Birth Defect Res B Dev Reprod Toxicol 2006; 80:18–27.
19. Einarson A, Pistelli A, DeSantis M, et al. Evaluation of risk of congenital cardiovascular defects associated with use of paroxetine during pregnancy. Am J Psychiatry 2008; 165:749–752.
20. Chambers CD, Hernandez-Diaz S, Van Marter LJ, et al. Selective serotonin-reuptake inhibitors and risk of persistent pulmonary hypertension of the newborn. N Engl J Med 2006; 354:579–587.
21. Gentille S. SSRIs in pregnancy and lactation: emphasis on neurodevelopmental outcome. CNS Drugs 2005; 19(7):623–633.
22. Nulman I, Rovet J, Stewart DE, et al. Child development following exposure to tricyclic antidepressants or fluoxetine throughout fetal life: a prospective controlled study. Am J Psychiatry 2002; 159:1889–1895.
23. Sanz EJ, De-las-Cuevas C, Kiuru A, et al. Selective serotonin reuptake inhibitors in pregnant women and neonatal withdrawal syndrome: a database analysis. Lancet 2005; 365:482–487.
24. Koren G. Discontinuation syndrome following late pregnancy exposure to antidepressants. Arch Pediatr Adolesc Med 2004; 158:307–308.
25. Jones I, Craddock N. Bipolar disorder and childbirth: the importance of recognising risk. Br J Psychiatry 2005; 186:453–454.
26. Munk-Olsen T, Laursen T, Pedersen C, et al. New parents and mental disorders: a population-based register study. J Am Med Assoc 2006; 296:2582–2589.
27. Munk-Olsen T. Postpartum Mental Disorders. Epidemiological Studies on Incidence, Selected Risk Factors and Readmissions. PhD thesis. University of Aarhus, 2008.
28. Jones I, Craddock N. Familiality of the puerperal trigger in bipolar disorder: results of a family study. Am J Psychiatry 2001; 158:913–917.
29. Jones I, Hamshere ML, Nangle JM, et al. Bipolar affective puerperal psychosis – genome-wide significant evidence for linkage to chromosome 16. Am J Psychiatry 2007; 164(7):1099–1104.
30. Yonkers KA, Wisner KL, Stowe Z, et al. Management of bipolar disorder during pregnancy and the postpartum period. Am J Psychiatry 2004; 161(4):608–620.

31. James L, Barnes TR, Lelliott P, et al. informing patients of the teratogenic potential of mood stabilising drugs: a case notes review of the practise of psychiatrists. J Psychopharmacol 2007; 21:815–819.

32. Meador K, Reynolds MW, Crean S, et al. Pregnancy outcomes in women with epilepsy: a systematic review and meta-analysis of published pregnancy registries and cohorts. Epilepsy Res 2008; 81 (1):1–13.

33. Holmes LB, Harvey EA, Coull BA, et al. The teratogenicity of anticonvulsant drugs. N Engl J Med 2001; 344:1132–1138.

34. Kennedy F, et al. PATH39 malformation risks of antiepileptic drugs in pregnancy: an update from the UK Epilepsy and Pregnancy Register. J Neurol Neurosurg Psychiatry 2010; 81:e18, doi:10.1136/jnnp.2010.226340.7.

35. Adab N. Therapeutic monitoring of antiepileptic drugs during the postpartum period: is it useful? CNS Drugs 2006; 20:791–800.

36. Gentile S. Prophylactic treatment of bipolar disorder in pregnancy and breastfeeding: focus on emerging mood stabilizers. Bipolar Disord 2006; 8(3):207–220.

37. Jablensky AV, Morgan V, Zubrick SR, et al. Pregnancy, delivery, and neonatal complications in a population cohort of women with schizophrenia and major affective disorders. Am J Psychiatry 2005; 162(1):79–91.

38. Oates M. Perinatal psychiatric disorders: a leading cause of maternal morbidity and mortality. Br Med Bull 2003; 67:219–229.

39. Seyfried LS, Marcus SM. Postpartum mood disorders. Int Rev Psychiatry 2003; 15(3):231–242.

40. Brockington I. Postpartum psychiatric disorders. Lancet 2004; 363(9405):303–310.

41. Nielsen Forman D, Videbech P, Hedegaard M, et al. Postpartum depression: identification of women at risk. BJOG 2000; 107 (10):1210–1217.

42. Pawlby S, Sharp D, Hay D, et al. Postnatal depression and child outcome at 11 years: the importance of accurate diagnosis. J Affect Disord 2008; 107(1–3):241–245.

43. Spinelli MG, ed. Infanticide: Psychological and Legal Perspectives on Mothers Who Kill. Washington, DC: American Psychiatric Publishing, 2003:272, 314–315.

44. Dennis C-L, Hodnett E, Kenton L, et al. Effect of peer support on prevention of postnatal depression among high-risk women: multi-site randomized controlled trial. Br Med J 2009; 338: a3064; doi: 10.1136/bmj.a3064.

45. Wieck A. Management of psychosis before, during and after pregnancy. In: O'Keane V, Marsh M, Seneviratne G, eds. Psychiatric Disorders and Pregnancy. London: Taylor and Francis, 2006:107–125.

46. Robertson E, Jones I, Haque S, et al. Risk of puerperal and non-puerperal recurrence of illness following bipolar affective puerperal (post-partum) psychosis. Br J Psychiatry 2005; 186:258–259.

47. Sit D, Rothschild AJ, Wisner KL. A review of postpartum psychosis. J Women's Health (Larchmt) 2006; 15(4):352–368.

48. Heron J, McGuinness M, Robertson E, et al. Early postpartum symptoms in puerperal psychosis. BJOG 2008; 115(3):348–353.

49. Jones JE, Hermann BP, Barry JJ, et al. Clinical assessment of axis I psychiatric morbidity in chronic epilepsy: a multicenter investigation. J Neuropsychiatry Clin Neurosci 2005; 17:172–179.

50. Gilliam F, Kuzniecky R, Faught E, et al. Patient-validated content of epilepsy-specific quality-of-life measurement. Epilepsia 1997; 38(2):233–236.

51. Lambert M, Schmitz EB, Ring H, et al. Neuropsychiatric aspects of epilepsy. In: Fogel BS, Schiffer RB, Rao SM, eds. Neuropsychiatry. Philadelphia: Lippincott Williams and Wilkins, 2003:1071–1131.

52. Pisani F, Oterl G, Costa C, et al. Effects of psychotropic drugs on seizure threshold. Drug Saf 2002; 25(2):91–110.

53. Jobe PC, Browning RA. The serotonergic and noradrenergic effects of antidepressant drugs are anticonvulsant, not proconvulsant. Epilepsy Behav 2005; 7(4):602–619.

54. Logsdail SJ, Toone BK. Post-ictal psychoses. A clinical and phenomenological description. Br J Psychiatry 1988; 152:246–252.

55. Devinsky O, Abramson H, Alper K, et al. Postictal psychosis: a case control series of 20 patients and 150 controls. Epilepsy Res 1995; 20:247–253.

56. Mendez MF, Grau R, Doss RC, et al. Schizophrenia in epilepsy: seizure and psychosis variables. Neurology 1993; 43:1073–1077.

57. Blumer D, Montouris G, Hermann B. Psychiatric morbidity in seizure patients on a neurodiagnostic monitoring unit. J Neuropsychiatry Clin Neurosci 1995; 7:445–456.

58. Shorvon S. The outcome of tonic-clonic status epilepticus. Curr Opin Neurol 1994; 7:93–95.

59. Reuber M, Fernandez G, Bauer J, et al. Diagnostic delay in psychogenic non-epileptic seizures. Neurology 2002; 58:493–495.

60. Smith PEM, Saunders J, Dawson A, et al. Intractable seizures in pregnancy. Lancet 1999; 354:1522.

61. Shen W, Bowman ES, Markand ON. Presenting the diagnosis of pseudoseizures. Neurology 1990; 40:756–759.

62. Goldstein LH, Deale A, Mitchell-O'Malley S, et al. An evaluation of cognitive behavioural therapy as a treatment of dissociative seizures. Cogn Behav Neurol 2004; 17:41–49.

63. Goldstein LH, Chalder T, Chigwedere C, et al. Cognitive-behavioral therapy for psychogenic nonepileptic seizures. A pilot RCT. Neurology 2010; 74:1986–1994.

64. Carson AJ, Ringbauer B, Stone J, et al. Do medically unexplained symptoms matter? A prospective cohort study of 300 new referrals to neurology outpatient clinics. J Neurol Neurosurg Psychiatry 2000; 68:207–210.

65. Kroenke K, Spitzer RL. Gender differences in the reporting of physical and somatoform symptoms. Psychosom Med 1998; 60 (2):150–155.

66. Smith VM, Farkas A. Dissociative disorder during pregnancy. J Obstet Gynaecol 2006; 26(8):810–811.

67. Stone J, Carson A, Sharp M. Functional symptoms and signs in neurology: assessment and diagnosis. J Neurol Neurosurg Psychiatry 2005; 76:2–12.

68. Confavreux C, Hutchinson M, Hours MM, et al. and the Pregnancy in Multiple Sclerosis Group. Rate of pregnancy-related relapse in multiple sclerosis. N Engl J Med 1998; 339:285–291.

69. Heaton RK, Nelson LM, Thompson DS, et al. Neuropsychological findings in relapsing-remitting and chronic-progressive multiple sclerosis. J Consult Clin Psychol 1985; 53:103–110.

70. Krupp LB, Christodoulou C, Melville P, et al. Donepezil improved memory in multiple sclerosis in a randomized clinical trial. Neurology 2004; 63:1579–1585.

71. Schiffer RB, Wineman M, Weitkamp LR. Association between bipolar affective disorder and multiple sclerosis. Am J Psychiatry 1986; 143:94–95.

72. Mattingley G, Baker K, Zorumski CF, et al. Multiple sclerosis and ECT: possible value of gadolinium enhanced magnetic resonance scans for identifying high risk patients. J Neuropsychiatry Clin Neurosci 1992; 4:145–151.

73. Rabins PV. Euphoria in multiple sclerosis. In: Rao SM, ed. Neurobehavioral Aspects of Multiple Sclerosis. New York: Oxford University Press, 1990:180–185.

74. Feinstein A. The neuropsychiatry of multiple sclerosis. Can J Psychiatry 2004; 49:157–163.

75. Aarsland D, Larsen JP, Karlsen K, et al. Mental symptoms in Parkinson's disease are important contributors to caregiver distress. Int J Geriatric Psychiatry 1999; 14(10):866–874.

76. Tandberg E, Larsen JP, Aarsland D, et al. The occurrence of depression in Parkinson's disease: a community-based study. Arch Neurol 1996; 53(2):175–179.

77. Cummings JL. Depression and Parkinson's disease: a review. Am J Psychiatry 1992; 149:443–454.

78. Voon V, Hassan K, Zurowski M, et al. Prevalence of repetitive and reward-seeking behaviors in Parkinson disease. Neurology 2006; 67:1254–1257.

79. Giovannoni G, O'Sullivan JD, Turner K, et al. Hedonistic homeostatic dysregulation in patients with Parkinson's disease on dopamine replacement. J Neurol Neurosurg Psychiatry 2000; 68:423–428.

80. Harper PS. The epidemiology of Huntington's disease. Hum Genet 1992; 89:365–376.

81. Hoskins KE, Tita AT, Biggio JR, et al. Pregnancy and active Huntington disease: a rare combination. J Perinatol 2008; 28 (2):156–157.

82. Robertson MM. Tourette syndrome, associated conditions and the complexities of treatment. Brain 2000; 123:425–462.

83. Roesler M, Fischer R, Ammer R, et al. A randomised, placebo-controlled, 24-week, study of low-dose extended-release methylphenidate in adults with attention-deficit/hyperactivity disorder. Eur Arch Psychiatry Clin Neurosci 2009; 259:120–129.

84. Michelson D, Adler L, Spencer T, et al. Atomoxetine in adults with ADHD: two randomized, placebo-controlled studies. Biol Psychiatry 2003; 53:112–120.

85. Humphreys C, Garcia-Bournissen F, Ito S, et al. Exposure to attention deficit hyperactivity medications during pregnancy. Can Fam Physician 2007; 53:1153.

FURTHER READING

O'Keane V, Marsh M and Seneviratne G. Psychiatric Disorders and Pregnancy. London: Taylor and Francis, 2006.

Taylor D, Paton C, Kapur S, eds. The Maudsley Prescribing Guidelines. 10th ed. London: Informa Healthcare, 2009.

9

Ethical and legal issues

Hannah Turton and Peter Haughton

INTRODUCTION

The vast majority of wanted pregnancies are unproblematic clinically, ethically and legally. With such pregnancies the doctors' role is at the periphery and marginal. The principal antenatal support for the woman is the midwife, together with other primary care services. The picture changes somewhat when a pregnant woman is also living with or affected by a neurological condition. For some women, pregnancy need not change their care and, in respect of their pregnancy, they can be treated as any other pregnant woman. For others, there will be additional concerns.

This chapter explores the potential ethical and legal conflicts that might arise in the health care management of such women. It first addresses the general ethical and legal principles to be borne in mind before looking at these in the context of the particular pitfalls that might arise in pregnancy. It will be emphasised that a positive approach to ethical and legal thinking will act as a constructive force for better health care management rather than merely a negative, defensive, avoidance approach that can plague certain practices of medicine.

Where specific legal principles are cited, these refer to U.K. law and other jurisdictions although similar will differ in their nuances.

GENERAL PRINCIPLES

Many tomes have been devoted to the minutiae of ethics and law and can be daunting to those unfamiliar with the area. One approach to making the ethical principles of medicine seem manageable is to simplify them into the four principles of what has become known among bioethicists as the 'Georgetown Mantra' (1) (see text box 1). Whilst these have become familiar and have their uses, these principles are often not sufficient in themselves.

Text Box 1
The four principles (1):

- Respect for autonomy
- Beneficence
- Non-maleficence
- Justice

Ethics is not merely the appropriate application of medical principles with the expectation of a justified decision; it goes deeper and further than this. An analogy might be made with the four medical ethical principles and do-it-yourself (DIY) with the four principles representing, say, a hammer, a screwdriver, a saw and a spanner. In unskilled hands much damage can be wrought with such devices and it soon becomes apparent that the DIY enthusiast needs more than one of each tool in the toolbox if s/he is to do a competent job.

A skilled craftsman recognises not only what the correct tool for a specified task is, but also acknowledges the need to modify both tools and technique according to the materials with which s/he is working. S/He has a detailed understanding of the mechanics involved but also an affinity for the materials themselves and how they feel.

If a craftsman's task is governed by the details of the object s/he is to create, a clinician's task is governed by the clinical details of the situation. The materials are the patients themselves and their circumstances. Like the craftsman, doctors in their ethical decision-making will need a reflective and responsive approach in their ethics in order to make appropriate decisions. There are certain foundational concepts in medical ethics and law without which the clinicians' 'tool kit' would be sorely deficient (see text box 2). Though most will be familiar with them, they are fundamental and it is thus worth revisiting them here.

Text Box 2
Foundational concepts:

- Autonomy
- Consent
- Capacity

FOUNDATIONAL CONCEPTS
Respect for Autonomy

The ethical principle of respect for autonomy dictates that people have the right to control what happens to their own person. This principle is robustly upheld in U.K. law (2) and other Western jurisdictions. The implication of this is that the task of doctors is not simply to obtain the best clinical outcome, but to enable patients to exercise their choice about what the best outcome will be for them and thus serve them in helping to achieve this. This has given rise to the emerging theme of 21st century of health care as 'patient-centred'. It should be noted that being 'patient-centred' does not mean 'doing whatever the patient wants'. A health practitioner cannot be compelled to offer a treatment that s/he believes to be clinically detrimental or unnecessary (3). Patient choice will, in general, be limited to a choice between a number of recommended interventions or deciding to do nothing.

Consent

Patient autonomy is legally protected by the requirement for valid consent before any clinical intervention. If an intervention is performed without valid consent, it may be deemed to be assault (4). For consent to be valid it must be a choice made freely, by a person with the capacity to do so and with all relevant information (5) (capacity is addressed below).

Regarding risks of treatment, relevant information can be considered as any risk with a likelihood of 1% or more, though the law does not put a precise percentage figure (6). Rather it looks to the quality of the information given and the particular circumstances of the individual patient (7). If the patient's choice is made freely and with all relevant information, then her/his choice is paramount (see text box 3).

Text Box 3
Requirements for valid consent:

• Sufficiently informed
• Voluntary (free from coercion)

Capacity

Capacity is closely linked with the notion of autonomy. In the United Kingdom, statute law makes the assumption that an adult patient will have capacity to make decisions for herself/himself until it is proven otherwise (8). Very little is required in order to have capacity. In general terms, patients must be able to understand and retain the information relevant to the decision, to use or weigh that information as part of the process of making the decision, and communicate their decision (9). That a decision may be irrational or clinically inadvisable is not proof of incapacity. It has been noted that in some cases irrationality may be symptomatic of incapacity, but it is not in itself diagnostic (see text box 4).

Text Box 4
Requirements for capacity:
The ability to

• Understand information
• Retain information
• Weigh information
• Communicate a decision

In cases where a patient obviously lacks capacity, such as when s/he is unconscious, it must be considered whether or not the person is likely to regain capacity and if this is likely to happen within a time frame which is compatible with deferring the decision until s/he can make it herself/himself. If this is not the case then decisions should be made in the best interests of the patient. Deciding what the best interests of the patient entail is a complex process involving a number of considerations. These will include the previously expressed wishes of the patient. If the previously expressed wishes of the patient have included the desire to refuse life-saving treatment, these must be recorded and witnessed in the form of an advanced directive in order for them to be binding. If the patient has not previously expressed a wish, then either the holder of lasting power of attorney, the court-appointed deputy or those close to the patient should be consulted regarding the wishes of the patient.

Having emphasised the importance of (free) patient choice, there will be some patients who desire a strong and informed figure of authority to help guide them through their very difficult decisions. A sense of care for their patients (beneficence) requires that doctors do help them when they require this, but this is best done by adopting an attitude of empowering the patient to make her/his choice rather than the paternalistic manner of simply stating and implementing what

should be done. That said, there are those within medical ethics who strongly recommend that given that medical practitioners will always be better informed than their patients, the doctor's sense of care actually requires that if patients are seeking to make detrimental choices doctors should do everything short of forced intervention to prevent a poor outcome (10). It is the view of the authors of this chapter that the power imbalance present within the doctor/patient relationship could result in a danger of attempts at persuasion acting as a form of forced intervention which then removes the all important elements of free choice.

If this were the extent of medical ethics and law, the task of behaving appropriately would be very simple; work out what the task is, choose the correct tool and carry out the work. The job would be algorithmic and could well be done by a machine. However, as with a craftsman, the materials worked with will be different each time and require careful assessment and empathy. The success of this endeavour relies wholly on the quality of the doctor/patient relationship. It is therefore worth exploring this further.

THE DOCTOR/PATIENT RELATIONSHIP

In general terms, the nature of the doctor/patient relationship is covenantal rather than contractual. By this it is meant that the doctor is in a covenantal relationship with her/his patient such that there are obligations that flow from the relationship that are not dependent on the other party (11). The clinician's role is primarily to meet the needs of the patient, thus fulfilling her/his duty of care.

Sometimes this gets lost in the language used, when the 'My' of 'My patient' slips into being the 'My' of possession rather than what it should rightly be, that is, the 'My' of relationship. Doctors easily and often inadvertently do this by moving from 'My patients' – those to whom I have a duty of care – to 'My cases' – those situations to which I have been assigned. This terminology often belies what has been forgotten: that appropriate behaviour is, to a great extent, dependant on the clinician's relationship with the patient.

Integral to the doctor/patient relationship are the duties that arise for the doctor. In the United Kingdom, the General Medical Council sets out in broad terms the duties of a doctor and these are given more substance and focus in their publication of Good Medical Practice (12). Likewise, the Royal College of Obstetricians and Gynaecologists have useful guidelines, in particular their 'green top' which 'provide systematically developed recommendations, ... assist[ing] clinicians and patients in making decisions about appropriate treatment for specific conditions' (13). Interestingly, whilst there is clinical guidance for pregnancy and women living with HIV or breast cancer, there is, at yet, none for chronic neurological diseases. Other jurisdictions will have similar guidelines.

The quality of the doctor/patient relationship is governed by both proximity and attentiveness. Where the quality is good or excellent, it is unlikely that ethical or legal conflict will occur. It is where the quality is poor or indifferent that problems may ensue.

The most common breakdown in the relationship (as with other relationships) is poor communication. Doctors who do not listen to their patients are storing up potential problems. If the patient's voice is not heard then decisions taken by doctors will inevitably be flawed. Clearly, failing to listen attentively to a patient is failing to respect the patient's autonomy. It is here that the importance of narrative ethics is evident. Active listening is not merely hearing what is being said but having an appreciation of the values of the speaker. This is not the same as holding the same values, merely recognising that the values expressed are those of the patient and are important to the patient.

Good communication requires not only active listening, but also time spent in explaining and then clarifying understanding. Often in a complex clinical setting there will be a lack of clarity and, sometimes contradictory messages will be forthcoming. To avoid subsequent confusion and misunderstanding, time spent in addressing the issues is time well-spent. For example, a woman's wish to become a mother is so strong that it blocks out the clinical information that she is sub-fertile or that for her to become pregnant would have life-threatening implications. The exasperation of doctors who say 'The number of times I've told the patient . . .' suggests that the patient is not yet willing to hear what has been said. Consequently, constructive progress is unlikely until the underlying problem has been addressed.

Good clinical practice is foundational to appropriate ethical and legal practice. To return to our craftsman's analogy, you could have wonderful technique with a screwdriver, and a natural affinity for the materials at hand, but if you create a shelf when the specification was for a cupboard, you cannot consider yourself to have been successful. There is thus the ethical requirement for clinicians to remain up to date in evidence-based best practice. We will now move on to consider the use of some of these tools in the specific context of pregnancy.

PRINCIPLES AS APPLIED TO PREGNANCY

The issues that may arise in pregnancy can be broadly divided into issues arising prior to conception, those arising during pregnancy and those arising after.

Preconception

Neurologists with patients of childbearing age should, in reviewing a patient's history, discuss with these patients their hopes and aspirations including the desire to start a family. For some women living with a neurological condition the desire for motherhood may be very strong, but the clinical implications could be catastrophic. It must be borne in mind that in many cases the most risk-prone time is not in fact during the pregnancy, but in the puerperium or post-partum. Giving women such information requires a certain amount of tact.

For some women, pregnancy and the puerperium have a direct impact on their disease progression (e.g., multiple sclerosis, during which the relapse rate falls during pregnancy and then rebounds in the puerperium – see chapter 21). For others, their pregnancy and the consideration that they wish to have for their unborn child will modify the treatment of their condition and it is this that leads to a changed prognosis (e.g., those women with epilepsy).

The main role of the doctor in such situations can be viewed as an information provider in helping the woman understand the various possible implications of a pregnancy such that she can make a choice. In some cases, there will be preparations to be made prior to conception such as when modifying the drug regime of women with epilepsy to attempt seizure control on monotherapy at the lowest possible dose (see chapter 12). In others, the main focus of the task is to attempt to help the woman address fully and comprehend the

implications of looking after a child whilst living with a neurological condition.

We now address three preconception domains in which the physician dealing with pregnancy and neurological disease is likely to encounter ethical or legal dilemmas, namely sub-fertility and neurological disease, conception and the avoidance of conception in those with limited capacity and preconception genetic counselling.

Sub-Fertility and Neurological Disease

The wish to become a mother is for many women a very strongly felt need of fulfilment. In embarking towards the goal of motherhood this desire raises an additional component, namely that of societal judgement. In the broader context, people make judgements, implicitly and sometimes explicitly, about the suitability of individual women to become mothers. Doctors are not immune from making these judgements. For the majority of women wishing to start a family, who have no fertility problems, judgements are still made both pre- and especially during pregnancy. Clearly there are many factors in what might determine 'a good mother', few of which might be deemed to be medical. It is worth noting that those couples who have a sub-fertility problem are subject to scrutiny concerning their fitness for parenting (14). It is important for the doctor to differentiate between medical professional opinion and personal prejudice as the latter is likely to be detrimental to the doctor/patient relationship.

> **Case Study 1**
> A 40-year-old woman who has a 7-year history of multiple sclerosis (MS) expresses her strong desire to become pregnant. She has limited use of her left hand due to spasticity and struggles to communicate verbally due to dysarthria. She has been attempting to conceive for 5 years. Her partner is very supportive. Investigations show that she will require in vitro fertilization (IVF) in order to conceive.

Commentary. In this case there are two areas that present ethical dilemma. The first is the challenge of helping this woman to understand the potential impact that the pregnancy could have on her condition. This is particularly significant given the degree of disability she already suffers. The doctor should be aware of her likely unfavourable response to the information and be ready to reiterate without frustration.

The second area that presents a significant challenge is the requirement of the Human Fertilisation and Embryology Act (HEFA) that no fertility treatment services should be provided without taking into account the welfare of any child to be born as a result (15). In the guidance provided by the HEFA's code of practice it is recommended that the welfare assessment should include any aspect of the patient's circumstances that might lead to an inability to look after the child. It is stated explicitly that this might include a physical condition (16). In this case a doctor may make the assessment that the welfare of the child would be adversely affected by the patient's neurological condition, however it is unlikely to lead to a complete inability to care to the child. The totality of her circumstances should be considered and this may include those who support her.

In practice, the responsibility for making this assessment lies with the centre providing the treatment. So, the primary duty of the neurologist is to discuss with her the impact of pregnancy on her condition, encourage her to consider her own capacity to enjoy the experience of parenting and then to refer her for treatment where they will make the appropriate assessment. That said, it may well be appropriate practice for the neurologist to offer to approach the local assisted conception unit (ACU) on behalf of her/his patient to determine what policy the ACU has with regard to treatment of women with her condition. If, in confidence, the neurologist learns that the ACU is unlikely to offer treatment, then it may well be more fitting for the neurologist to discuss this matter with her/his patient rather than expose the woman to rejection from the ACU. This is because the neurologist will have an ongoing relationship with her/his patient and may be in a better position to limit any harm felt by the woman through applying and being rejected by the ACU. Clearly, if the ACU is prepared to accept her as a patient, then the proper referral should be made.

Conception and the Avoidance of Conception in Those with Limited Capacity

In some cases neurological conditions will affect a woman's capacity by limiting her ability to understand, weigh or retain information (e.g., epilepsy leading to brain damage). In these cases the physician must be guided by the principle that capacity is decision specific and commensurate to the gravity of the decision being made (17). The result is that whilst a woman may not have the ability to look after a child a full assessment of her capacity remains necessary regarding each decision. Where it is judged that a patient does not have the capacity to make a decision then a decision must be made in her best interests, with the maximum involvement possible of the patient and it must be the least restrictive option available (18). The issue of capacity and termination is dealt with below.

Preconception Genetic Counselling

In some cases the neurological condition from which a woman suffers may be hereditary. It may only be possible to provide counselling as to the risks involved, in other situations it may be possible to provide testing of the offspring. The options for this may include undergoing IVF followed by pre-implantation genetic diagnosis or post-implantation diagnosis using amniocentesis or chorionic villus sampling. Currently in the United Kingdom, the availability of pre-implantation genetic diagnosis is limited both by resources and legal restrictions. It is worthy of note that clinicians in the United Kingdom are protected from the charge of 'wrongful birth' provided that the pregnant woman was aware of the risk to the child she carries (this is discussed further below).

At present, the reasons why some people are afflicted are poorly understood, but it may well be that there could be a genetic predisposition. Whether or not this is the case, there will be those who have already become mothers before the onset of a neurological condition who may wish to discuss the genetic implications for their children with their doctor. Clearly, openness and honesty are the most appropriate response of the doctor to these concerns. Whilst the doctor may have limited knowledge of these matters, the fact that the woman has these worries should not be dismissed. Referral to genetic counselling might be appropriate or it may be sufficient to acknowledge the patient's anxieties and help the patient to live with this uncertainty. None of us choose our parents nor our genetic make-up. None of us, as a matter of choice, would wish to live with a neurological condition, be it MS, Parkinson disease or motor neurone disease. The fact is that this is a reality for a number of people and the onset and development of their illness limit the choices open to them.

It is important to re-emphasise the concept of autonomy. The choice to proceed to pregnancy may be difficult to accept

by some doctors. The anticipation of complications resulting from a patient's choice can be for some doctors personally distressing, particularly when the doctor has witnessed previous poor outcomes resulting from similar choices. In spite of this, provided the choice is made freely, with sufficient information and the woman has capacity, it is important for the doctor to remain an ally in her choice and stay ready and willing to reassess her clinical situation with her.

During Pregnancy

Once the choice has been made to conceive and this has successfully occurred, there is a new set of dilemmas. Many of these stem from the view that rather than there being a single patient, there are now two, one of whom does not have a voice (19). Obstetricians will be familiar with this, but for some neurologists this might be fresh territory. Whilst it is possible to regard pregnancy as having two patients in one, this is not a helpful or legally accurate view to take. Both ethically and legally the fetus may be recognised as deserving of consideration, but is not of equal legal standing to the mother. Indeed the fetus, *qua* fetus has no legal identity at least under the law in the United Kingdom (20). Legal status is acquired at birth. The result of this is that at any stage in the pregnancy if the mother's life is threatened by the continuation of the pregnancy it is legally acceptable to terminate the pregnancy (with the mother's consent) (21). The dominant status of the pregnant woman is not only evidenced by the legal acceptability of termination, but it is also confirmed in that under U.K. law the doctor's duty to the fetus only extends so far as her/his duty to the mother (22). This is particularly significant in cases where adequate treatment of the mother poses a risk to the fetus. A good example of this would be where the adequate treatment of a woman with epilepsy requires that she take an anti-epileptic drug regime that is known to carry a risk of teratogenicity. If the mother understands the risks of the treatment but decides to proceed with the regime, then even if the fetus is damaged as a result, no action can be brought against the doctor, provided that the mother understood the risk at the time of treatment.

Case Study 2

A 26-year-old woman with severe epilepsy with a history of tonic-clonic seizures expresses a wish to have a child. In collaboration with her neurologist she attempts to gain good seizure control on monotherapy prior to conception. This is very difficult and in the process she experiences a number of seizures. Eventually it is decided that for her health it is best to remain on dual therapy. Six months after this decision is made she conceives. Seven weeks into her pregnancy she suffers a seizure and she comes in to discuss the option of changing her treatment regime.

Commentary

In this case the key things to consider are the following: the likely impact any new regime on the patient and the impact on the fetus as compared to the old regime and the understanding of the patient regarding this information. If the regime the patient is requesting would be beneficial to the patient but is potentially detrimental to the fetus (e.g., if she wants to be returned to a high-dose dual therapy), then the main concern is that she understands the potential risks to the fetus. If she understands them but decides to go ahead with the treatment, this is her choice to make in spite of any additional risk to the fetus.

If the regime that she is suggesting is one that she imagines will beneficial to the fetus but is potentially detrimental to the patient (e.g., if she wishes to attempt seizure control on the same monotherapy that had previously been unsuccessful), then it is vital for the doctor to ensure that her understanding of the facts is correct. She should be reminded that the health of the fetus is dependant of her remaining healthy and that her suffering future seizures will not be beneficial to the fetus. This communication should be handled carefully to ensure that the patient understands that her opinion is valued and that her concern for the fetus is not dismissed as this could lead to a breakdown in the doctor/patient relationship and potentially put the patient's and the fetus's health at risk. Ultimately if she decides that she wants to reduce or refuse her treatment altogether then she is at liberty to do so in spite of any potential harm to the fetus (23).

Another issue that may arise in pregnancy is where the health of the mother requires hasty delivery of the child. This may cause issues both where the delivery is premature and thus the risk of poor outcome for the child must be weighed against the risk of continued pregnancy to the mother, or it may cause an issue where caesarean section is needed but this is unacceptable to the mother. An example of this might be in the case of a patient with severe pre-eclampsia worsening to eclampsia, for which the only definitive treatment is delivery of the fetus (see chapter 10). There may be some cases where in spite of the danger posed to the mother through the continuance of the pregnancy she does not wish to undergo caesarean section. It is important to re-emphasise that although some medical conditions may interfere with a person's capacity to make a decision, this is not necessarily the case and it must be assumed until proven otherwise that a woman has capacity to refuse treatment. In cases of conflicting interests it is worth bearing in mind that the woman herself may be ambivalent as to what decision to make. Creating an adversarial environment may cause her to defend robustly a decision of which she herself is unsure.

Case Study 3

A 35-year-old woman presents in the 30th week of her pregnancy with recurrent visual disturbances and headaches. On investigation she has +++protein in her urine and her blood pressure (BP) is 180/110. She has previously had three miscarriages and is desperate for a child. It is explained to her that if her BP remains above 170/110 in spite of treatment and the fetus shows signs of distress, it is recommended that she is delivered by caesarean section for her own health. After consulting with her husband she explains that they wish to continue with the pregnancy regardless of the risk to her health as this child is too precious to risk losing. Shortly after this conversation her BP rises steeply, she has a convulsion and falls unconscious. The fetus continues to show signs of distress.

Commentary

In this case although her previously expressed wish was to continue with the pregnancy in spite of the risk to her health, at this stage her refusal of delivery presents a severe danger to her health and even her life. In order for a refusal of life-saving treatment to be valid it must be a witnessed legal refusal (24). In this situation it is important to consider the views of the husband, but ultimately the treating team must act in the best interests of the patient. It is important to ensure that the partner understands why the delivery is necessary and it

would be prudent to cultivate the relationship of an ally rather than an adversary.

There have been cases reported of pregnant women who have had their lives artificially prolonged in intensive care unit (ICU) in order that the fetus might reach viability. These tend to be tragic cases of trauma where the woman is assessed by the neurologist as being brainstem dead. Whilst it might be laudable to save the life of the unborn child, each case would need to be judged on its merits. There is an element here of 'can do' and therefore 'will do'. Clearly the welfare situation of the unborn child together with the quality of life would be the primary considerations. The wishes of the grieving family would form a major component in the decision-making process and great sensitivity will need to be exercised by the health care team.

Termination

Thus far we have discussed only wanted pregnancies and those yet to come about but it is necessary here to address briefly unwanted pregnancies. Abortion law varies considerably internationally with some jurisdictions being much more restrictive than others. Different issues arise according to whether the pregnant woman has capacity. In the United Kingdom where a woman has capacity then termination is guided by her desire and the requirements of the Abortion Act 1967 (25). When a patient lacks capacity the decision must be made in her best interests. In these cases it is worthy of note that the earlier the termination, the less invasive the termination and the more likely it is to be found to be in the best interests of the patient (26).

CONCLUSION

The potential for ethical and legal problems in this combined field of medical practice is enormous. Our case studies have acted as a way of illustrating how such matters may or may not be approached and the pitfalls that trap the unwary. Key to navigating through the potential ethical and legal problems is an awareness of where likely conflicts of interests and values may occur. Some of this is gained by experience and from learning and reflecting on situations that have proved unsatisfactory. To end on a positive note, the doctor who is attentive to the potential problems that are part and parcel of clinical practice will be better equipped to deal with such situations when they arise and act appropriately.

REFERENCES

1. Beauchamp TL, Childress JF. Principles of Biomedical Ethics. 5th ed. New York: Oxford University Press, 2001. Popularised in the UK by Professor Raanan Gillon – see Principles of Health Care Ethics. In: Gillon R, ed. Chichester: Wiley, 1996, and Gillon R. Medical ethics: four principles plus attention to scope. BMJ 1994; 309:184 and online at http://www.bmj.com/cgi/content/full/309/6948/184?eaf.

2. 'An adult patient who suffers no mental incapacity has an absolute right to choose whether to consent to medical treatment, to refuse it or to chose one rather than another of the treatments being offered' Lord Donaldson MR Re T [1993] Fam 95.

3. 'Autonomy and the right to self determination do not entitle the patient to insist on receiving a particular medical treatment regardless of the nature of the treatment ultimately a patient cannot demand that a doctor administer a treatment which the doctor considers is adverse to the patient's clinical needs' Lord Phillips R (on the application of Burke) v The General Medical Council [2005] EWCA Civ 1003.

4. 'It is trite law that in general a doctor is not entitled to treat a patient without the consent of someone who is authorised to give that consent. If he does so, he will be liable in damages for trespass to the person and may be guilty of criminal assault' Lord Donaldson MR Re R (Wardship) (A Minor: Consent to treatment) [1992] Fam 11.

5. The need for informed consent was established by the land mark Sidaway case 'If one considers the scope of the doctor's duty by beginning with the right of the patient to make his own decision whether he will or will not undergo the treatment proposed, the right of the patient to be informed of significant risk and the doctor's corresponding duty are easy to understand: for the proper implementation of the right requires that the doctor be under a duty to inform his patient of the material risks inherent in the treatment' Lord Scarman Sidaway v Board of Governors of the Bethlem Royal Hospital and the Maudsley Hospital [1985] AC 871 (HL).

6. Chester v Afshar [2004] UKHL 41.

7. Chatterton v Gerson [1981] QB 432.

8. Mental Capacity Act 2005 Section 1 (2).

9. Mental Capacity Act 2005 Section 3 (1).

10. Savulescu J. Rational non-interventional paternalism: why doctors ought to make judgments of what is best for their patients. J Med Ethics 1995; 21:327–331.

11. A parallel paradigm is the parent/child relationship. A parent will talk of 'This is my child' where clearly the 'my' is one of relationship and not of possession. The parents will have duties towards their children that are covenantal rather than contractual. How well they fulfil those duties within the covenant is a separate issue.

12. See the GMC's website http://www.gmc-uk.org/guidance/good_medical_practice.asp. Accessed 13/11/11.

13. See the RCOG's website http://www.rcog.org.uk/womens-health. Accessed 13/11/11.

14. Human Fertilisation and Embryology Act 1990 c.37. 13 (4): 'A woman shall not be provided with treatment services unless account has been taken of the welfare of any child' Guidance on how to carry out this assessment is provided by the HFEA Code of practice 7th edition (2007) at G3.3.1. Please see case study 1 for further discussion.

15. Ibid.

16. G 3.3.2 (b) i, S 7.1.2 HFEA code of practice, 7th ed. 2007, at pp. 104–105, p. 55 of 262. Available at: http://cop.hfea.gov.uk/cop/pdf/CodeOfPracticeVR_3.pdf. Accessed 03/09/08.G 3.3.2 (b)
In order to take into account the welfare of the child, the centre should consider factors which are likely to cause serious physical, psychological or medical harm, either to the child to be born or to any existing child of the family. These factors include: any aspect of the patient's (or, where applicable, their partner's) past or current circumstances which is likely to lead to an inability to care for the child to be born throughout its childhood or which are already seriously impairing the care of any existing child of the family. Such aspects might include:
(i) mental or physical conditions

S.7.1.2 The Centre shall ensure that all assisted conception Processes are conducted in a manner that takes into account the welfare of any child that may be born as a result of treatment services.

17. Mental Capacity Act 2005 Section 1 (5).

18. Mental Capacity Act 2005 Section 1 (6).

19. Chervenak FA, McCulloug. LB. The fetus as a patient: an essential ethical concept for maternal-fetal medicine. J Matern Fetal Neonatal Med 1996; 5(3):115–119.

20. 'Although human and protected by the law in a number of different ways..., an unborn child is not a separate person from its mother. Its need for medical assistance does not prevail over her rights'. Judge LJ St Georges NHS Trust v S [1999] Fam 26.

21. Abortion Act 1967.

22. Congenital Disability Act 1974.

23. Butler-Sloss LJ. 'A competent woman who has the capacity to decide may, for religious reasons, other reasons, for rational or irrational reasons or for no reason at all, choose not to have a medical intervention, even though the consequence may be the death or serious handicap of the child she bears, or even her own death'. Re MB (An Adult: Medical Treatment) [1999] Fam 26.

24. Mental Capacity Act 2005 Section 25 (6).

25. Abortion Act 1967 Section 1 (1).

26. 'The nature of the procedure required to terminate the pregnancy required at 23+ weeks has been a powerful factor in my decision. Had the case been heard at an earlier stage in the pregnancy, the balance might well have shifted the other way' Wall J Re SS (An Adult: Medical Treatment) [2006] 1 FLR 445 – In this case the judge found that termination was not in the best interests of the patient.

10

Pre-eclampsia/eclampsia and peri-partum convulsions

Michael S. Marsh

INTRODUCTION

Hypertensive disorders are the most common medical complication of pregnancy, found in about 6% to 8% of all pregnancies. Approximately one half of hypertensive disorders in pregnancy are caused by chronic hypertension, and the remainder are due to pre-eclampsia, giving an incidence of pre-eclampsia of around 2% to 8%, depending on the definition used. The spectrum of pre-eclampsia ranges from mildly elevated blood pressures (BP) with little clinical significance (which has been termed pregnancy-induced hypertension) to severe hypertension and multi-organ dysfunction.

Risk factors for pre-eclampsia include a previous history of pre-eclampsia, primiparity, obesity, family history of pre-eclampsia, multiple pregnancies and chronic medical conditions such as long-term hypertension or diabetes (1). Some of these factors, such as obesity and diabetes, are steadily increasing in the obstetric population in the developed world, so pre-eclampsia is a condition that is likely to become even more common in future.

There is increasing evidence that pre-eclampsia is not a single disease entity, but two different conditions which have different times of onset, pathophysiology and maternal and fetal effects. The early form, with onset before 34 weeks, is more severe and associated with worse perinatal and maternal outcomes during the pregnancy and more likely to recur in the next pregnancy. Early-onset pre-eclampsia is also linked with an increased risk of long-term maternal hypertension, heart disease and associated metabolic disturbances, including higher insulin levels and evidence of endothelial dysfunction (2).

Pre-eclampsia is responsible for the deaths of 60,000 women per year worldwide (3). The acute cerebral complications, such as eclampsia, intracranial haemorrhage and cerebral oedema are responsible for around two-thirds of these fatalities (4,5). In the United Kingdom, eclampsia accounts for 6% of direct maternal deaths (6), for nearly 50% of pregnancy-related ischaemic strokes and around 40% of pregnancy-related haemorrhagic strokes (7,8).

PRE-ECLAMPSIA – AN OVERVIEW

Although pre-eclampsia is most often recognised by new-onset hypertension and proteinuria appearing after 20 weeks of pregnancy, pre-eclampsia may occur in women with hypertension who do not have proteinuria and in women who are proteinuric without hypertension. In such cases, the diagnosis will be based on the presence of other features such as fetal compromise, liver dysfunction, eclampsia, renal impairment without proteinuria or thrombocytopaenia and consumption of clotting factors. Although the criteria for the diagnosis of pre-eclampsia have been defined as hypertension after 20 weeks of gestation in a woman with previously normal BP and significant proteinuria (9) a more clinically useful definition, which will avoid missing clinical cases and subsequent adverse outcomes, is the more general 'a multisystem disorder peculiar to pregnancy that usually presents after 20 weeks' gestation which is characterised by hypertension and proteinuria but which may clinically affect the foetoplacental unit, coagulation and the function of the liver, kidney and nervous system'.

Hypertension in pregnancy is widely defined as a systolic BP of 140 mmHg or greater or a diastolic BP of 90 mmHg or greater present on at least two occasions at least 4 hours apart (10). Significant proteinuria in pregnancy is defined as the presence of 0.3 g or more protein in a 24-hour urine specimen (9).

PATHOPHYSIOLOGY OF PRE-ECLAMPSIA

The aetiology of pre-eclampsia remains largely unclear, and the mechanism for the interaction of the known abnormalities of placental development, autoimmune disorders and endothelial cell damage in pre-eclampsia remains poorly understood. Vascular endothelial cell damage is a common end point in a number of organs affected in pre-eclampsia.

The hypertensive changes seen in pre-eclampsia are thought to be due to vasospasm caused by increased vascular reactivity secondary to endothelial inflammatory damage related to alterations of factors that cause vasodilatation, such as prostacyclin and nitric oxide, and factors causing vasoconstrictive such as thromboxane A2 and endothelin. A current strong candidate implicated in the process is the soluble receptor for vascular endothelial growth factor (VEGF)-1 which binds VEGFs and placental growth factors (11). Another hallmark of the vascular effects of pre-eclampsia is haemoconcentration. Women with pre-eclampsia have lower intravascular volumes, partly due to endothelial damage allowing distribution of fluid into the peripheral tissues.

The pathognomonic renal lesion in pre-eclampsia is glomerular capillary endotheliosis, which on histology is seen as swelling of the glomerular capillary endothelial and mesangial cells (12). This change is thought to be due to endothelial damage affecting the glomerulus, leading to proteinuria. The same endothelial damage process may affect tubular function, although this is less common and seldom severe. Renal failure directly as a result of pre-eclampsia is uncommon. Serum uric acid is often raised in pre-eclampsia and believed to result primarily from the decreased renal excretion that occurs as a consequence of the pre-eclampsia, although there is also evidence that there is increased generation of uric acid from the ischaemic placenta (13).

The most common haematologic abnormality in pre-eclampsia is thrombocytopaenia (<100,000/mL), probably as a result of consumption during the associated low-grade disseminated intravascular coagulation in the microvasculature. As platelet count falls in normal pregnancy, serial platelet measurements are often needed to confirm an effect. If the platelet count remains stable then more severe clotting abnormalities are seldom seen (14). However, pre-eclamptic consumptive coagulopathy can become more severe leading to factor-VIII consumption (15) and consumption of vitamin K clotting factors causing elevation of prothrombin time and partial thromboplastin time and clinical sings of coagulopathy.

HELLP syndrome [haemolysis (H), elevated liver enzymes (EL), and low platelet count (LP)] is diagnosed by laboratory findings consistent with haemolysis, elevated levels of liver function tests and thrombocytopaenia. The BP may be normal or only marginally elevated. HELLP syndrome is considered a manifestation of severe pre-eclampsia and not distinct from this condition. Acronyms for other combinations of effects of pre-eclampsia on different organ systems have not been developed to date.

Hepatic effects of pre-eclampsia range from mildly elevated transaminase levels to subcapsular liver haematomas and hepatic rupture. The last is commonly associated with HELLP syndrome. Histopathology shows periportal haemorrhages, ischaemic areas and fibrin deposition, and are a result of endothelial damage. Women with liver oedema or haemorrhages may complain of epigastric discomfort.

The foetoplacental unit is affected to varying degrees in pre-eclampsia, from no obvious clinical effects on fetal growth to intrauterine growth restriction, placental abruption, fetal distress or fetal demise. It is clear that in women who develop severe pre-eclampsia these effects are in part caused by the abnormal adaptation of the spiral artery/cytotrophoblast interface in the second trimester of pregnancy which results in high resistance to flow in the placental circulation and poor placental perfusion.

MANAGEMENT OF PRE-ECLAMPSIA

Delivery of the placenta is the only treatment for pre-eclampsia. The maternal condition usually improves soon after delivery, although in severe cases there may be further clinical deterioration for a few days, and during this period occasionally new severe manifestations such as liver abnormalities or eclampsia may occur. The decision to deliver a patient with pre-eclampsia is to be made by balancing the maternal and fetal risks by ongoing assessment of the effects of pre-eclampsia on each organ system and the likely chance of these worsening to critical levels for the fetus or mother. For example, women with heavy proteinuria may be managed conservatively if serum proteins are maintained (16). In contrast, significant abnormalities of liver transaminases, with or without HELLP syndrome, usually prompt delivery, as deterioration of liver function with pre-eclampsia is usually rapid. Fetal assessment and the timing of delivery for fetal concerns rely on serial ultrasound assessment of fetal well-being by measurement of growth, liquor volume, fetal movement and Doppler measures of fetal circulatory changes.

The two main goals of drug treatment of women with pre-eclampsia are prevention of eclampsia and the control of hypertension to avoid early delivery because of concerns about severe hypertension and consequent haemorrhagic stroke. In the non-acute setting, oral labetalol, nifedipine or alpha-methyldopa are commonly used. Drugs used in the acute treatment of severe hypertension (mean arterial pressure >125 mmHg) include intravenous (IV) hydrallazine, labetalol or nitric oxide. The prevention and termination of eclamptic seizures are discussed below.

NEUROLOGICAL ASPECTS OF PRE-ECLAMPSIA AND ECLAMPSIA
Neurological Symptoms and Signs of Pre-Eclampsia

Cerebral symptoms in pre-eclampsia include headache, dizziness, tinnitus, hyperreflexia and clonus, drowsiness, altered mental status, visual disturbances and seizures (17). Severe disease can lead to cortical blindness or coma. Symptoms and signs of cerebral disease can be used as warning signs of impending eclampsia, although isolated symptoms are quite common in the normal obstetric population.

The headache of pre-eclampsia is persistent, unrelieved by analgesics such as paracetamol and is often described by the patient as 'throbbing'. Headache is reported by 82.5% of patients prior to seizures (17). However, headache also remains the most common neurological symptom in pregnancy, commonly of the tension-type.

The visual disturbances which can occur in pre-eclampsia have been compared to the aura of a migraine and include flashing and multicoloured lights, blurring and scotomata. They have been reported in around 45% of women who have an eclamptic seizure (17). Temporary amaurosis has occasionally been reported in women with eclampsia. It usually resolves within 7 days (18). Retinal detachment has been reported to occur in 1% to 2% of eclamptic patients (19). Cortical blindness can result from microinfarction, microhaemorrhages and oedema in the occipital cortex and is often a manifestation of the posterior reversible encephalopathy syndrome (PRES) (20).

Deep tendon reflexes are increased in many women prior to seizures (17) but mild to moderate hyperreflexia is not a reliable predictor of eclampsia. Physiological hyperreflexia can occur in an understandably anxious woman who is admitted with pre-eclampsia, and conversely seizures often occur in the absence of hyperreflexia (17). Three or more beats of clonus is considered to be pathological and may have more prognostic significance.

Eclampsia

The seizures of eclampsia are classical generalised tonic-clonic seizures, although focal seizures have occasionally been described (17). In women within a hospital setting where treatment to terminate the seizure is readily available, about two-third of women who develop eclampsia will have a single seizure and the remaining third will have two seizures. The risk of three or more seizures is around 8% (21).

Prediction of Eclampsia

Eclamptic seizures occur in less than 1% of women with severe pre-eclampsia. Around one-third of eclamptic seizures will occur post-delivery. In general, it appears that prediction of an eclamptic seizure is difficult using neurological symptoms and signs, as evidenced by older case series, before the widespread use of preventative treatment, which report that 43% to 83% of women who have eclampsia are inpatients prior to the onset of seizure (22,23). Headache and visual disturbances are absent in up to 30% of women immediately before a seizure, hyperreflexia is absent in up to 20% and more than half show no ankle clonus (23). This difficulty is confirmed by a more recent study of 445 women with pre-eclampsia and eclampsia which examined the factors that were associated with eclamptic seizures (24). With univariate analysis, the following variables were found to have a statistically significant association with eclampsia: elevated uric acid, proteinuria >3+, headache, visual symptoms and deep tendon reflexes >3+; low serum albumin and raised serum creatinine. However, with multivariate analysis only headache and deep tendon reflexes >3+ remained significant predictors. There was no association of eclampsia with systolic, diastolic or mean arterial BP, quantitative proteinuria, epigastric pain, bleeding, gestational age at delivery, history of pre-eclampsia or chronic hypertension. In this study, the greatest morbidity associated with eclampsia occurred in women with preterm gestations not receiving medical attention.

In another smaller retrospective study of 53 women with eclampsia, headache preceded seizures in two-third of cases and visual disturbance preceded seizures in one-third of cases. Uric acid levels were significantly elevated in around 80% of women. In 60% of cases, seizures were the first sign of pre-eclampsia and only nine cases were deemed to be potentially preventable with current standards of practice (25). The difficulty in predicting eclampsia is chiefly because there is no satisfactory objective method of assessing the neurological effects of pre-eclampsia.

Further diagnostic confusion may occur because visual disturbance may be a common neuro-ophthalmic side effect of treatment with IV magnesium sulphate ($MgSO_4$). However, it may be possible to distinguish between symptom and side effect as pre-eclampsia/eclampsia is more associated with scotomata and blurring, whereas IV $MgSO_4$ use is associated with diplopia and blurring (26).

Neurological symptoms associated with pre-eclampsia can also be elicited in the peripheral nervous system. Paraesthesia can occur due to compression of the medial and ulnar nerves (17). However, this is likely to be due to compression secondary to oedema and may also be found in normal pregnancy.

NEUROLOGICAL INVESTIGATIONS IN PRE-ECLAMPSIA AND ECLAMPSIA
Computed Axial Tomography (CT) Scan
Nearly half of women who have had an eclamptic seizure have abnormal CT findings (27). The most common abnormality is the appearance of hypodense areas, which can be found in women without any neurological symptoms or signs. There appears to be little correlation between the extent of the lesions with either the rise in BP or the number of seizures (28). The hypodensity is likely to be due cerebral oedema. The presence of cerebral oedema can also be suggested by loss of sulci and reduced ventricular size seen in some post-eclamptic women. These findings on imaging are similar to those of the PRES syndrome. The hypodense lesions at the grey-white matter junction are typically found primarily in the parieto-occipital lobes. Less commonly, such lesions may be found in the frontal and inferior temporal lobes, basal ganglia and thalamus (27). Other CT findings in eclampsia include parenchymal and intraventricular haemorrhage and cerebral infarction.

Magnetic Resonance Imaging
Magnetic resonance imaging (MRI) is more sensitive than CT in detecting cerebral changes in eclampsia. Areas of hyperintensity are seen on T2-weighted images (29). These lesions represent cerebral oedema and tend to be preferentially located in the posterior brain. This posterior brain predominance may be related to innervation of blood vessels supplying this area. In hypertensive states such as pre-eclampsia, cerebral autoregulation is maintained due to the autonomic response of the blood vessels supplying the brain (30). The vertebrobasilar

vessels that supply the posterior brain have a relatively reduced sympathetic innervation and therefore respond less to hypertension. The hyperintense lesions in most cases resolve, but around a quarter of eclamptic women may demonstrate persistent lesions several weeks post-partum. It is uncertain whether these areas represent permanent brain ischaemia (31,32). The role of neuroimaging in the clinical management of pre-eclampsia/eclampsia is to confirm the diagnosis in women with unusual or uncommon neurological signs and symptoms, to exclude intraventricular haemorrhage and cerebral infarction in women with prolonged coma or for those with prolonged recovery (33).

Neurophysiological Tests
The electroencephalogram (EEG) is abnormal in almost all eclamptic patients, showing slow delta or theta waves and intermittent generalised epileptiform seizure activity. Between 15% and 35% of pre-eclamptic patients will show evidence of slow EEG activity (17). There is a correlation between the slowing of background activity and the drowsiness of the mother (28). However, BP does not appear to be correlated with EEG abnormalities (34). Visual evoked potential (VEP) latency has been reported to be related to systolic BP in pre-eclamptic but not in normotensive pregnant women (35). After eclamptic seizures, the EEG may remain abnormal for 3 to 6 months. This implies a prolonged state of cortical irritation after the acute eclampsia (28).

Angiography
Cerebral angiography shows widespread vasoconstriction of the intracranial circulation in eclampsia (36). However, angiography has a limited role in the management and investigation of pre-eclampsia due to its invasive nature and radiation exposure.

Doppler Ultrasound Studies
Doppler ultrasound measurement can be used to detect changes in cerebral blood flow. Transcranial Doppler can be used to examine the basal arteries of the brain, and colour Doppler ultrasound to measure the orbital circulation. The latter is embryologically, anatomically and functionally similar to the small-diameter cerebral arteries, so blood flow changes in orbital arteries may reflect similar changes are occurring in resistance vessels in parenchyma of the brain (37).

Most eclamptic seizure activity occurs in middle cerebral artery (MCA) territory (37) and it is possible that eclamptic seizures occur due to a failure of autoregulation in this vessel. Increased blood flow velocities in the MCA are found in eclamptic women when compared to non-eclamptic women, suggesting that cerebral vasospasm is important in the pathophysiology of eclampsia (38,39). This increase in blood flow varies with posture (39) and can be detected in pre-eclamptic women even when there is very little change in BP (38). This offers some explanation for the 23% of eclamptic women who have minimal or absent hypertension at the onset of seizures (41). In contrast, a closer correlation has been reported between systemic BP and blood flow in the orbital arteries (41).

Cerebral perfusion pressure (CPP) may be estimated from Doppler measurements and it has been suggested that CPP measurements may have a role to play in selecting the most appropriate treatment for pre-eclamptic patients (37). In patients with mild pre-eclampsia the CPP is lower than in severe cases (41). It may be that in mild pre-eclampsia there is vasospasm leading to an initial decrease in CPP and that the resulting pathophysiology in mild pre-eclampsia is ischaemia. In more severe cases, vasospasm becomes more prolonged, the systemic BP increases to improve perfusion and the CPP increases and produces cerebral damage via a hypertensive encephalopathy (37).

It has been suggested that pre-eclamptic women with a low CPP should have their BP reduced and the cerebral vasculature dilated to reduce ischaemic damage. Nifedipine would be appropriate. In contrast, in patients with a high CPP the mechanism of cerebral damage is overperfusion leading to a hypertensive encephalopathy. These women therefore need to have the BP reduced without cerebral vasodilatation, which could increase hyperperfusive damage, and a beta-blocker such as labetalol may be the optimal pharmaceutical agent. Such management principles have not yet been the subject of detailed study.

Changes seen on Doppler flow have also been reported to be related to some of the neurological symptoms of pre-eclampsia. Visual symptoms are associated with vasospasm of the central retinal artery (38). A significantly higher CPP has been found in women with pre-eclamptic headaches than without (37).

MAGNESIUM SULPHATE

$MgSO_4$ has been used to prevent eclamptic seizures since 1906. It significantly reduces the incidence of seizures in women with severe pre-eclampsia and has been shown to be superior to other anticonvulsants in the treatment of recurrent eclamptic seizures (42,43). There have also been suggested benefits for the fetus, with a possible protective effect against cerebral palsy (44).

At present, $MgSO_4$ is the clear current first choice drug used to terminate eclamptic seizures in the developed world. However, its use and the criteria for its use in women with pre-eclampsia remain controversial. There is no evidence for benefit in women with mild pre-eclampsia. In women with severe pre-eclampsia, it is common practice to give parenteral $MgSO_4$ around the time of delivery and to continue the infusion for at least 24 hours post-delivery. This is chiefly because clinical signs, symptoms or investigations are poor predictors of the 1% of women with severe pre-eclampsia who will have an eclamptic seizure. The largest randomised trial to date, the Magpie trial, enrolled 10,141 women with pre-eclampsia in 33 nations (largely in the developing world) (21). The majority of women enrolled as patients had severe disease. Among all women, the rate of eclampsia was significantly lower in those assigned to $MgSO_4$ (0.8% vs. 1.9%; relative risk (RR): 0.42; 95% confidence interval (CI), 0.29–0.60). Overall, 11 per 1000 fewer women allocated $MgSO_4$ had an eclamptic convulsion. However, among the 1560 women enrolled in the Western world, the rates of eclampsia were 0.5% in the magnesium group versus 0.8% in the placebo, a difference that was not significant (RR: 0.67; 95% CI: 1.19–2.37). Most women recruited in unit in the West had less severe pre-eclampsia, presumably because women within units recruiting in the West were given $MgSO_4$ rather than being recruited to the trial. Side effects of $MgSO_4$ include flushing (in around 20%) and nausea and vomiting (in around 4%). More serious side effects as a result of overdose include, in order of development, absent tendon reflexes, respiratory depression and cardiac arrest, but these problems are unlikely to occur if vital signs are monitored. In the Magpie trial, respiratory depression or absent tendon reflexes was the reason for stopping treatment in 1.4% of women allocated $MgSO_4$ and 1.3% allocated to placebo infusion.

MECHANISM OF ACTION OF MgSO$_4$

The vasospasm seen in pre-eclampsia may be due to endothelial dysfunction which makes the vessel more susceptible to free radical damage (45) and lower the threshold for eclamptic seizures (46). The mechanism by which $MgSO_4$ acts in the treatment of pre-eclampsia is uncertain, but may include cerebrovascular effects to prevent vasospasm, direct action on neural conduction or effects on the general cardiovascular system.

Cerebrovascular Effects

$MgSO_4$ produces vasodilatation of the cerebral vessels. Pre-eclamptic women treated with $MgSO_4$ have been reported to show reduced vasospasm of the middle cerebral and internal carotid arteries (45). This vasodilatation may be produced by an inhibition of the calcium required for smooth muscle contraction. Magnesium competes with calcium for binding sites and may alter the flux of calcium ions across cell membranes (47). $MgSO_4$ also increases levels of prostacyclin, which has vasodilatory properties (48). In vitro studies suggest that $MgSO_4$ may protect against free radical–induced vasospasm (49).

However, $MgSO_4$ also produces peripheral vasodilatation. In some women, this peripheral effect may dominate and the overall effect of $MgSO_4$ might be a decrease in cerebral perfusion (37). $MgSO_4$ will have no therapeutic effect if it produces a further decrease in cerebral perfusion in pre-eclampsia due to vasospasm and underperfusion. This may explain the cases of pre-eclampsia that are resistant to $MgSO_4$. Drugs with more selective cerebral vasodilatory effects such as nifedipine may be more effective in pre-eclampsia associated with a reduced CPP (37).

A decrease in cerebral perfusion may, however, be therapeutic for some pre-eclamptic women. As discussed above, overperfusion and hypertensive encephalopathy may be important in severe pre-eclampsia. If $MgSO_4$ leads to a decrease in CPP, it reverses or prevents overperfusive cerebral damage.

Trials of pre-eclampsia treatment based on CPP findings may help to define a role for $MgSO_4$ in the treatment of pre-eclampsia.

Direct Central Nervous System Effects

It had been hypothesised that $MgSO_4$ has a direct effect on the central nervous system (CNS) as a consequence of disruption to the blood-brain barrier and leakage of Mg^{2+} into the brain (50). Mg^{2+} can block the action of N-methyl-D-aspartate which is an excitatory neurotransmitter in the CNS. $MgSO_4$ may prevent seizures by inhibiting excitatory impulses in the brain (51).

However, one report revealed that there is no difference in the permeability of the blood-brain barrier to Mg^{2+} in pre-eclamptic women compared to normotensive pregnant women (52). Furthermore, abnormal EEG traces have been seen in pre-eclamptic and eclamptic women despite maternal therapeutic magnesium levels (34), suggesting that direct effects may not be important.

Cardiovascular Effects

As well as acting as an anticonvulsant, $MgSO_4$ can also act as an antihypertensive and significant decreases in BP have been reported (53).

The hypotensive effect of $MgSO_4$ may be mediated by inhibition of calcium transport between cells and across the vascular membranes (45). MgSO$_4$ also produces a decrease in levels of endothelin-1, which is a potent vasoconstrictor (54). Nitric oxide mediates vasodilatation via cyclic guanosine monophosphate (cGMP), the secretion of which increases in pre-eclamptic women treated with infusions of MgSO$_4$ (55).

However, the hypotensive effects of MgSO$_4$ are only transient, partly because MgSO$_4$ is rapidly secreted by the kidney (45) and partly because MgSO$_4$ produces an increase in stroke volume and cardiac output which counteracts the vasodilatation and maintains BP (56). The therapeutic role of MgSO$_4$ in decreasing BP in pre-eclampsia is limited, and this effect is probably not an important mechanism of anti-eclamptic action.

STROKE

Cerebral haemorrhage has been reported to be the most common cause of death in patients with eclampsia (57,58), and stroke is known to be the most common cause of death (45%) in women with HELLP syndrome (5). Although the majority of pre-eclampsia–related strokes are haemorrhagic, eclampsia is also the commonest associated condition with non-haemorrhagic stroke in the pregnant patient (7,8). Up to 40% of eclamptic deaths show evidence of cerebral haemorrhage at autopsy (59). The range of haemorrhage varies from small petechiae to intraventricular and subarachnoid bleeds.

In contrast to the weak relationship between risk of eclampsia and BP, the risk of haemorrhagic stroke in women with pre-eclampsia is closely related to BP. The mechanism for the haemorrhage is likely due to a combination of loss of intracrebral autoregulation as a result of hypertension and a damaged vasculature. There is evidence that cerebral blood flow is increased in patients with severe pre-eclampsia and that women with severe pre-eclampsia have high CPP compared with controls. This combined with damaged endothelium may mean that the cerebral vasculature is at greater risk for barotrauma and vessel damage than in a woman without pre-eclampsia (60–62). Coagulation disorders may also play a part (63). The risk appears to be related more closely to systolic rather than diastolic BP. In a recent report of 24 haemorrhagic strokes associated with severe pre-eclampsia and eclampsia, in 23 cases the systolic BP was more than 160 mmHg and this has been proposed at a target level to instigate urgent hypertensive treatment in women with pre-eclampsia to prevent stroke (64).

The prognosis for stroke in pregnancy, in general, is poor, with an estimated mortality of 8% to 15% (65), with many survivors suffering profound and permanent disability (66,67). Eclampsia complicated by haemorrhagic stroke has a poor prognosis (59,68).

Loss of cerebral vessel autoregulation and vasospasm and a consequential increase in CPP may be the cause of subsequent hypertensive encephalopathy and haemorrhage (37).

PERI-PARTUM CONVULSIONS

Possible causes of peri-partum convulsions are listed in Table 10.1. The individual management of these conditions is dealt within the other chapters in this book. Aside from pre-eclampsia/eclampsia, other conditions causing convulsions that are peculiar to pregnancy include amniotic fluid embolism and acute fatty liver of pregnancy.

Amniotic Fluid Embolism

Amniotic fluid embolism (AFE), although uncommon, has high maternal morbidity and mortality rates and is a leading

Table 10.1   Causes of Peri-partum Convulsions

Epilepsy
  Idiopathic
  Causal condition
Hypertension
  Eclampsia
  Hypertensive encephalopathy
  Posterior reversible encephalopathy syndrome (PRES)
Vascular
  Ischaemic or haemorrhagic stroke
  Subarachnoid haemorrhage
  Cortical venous thrombosis
  Susac syndrome (retinocochleocerebral vasculopathy)
Thrombotic
  Pulmonary embolism
Structural
  Tumour, primary or metastatic
  Abscess
  Arteriovenous (AV) malformations
Infection
  Subdural empyema
  Abscess
  Meningo-encephlalitis
Migraine
  Migranous infarction
Toxins
  Amphetamine
  Cocaine
  Atypical antipsychotic drugs
Obstetric
  Hypovolaemia (haemorrhage)
  Amniotic fluid embolism (AFE)
  Acute fatty liver of pregnancy
Metabolic
  Hyponatraemia
  Hypocalcaemia
  Hypoglycaemia
  Hyperglycaemia
  Hypomagnesaemia

cause of maternal death in the developed world. Over the past five triennia AFE has been responsible for 8.4% of maternal deaths in the United Kingdom (69) and 7.5% to 10% of maternal deaths in the United States (70). Maternal mortality in AFE is around 20% (71,72) and has improved since the 1970s, probably because intensive care facilities have improved alongside a higher index of suspicion for the condition. Clinical presentation ranges from severe cases with maternal collapse, breathlessness, cyanosis, cardiac dysrhythymia, hypotension, convulsions and haemorrhage secondary to disseminated intravascular coagulation (DIC) to milder cases where maternal symptoms may be mild but the fetus shows evidence of fetal distress. A recent case report described AFE presenting as maternal abdominal pain and weakness (73). The condition is caused by a maternal anaphylactic response, probably due to fetal squamous cells being extruded with amniotic fluid into the maternal circulation. Cases can occur during labour, at the time of delivery or immediately post-partum. There is no diagnostic test that has been shown to be reliable, so diagnosis is based on clinical presentation and exclusion of other causes. Management relies on resuscitation, replacement of blood, correction of clotting abnormalities, maintenance of cardiovascular output and prompt delivery of the fetus. It has been suggested that haemodiafiltration could be used to remove cytokines which may be responsible for multi-organ failure in this condition (74).

Acute Fatty Liver of Pregnancy

Acute fatty liver of pregnancy is a rare condition (1 in 20,000 pregnancies), characterised by liver failure of varying degrees due to microvacuolar fatty transformation of hepatocytes. It is identified by the U.K. Confidential Enquiry into Maternal Deaths as a leading cause of maternal mortality. It usually presents in the third trimester of pregnancy with abdominal pain, vomiting and weakness. These symptoms are present in 60% to 80% of cases (75,76). Symptoms can progress as a result of abnormal coagulation [prolonged prothrombin time (PT) and activated partial thromboplastin time (APTT), low fibrinogen] and liver and renal failure to confusion and seizures secondary to encephalopathy and hypoglycaemia. In the acute phase the condition has clinical and diagnostic features similar to HELLP syndrome and management may be similar. When the exact diagnosis remains unclear in the acute phase the treatment for both is similar and the two conditions have been grouped together as 'acute hepatic dysfunction of pregnancy' (AHDOP). As with HELLP syndrome management relies on early diagnosis, prompt delivery, correction of coagulopathy and intensive supportive care. Liver biopsy is seldom performed to confirm the diagnosis because of the risk of bleeding secondary to coagulopathy. Recent studies report a maternal mortality around 13% and a fetal mortality around 17% (77–79). A recent U.K. survey studied outcomes in 61 cases and reported no maternal mortality and a 13% fetal mortality (80).

REFERENCES

1. Duckitt K, Harrington D. Risk factors for pre-eclampsia at antenatal booking: systematic review of controlled studies. BMJ 2005; 330:565.
2. Marsh M. Editor's choice. BJOG 2010; 117(8):i–ii.
3. World Health Organisation. Maternal mortality in 2000: estimates developed by WHO, UNICEF and UNFPA. Geneva: World Health Organisation, 2004.
4. Okanloma KA, Moodley J. Neurological complications associated with the pre-eclampsia/eclampsia syndrome. Int J Gynaecol Obstet 1989; 71:223–225.
5. Isler CM, Rinehart BK, Terrone DA, et al. Maternal mortality associated with HELLP (hemolysis, elevated liver enzymes and low platelets) syndrome. Am J Obstet Gynecol 1999; 181:924–928.
6. Why Mothers Die 2000-2002: The Sixth Report of Confidential Enquiries into Maternal Deaths in the United Kingdom. London: RCOG Press, 2004.
7. Sharshar T, Lamy C, Mas JL. Incidence and causes of strokes associated with pregnancy and puerperium. Stroke 1995; 26: 930–936.
8. Kittner SJ, Stern BJ, Feeser BR, et al. Pregnancy and the risk of stroke. N Engl J Med 1999; 335:674–768.
9. Report of the National High Blood Pressure Education Program Working Group on High Blood Pressure in Pregnancy. Am J Obstet Gynecol 2000; 183:S1–S22.
10. RCOG. Pre-eclampsia – study group consensus statement 01/09/2003.
11. Karumanchi SA, Bdolah Y. Hypoxia and sFlt-1 in preeclampsia: the "chicken-and-egg" question. Endocrinology 2004; 145:4835.
12. Spargo BH, McCartney C, Winemiller R. Glomerular capillary endotheliosis in toxaemia of pregnancy. Arch Pathol 1959; 13: 593–599.
13. Kang D-H, Finch J, Nakagawa T, et al. Uric acid, endothelial dysfunction and pre-eclampsia: searching for a pathogenetic link. J Hypertens 2004; 22(2): 229–235.
14. Leduc L, Wheeler JM, Kirshon B, et al. Coagulation profile in severe preeclampsia. Obstet Gynaecol 1992; 79(1):14–18.
15. Redman CWG, Denson KWE, Beilin LJ, et al. Factor-VIII consumption in pre-eclampsia. Lancet 1977; 310(8051):1249–1252.
16. Schiff E, Friedman SA, Lu Kao RN, et al. The importance of urinary protein excretion during conservative management of severe preeclampsia. Am J Obstet Gynecol 1996; 175(5): 1313–1316.
17. Dekker GA, Walker JJ. Maternal assessment in pregnancy-induced hypertensive disorders: special investigations and their pathological basis; Hypertension in pregnancy. Chapman and Hall: London, 1997.
18. Chesley LC. Hypertensive disorders in pregnancy. New York: Appleton-Century-Crofts, 1978.
19. Donaldson JO. Neurology of Pregnancy. 2nd ed. London: WB Saunders, 1989.
20. Bartynski WS. Posterior reversible encephalopathy syndrome, part 1: fundamental imaging and clinical features. AJNR Am J Neuroradiol 2008; 29:1036–1042.
21. The Magpie Trial Collaborative Group: Do women with preeclampsia, and their babies, benefit from magnesium sulfate? The Magpie trial: a randomized placebo-controlled trial. Lancet 2002; 359:1877–1890.
22. Templeton A, Campbell DM. A retrospective study of eclampsia in the Grampian Region 1965-1977. Health Bull 1979; 37:55–59.
23. Porapakkham S. An epidemiological study of eclampsia. Obstet Gynecol 1979; 54:26–30.
24. Witlin AG, Saade GR, Mattar F, et al. Risk factors for abruptio placentae and eclampsia: analysis of 445 consecutively managed women with severe pre-eclampsia and eclampsia. Am J Obstet Gynecol 1999; 180:1322–1329.
25. Katz VL, Farmer R, Kuller JA. Pre-eclampsia: towards a new paradigm. Am J Obstet Gynecol 2000; 182:1389–1396.
26. Digre KB, Varner MW, Schiffman JS. Neuroophthalmologic effects of intravenous magnesium sulfate. Am J Obstet Gynecol 1990; 163:1848–1852.
27. Brown CE, Purdy P, Cunningham FG. Head computed tomographic scans in women with eclampsia. Am J Obstet Gynecol 1988; 159:915–920.
28. Thomas SV. Neurological aspects of eclampsia. J Neurol Sci 1998; 155:37–43.
29. Sanders TG, Clayman DA, Sanches-Ramos L, et al. Brain in eclampsia: MR imaging with clinical correlations. Radiology 1991; 180:475–478.
30. Schwartz RB, Jones KM, Kalina P, et al. Hypertensive encephalopathy: findings on CT, MR imaging, and SPECT imaging in 14 cases. Am J Roentgenol 1992; 159:379–383.
31. Zeeman GG, Fleckenstein JL, Twickler DM, et al. Cerebral infarction in eclampsia. Am J Obstet Gynecol 2004; 190:714–720.
32. Loureiro R, Leite CC, Kahhale S, et al. Diffusion imaging may predict reversible brain lesions in eclampsia and severe preeclampsia: initial experience. Am J Obstet Gynecol 2003; 189: 1350–1355.
33. Konstantinopoulos PA, Mousa S, Khairallah R, et al. Postpartum cerebral angiopathy: an important diagnostic consideration in the postpartum period. Am J Obstet Gynecol 2004; 191:375–377.
34. Sibai BM, Spinnato JA, Watson DL, et al. Effect of magnesium sulfate on electroencephalographic findings in preeclampsia-eclampsia. Obstetrics Gynecol 1984; 64:261–266.
35. Marsh MS, Smith S. The visual evoked potential in the assessment of central nervous system effects of pre-eclampsia: a pilot study. Br J Obstet Gynaecol 1994; 101:343–346.
36. Will AD, Lewis KL, Hinshaw DB, et al. Cerebral vasoconstriction in toxemia. Neurology 1987; 37:1555–1557.
37. Belfort MA, Giannina G, Herd JA. Transcranial and orbital Doppler ultrasound in normal pregnancy and pre-eclampsia. Clin Obstet Gynecol 1999; 42:479–506.
38. Williams K, MacLean C. Maternal cerebral vasospasm in eclampsia assessed by transcranial Doppler. Am J Perinatol 1993; 10:243–244.
39. Williams K, MacLean C. Transcranial assessment of maternal cerebral blood flow velocity in normal versus hypertensive states: variations with maternal posture. J Reprod Med 1994; 39:685–688.
40. Sibai BM. Eclampsia VI: maternal–perinatal outcome in 254 consecutive cases. Am J Obstet Gynecol 1990; 163:1049–1055.

41. Belfort MA, West SM, Giannina G, et al. Cerebral perfusion pressure is significantly lower in mild pre-eclampsia than in severe pre-eclampsia: pathophysiological implications for eclampsia. J Soc Gynecol Investig 1997; 4:162A.

42. Lucas MJ, Levene KJ, Cunningham FG. A comparison of magnesium sulphate with phenytoin for the prevention of eclampsia. N Engl J Med 1995; 333:201–205.

43. The Eclampsia Trial Collaborative Group: Which anticonvulsant for women with eclampsia? Lancet 1995; 345:1455–1463.

44. Nelson KB, Grether JK. Can magnesium sulphate reduce the risk of cerebral palsy in low birth weight infants? Pediatrics 1995; 95:263–269.

45. Idama TO, Lindow SW. Magnesium sulphate: a review of clinical pharmacology applied to obstetrics. BJOG 1998; 105(3):260–268.

46. Naidu S, Payne AJ, Moodley J, et al. Randomised study assessing the effect of phenytoin and magnesium sulphate on maternal cerebral circulation in eclampsia using transcranial Doppler ultrasound. Br J Obstet Gynaecol 1996; 103:111–116.

47. Levine BS, Coburn JW. Magnesium, the mimic/antagonist of calcium. N Engl J Med 1984; 310:1253–1255.

48. Sipes LS, Weiner CP, Gellhaus TM, et al. Effect of magnesium sulphate infusion upon plasma prostaglandins in pre-eclamptic and pre-term labour. Hypertens Pregnancy 1994; 13:293–302.

49. Dickens BF, Weglicki WB, Li YS, et al. Magnesium deficiency in vitro enhances free radical induced intracellular oxidation and cytotoxicity in endothelial cells. FEBS Lett 1992; 311(3):187–191.

50. Donaldson JD. Does magnesium sulphate treat eclamptic convulsions? Clin Neuropharmacol 1996; 9:37–45.

51. Cotton DB, Hallak M, Janusz C, et al. Central anticonvulsant effects of magnesium sulphate on N-methyl-D-aspartate-induced seizures. Am J Obstet Gynecol 1993; 168:974–978.

52. Fong J, Gurewitsch ED, Volpe L, et al. Baseline serum and cerebrospinal fluid magnesium levels in normal pregnancy and pre-eclampsia. Obstet Gynecol 1995; 85:444–448.

53. Cotton DB, Gonik B, Dorman KF. Cardiovascular alterations in severe pregnancy-induced hypertension: acute effects of intravenous magnesium sulfate. Am J Obstet Gynecol 1984; 148(2):162–165.

54. Mastrogiannis DS, Kalter CS, O'Brien WF, et al. Effect of magnesium sulphate on plasma endothelin-1 levels in normal and pre-eclamptic pregnancies. Am J Obstet Gynecol 1992; 167:1554–1559.

55. Barton JR, Sibai BM, Ahokas RA, et al. Magnesium sulphate therapy is associated with increased urinary cyclic guanosine monophosphate excretion. Am J Obstet Gynecol 1992; 167:931–934.

56. James MFM, Cork RC, Dennet JE. Cardiovascular effects of magnesium sulphate in the baboon. Magnesium 1987; 6:314–324.

57. Okanloma KA, Moodley J. Neurological complications associated with the pre-eclampsia/eclampsia syndrome. Int J Gynaecol Obstet 2000; 71:223–225.

58. Moodley J. Preeclampsia/eclampsia syndrome. S Afr J Contin Med Educ 1997; 15:31–41.

59. Mas J-L, Lamy C. Stroke in pregnancy and the puerperium. J Neurol 1998; 245:305–313.

60. Zeeman GG, Hatab MR, Twickler DM. Increased cerebral blood flow in preeclampsia with magnetic resonance imaging. Am J Obstet Gynecol 2004; 191:1425–1429.

61. Riskin-Mashiah S, Belfort MA, Saade GR, et al. Cerebrovascular reactivity is different in normal pregnancy and preeclampsia. Obstet Gynecol 2001; 98:827–832.

62. Williams KP, Wilson S. Variation in cerebral perfusion pressure with different hypertensive states of pregnancy. Am J Obstet Gynecol 1998; 179:1200–1203.

63. Richards A, Graham D, Bullock R. Clinicopathological study of neurological complications due to hypertensive disorders of pregnancy. J Neurol Neurosurg Psychiatry 1988; 51:416–421.

64. Martin JN Jr., Thigpen BD, Moore RC, et al. Stroke and severe preeclampsia and eclampsia: a paradigm shift focusing on systolic blood pressure. Obstet Gynecol 2005; 105(2):246–254.

65. Jaigobin C, Silver FL. Stroke and pregnancy. Stroke 2000; 31: 2948–2951.

66. Kappelle LJ, Adams HP Jr, Heffner ML, et al. Prognosis of young adults with ischemic stroke: a long-term follow-up study assessing recurrent vascular events and functional outcome in the Iowa Registry of Stroke in Young Adults. Stroke 1994; 25:1360–1365.

67. Hankey GJ, Jamrozik K, Broadhurst RJ, et al. Long-term disability after first-ever stroke and related prognostic factors in the Perth Community Stroke Study, 1989–1990. Stroke 2002; 33:1034–1040.

68. Horton JC, Chambers WA, Lyons SL, et al. Pregnancy and the risk of haemorrhage from cerebral arteriovenous malformations. Neurosurgery 1990; 27:867–872.

69. Department of Health, Welsh Office, Scottish Office Department of Health, Department of Health and Social Services, Northern Ireland. Why mothers die. Report on confidential enquiries into maternal deaths in the United Kingdom, 1997–1999. London: The Stationery Office, 2001:104–110.

70. Atrash HK, Koonin LM, Lawson HW, et al. Maternal mortality in the United States, 1979–1986. Obstet Gynecol 1990; 76: 1055–1060.

71. Burrows A, Khoo SK. The amniotic fluid embolism syndrome: 10 years' experience at a major teaching hospital. Aust N Z J Obstet Gynaecol 1995; 35:245–250.

72. Morgan M. Amniotic fluid embolism. Anaesthesia 1979; 34:20–32.

73. Awad IT, Shorten GD. Amniotic fluid embolism and isolated coagulopathy: atypical presentation of amniotic fluid embolism. Eur J Anaesthesiol 2001; 18:410–413.

74. Tuffnell DJ. Amniotic fluid embolism. Curr Opin Obstet Gynecol 2003; 15(2):119–122.

75. Reyes H. Acute fatty liver of pregnancy: a cryptic disease threatening mother and child. Clin Liver Dis 1999; 3:70–81.

76. Castro MA, Fassett MJ, Reynolds TB, et al. Reversible peripartum liver failure: a new perspective on the diagnosis, treatment and cause of acute fatty liver of pregnancy, based on 28 consecutive cases. Am J Obstet Gynecol 1999; 181:389–395.

77. Knox TA, Olans LB. Liver disease in pregnancy. N Eng J Med. 1996; 335:569–576(s).

78. Castro MA, Fassett MJ, Reynolds TB, et al. Disseminated intravascular coagulation and antithrombin III depression in acute fatty liver of pregnancy. Am J Obstet Gynaecol 1996; 174:211–216 (s).

79. Wanders RJ, IJlst L, Poggi F, et al. Human trifunctional protein deficiency: a new disorder of mitochondrial fatty acid beta-oxidation. Biochem Biophys Res Commun 1992; 188:1139–1145 (s).

80. Knight M, Nelson-piercy C, Kurinczuk J, et al. A prospective national study of acute fatty liver of pregnancy in the UK. Gut 2008; 57:951–956.

11

Blackouts arising in pregnancy

Robert Delamont and Nicholas Gall

INTRODUCTION

The word 'blackout' means many different things to many different people. The dictionary definition is that it represents a temporary loss of consciousness, memory or sight. In clinical practice, the lay definition expands to include collapses, faints, fits, dizzy spells and attacks of undetermined cause. The unifying process is an impairment in generalised cerebral function leading to a loss of the consciousness continuity; the causes are many and various, and characterising the features can be a significant challenge.

In practice, it is useful to divide the causes of such temporary dysfunction into several broad categories, the first three being the most important in numerical terms both in and outside of pregnancy:

- An interruption in cerebral perfusion or syncope
- An electrical discharge or seizure
- Psychological events such as panic episodes or dissociative events
- Dysfunction of sleep regulatory control
- Cerebrovascular events

In the general population syncope is the commonest cause; perhaps up to 30% of the population will pass out at some stage (1). The majority do not seek medical attention and of those that do, a significant proportion (40–85%) will not suffer a recurrence (2). The frequency of syncope in the upright position in the pregnant population is poorly described but given the cardiovascular physiological changes it is not surprising that syncope and presyncope occur quite frequently in pregnancy. The supine hypotensive syndrome is well recognised, affecting up to 11% of women after the 20th week of gestation (3).

Epileptic seizures affect 1% of the population. About 60% of these events either will not recur or are easily controlled with medication. In some cases patients may forget or even be unaware that they have had seizures, particularly if occurring in childhood. Seizures may recur with the changes induced by pregnancy, for example, alterations in life circumstances, reduced sleep and altered eating habits. For those with an established diagnosis of epilepsy, the pregnant state will have variable effects on seizure frequency (see chapter 12). The causes for this are only partly understood. Alteration in drug compliance is a factor and this change may not be reported (4); pharmacodynamic changes will also be important although, with the notable exception of lamotrigine, there is a poor correlation between serum drug levels and seizure frequency.

The incidence of psychological non-epileptic attacks during pregnancy is unknown. However, estimates of between 2 and 33 per 100,000 population have been made (5). There is little evidence to suggest an alteration in the frequency between the pregnant and non-pregnant state. The attacks commonly present in the third decade (6) and three-quarters of them are women (7).

Psychogenic pseudosyncope is also recognised, affecting 24% to 31% of patients with recurrent undiagnosed syncope (8). There is a clear association with depression and panic disorder. Strong emotion is a definite trigger for syncope suggesting that these disorders may be intertwined in a complex fashion.

Subarachnoid haemorrhage may present during pregnancy, and there is a greater incidence during pregnancy, of 1 in 10,000 pregnancies, as a result of increased ruptures of berry aneurysms and arteriovenous malformations (9) (see chapter 6c).

Haemorrhage of the pituitary gland can also be associated with a blackout, though rarely repeated blackouts unless there is pituitary hypofunction.

SYNCOPE
Cardiovascular Changes in Pregnancy

It is well established that there are profound changes in the cardiovascular system during pregnancy. In healthy women, there is a 50% increase in cardiac output; the initial rise is seen as early as by 5 weeks, with half of the total rise seen by 8 weeks. Peripheral vascular resistance falls by one-third by the 16th week and persists thereafter (10,11). This mostly relates to the direct effects of oestrogen and progesterone on resistance vessels, although other hormones such as prostaglandins, atrial natriuretic hormone and endothelial nitric oxide probably contribute. The low-resistance uterine circulation also plays a role. After 20 weeks, cardiac output becomes increasingly susceptible to maternal position; in particular, lying flat can lead to compression of the inferior vena cava and distal aorta with a subsequent fall in venous return and cardiac output (12).

There is an initial slight increase in heart rate during early pregnancy with later increases reaching a maximum of 10% to 15% by the end of gestation. However, this increase contributes little to the increase in cardiac output in the first and second trimesters which is mostly due to an increase in stroke volume.

Blood pressure initially falls in the first trimester, reaching its nadir half way through pregnancy, which correlates to the fall in peripheral resistance. It subsequently returns to preconceptual levels by term.

Blood volume begins to increase during the 6th week and will rise by about 50% although this can vary depending on the pregnancy. There is a greater increase in plasma volume than red cell mass, which largely explains the fall in haemoglobin in pregnancy, although iron and folate deficiency may coexist (13,14).

Pathophysiology of Syncope

The underlying mechanism is transient global cerebral hypoperfusion due to a reduction in cerebral perfusion. This is always associated with a loss of postural tone. Cerebral blood flow is approximately 50 to 60 mL/100 g of brain tissue/min in normal young adults. Whilst homoeostatic mechanisms allow consciousness to be maintained in the face of fairly significant changes in perfusion pressure, this may be impaired in illness and aging.

It has been estimated that as little as a 20% drop in oxygen delivery to the brain can cause a loss of consciousness. While there is a slight reduction in the oxygen-carrying capacity of blood in late pregnancy from 18 to 16 mL/dL of arterial and 13.5 to 12 mL/dL in mixed venous blood, oxygen delivery is not significantly different (868 and 806 mL/min) (15). Several mechanisms maintain adequate cerebral oxygenation and these can be affected by pregnancy.

Cerebral perfusion pressure is largely dependant on systemic arterial blood pressure which in turn depends on cardiac output (the product of heart rate and stroke volume) and peripheral resistance. Arterial baroreceptors are key players in influencing heart rate, cardiac contractility and systemic vascular resistance in order to protect cerebral blood flow. Intravascular volume regulation, largely under renal and endocrine control, ensures an adequate blood volume, and cerebrovascular autoregulation provides a stable cerebral blood flow over a wide range of systemic arterial perfusion pressures. Failure in any one of these control mechanisms leads to a greater chance of syncope.

Venous return influences cardiac output significantly and anything that interferes with it risks a fall in cardiac output and syncope. Blood pooling in the legs on standing is an obvious cause. In the non-pregnant state on standing there is a shift away from the thoracic cavity to the capacitance vessels below the diaphragm of between 0.5 and 1.0 L of thoracic blood. This largely occurs within 10 seconds of standing and is subsequently counteracted by sympathetically mediated contraction of these vessels. With prolonged standing there is a further filtration of protein-free fluid from the vascular compartment into the interstitial spaces due to high capillary transmural pressure. This can be as much as 0.7 L, and further contributes to reduced cardiac filling.

The commonest cause of hypoperfusion leading to syncope relates to an excessive fall in peripheral resistance due to vasodilatation. This can be a sudden event in an intact nervous system, for example, in vasovagal syncope, or a slower event as with autonomic failure. The natural vasodilatation occurring in pregnancy increases the susceptibility to syncope.

Arrhythmia, impaired cardiac pump function or other structural diseases can also reduce cardiac output. Cardiac output rarely falls significantly with changes in heart rate, unless it is profound (to less than 30 or more than 200 beats/min). In the face of associated structural heart disease, however, significant falls in cardiac output can occur at more normal heart rates.

Obstruction to cerebral blood flow itself may also lead to syncope. For instance, increased resistance to cerebral blood flow is seen with hypocapnia due to hyperventilation, although this is rarely seen in pregnancy.

Cardiac Causes of Syncope
Cardiac causes can be further divided into four broad groups:

- Neural reflex syncope or vasovagal syncope
  - Situational syncope
    - emotion related
    - swallowing
    - post-micturition
    - defecation
    - due to increased intrathoracic pressure (cough, sneeze)
  - Prolonged standing or sitting
- Orthostatic hypotension
  - Medication related
  - Autonomic dysfunction such as postural orthostatic tachycardia syndrome (POTS)
  - Related to blood volume change, for example, dehydration
- Arrhythmia related
  - Bradycardias
    - Sinus node disease
    - Atrioventricular conduction disease, including nodal disease and infranodal bundle branch disease
  - Tachycardias
    - Benign supraventricular tachycardias (SVTs)
    - Benign ventricular tachycardias (associated with a normal heart)
    - Rhythms due to accessory pathways (Wolff–Parkinson–White syndrome)
    - Life-threatening ventricular arrhythmias (e.g., dilated or restrictive cardiomyopathies, peri-partum cardiomyopathy, arrhythmogenic right ventricular cardiomyopathy, Brugada syndrome, long QT syndrome, short QT syndrome, early repolarisation syndrome and catecholaminergic polymorphic ventricular tachycardia)
- Cardiac structural disease, particularly obstruction
  - Valve disease, especially aortic and mitral stenosis
  - Other obstructive lesions including atrial myxoma and hypertrophic cardiomyopathy
  - Coronary disease, especially congenital coronary anomalies
  - Pulmonary emboli

As with non-pregnant patients, most blackouts in pregnancy relate to neurocardiogenic mechanisms. Orthostatic hypotension while uncommon in normal young people is more likely to occur due to the vascular changes associated with pregnancy with the additional contribution of uterine pressure on the inferior vena cava. There is a group of patients with orthostatic intolerance with POTS who may have syncope as part of their clinical picture. In established cases, a worsening of symptoms may be expected in the first trimester with an improvement in the second (16). Any arrhythmia can be associated with hypotension, either at its onset prior to vascular compensatory mechanisms or sometimes as part of a neurocardiogenic mechanism initiated during the arrhythmia. In aterioventricular (AV) nodal-dependent arrhythmias (e.g., many SVTs), the vagal excess of a faint may even terminate the rhythm disturbance. Pregnancy is associated with an increase in the frequency of arrhythmias in susceptible patients, particularly SVTs and other cardiac ventricular tachycardias (17). Medications, electrolyte abnormalities (hyperemesis gravidarum) or pre-eclampsia may also increase the risk of ventricular arrhythmia in the susceptible. Heart block is rare in young people; high-grade AV block does not seem to be a bar to a successful pregnancy and there are variable reports of improvement or a deterioration associated with pregnancy (13). Structural lesions may become more significant due to the circulatory changes of pregnancy, particularly valvular stenotic lesions.

NEUROLOGICAL CAUSES OF BLACKOUTS

In quantitative terms, syncope is seen more frequently than neurological blackouts, but the latter carries a greater proportional risk of significant disability. A seizure is the commonest neurological cause seen.

The annual incidence of epilepsy in women of a child-bearing age is 20 to 30 cases per 100,000 persons. Thus, a first presentation during pregnancy by chance alone is not uncommon (18).

Symptomatic seizures may also be due to a structural lesion or a metabolic disturbance but the most likely cause in the second half of pregnancy is eclampsia.

Structural lesions are commonly due to tumours or vascular abnormalities. The commonest tumours are meningiomas, which may expand because of oestrogenic stimulation and this expansion may lead to seizures and increasing mass effect in some cases. Vascular lesions include arteriovenous malformations which may bleed and present with seizures or bleeding with collapse, again because of hormonal changes associated with pregnancy. The prothrombotic state increases the risk of thrombotic stroke both arterial and venous and, paradoxically, bleeding with a higher incidence of subarachnoid haemorrhage. Alterations in immune function are associated with cerebral angiitis, arteritis and cerebral infections, all of which can present with a blackout.

The commonest symptomatic cause of seizures after 20 weeks' gestation is eclampsia. It may also present after delivery. It may not be associated with other manifestations of pre-eclampsias such as hypertension, proteinuria, oedema, abnormalities in clotting and hepatic function. The incidence of eclampsia varies from 1 in 100 pregnancies in some developing countries to 1 in 2000 pregnancies in western Europe.

MANAGEMENT OF BLACKOUTS IN PREGNANCY
The Clinical History

As is often the case in medicine, the initial and most important key to unravelling the diagnosis is a detailed history, which in the case of blackouts should include an account from an eyewitness.

A history of blackouts before the pregnancy and the results of their investigation are of great importance. In this situation it may be that the current events represent a continuation of a known illness, exacerbated and perhaps altered by the pregnant state. While de novo events occurring during pregnancy may reflect an underlying asymptomatic process made symptomatic with pregnancy or they may be due to a cause purely related to the pregnant state.

The most common cause of blackouts presenting in pregnancy is likely to be syncope. The detailed pathogenesis of neural reflex syncope remains incompletely understood. However, sympathetic stimulation and subsequent withdrawal and vagal excess are important. They produce a varied combination of vasodilatation and bradycardia. As the vascular changes develop slowly there is usually some warning, perhaps lasting from seconds to minutes, although this may be less prominent in the pregnant state. The autonomic changes lead to associated symptoms; with sympathetic overactivity, there may be tachycardia, palpitations, pallor and sweating. With vagal overactivity, nausea or epigastric discomfort may occur. As the event progresses, particularly if the symptoms are ignored or if the subject stands up for fear of being ill in public, further strain is put on the circulation.

Patients may develop symptoms including fatigue, poor concentration and visual disturbances including blurring, fading and altered colour perception in association with blackouts. Witness accounts often note facial pallor, sweating, yawning, deep and sighing respiration and dilated pupils. With persisting hypotension, patients may lose awareness of their surroundings and may be unable to move or respond although they may still be able to hear. Soon after, loss of consciousness ensues.

While standing or sitting, the initial component of the faint consists of loss of tone. Myoclonus is seen less frequently and occurs *after* the collapse. The movements have been elegantly described by Lempert (19). They last for no more than 16 seconds and may be symmetrical or asymmetrical involving jaw, arms and legs in varying combinations. Myoclonus is thought to be secondary to brainstem ischaemia. These contrast with tonic-clonic seizures where there is a clear tonic phase and clonus is not dependent on the patient's body position.

In the gravid state, syncope can occur even if semi-recumbant or even while supine, due to inferior vena cava pressure. In this more horizontal position, the prodrome may be shortened. While a collapse from the upright position will normally re-establish cerebral circulation, a collapse while already supine is associated with less opportunity for spontaneous recovery. Lying on the left side allows the gravid uterus to fall away from the inferior vena cava and distal aorta.

Syncope associated with sudden-onset cardiac arrhythmias or cardiac obstruction may be associated with few premonitory symptoms, although with tachycardias palpitations of varying forms, chest pain or breathlessness can occur. With the more pure cardiological causes, exertional syncope may occur, whereas neural reflex syncope tends not to occur in this situation. Syncope will be independent of position. Because of the shortened prodrome, injury is more likely. With recovery, there is often a hypertensive overshoot during recovery with facial flushing. Recovery is usually rapid which may differentiate these events from other forms. A preceding history of cardiac disease may be found, and a family history of collapses and particularly of sudden cardiac death under the age of 40 are particularly relevant findings (20).

It is uncommon for patients with significant autonomic failure to fall pregnant, but pregnancy is probably commoner in milder forms. The primary symptoms occur in the upright posture and consist of light-headedness, blurred vision and neck ache, the so-called coat hanger headache. This usually occurs within a few minutes of being upright and will tend to be reproducible, whereas the other forms of syncope will be more random.

Epileptic seizures can consist of simple partial, complex partial seizures, myoclonus and absence blank spells as well as generalised tonic-clonic seizures. Pre-blackout aura symptoms are relevant. Events may display a pattern with circadian features or with certain precipitants, for example, alcohol, fatigue or stress. Tongue biting, particularly laterally, head turning and the presence of central cyanosis are frequent associations of seizures. Confusion, profound tiredness and muscle pain are important markers of tonic-clonic seizures as compared to syncope (21). Faecal incontinence is also more common with seizures than with syncope, although may occur with either.

Some aspects of the history may suggest non-epileptic rather than epileptic seizures (22). In many ways these components of the history should be considered risk factors for the condition and then supplemented with a more detailed description of what happens during the attack (15). Plug and Reuber draw attention to the importance of listening to more than just the content of the interview with the patient. They propose a structured interview starting with an open phase letting the patient drive the conversation with a detailed account of the events, then a 'challenging' or clarifying phase followed by a spectrum of other questions. The importance of letting patients describe their symptoms in their own words has always been an essential component of history taking. Combining that with listening to what patients say and how they say it does require a high degree of intellectual discipline, and is particularly relevant for the pregnant woman who may be under additional stress because of concerns about effects on the fetus.

Apparent blackouts occurring repeatedly without definite injury and with symptoms referable to multiple organ systems should raise the possibility of psychogenic attacks. It also needs to be remembered that patients may suffer events of differing aetiologies during the course of the pregnancy.

Investigations

Concern always surrounds blackouts due to the perception in patients that they may presage a risk of imminent sudden death. Their investigation is therefore of the utmost importance and can be particularly pressurised during a pregnancy, not least due to concerns for both the mother and the fetus. In addition, the treating physician must consider the potential effects of any investigations on the fetus as well as the mother, balancing this against the potential effects of continued blackouts on both 'patients'.

As discussed above, much of the diagnosis rests with a detailed history and careful examination. This is particularly relevant during pregnancy because of the constraints of applying diagnostic tests in this state. The history from the patient and any eyewitnesses should be obtained directly by the doctor. It should be appreciated that eyewitness reports are often clouded by the reporter's own anxieties at the time of the event. Visual records of events such as video telemetry or even CCTV can be of great value.

In differentiating cardiac syncope from seizures a detailed cardiological examination may assist in the diagnosis by revealing evidence of cardiac failure, rhythm disturbances or murmurs. However, flow murmurs are common in pregnancy and can cause confusion. An electrocardiogram (ECG) and an echocardiogram are important. While not an absolute guarantee, a normal ECG can be very reassuring; a normal echo will exclude the obstructive cardiac lesions and, if there is normal left-ventricular function, serious ventricular arrhythmia is unlikely (13). Where syncope is likely, a cardiological referral should be considered. Assessing blood pressure in the upright position over several minutes will define a tendency to orthostatic hypotension and in the left lateral position it may provide evidence for the supine hypotensive syndrome. Unless the diagnosis is certain, some form of prolonged rhythm monitoring may be required to exclude both brady- and tachyarrhythmias. These monitors can be external, recording as much as 7 days of ECG; implantable monitors able to record over half an hour of ECG retrospectively are also available with battery lives of up to 3 years. These are similar in size to a USB stick and are implanted under local anaesthetic subcutaneously. The diagnosis of neural reflex syncope can be difficult, often relying on the history and the exclusion of other causes of syncope; tilt testing is often used in clinical practice but is not appropriate in pregnancy (23).

Differentiating epileptic from non-epileptic seizures can be difficult. The current gold standard for their identification is video telemetry. Access to such sophisticated investigational tools is, however, variable. Careful clinical examination is mandatory, with particular attention paid to evidence of pre-eclampsia and focal neurological deficits. The essential aspects of the neurological examination should include fundi, weakness, reflexes, coordination and plantar responses.

With regard to neurological investigations, EEG is safe and may identify focal slowing, epileptiform discharges and diffuse background slowing, all of which may prompt further investigation. Drug-induced sleep EEGs are usually avoided, but allowing the patient to drowse may confirm epileptiform abnormalities. Activation procedures are usually avoided.

Imaging with MRI is regarded as relatively safe for the fetus and is the modality of choice. No adverse reports in humans after exposure to MRI have been reported. There are reports of structural abnormalities in mice and rabbits (24). There are reports of gadolinium contrast agents being given to pregnant patients without adverse effects on the fetus. However, high and repeated doses given to animals have been associated with teratogenesis, so the use of gadolinium is not recommended during organogenesis in the first trimester (25). There is also the risk of nephrogenic systemic fibrosis from gadolinium and in the fetus excreting it into the amniotic sac, the long-term effect of which is unknown (26). As a result, the American College of Radiology (ACR) 2007 guidance document recommends the avoidance of intravenous gadolinium during pregnancy and that it should only be used if clinically essential and after the risks and benefits explained to patient and treating clinician (27). The safety of MRI in pregnancy is discussed further in chapter 2.

The presence of focal features to the seizure, focal neurological signs or unexplained diffuse cerebral dysfunction should prompt imaging as soon as possible.

Treatment

The importance of an accurate diagnosis in pregnancy cannot be overemphasised. Treatment of any condition in pregnant women may be complex, with a mother whose physiology has changed and the presence of a developing fetus.

The most frequent cause of blackouts is syncope related to the cardiovascular changes brought about by pregnancy. For blackouts related to positioning, particularly recumbency, education of the patient is often all that is needed. Avoiding prolonged standing and avoiding rapid rising from sitting, particularly after a heavy meal, are likely to reduce the risk of syncope. Ensuring adequate hydration, maintaining cardiovascular fitness and iron and folate supplements all contribute to a reduction in faint frequency. Compression garments to prevent venous pooling can be helpful but are limited in their usefulness due to discomfort.

Seizures and their management in pregnancy are discussed in more detail in chapter 12 'Epilepsy and Pregnancy' and chapter 10 'Pre-eclampsia/Eclampsia and Peri-partum Convulsions'. The invasive treatment of arrhythmias with radiofrequency ablation or the implantation of pacemakers or defibrillators is possible if needed and can be achieved with non-radiological imaging methods, although this is very rarely necessary. Drug treatment of arrhythmias is possible, tailored to reduce the risk of teratogenic effects. Major structural heart disease is usually more serious and should prompt early involvement of cardiologists with an expertise in rhythm management and/or cardiovascular problems in pregnancy. Psychogenic blackouts remain as problematic within pregnancy as they are without, but involvement of the perinatal psychiatric or neuropsychiatric teams once the diagnosis is clear may be helpful.

Women with POTS during pregnancy are managed conservatively by reducing their medication to the minimum needed and close monitoring of their cardiovascular state (28,29).

REFERENCES

1. Kapoor WN. Evaluation and outcome of patients with syncope. Medicine (Baltimore) 1990; 69:160–175.
2. Kapoor WN, Peterson J, Wiend HS, et al. Diagnostic and prognostic implications of recurrences in patients with syncope. Am J Med 1987; 83:700–708.
3. Kinsella SM, Lohmann G. Supine hypotensive syndrome. Obstet Gynecol 1994; 83(5):774–788.
4. Williams J, Myson V, Sterard S, et al. Self-discontinuation of anti-epileptic medication in pregnancy: detection by hair analysis. Epilepsia 2002; 43:824–831.
5. Benbadis SR, Allen HW. An estimate of the prevalence of psychogenic non-epileptic seizures. Seizure 2000; 9:280–281.
6. Meierkord H, Will B, Fish D, et al. The clinical features and prognosis of pseudoseizures diagnosed using video-telemetry. Neurology 1991; 41:1643–1646.
7. Lesser RP. Psychogenic seizures. Neurology 1996; 46:1499–1507.
8. Linzer M, Felder A, Hackel A, et al. Psychiatric syncope: a new look at an old disease. Psychosomatics 1990; 31:181–188.
9. Robinson JL, Chir B, Hall CJ, et al. Subarachnoid hemorrhage in pregnancy. J Neurosurg 1972; 36:27–33.
10. Capeless EL, Clapp JF. Maternal cardiovaacular changes in early phase of pregnancy. Am J Obstet Gynecol 1989; 161(6):1449–1453.
11. Duvekot JJ, Peeters LL. Maternal cardiovascular hemodynamic adaptations to pregnancy. Obstet Gynecol Surv 1994; 49(12 suppl):S1–S14.
12. Clapp JK III, Capeless EL. Cardiovascular function before, during and after the first and subsequent pregnancies. Am J Cardiol 1997; 80(11):1469–1473.
13. Mushlin PS, Davidson KM. Cardiovascular disease in pregnancy. In: Datta S, ed. Anesthetic and Obstetric Management of High-Risk Pregnancy. 3rd ed. New York: Springer-Verlag, 2004:155–195.
14. Clark SL, Cotton DB, Lee W, et al. Central hemodynamic assessment of normal pregnancy. Am J Obstet Gynecol 1989; 161(6):1439–1442.
15. Hankins GD, Clark SL, Uckan E, et al. Maternal oxygen transport variables during the third trimester of normal pregnancy. Am J Obstet Gynecol 1999; 180(2):406–409.
16. Grubb BP, Calkins H, Rowe PC. Postural tachycardia, orthostatic intolerance, and the chronic fatigue syndrome. In: Grubb BP, Olshansky B, eds. Syncope Mechanisms and Management. 2nd ed. Malden: Blackwell, 2005:225–244. ISBN 1-4051-2207-2.
17. Kounis N, Zawras G, Papadaki P, et al. Pregnancy-Induced increase of Supraventrciular Tachycardia in Wolf-Parkinson-White Syndrome. Clin Cardiol 1995; 18:137–140.
18. Schmidt D, Canger R, Avanzi G, et al. Changes of seizure frequency in pregnant epileptic women. J Neurol Neurosurg Psychiatry 1983; 46:751–755.
19. Lempert T, Bauer M, Schmidt D. Syncope: a videometric analysis of 56 episodes of transient cerebral hypoxia. Ann Neurol 1994; 36:233–237.
20. Ekholm EMK, Erkkola RU, Piha SJ, et al. Changes in autonomic cardiovascular control in mid-pregnancy. Clin Physiol Funct Imaging 1992; 12(5):527–536.
21. Sheldon R, Rose S, Ritchie D, et al. Historical criteria that distinguish syncope from seizures. J Am Coll Cardiol 2002; 40:142–148.
22. Plug L, Reuber M. Making the diagnosis in patients with blackouts: it's all in the history. Pract Neurol 2009; 9:4–15.
23. Powless CA, Harms RW, Watson WJ. Postural tachycardia syndrome complicating pregnancy. J Matern Fetal Neonatal Med 2010; 23:850–853.
24. Tyndall DA, Sulik KK. Effects of magnetic resonance imaging on eye development in the C57BL/6J mouse. Teratology 1991; 43:263–275.
25. Webb JA, Thomsen HS, Morcos SK. The use of iodinated and gadolinium contrast media during pregnancy and lactation. Eur Radiol 2005; 15:1234–1240.
26. Spencer JA, Tomlinson AJ, Weston MJ, et al. Early report: comparison of breath-hold MR excretory urography, Doppler ultrasound and isotope renography in evaluation of symptomatic hydronephrosis in pregnancy. Clin Radiol 2000; 55:446–453.
27. Kanal E, Barkovich AJ, Bell C, et al. ACR guidance document for safe MR practices: 2007. AJR Am J Roentgenol 2007; 188:1447–1474.
28. Kanjwal K, Karabin B, Kanjwal Y, et al. Outcomes of pregnancy in patients with preexisting postural tachycardia syndrome. Pacing Clin Electrophysiol 2009; 32(8):1000–1003.
29. Glatter KA, Tuteja D, Chiamvimonvat N, et al. Pregnancy in postural orthostatic tachycardia syndrome. Pacing Clin Electrophysiol 2005; 28(6):591–593.

12

Epilepsy and pregnancy

Lina A. M. Nashef, Nicholas Moran, Sara Lailey, and Mark P. Richardson

INTRODUCTION

The management of epilepsy in pregnancy needs to be based not only on available evidence but also on a good knowledge of the woman's epilepsy, medical and social history, previous pregnancy outcomes and anti-epileptic drug (AED) treatment as well as an appreciation of her attitudes, beliefs, concerns and priorities. It calls for judgement and experience and is as much an art as it is a science. It requires balancing conflicting interests and supporting the patient and her partner in making important, potentially far-reaching decisions, often based on insufficient evidence, the outcomes of which for her child may not be apparent for years. It requires sharing the decision-making process, aimed at minimising risk to both mother and child, so that the woman does not feel she alone carries the burden of a potential adverse outcome. It involves individual assessment and regular review within a prompt responsive multidisciplinary service, all while reassuring her that the majority of pregnant women have healthy children. This chapter addresses the evidence available in relation to epidemiology, teratogenicity, genetics and AED levels and provides some clinical guidance which draws on this evidence. The contribution of the epilepsy nurse, within a multidisciplinary neurology and obstetric team is then outlined, with a checklist of discussion points.

EPIDEMIOLOGY

This subject has been reviewed with a focus on primary neurological mechanisms (1), effect of AEDs (2) and animal studies (3).

Fertility is reduced in people with epilepsy and this is likely to be due to a number of factors, social and biological, including the effect of AEDs (1, 4–10). In the Rochester–Olmsted County Medical Records Linkage study, covering 1935–1974, fertility rates were significantly reduced to 80% of expected for affected males and 85% for females (10). In a U.K. population-based study, fertility rates among women in the general population were significantly higher by 33% compared to AED-treated women with epilepsy (WWE). In the treated WWE group an overall rate of 47.1 (42.3–52.2) live births per 1000 women aged 15 to 44 per year was observed, compared with a national rate of 62.6 (8). In population-based Finnish study (7) comparing 14,077 patients against 29,828 controls, significantly lower fertility rates were seen in men (hazard ratio 0.58) and women (0.88). In a study of 863 married people with epilepsy recruited through voluntary-sector groups, fertility rates were lower in both men and women compared with their siblings (11).

Menstrual irregularities occur relatively frequently in WWE and, in some studies, polycystic ovaries in women on valproate are reported to be more common than in the general population and than in WWE taking other AEDs (2,12,13), particularly in younger women. The polycystic ovary syndrome (PCOS) is characterised by polycystic ovaries on ultrasound scanning, infrequent periods, anovulation, hyperandrogenism, and is associated with obesity and insulin resistance. Enzyme-inducing AEDs reduce androgen levels and increase sex hormone binding globulin (SHBG) which may contribute to decreased libido and increased incidence of erectile dysfunction in men with epilepsy (2). Other factors, such as the epilepsy itself, particularly if the temporo-limbic system is involved (1), may also contribute to disorders of reproduction.

The proportion of all pregnancies occurring in WWE is, nevertheless, broadly in keeping with the incidence of epilepsy in the general population: in a region of the United Kingdom, 0.61% of all pregnancies over a 2-year period were in WWE (14); over a 19-year period, 0.33% of all pregnancies in Iceland were in WWE (15). Guidelines for the management of WWE emphasise the need for preconception advice, including the need to plan pregnancies, take folate and maintain appropriate contact with an epilepsy specialist. In a U.K. population-based series, only about half the WWE planned their pregnancies and 38% recalled preconception counselling (14); in a U.S. tertiary centre-based series, there was lack of preconception contact with a neurologist in 85%, and lack of contact with a neurologist during pregnancy in 36% (16).

WWE may be concerned that seizure control could deteriorate during pregnancy. In a U.K. regional population-based series, 71% had ongoing seizures during pregnancy (14). In a series from a single Finnish centre, 64% were seizure-free during pregnancy; seizure control remained unchanged during pregnancy in 56%, worsened in 27% and improved in 18% (17). The EURAP collaboration reported 1956 pregnancies in WWE from several European countries; 58.3% were seizure-free during pregnancy, and seizures were more frequent in focal epilepsy, in WWE on polytherapy and in WWE with generalised tonic-clonic seizures taking oxcarbazepine. Seizure control remained unchanged during pregnancy in 63.6%, worsened in 17.3% and improved in 15.9%. Seizures occurred during delivery in 3.5%; having seizures during pregnancy was a risk factor for seizures in labour. Convulsive status occurred in 0.61% with one stillbirth but no maternal deaths (18). There have been several reports suggesting that the seizure frequency before pregnancy to some extent predicts the likelihood of seizures occurring or worsening in pregnancy. The study of Knight and Rhind (19) reported that in women who were having seizures more than once a month prior to pregnancy, 100% had an increased seizure frequency during pregnancy, whilst only 60% of those women who had seizures every 9 months prior to pregnancy showed an increased seizure frequency. Only around 20% of those women who had seizures less frequently than once every 9 months prior to pregnancy had a worsening of seizure frequency during pregnancy. Richmond et al. (20) compared the frequency of seizures in the antenatal period, labour and puerperium between women who had seizures within the last 2 years prior to pregnancy (*n* = 185) and those women who had not (*n* = 160). In those women who had not a had a seizure for 2 years, the percentages of women who had had a seizure during the antenatal period, labour and puerperium were 9.4%, 0% and 1.9%, respectively. The corresponding figures for women who had a seizure within the 2 years prior to pregnancy were 54%, 2.7% and 6.5%.

More recently, in an analysis of 7 years outcome data from the Australian Register of Antiepileptic Drugs in Pregnancy, in 418 of the 841 (49.7%) AED-treated pregnancies at least one seizure occurred. In close to half, seizures were generalised tonic-clonic. The risk of seizures during pregnancy was 50% to 70% less if the pre-pregnancy year was seizure-free, decreasing relatively little with longer periods of seizure control. Of the 391 pregnant WWE with seizures in the pre-pregnancy year, 75.2% had seizures during pregnancy and labour compared to 19.8% of those 450 women without seizures in the pre-pregnancy year (21).

Despite extensive study of AED effects in pregnancy, and numerous clinical guidelines on the management of pregnancy in WWE, there are few studies examining maternal complications of pregnancy and labour in WWE. WWE are often regarded as at increased risk of adverse obstetric outcomes of pregnancy and labour, but recent data do not generally support this. Published evidence was evaluated in the Report of the Quality Standards Subcommittee and Therapeutics and Technology Assessment Subcommittee of the American Academy of Neurology and the American Epilepsy Society (22). The report concluded that for WWE on AEDS, there was probably no substantially increased risk (>2 times expected) of caesarean delivery or late pregnancy bleeding although there was possibly a moderately increased risk (up to 1.5 times expected) of caesarean delivery. The report also concluded that the risk of contractions or premature labour and delivery was probably not increased by more than 1.5 times expected, but it was possible that this risk was substantially increased in WWE who smoke. Another conclusion of the report was that there was insufficient evidence to support or refute an increased risk of pre-eclampsia, pregnancy-related hypertension, spontaneous abortion, a change in seizure frequency or status epilepticus.

In a population study from Iceland of adverse events in pregnancies in WWE, only caesarean section was shown to be more frequent in WWE compared to the general population, being performed twice as often (15). Caesarean section was performed in 35 (13%, 35 of 266 deliveries as compared with 8.8%, 7139 of 81,473, *p* = 0.01). Indications for caesarean sections were diverse but included seizure during delivery (3 patients), status epilepticus during delivery (1) and 'epilepsy' (4). Comparing 414 births to 313 women with a pre-pregnancy diagnosis of epilepsy attending a single Canadian centre over a 22-year period with 81,759 pregnancies in women without epilepsy from the same centre and period of time, non-proteinuric hypertension (11.4% vs. 8.2%) and induced labour (32.6% vs. 20.7%, *p* = 0.001) were commoner in WWE, with fewer instrumental vaginal deliveries in this group. Rates of other complications were similar, with rates of caesarean section 24% in the epilepsy group compared to 20.5% in the control group. Generalised tonic-clonic seizures were not associated with increased adverse outcomes (20). In a series from Finland, there was no increased risk in WWE for pre-eclampsia, preterm labour, caesarean section or perinatal mortality (23). However, in a population-based study from

Norway (24), complication rates were similar in WWE or women with a past history of epilepsy who were not taking AEDs compared to the general population (with only a slight increased risk of caesarean delivery), whereas in those WWE on AEDs, risks were increased for induction [odds ratio (OR), 1.6; 95% confidence interval (CI), 1.4–1.9], caesarean section (OR, 1.6; 95% CI, 1.4–1.9), post-partum haemorrhage (OR, 1.5; 95% CI, 1.3–1.9), with an increases risk of an Apgar score in the infant of <7 (OR, 1.6; 95% CI, 1.1–2.4). Whether this was related to more severe epilepsy or AEDs was uncertain. A later study from the same group of a hospital-based cohort (25) also reported an increased risk of complications in WWE on AEDs of severe pre-eclampsia (OR, 5.0; 95% CI, 1.3–19.9), bleeding in early pregnancy (OR, 6.4; 95% CI, 2.7–15.2), induction (OR, 2.3; 95% CI, 1.2–4.3), caesarean section (OR, 2.5; 95% CI, 1.4–4.7) and malformations in the offspring (OR, 7.1; 95% CI, 1.4–36.6). In this study, active epilepsy (seizures during the last 5 years) versus non-active epilepsy did not discriminate for any of these complications.

To assess mortality from epilepsy in pregnancy, large cohorts are required and limited data are available. Adab pointed out that, in the UK, there appears to be a 10 fold higher mortality in pregnant WWE (Adab et al 2004). In the United Kingdom, it is a government requirement that all maternal deaths be subject to a confidential enquiry. This process of careful surveillance began more than 50 years ago and continues to this day. Reports are published to cover 3-year periods with the latest report relating to 2006–2008 (26). Deaths are classified as directly due to the pregnancy, indirectly related, apparently unrelated, coincidental (previously 'fortuitous') or late (between 42 days and 1 year after the end of pregnancy, also subclassified into direct and indirect). Epilepsy falls under the indirectly related deaths. In the most recent report, there were 107 direct deaths and 154 indirectly related deaths giving a total of 261 deaths amongst 2,291,493 maternities, with a rate of 11.39/100,000 (95% CI, 10.09–12.86). There were 50 coincidental deaths during pregnancy and 33 late deaths occurring within 6 months of delivery, 9 classified as late direct and 24 late indirect.

Fourteen women in total died of epilepsy, nine while pregnant, one not yet knowingly so, one shortly after a miscarriage and four in the postpartum period. The rate was 0.61 per 100,000 maternities. Nine were treated with lamotrigine and two were on polytherapy [one with levetiracetam and one with carbamazepine (CBZ), antipsychotic and antidepressant medication]. One woman stopped lamotrigine before conception. The other AEDS used in monotherapy were CBZ (2 patients), phenytoin (1) and sodium valproate (1). While this may reflect current preferential prescribing of lamotrigine in young women of childbearing age because of perceived lower teratogenic risk, the report emphasises the need to monitor levels of lamotrigine in pregnancy. The 'assessors considered that all those caring for WWE in pregnancy should be aware of the likely fall in lamotrigine levels in pregnancy and that they should take account of this in their management plans' adding more generally that 'A management strategy that aims to reduce the dose of anticonvulsant in pregnancy to reduce effects on the fetus should be tempered by the knowledge that a pregnancy induced reduction in blood levels of some anticonvulsant drugs will increase the risk of seizure'. Eleven of the 14 epilepsy deaths were classified as sudden unexpected death in epilepsy (SUDEP). The remaining deaths were secondary to seizures [secondary hypoxic brain damage (1 patient), complications of chest trauma (1) and death in the bath (1)]. Only six were referred to a health care provider with an interest in epilepsy and only six had received pre-pregnancy counselling. The report stated that 'It is of paramount importance that women with epilepsy are seen by health care providers with expertise in the management of the condition' and that 'Several women might not have died if they had been advised about the maternal risks in pregnancies complicated by epilepsy.' One of the top 10 recommendations of the report was pre-pregnancy counselling in women of childbearing age with pre-existing medical illness, the most common conditions requiring this, in addition to epilepsy, were diabetes, asthma, congenital or known acquired cardiac disease, autoimmune disorders, renal or liver disease, obesity, severe pre-existing or past mental illness and HIV infection.

Without knowing how many of the 2,291,493 maternities were in WWE, it is difficult to accurately arrive at the risk of death from epilepsy for any woman with this diagnosis contemplating pregnancy. If we assume the U.K. regional study, where 0.61% of all pregnancies were in WWE (14), to be representative of the country as whole, 14 epilepsy-related deaths amongst about 13,978 maternities with epilepsy, gives a rate of death from epilepsy (mostly SUDEP) during or shortly after pregnancy of the order of 1:1000. This would need to be compared to the background risk of dying of epilepsy over a similar period in otherwise well non-pregnant WWE in the general population.

THE RISK OF INHERITING EPILEPSY TO OFFSPRING AND SIBLINGS

Epilepsy aggregates in families with two to fourfold increased risk in first-degree relatives of people with idiopathic or cryptogenic epilepsy, compared with population incidence (27). Potential parents with epilepsy or with a family history of epilepsy often seek to know the risk of passing the epilepsy on. Epilepsy is a heterogeneous disorder resulting from multiple genetic and non-genetic causes, and estimating this risk depends on a number of factors including the epilepsy diagnosis/classification as well as the family history. Basic principles and approaches are presented here. The topic is also discussed in chapter 1, 'Neurogenetics and Pregnancy'.

Recognising limitations and variable interpretations of the terms idiopathic, symptomatic and cryptogenic in the classification of epilepsy, the recent International League Against Epilepsy (ILAE) commission recommended classification by underlying type of cause (aetiology) as follows: (a) genetic, where the epilepsy is the direct result of a known or presumed genetic defect(s) in which seizures are the core symptom of the disorder (this replaces the idiopathic category); (b) structural/metabolic, this replaces the symptomatic category and may be acquired or genetic, but with a separate disorder interposed between the genetic defect and the epilepsy and (c) unknown cause (28). In the 'structural/metabolic' category, and where the epilepsy is acquired due to a significant brain insult, for example, severe head injury or brain abscess, the genetic contribution to the epilepsy is likely to be small. Within this category, there are also many diverse genetic diseases with epilepsy, where the epilepsy is often a frequent or predominant feature, but usually with other manifestations of a complex syndrome: Examples include tuberous sclerosis, X-linked periventricular heterotopias and other neuronal migration disorders, Down syndrome, neurofibromatosis, mitochondrial disorders, familial cerebral cavernomas and Angelman syndrome. In such disorders, counselling and management will depend on the genetics of the individual condition which is outside the scope of this chapter (see chapter 1).

The focus of this section is on presentations where epilepsy is the main phenotype (previously idiopathic, currently classified as genetic).

Genetic susceptibility may be due to new mutations or be inherited. In those with suspected or proven de novo mutations (such as in the sodium channel gene, SCN1A, in Dravet syndrome), the risk of recurrence in siblings is low and estimated at 1% allowing for germline mosaicism. If inherited, inheritance may be polygenic or Mendelian. A careful family history is a prerequisite to giving genetic advice. Some caution is needed here. Some inherited epilepsies, for example, those associated with microdeletions, diagnosed using the molecular cytogenetic technique of array comparative genomic hybridisation (CGH), may be associated with a personal or family history of learning disability or mental health problems and may be missed if the focus of the history is only on epilepsy. Dysmorphic features may also be present. Array CGH can be a very useful test, carried out after counselling, to identify microdeletions or duplications (copy number variants, CNVs), not identified by much less sensitive standard cytogenetic techniques. CNVs may be found in regions known to be associated with well-defined clinical presentations (such as 15q13.3 and 16p13.11) or be of uncertain significance, sometimes considered 'benign variants'. CNVs constitute the commonest known genetic cause of the epilepsies (29).

A number of mutations in specific genes causing epilepsy have been described (Table 12.1) in a small proportion of the epilepsy population, generally in those with Mendelian pedigrees. Recurrence risk of the genotype in those with a clear Mendelian family history depends on the mode of inheritance (see chapter 1). Even with Mendelian autosomal-dominant pedigrees, penetrance is often reduced and variable within and between families, as has been clearly demonstrated in genetic (formerly generalized) epilepsy with febrile seizures plus (GEFS plus) families, this being due to the influence of modifier genes and/or environmental factors. Thus, while genetic testing can be very useful with certain genetic epilepsies, it is not always possible to accurately predict the occurrence or severity of epilepsy in offspring with the genotype. For guidance on where genetic testing is considered helpful, the reader is referred to the recommendations outlined in a report on genetic testing by the ILAE Genetics commission (27) (Table 12.2).

Genetically complex epilepsies (without a clear cause and without a known mutation or Mendelian pedigree) constitute a significant proportion of patients with epilepsy, usually presenting in childhood or early adulthood. Risk prediction for offspring or siblings is based on results of epidemiological studies looking at risk of epilepsy in family members of the proband compared to the baseline risk in the general population estimated at 1% by age 20 (30).

Winawar and Shinnar (30) quote data from older studies. These show that between 2.4% and 4.6% of offspring of a parent with epilepsy also develop epilepsy. The risk is above that of the general population but relatively low. Siblings of individuals with epilepsy carry a similar risk. Risk is higher with idiopathic than acquired epilepsies. Where there is a clear exogenous post-natal insult causing epilepsy (excluding alcohol), there is no significantly increased risk. Some, but not all studies, observed a greater risk in offspring if the mother has epilepsy (2.8–8.7%) compared to the father (1.0–3.6%). The risk of epilepsy to a sibling of a proband with epilepsy rises from approximately 3% to 8% if the parent also has epilepsy. Seizure type can affect risk. A 4% to 8% risk of any epilepsy has been observed in offspring of individuals with myoclonic seizures,

Table 12.1 Genes Identified in Idiopathic Epilepsy Syndromes

	Locus	Gene	Product	References
Syndromes beginning in the first year of life				
Benign familial neonatal seizures	20q13.3	KCNQ2	$K_V7.2$ (K+ channel)	(Biervert et al., 1998; Singh et al., 1998)
	8q24	KCNQ3	$K_V7.3$ (K^+ channel)	(Charlier et al., 1998)
Benign familial neonatal-infantile seizures	2q23–q24.3	SCN2A	$Na_V1.2$ (Na^+ channel)	(Heron et al., 2002; Berkovic et al., 2004; Striano et al., 2006; Herlenius et al., 2007)
Ohtahara syndrome	9q34. 1	STXBP1	Syntaxin binding protein 1	(Saitsu et al., 2008)
	Xp22. 13	ARX	Aristaless-related homeobox protein	(Kato et al., 2007; Fullston et al., 2009)
Early-onset spasms	Xp22	STK9/CDKL5	Cyclin-dependent kinase-like 5	(Kalscheuer et al., 2003)
X-linked infantile spasms	Xp22.13	ARX	Aristaless-related homeobox protein	(Stromme et al., 2002; Gecz et al., 2006)
Syndromes with prominent febrile seizures				
Dravet syndrome (severe myoclonic epilepsy of infancy)	2q24	SCN1A	$Na_V1.1$ (Na^+ channel)	(Claes et al., 2001; Nabbout et al., 2003; Wallace et al., 2003; Harkin et al., 2007)
Genetic (generalised) epilepsy with febrile seizures plus (GEFS+)	2q24	SCN1A	$Na_V1.1$ (Na^+ channel)	(Escayg et al., 2000b; Sugawara et al., 2001; Wallace et al., 2001b)
	19q13.1	SCN1B	β_1 subunit (Na^+ channel)	(Wallace et al., 1998, 2002; Audenaert et al., 2003; Scheffer et al., 2007)
	5q34	GABRG2	γ_2 subunit ($GABA_A$ receptor)	(Baulac et al., 2001; Harkin et al., 2002)
Childhood absence epilepsy with febrile seizures	5q34	GABRG2	γ_2 subunit ($GABA_A$ receptor)	(Wallace et al., 2001a; Kananura et al., 2002)
Epilepsy and mental retardation limited to females	Xq22	PCDH19	Protocadherin	(Dibbens et al., 2008)
Idiopathic generalized epilepsies				
Early-onset absence epilepsy	1p35–p31.1	SLC2A 1	GLUT 1 (glucose transporter type 1)	(Suls et al., 2009)
Juvenile myoclonic epilepsy	5q34–q35	GABRA 1	α_1 subunit ($GABA_A$ receptor)	(Cossette et al., 2002)
	6p12–p11	EFHC1	EF hand motif protein	(Suzuki et al., 2004)
Focal epilepsies				
Autosomal-dominant nocturnal frontal lobe epilepsy	20q13.2–q13.3	CHRNA4	α_4 subunit (nACh receptor)	(Steinlein et al., 1995; Phillips et al., 2000)
	1 q21	CHRNB2	β_2 subunit (nACh receptor)	(De Fusco et al., 2000; Phillips et al., 2001)
	8p21	CHRNA2	α_2 subunit (nACh receptor)	(Aridon et al., 2006)
Autosomal-dominant partial epilepsy with auditory features (Autosomal-dominant lateral temporal epilepsy)	10q24	LGI1	Leucine-rich repeat protein	(Gu et al., 2002; Kalachikov et al., 2002; Morante-Redolat et al., 2002)
Generalised epilepsy and paroxysmal dyskinesia	10q22	KCNMA1	K_{Ca} 1.1 (K^+ channel)	(Du et al., 2005)
Epilepsy with paroxysmal exercise-induced dyskinesia	1p35–p31.3	SLC2A 1	GLUT 1 (glucose transporter type 1)	(Suls et al., 2008; Weber et al., 2008)
Absence epilepsy and episodic ataxia	19p13	CACNA1A	$Ca_V2.$ 1 (Ca^{2+} channel)	(Jouvenceau et al., 2001; Imbrici et al., 2004)
Focal epilepsy and episodic ataxia	12p13	KCNA1	$K_v1.1$ (K^+ channel)	(Spauschus et al., 1999; Zuberi et al., 1999; Eunson et al., 2000)
Familial hemiplegic migraine and epilepsy	1 q21–23	ATP1A2	Sodium-potassium ATPase	(Vanmolkot et al., 2003; Deprez et al., 2008)

Source: From Ref. 27.
Note: References cited in this table belong to Ref. 27, and are not listed in this chapter.

and a 5% to 9% risk of any epilepsy in offspring of individuals with absence seizures. In general, the risk is considered greater in relatives of individuals with generalised compared to focal epilepsy. The risk to offspring is also greater if the parent's epilepsy presents early. Parents whose epilepsy presents before age 20 years carry an offspring epilepsy risk of 2.3% to 6% compared to a risk of 1.0% to 3.6% if older, with no increased risk observed over the age of 35. The presence of specific electroencephalogram (EEG) abnormalities [generalised spike-wave discharges (GSW), photoparoxysmal response (PPR), and multifocal spikes] confers an increase risk. Sibling risk rises to 6% if the proband has GSW, and 8% if both GSW and PPR, or GSW and multifocal spikes. Photosensitivity on EEG (or PPR) is a familial genetically determined trait, with age-related manifestations, which though associated with epilepsy can segregate separately. Familial clustering of the four

Table 12.2 Examples of Assessment of Clinical Validity and Clinical Utility for Diagnostic Testing in an Affected Individual[a]

	Gene(s)	Proportion of patients/families with mutations[b]	How accurate is a positive mutation test for confirming the diagnosis?	Clinical utility: In an affected individual, how useful is knowledge of mutation status for clinical management?
Syndromes beginning in first year of life				
Benign familial neonatal seizures	KCNQ2	>50% of families	Highly accurate in correct clinical context (but most cases have clear AD inheritance so diagnosis is usually clear without testing)	Somewhat useful Outcome usually benign (although severe outcome has been reported) Mutation status predicts favourable outcome; hence less aggressive management may be warranted
	KCNQ3	7% of families		De novo KCNQ2 mutations reported in rare isolated cases. Finding of de novo mutation informs diagnosis and has management implications Genetic counselling implications
Benign familial neonatal-infantile seizures	SCN2A	unknown	Highly accurate in correct clinical context (but most cases have clear AD inheritance so diagnosis is usually clear without testing)	Somewhat useful Outcome is usually benign Mutation status predicts favourable outcome, hence less aggressive management may be warranted Genetic counselling implications
Ohtahara syndrome	STXBP1	~35% of patients	Highly accurate in correct clinical context	Very useful
	ARX	Unknown		Establishes aetiology so avoids further diagnostic test procedures Genetic counselling implications Usually de novo
Early-onset spasms	STK9/CDKL5	10–17% of patients	Highly accurate in correct clinical context	Very useful Establishes aetiology so avoids further diagnostic test procedures Genetic counselling implications Usually de novo
X-linked infantile spasms (usually in boys)	ARX	<5% of male patients	Highly accurate in correct clinical context	Very useful Establishes aetiology so avoids further diagnostic test procedures Genetic counselling implications De novo cases reported in rare isolated cases. Finding of de novo mutation informs diagnosis and may alter clinical management
Syndromes with prominent febrile seizures				
Dravet syndrome (Severe myoclonic epilepsy of infancy)	SCN1A	70–80% of patients	Truncation mutations: highly accurate in correct clinical context Missense mutations: less clear and depends on electroclinical context	Very useful Establishes aetiology so avoids further diagnostic test procedures Allows early optimisation of antiepileptic therapy Most mutations de novo Mutations rarely identified in parent, sometimes with somatic mosaicism Genetic counselling implications

Table 12.2 Examples of Assessment of Clinical Validity and Clinical Utility for Diagnostic Testing in an Affected Individual[a] (*Continued*)

	Gene(s)	Proportion of patients/ families with mutations[b]	How accurate is a positive mutation test for confirming the diagnosis?	Clinical utility: In an affected individual, how useful is knowledge of mutation status for clinical management?
Genetic (formerly generalised) epilepsy with febrile seizures plus	SCN1A	5–10% of families	Missense mutations: highly accurate in correct clinical context	Not useful
	SCN1B	<5% of families		Because of extensive phenotypic heterogeneity, mutation status does not predict prognosis or treatment
	GABRG2	<1% of families		
Epilepsy and mental retardation limited to females	PCDH19	Unknown	Highly accurate in correct clinical context	Very useful
				Establishes aetiology, especially in isolated cases or smaller families where mode of inheritance is unclear
				Genetic counselling implications
Idiopathic generalized epilepsy				
Early-onset absence epilepsy	SLC2A 1	~10% of patients	Highly accurate in correct clinical context	Very useful
				Establishes aetiology so avoids further diagnostic test procedures
				May alter clinical management decisions (ketogenic diet found to be effective)
				Genetic counselling implications
Focal epilepsies				
Autosomal-dominant nocturnal frontal lobe epilepsy	CHRNA4	<10% of families	Highly accurate in correct clinical context	Very useful
	CHRNB2	<5% of families		Variable outcome; some cases highly refractory
	CHRNA2	unknown, probably rare		Establishes aetiology so no need to pursue structural lesion with repeated imaging
				Not known if optimal antiepileptic drug therapy or outcome of surgery will differ by mutation status
				Genetic counselling implications
				De novo mutations reported in rare isolated cases. Finding of de novo mutation informs diagnosis, and may alter clinical management if surgery is being considered
Autosomal-dominant partial epilepsy with auditory features	LGI1	~50% of families	Highly accurate in correct clinical context	Not very useful
				Most cases have favourable course
				Establishes aetiology so no need to pursue structural lesion with repeated imaging in rare severe cases
				Mutation status unlikely to alter management decisions (unknown if optimal antiepileptic drug therapy or surgery outcome will differ by mutation status)
				Genetic counselling implications
				De novo cases reported in rare isolated cases. Finding of de novo mutation informs diagnosis, but is unlikely to alter clinical management unless surgery is being considered

(*Continued*)

Table 12.2 Examples of Assessment of Clinical Validity and Clinical Utility for Diagnostic Testing in an Affected Individual[a] (*Continued*)

	Gene(s)	Proportion of patients/ families with mutations[b]	How accurate is a positive mutation test for confirming the diagnosis?	Clinical utility: In an affected individual, how useful is knowledge of mutation status for clinical management?
Epilepsies associated with other paroxysmal disorders				
Epilepsy with paroxysmal exercise-induced dyskinesia	SLC2A1	unknown	Highly accurate in correct clinical context	Very useful
				Establishes aetiology so avoids further diagnostic test procedures
				May alter clinical management decisions (ketogenic diet found to be effective)
				Genetic counselling implications

[a]AD, autosomal dominant; Clinical context: includes syndrome, age at onset, seizure types and frequency, clinical course, electroencephalography (EEG), neuroimaging and family history.
[b]Estimates of mutation frequency from Combi et al., 2004; Ottman et al., 2004; Deprez et al., 2009.
Source: From Ref. 27.
Note: References cited in this table belong to Ref. 27, and are not listed in this chapter.

different PPR types, from occipital spikes to GSW, suggests that they share a common genetic predisposition. Type 4 PPR (GSW) is particularly associated with epilepsy (31–33).

Twin studies show greater concordance for the presence and type of epilepsy in monozygotic (MZ) compared to dizygotic (DZ) twins (34,35). Berkovic et al. (35) found 48/ 108 MZ pairs concordant for seizures compared to 14/145 DZ pairs. Casewise concordance for the major epilepsy syndrome was as follows: generalised epilepsy, MZ = 0.82, DZ = 0.26; febrile seizures (FS), MZ = 0.58, DZ = 0.14; partial epilepsies, MZ = 0.36, DZ = 0.05. This and other reports (36,37) suggest syndrome-specific genetic determinants. In one study, however, the increased risk in family members was not restricted to the same broad epilepsy type (generalised or focal) suggesting some shared genetic mechanisms (38). Different idiopathic generalised epilepsy (IGE) subsyndromes may be observed within families. Fifty-five families were grouped according to the probands' subsyndrome and seizures analysed in relatives (39). Phenotypic concordance for the subsyndrome within families of childhood absence epilepsy (CAE) and juvenile myoclonic epilepsy (JME) probands was 28% and 27%, respectively, but was lower in juvenile absence epilepsy (JAE) and IGE with tonic-clonic seizures only (IGE-TCS) at 10% and 13%. As with a previous Italian study (40), JME and absence epilepsies tended to segregate separately. FS and epilepsy with unclassified tonic-clonic seizures were frequent in affected relatives of all IGE individuals.

Information on risk to offspring when both parents have epilepsy is scarce. One report suggested that the risk of having epilepsy may be higher (41), and another reported a proband with a milder phenotype than either parent (42).

A history of FS also confers an increased risk of passing the epilepsy on. FS are not a homogenous disorder. A useful estimate of risk is provided by a study of 179 offspring of 120 probands with a history of FS, where the seizure incidence in the offspring was 10% (64% of the affected offspring had FS only). The risk was highest if the mother of the proband had experienced seizures (20% vs. 9% in offspring of probands with non-affected parents). Offspring of probands with affected mothers had a much higher risk (27%) than offspring of probands with affected fathers (7%) (43).

In summary, in most patients with epilepsy, excluding those with Mendelian pedigrees or known mutations, the risk to off-spring when one parent has epilepsy is less than 10% and in many cases less than 5%. Despite this, the risk of passing the epilepsy on may be overestimated by patients and is one of the factors influencing decisions regarding family size in this setting (44).

AEDs IN PREGNANCY: STRUCTURAL AND FUNCTIONAL TERATOGENESIS
Overview, General Considerations and Limitations of Available Evidence

There are various definitions of teratogenesis; a reasonable one is as follows: the induction of non-hereditary congenital malformations (birth defects) in an embryo or fetus by interference with normal embryonic development due to the action of exogenous factors (based on a definition by the National Safety council, United States). However, the term is commonly used more expansively to embrace the following:

- Non-hereditary, endogenous factors as structural teratogens, for example, maternal diabetes
- Functional teratogenesis: dysfunction or disease without malformation that may not be evident at birth, for example, reduced IQ due to exposure to drugs in utero; adult obesity in the offspring of diabetic mothers
- Abnormal growth: macrosomia in maternal diabetes; reduced intrauterine or neonatal growth due to exposure to drugs in utero (in fact, the commonest form of teratogenesis if accepted within the definition)
- Intrauterine death and neonatal death unrelated to a malformation

There is no doubt that maternal epilepsy is associated with increased teratogenicity. This is manifested by the following:

- Structural malformations, for example, congenital heart defects
- Impaired neuropsychological development (a form of functional teratogenesis)
- Reduced intrauterine growth

The clinician wishes to provide optimal counselling and medical management to minimise the risks of teratogenesis in the offspring of WWE. However, there are many unanswered questions in this field. Although the literature on epilepsy and teratogenesis is quite extensive (see review in Ref. 45), until recently, it has yielded few robust findings that can be used clinically and, despite recent advances remains insufficient. In order to provide valid counselling it is important to be familiar with the unresolved questions. The principal question, of course, is which factors are the most powerful teratogens and how might they be ameliorated. The focus in research has been very much upon AED treatment as the most obviously modifiable factor. However, it can be difficult to tease out the relative importance of AEDs from that of other plausible influences, particularly as studies of teratogenesis in humans are necessarily observational. In addition to AEDs, the factors below, amongst others, need to be considered.

- Maternal genetic predisposition to epilepsy
- Parental IQ
- Occurrence of seizures during gestation

Many studies of AED and teratogenesis are flawed, for example, by the use of too few subjects or absence of a control group. In studies of functional teratogenesis, subjects of widely different ages are often included requiring the use of multiple age-appropriate neuropsychological measurement tests that are not directly comparable. Neuropsychological deficit (particularly in the verbal domain which is most vulnerable to teratogens) becomes more readily detectable with increasing age and so studies of very young children may underestimate any effects; conversely, studies of children cannot address the possibility that there may be later life catch-up in development. There may also be bias in subject recruitment. For example, families that suspect a problem in their child are more likely to agree to participate in studies; children in higher socioeconomic groups are more likely to participate in studies but ameliorating factors may be more prevalent, for example, less maternal smoking (reduced probability of malformation) or higher maternal educational level (possibly reduced probability of neuropsychological deficit). Reflecting on the above, it is not surprising that there is a great deal of uncertainty in this area.

The Effects of Maternal Seizures on the Fetus

A central question in the management of epilepsy in reproductive females is how pregnancy or the possibility of pregnancy should influence AED selection and dose and, in some cases, whether the benefit of AED use outweighs potential harm. Outside of this situation, the control of seizures is the patient's principal concern. In reproductive women, however, the well-being of the fetus is also a principal concern. A woman unilaterally stopping her AED on discovering she is pregnant is not an uncommon scenario. Most clinicians hold that the risk to the mother and the fetus of seizures outweighs the risks of AED exposure. Whilst this may be generally valid, it is important to examine this premise and attempt to define the magnitude of the risks to the fetus from both factors, either due to miscarriage/spontaneous abortion or cognitive teratogenesis, there being no indications/evidence that seizures increase the risk of obvious structural malformation.

It seems clear that hypoxia in Generalised Tonic Clonic Seizures (GTCS) can cause fetal organ damage and, if prolonged, death. The EURAP Epilepsy Pregnancy Registry identified 36 cases of status epilepticus in pregnancy, including 12 convulsive; there was a single stillbirth but no cases of miscarriage or maternal mortality. Long-term follow-up of the offspring in this study, however, is not available. Adab (46) found that the occurrence of five or more generalized convulsive seizures in pregnancy was associated with a significantly reduced verbal IQ in the child (VIQ 84.4 vs. 90.2 where no convulsive seizures occurred). Mechanical injury consequent to a seizure may directly damage the fetus or its supporting apparatus. However, it should also be recognised that around 40% of WWE will not be seizure-free in pregnancy (18) and it is common clinical experience that a healthy child is born despite convulsive seizures in pregnancy. The regulatory body in the United Kingdom, National Institute for Health and Clinical Excellence (NICE), strikes a reasonable balance with its conclusion that '*Women with generalised tonic–clonic seizures should be informed that the fetus may be at relatively higher risk of harm during a seizure, although the absolute risk remains very low, and the level of risk may depend on seizure frequency*' (http://www.nice.org.uk/nicemedia/live/10954/29532/29532.pdf).

It is not known to what extent non-convulsive, non-falling seizures might be detrimental. There is very little data available on the effects of complex partial seizures on the fetus. However, it is clear that even where prominent motor activity does not occur, there may be significant cardiorespiratory disturbance. Bradycardia and asystole, though uncommon, are well documented in complex partial seizures (ictal bradycardia syndrome). Significant apnoea sometimes associated with hypoxia, however, was observed relatively frequently in ictal recordings during EEG video monitoring in complex partial seizures (47,48). Sahoo and Klein (49) observed maternal oxygen desaturation to 75% and heart rate acceleration to 125/m in a complex partial (hemimotor) seizure in a woman 7 months pregnant; the fetal heart rate decelerated as low as 70 beats/min for 2.5 minutes (a healthy baby was born at term). There is little data on minor seizures, principally absence seizures and myoclonic jerks, and it seems unlikely that these seizure types are associated with significant cardiorespiratory effects of any duration or severity.

Malformations: Structural Teratogenesis

It is generally accepted that AEDs cause malformations. This is supported by five observations listed below.

- Most studies have found the offspring of WWE taking AEDs have an overall 3% to 14% rate of malformations compared to around 3% or less in the general population without epilepsy.
- Children born to mothers taking AEDs have a higher risk of malformations compared to drug-free WWE.
- A higher risk of malformations with polytherapy is observed compared to monotherapy, with recent studies emphasising that this varies considerably depending on the combination.
- Some studies identified a dose-response effect in mothers with children with a malformation.
- Animal studies demonstrate teratogenesis of AED independent of confounding factors inherent in human studies.

Phenytoin was in clinical use for 30 years before it was suspected to cause malformations. Subsequently, the other commonly used AEDs, phenobarbital, valproate and CBZ fell under suspicion. Information on the newer AEDs (except lamotrigine) remains limited. There is a spectrum of seriousness in the range of malformations reported and it is usual practice to divide them into major, for example spina bifida and congenital heart disease, and minor, for example hypoplastic nails and epicanthic folds. However, there is no universally accepted definition of major and minor. Some authors classify major malformations as those requiring intervention in the first year of life, but the need for this may vary between individuals with similar malformations. Both malformations restricted to a single organ and characteristic constellations of malformations have been recognised. Neural tube defects (NTDs) have been most strongly associated with valproate,

Table 12.3 Major Malformation Rates from the UK Epilepsy and Pregnancy Register (Data, to April 2010, Personal Communication, J Craig)

	Major Malformation Rate (%)	95% Confidence Intervals (%)
No AED	2.5	1.4-4.3
AED monotherapy	3.3	2.8-3.9
Valproate monotherapy	6.2	4.9-7.8
Lamotrigine monotherapy	2.2	1.6-3
Carbamazepine monotherapy	2.4	1.7-3.3
AED polytherapy	5.2	4.1-6.5
Levetiracetam*	0/195	− 1.6%

*Update from UK pregnancy register presented at the 2011 American Epilepsy Society meeting, Baltimore: Levetiracetam monotherapy, 304 pregnancies, 286 livebirths; 2 major malformations (13 minor); major malformation rate = 0.7% (0.2–2.5%).

CBZ and barbiturates, while congenital heart disease and cleft lip and palate, for example, have been most strongly associated with phenytoin. However, many other malformations have been reported including of the urogenital system, skeleton and gut. Various constellations of major and minor malformations, the latter including various proposed characteristic dysmorphic facial appearances, have been attributed to particular drugs, for example fetal hydantoin or valproate syndrome, but the validity of some of these observations is controversial.

Once the decision to treat with an AED has been made, the aim is then to choose the safest drug that is likely to be efficacious in relation to the epilepsy syndrome. This requires data on the relative risks of the many AEDs available. Comparative data are limited and are generally more available for those 'old' AEDs most in use in recent decades, namely CBZ, valproate, phenytoin and phenobarbital, and lamotrigine, the oldest of the 'new' commonly used AEDs. The findings on the relative teratogenicity of 'old' AED varied so much between older studies that the clinician could easily reach a state of despair on reviewing them. This seemed to have befallen Delgado-Escueta who stated in 1992: *'each of the four major AEDs has been considered more teratogenic than the other three AEDs, depending on the author cited …. Since no agreement has been reached regarding which AED is the most teratogenic, the present consensus opinion is that the AED that stops seizures in a given patient should be used'* (50). Tomson and Battino collected data from seven studies of AEDs and teratogenesis from 1978 onwards with widely different study designs in different countries and settings (51). The AED monotherapy major congenital malformation (MCM) rates varied widely: CBZ 2.8% to 12.5%; phenobarbital 0% to 20.0%; phenytoin 0% to 6.8%; oxcarbazepine 0% to 11.1%; there was no consistency in the rank order of AED teratogenicity between the studies. Hence a number of prospective pregnancy epilepsy registers, using different methodologies, were set up around the world with the aim of collecting prospective data on large numbers of patients. These major endeavours have begun to yield useful results which are already guiding clinical practice. An acknowledgment is due to those clinicians and researchers for their foresight and dedication for setting up these prospective registers to collect essential and overdue data (18,52–56). It has to be recognised, however, that limitations still apply to these registers particularly with respect to recruitment bias, case ascertainment and age of assessment of the infant. Despite the U.K. Epilepsy and Pregnancy register having the highest ascertainment rate, it only captures an estimated 25% to 33% of U.K. pregnancies (57).

The following *published* observations from the U.K. register pertain to *treatment with monotherapy* (54). The risk of malformations appears to be statistically significantly higher from in utero exposure to valproate in comparison to CBZ. In Morrow's study, the risk of MCM with valproate was 6.2%, significantly different when compared to 2.2% with CBZ. In the U.K. register, the malformation rate is ascertained routinely at

3 months. Some malformations may be missed if ascertainment is only based on early reporting as shown in the EURAP and Australian Registries (57,58). There is less robust evidence in the published paper (54) that the risk is lower with lamotrigine compared to valproate. The risk of MCM associated with lamotrigine was 3.2% but not statistically significantly less than that for valproate (6.2%), although additional data have been presented since from this (Table 12.3) and several other studies supporting a significant difference in malformation rates between these two medications, and showing valproate to have a relatively high teratogenic effect. The North American AED Pregnancy Registry identified 16 MCM among 149 children exposed to valproate monotherapy in utero (10.7%; 95% CI, 6.3–16.9%) as compared to 2.9% in a control group (95% CI, 2.0–4.1%; OR, 4.0; 95% CI, 2.1–7.4; $p = 0.001$); a relative risk of MCM of 7.3 (95% CI, 4.4–12.2; $p = 0.001$) was estimated (59). The Australian Register of AED in Pregnancy reported an incidence of fetal malformations (including minor) of 16% where there had been valproate exposure in monotherapy or polytherapy. This was in contrast to exposure to other AED where the incidence was similar to that in WWE not taking AED (53). An older meta-analysis of prospective European studies found a relative risk of MCM of 3.7 (95% CI, 1.2–11.8) with valproate monotherapy exposure (60) compared to a matched control group without epilepsy. A dose-response relationship for valproate and MCM was observed in two of the above studies, the risk being considerably less with doses below 1000 mg/day. A dose effect was also reported on for lamotrigine by the U.K. Pregnancy Register (54). More recently, EURAP reported on malformation rates in relation to dose after the exclusion of cases with potential confounding factors (61). A relationship between dose and malformation rate was found for each of CBZ, lamotrigine, valproate and phenobarbital (Table 12.4).

Many studies have found much higher risks of MCM with AED polytherapy but this did not reach statistical significance in Morrow's paper: 3.5% of WWE not taking AED had a child with an MCM compared to 6.0% in WWE on polytherapy; $p = 0.16$. The risk with polytherapy may be more related to the AEDS in question rather than polytherapy per se. The North American AED Pregnancy Registry reported on risk of malformations in WWE exposed to lamotrigine or CBZ alone or in polytherapy. For lamotrigine, the risk of malformations was 1.9% in monotherapy, 9.1% for lamotrigine plus valproate (OR, 5.0; 95% CI, 1.5–14.0) and 2.9% for lamotrigine plus any other AEDs (OR, 1.5; 95% CI, 0.7–3.0). For CBZ, the risk of malformations was 2.9% in monotherapy, 15.4% for CBZ plus valproate (OR, 6.2; 95% CI, 2.0–16.5) and 2.5% for CBZ plus any other AEDs (OR, 0.8; 95% CI, 0.3–1.9) (62).

In addition to data on lamotrigine already presented above, Holmes et al. summarised the findings on MCMs and lamotrigine monotherapy exposure in the first trimester. Of 1623 pregnancies, MCMs occurred in 2.8%. The range

Table 12.4 Number of Offspring with Malformations for the Four Monotherapies at Different Doses at Conception (mg/day)

	Sample size	Congenital malformation up to birth to 2 months	Congenital malformation up to 1 year	Number seizure-free (%)
Carbamazepine				
<400	148	2 (1.3%, 0.16–4.80)	5 (3.4%, 1.11–7.71)	95 (64%)
≥400 to <1000	1047	34 (3.2%, 2.26–4.51)	56 (5.3%, 4.07–6.89)	699 (67%)
≥1000	207	16 (7.7%, 4.48–12.25)	18 (8.7%, 5.24–13.39)	129 (62%)
Lamotrigine				
<300	836	14 (1.7%, 0.92–2.79)	17 (2.0%, 1.19–3.24)	562 (67%)
≥300	444	16 (3.6%, 2.07–5.79)	20 (4.5%, 2.77–6.87)	303 (68%)
Phenobarbital				
<150	166	7 (4.2%, 1.71–8.05)	9 (5.4%, 2.51–10.04)	117 (71%)
≥150	51	7 (13.7%, 5.70–26.26)	7 (13.7%, 5.70–26.26)	35 (69%)
Valproic acid				
<700	431	18 (4.2%, 2.49–6.52)	24 (5.6%, 3.60–8.17)	306 (71%)
≥700 to <1500	480	43 (9.0%, 6.65–11.88)	50 (10.4%, 7.83–13.50)	316 (66%)
≥1500	99	23 (23.2%, 15.33–32.79)	24 (24.2%, 16.19–33.89)	63 (63%)

Data are events (rate, 95% CI) unless otherwise stated.
Source: From Ref. 61.

amongst these studies was 0% to 4.4% although the lowest and highest resulted from the smallest studies. The North American AED Pregnancy Registry found a particular risk of isolated cleft palate or cleft lip (63,64) which does not appear to be observed in other studies. Sixteen of 684 (2.3%) infants exposed to lamotrigine had major malformations identified at birth, five of whom had (7.3/1000) oral clefts. They compared this to a prevalence of isolated oral clefts of 0.7/1000 amongst 206,224 unexposed infants at Brigham and Women's Hospital in Boston. The authors compared their data to the rate in 1623 infants exposed to lamotrigine as monotherapy in five other registries with four infants with oral clefts observed and a prevalence 2.5/1000 (RR, 3.8; 95% CI, 1.4–10.0).

Other New AEDs: Teratogenesis

A population-based cohort from Denmark reported results in relation to the risk of malformation associated with some newer-generation AEDs (65). Using nationwide health registries, and compared with 2.4% major malformations amongst unexposed infants, 49 of 1532 infants (3.2%) exposed to new AEDs during the first trimester were diagnosed with a major malformation – lamotrigine (38/1019, 3.7%), oxcarbazepine (11/393, 2.8%), topiramate (5/108, 4.6%), gabapentin (1/59, 1.7%) and levetiracetam (0/58). A significant association was found in unadjusted estimates between exposure to newer-generation AEDs or lamotrigine alone during the first trimester; the risk was also elevated but not significantly so for oxcarbazepine, topiramate and gabapentin. However, after adjustment for older-generation AED use and epilepsy, no associations remained. The authors concluded that among live-born infants in Denmark, first-trimester exposure to these newer-generation AEDS compared with no exposure was not associated with an increased risk of major birth defects. It is important to keep in mind that, apart from with lamotrigine, where data available are comparable to older AEDs such as CBZ and valproate, data for other newly introduced AED are limited. Further data on levetiracetam and topiramate are presented below.

Levetiracetam
In animal studies, levetiracetam causes minor skeletal anomalies and growth restriction. In the U.K. Epilepsy and Pregnancy Register (54), there were 117 levetiracetam-exposed pregnancies, all as polytherapy, with three cases of MCM (2.7%; 95% CI, 0.9–7.7%). In a Danish study of 58 levetirace-

tam-exposed live births, there were no MCM (65). In a study of nine live births, there were no MCM but two cases of low birth weight (66). The U.K. Epilepsy Pregnancy Register found no risk of delayed cognitive development in children exposed to levetiracetam in utero, but the oldest age of assessment was 2 years (67).

Topiramate
In animal studies, topiramate causes craniofacial and limb anomalies and reduced birth weight. The U.K. Epilepsy and Pregnancy Register (54) reported 70 live births following topiramate monotherapy exposure. There were three MCMs (4.8%; 95% CI, 1.7–13.3%). In 108 cases of polytherapy exposure including topiramate, there were 13 MCMs (9.0%; 95% CI, 5.6–14.1%). The latter included an unexpectedly high number of oral clefts (68). A study of 52 pregnancies found no increase in MCM but an increased rate of low birth weight. Weight loss in patients taking topiramate is well recognised outside of pregnancy, possible due to inhibition of lipogenesis as well as appetite suppression (69). A study in Denmark identified an MCM in 4.6% (of 57) topiramate exposures (monotherapy and polytherapy); following adjustment for confounding factors, the relative risk of MCM was 1.44; the authors concluded that a relative risk of 3.6 could not be excluded with any certainty (65).

Growth: Intrauterine and Subsequent

There is no consensus between studies but the weight of evidence suggests that intrauterine growth tends to be reduced in WWE. There is some but not conclusive evidence that AED may play a major role. In a Norwegian study of military conscripts in 1605 male infants born to WWE the mean birth was 53 g below and the mean birth length was 0.2 cm below those in a control group (both differences were highly statistically significant). Height remained significantly reduced at conscription (70).

Functional Teratogenesis

While there may be some theoretical concern that the occurrence of seizures in pregnancy might confer a higher risk of epilepsy on the child beyond any genetic influence, most interest in functional teratogenesis and AEDs has focused on neuropsychological impairment. In experimental animals in utero exposure to AED including phenobarbital, phenytoin, primidone and valproate may cause neurodevelopmental and behavioural problems. This effect occurs at maternal plasma drug concentrations similar to human therapeutic ranges and below those associated with structural teratogenesis (71,72). Exposure to AEDs whilst in utero is associated with reduction in IQ, minimal neurological dysfunction and abnormal EEG in childhood and adolescence. There are many confounders such as the effects of having a chronically unwell mother, socioeconomic group and genetic factors. The precise pathogenesis of neurodevelopmental problems is rather unclear. Factors that may influence neurocognitive development in infants include maternal epilepsy syndrome, seizures during pregnancy, folate and other nutritional deficiency states, exposure to AEDs in utero, maternal IQ and the social environment in which the children grow up. Mothers on polytherapy will in general have more difficulty to control epilepsy and more seizures during pregnancy. Although studies have been conflicting, and as already cited, Adab (46) found that generalised tonic-clonic seizures in pregnancy were a risk factor for lower IQ in childhood. Adab also observed that, in children exposed to valproate in utero, VIQ was lower in all age groups (encompassing 6 months to 8 years) although different neuropsychological tools were employed to suite age. A dose effect was also observed. The VIQ of children exposed to 800 mg or below was similar to unexposed children. One is hard-pressed to identify a pair of studies with entirely concordant findings. For example, both Adab et al. and Dean et al. (73) found verbal but not performance IQ deficits in children with exposure to valproate; however, Dean et al. found significant association between verbal deficit and CBZ or phenytoin exposure while Adab et al. found a dosage effect for valproate, findings not confirmed in the other study. In studies of IQ in children with mothers with epilepsy, confounding factors are legion, including age at testing and a wide range of intelligence testing tools. In several studies, mothers taking valproate had significantly lower mean neuropsychological scores, for example, in a study by Eriksson (74), mean maternal full scale IQ (FIQ) was 109 in both WWE not prescribed AED or prescribed CBZ but 96 in those prescribed valproate ($p = 0.003$); the findings for VIQ and Performance IQ (PIQ) subsets were similar. WWE prescribed valproate also had significantly fewer years in education. WWE taking multiple AEDs and/or AEDs at higher doses may be less likely to have satisfactory interaction with their child due to adverse effects and underlying more severe chronic epilepsy; additionally their IQ and educational levels may be lower due to chronic disease and its treatment as well as underlying central nervous system (CNS) abnormalities. Neonates exposed to AED in utero are prone to a withdrawal syndrome (jitteriness, seizures, apnoea, feeding difficulties and hypoglycaemia). Conjecturally, this syndrome might cause cerebral damage and contribute to neurodevelopmental delay although there are no data to support this.

Verbal development seems more vulnerable to teratogens compared to motor/performance aspects. Verbal development appears to be particularly more liable to interference by environmental factors, for example, in utero cigarette or marijuana exposure or shorter duration of breastfeeding (74). Published studies inevitably lag behind current practice given the shifts in AED use with respect to long-standing AED, changes with respect to doses used and dose individualisation and the use of newly introduced ones. For example, with respect to the study by Øyen et al. 2007 (70), of army conscripts, the widely used AEDs at the time of the subjects' gestations (1973–1979) were phenytoin and phenobarbital; valproate was not introduced in Norway until 1981. Table 12.5 collects together the details and findings of the most useful studies in this area. For reasons discussed, it is not possible to pool the available studies to provide a quantitative meta-analysis.

Table 12.5 Studies of Neuropsychological Development in the Offspring of WWE

Author	Publication year	N (subjects)[a]	N (controls)[b]	Mean follow-up from birth/years	Findings
Speidel B, Meadow (77)	1972	427	448	NS	Of 23 children with malformations and other abnormalities: 6 'mentally handicapped', 4 of these 'severely subnormal'.
Jones et al. (80)	1989	48	0	NS	20% of children exposed to CBZ monotherapy had developmental delay.
Gaily et al. (78)	1990	104	105	6	Significantly more exposed children had deficits on specific neuropsychological tasks but not associated with exposure.
Vanoverloop et al. (86)	1992	20	0	98	Significantly lower FSIQ in AED exposed children compared to controls; the greatest differences were in performance tasks.
Skolnik et al. (81)	1994	70	70		PTH exposed children had mean FSIQ 10 points lower than controls; CBZ exposed children did not significantly differ from controls.
Reinisch (79)	1995	114	153	adult	Men exposed to PB in utero had significantly lower IQ scores: about 0.5 SD below controls.
Ornoy (83)	1996	47	47	3	CBZ monotherapy exposed children significantly lower mental development scores compared to controls; no difference in motor development scores.

(Continued)

Table 12.5 Studies of Neuropsychological Development in the Offspring of WWE (*Continued*)

Author	Publication year	N (subjects)[a]	N (controls)[b]	Mean follow-up from birth/years	Findings
Koch et al. (76) (later follow-up of subjects in study by Titze et al.)	1999	67	49	15	Mean IQ: control 105; epilepsy no AED 102; monotherapy 100; polytherapy 92. Higher proportion with abnormal EEG and/or minimal neurological dysfunction compared to control group.
Holmes (87)	2000	57	57		No difference in FSIQ or subsets between children of WWE but not exposed to AED in utero compared to controls.
Wide et al. (82)	2000	100	100	1	Global development testing not significantly different in CBZ or PTH exposed infants compared to controls.
Dean (73)	2002	261	0	9	In exposed children: developmental delay 24% (statistically significant compared to non-exposed), behaviour disorders 11% (not statistically significant).
Parisi (91)	2003	20	0	3	Neurological examination scores (at 7 days and 4, 13 weeks and 6 months) and global development scores at 30 months 'markedly lower than optimal'
Adab et al. (46)	2004	375	0	8	No significant difference IQ between unexposed and monotherapy or between unexposed and polytherapy; no significant differences in PIQ between any group; VIQ significantly lower in those exposed to valproate compared to unexposed (7 points difference) or other monotherapies (CBZ 11 points; PTH 15).
Gaily et al. (84)	2004	182	141		No significant difference in VIQ or PIQ in CBZ exposed children compared to controls. Valproate or polytherapy exposed children mean VIQ significantly lower than controls valproate 13 points difference; polytherapy 12 points).
Hirano et al. (90)	2004	71	99	2	Exposed children had significantly lower scores in most performance and verbal tests.
Eriksson et al. (74)	2005	39	0	10	FIQ, VIQ and PIQ similar in children of WWE not exposed to AED and exposed to CBZ; FIQ, VIQ and PIQ lower in children of WWE exposed to valproate compared to not exposed or CBZ exposed but not statistically significant.
Viinikainen et al. (17)	2006	39	13		62% of SVP exposed required educational support vs 15% CBZ exposed or non-exposed (the national average) ($p = 0.02$)
Kantola-Sorsa (85)	2007	154	130		Offspring of mother with epilepsy scored significantly lower vs controls measures of attention, memory, and free-motor function, valproate exposed children had significantly lower VIQ (mean 83) vs those exposed to other AED (97) or non-exposed (98) ($p = 0.001$)

(*Continued*)

Table 12.5 Studies of Neuropsychological Development in the Offspring of WWE (*Continued*)

Author	Publication year	N (subjects)[a]	N (controls)[b]	Mean follow-up from birth/years	Findings
Øyen et al. (70)	2007	1207	316554	20	Adult IQ (120 question test on military conscription) significantly reduced in offspring of WWE
Thomas (55)	2008	395	0	1	Valproate exposed children had significantly lower scores in assessments of motor (but not mental) development compared to CBZ exposed children. One-third of all AED-exposed children had developmental quotients below normal.
Titze et al. (75)	2008	67	49	14	19 prenatally exposed children had lower IQ than control children; monotherapy 6 IQ points lower; polytherapy 12 IQ points lower.
Nadebaum et al. (93,94)	2011	102	0		Language scores in SVP exposed either monotherapy {mean 92) or in polytherapy (mean 73) significantly below population mean (100) (*p* < 0.05). Mean scores in CBZ or LTG monotherapy or poiytherapy without SVP not significantly different from normal. 1st trimester SVP dose negatively correlated with language scores.
Cummings (95)	2011	108	44		SVP and CBZ exposure significantly associated with developmental delay: odds ratios 26 for SVP, 8 for CBZ compared to normals. LTG exposure no evidence of delay.
Meador et al. (96)	2011	229	0		Exposure to higher doses of SVP or CBZ monotherapy significantly associated with lower score for motor function; SVP exposure at higher doses significantly associated with lower score for adaptive function. No effect from PTH or LTG.
Shallcross et al. (67)	2011	95	97		Compared LEV to SVP exposure. LEV exposed did not differ from normals. 8% of LEV exposed were below average compared to 40% of SVP exposed (*p* < 0.001).

NS = not stated.

[a]This refers to the number of children not the number of mothers. Not all mothers were taking AEDs at the time of conception or during pregnancy. In some studies, a small number of subjects were taking AEDs for conditions other than epilepsy.

[b]For the purposes of this table, 'controls' refers to individuals born to mothers without a history of epilepsy or exposure to AED.

A significant study in this field prospectively examined 309 children exposed to AED in utero. An analysis of cognitive development at 3 years of age strongly implicated valproate in leading to reduced IQ in comparison to other AEDs and controls. After correction for confounding factors, the mean IQ was 92 for those exposed to valproate compared to between 98 and 101 for other AEDs and, on average, children exposed to valproate had an IQ between 6 and 9 points lower than for other AEDs. In the case of valproate only, the correlation between the maternal and child IQ was lost, indicating a biological disruption. At 3 years of age, children who had been exposed to valproate in utero had significantly lower IQ scores than those who had been exposed to other AEDS. After adjustment for maternal IQ, maternal age, AED dose, gestational age at birth and maternal preconception use of folate, the mean IQ was 101 for children exposed to lamotrigine, 99 to phenytoin, 98 to CBZ and 92 to valproate (97). A significant inverse correlation was found between the average dose of the AED in pregnancy and a child's IQ at the age of 3 years only with valproate. The worse outcome was associated with higher doses of valproate. Another more recent publication from the same group reported on cognitive outcome in 216 children, born to mothers with a diagnosis of epilepsy, who were exposed in utero to CBZ, lamotrigine, phenytoin and valproate in monotherapy and who completed testing at the age of 3 years. Pre-conceptional folate use was associated with higher verbal outcomes. Valproate was associated with poorer cognitive outcomes and this was negatively associated with valproate dose for both verbal and non-verbal domains. There was a negative association with CBZ dose only for verbal performance, but no dose effects were observed for lamotrigine and phenytoin (96). Other recent studies include a prospective study comparing children born to WWE exposed in utero to levetiracetam, valproate or neither. Children exposed to levetiracetam did not differ from control children on overall development. Eight percent of levetiracetam-exposed children fell within the below-average range compared with 40% of those exposed to valproate in utero. After controlling for confounding factors, exposure to levetiracetam was not associated with outcome ($p = 0.67$), unlike with valproate (67). Another recent study compared in utero exposure to lamotrigine, valproate and CBZ monotherapy compared to a control group and found that, after multivariable analysis, in utero exposure to valproate (OR, 26.1; 95% CI, 4.9–139; $p < 0.001$) and to CBZ (OR, 7.7; 95% CI, 1.4–43.1; $p<0.01$) but not to lamotrigine had a significant detrimental effect on neurodevelopment (95).

Summary: Although most WWE give birth to a child within normal limits, AEDs, which are known to cross the placenta, increase the risk of congenital malformations, both minor and major. There is also an increased incidence of developmental delay, likely due to a number of risk factors. Although many of these factors are unrelated to treatment, they include possible effect of seizures and medication. Studies in particular implicate valproate, in monotherapy and polytherapy, amongst the old AEDs. Data are limited for many new AEDs. The increased risk associated with many AEDS, particularly in monotherapy, appears small and needs to be weighed against the risk to the mother and the unborn child of uncontrolled epilepsy. The risk, with at least some drugs, is dose related. Certain drugs, again notably valproate, more so the higher the dose, appear to carry a greater risk and, wherever possible, should be avoided. Valproate should not be a first-line drug for WWE considering pregnancy and female children (98). While major malformations can be screened for and, termination considered, minor malformations are not adequately screened for but would not generally be grounds for termination. Developmental outcome may take years to become clear. In a proportion, there may be early indications that could guide the mother with future pregnancies. A healthy diet, avoidance of other teratogenic agents including alcohol and tobacco, and folic acid supplementation, started preconception, reduce background risk. Management in practice is discussed below.

AEDs DOSES AND PHARMACOKINETICS DURING PREGNANCY
Overview

As discussed in chapter 4, 'Disposition of Drugs in Pregnancy: Anti-Epileptic Drugs', many changes occur during pregnancy which can affect AED metabolism and, potentially, seizure control. These include change in adherence to prescribed medication, change in seizure threshold, hyperemesis, reduced gastric motility, altered absorption, for example, due to antacid ingestion with phenytoin, increased body weight, increased hepatic elimination, reduced albumin/protein binding and increased cardiac output and renal drug clearance. Several of

these factors combine to reduce serum AED levels. Hyperemesis is more likely in the first trimester and changing the timing of taking AEDs can help maintain cover. In general, however, and although changes in serum levels may start before, more significant decreases in serum AED levels occur in the second and, particularly, the third trimester. Although the relationship between serum levels and seizure control in non-pregnant or pregnant women is not clear-cut, individual patients may have a well-defined therapeutic level. Thus, preconception or, if not available, early pregnancy pre-dose AED serum levels can be useful as a baseline to which later measurements are compared. Where a decrease in levels is due to reduced protein binding, measuring total levels does not accurately reflect free unbound active drug levels. Protein binding of different AEDs is listed below (see text box 1). Changes due to increased metabolism and elimination, however, are more likely to be of clinical relevance. In general, dose adjustments are made on clinical grounds; however, with certain drugs, levels are known to drop to such an extent that it is advisable to aim to maintain serum levels during pregnancy to prevent an increase in seizures as, for example, with lamotrigine. Current published guidelines and the effect of pregnancy on levels of individual AEDs are discussed further below. Most studies follow a relatively small number of women in pregnancy for information on seizure frequency, serum concentration/dose ratio (C/D ratio) and seizure frequency. Of particular interest are the results of the prospective EURAP study, already cited, of 1956 pregnancies in 1882 WWE (18). While 58% of cases were seizure-free throughout pregnancy, a number of associations with the occurrence of seizures emerged, including focal epilepsy (OR, 2.5; 1.7–3.9), polytherapy (OR, 9.0; 5.6–14.8) (any seizures) and oxcarbazepine monotherapy (OR, 5.4; 1.6–17.1) (tonic-clonic seizures only). AED treatment remained unchanged in 62.7% of pregnancies. The number or dosage of AEDs were more often increased in pregnancies with seizures (OR, 3.6; 2.8–4.7) and with monotherapy with lamotrigine (OR, 3.8; 2.1–6.9) or oxcarbazepine (OR, 3.7; 1.1–12.9). Amongst patients included in this study, there were 1367 (78.7%) on monotherapy, of whom 498 (28.7%) were on CBZ, 345 (19.9%) on valproate, 238 (13.7%) on lamotrigine, 117 (6.7%) on phenobarbital, 44 (2.5%) on phenytoin and 41 (2.4%) on oxcarbazepine. This large study suggests that changes in seizure control may, to some extent, relate to the AED taken, one explanation for which being more pronounced changes in levels during pregnancy.

> **Text box 1: Percentage serum protein binding for different AEDs (derived from Ref. 99)**
> Carbamazepine = 75, Clobazam = 85, Clonazepam = 85, Ethosuximide = 0, Felbamate = 25, Gabapentin = 0, Lamotrigine = 55, Levetiracetam = 0, Oxcarbazepine (active metabolite) = 40, Phenobarbital = 55, Phenytoin = 90, Pregabalin = 0, Primidone = 10 (note: phenobarbital is one of its metabolites), Tiagabine = 96, Topiramate = 15, Valproic acid = 90 (bound fraction decreases with higher concentrations), Vigabatrin = 0, Zonisamide = 50

Published Guidelines on AEDs Levels in Pregnancy

Guidance from different official bodies is to some extent conflicting reflecting the limited evidence available. This section mentions some of the published recommendations. The reader is advised to regularly seek up-to-date information, particularly in relation to newer drugs. At the time of writing, the U.K. new NICE *draft* revised guidelines state the following: '*Do not routinely monitor AED levels during pregnancy. If seizures increase or are likely to increase, monitoring AED levels (particularly levels of lamotrigine and phenytoin which may be particularly affected in pregnancy) may be useful when making dose adjustments*'. This guidance is not yet finalised and may yet change. We believe this advice, as it stands, is suboptimal and needs further clarification. The phrase '*or are likely to increase*' would be expected to include situations where there is an expected significant drop in serum levels with certain AEDs known to be associated with more seizures. A recommendation to monitor AED levels in such circumstances, in our view, should be more explicitly stated.

Studies reporting on changes in AED levels in pregnancy were reviewed in 2009 in the Report of the Quality Standards Subcommittee and Therapeutics and Technology Assessment Subcommittee of the American Academy of Neurology and the American Epilepsy Society (100). In summary, the report stated, '*Pregnancy probably causes an increase in the clearance and a decrease in the concentrations of lamotrigine, phenytoin, and, to a lesser extent carbamazepine, and possibly decreases the level of levetiracetam and the active oxcarbazepine metabolite, the monohydroxyderivative (MHD)*'. The report concluded, '*Monitoring of lamotrigine, carbamazepine, and phenytoin levels during pregnancy should be considered, and monitoring of levetiracetam and oxcarbazepine (as MHD) levels may be considered*' declaring that a '*paucity of evidence limited the strength of many recommendations.*'

Best practice guidelines for therapeutic anti-epileptic drug monitoring (TDM) in epilepsy is addressed in a 2008 position paper by the ILAE subcommission in which the relevance of TDM for individual drugs is discussed both in general and in relation to pregnancy (99) The reader is referred to this document for a detailed account of pharmacokinetics of individual AEDs including available information in pregnancy. The effect of pregnancy on AED levels varies and, importantly, the extent of change varies between patients, the decline being insignificant in some and pronounced in others, making it difficult to predict the drop in an individual patient or give a standard recommendation for dose adjustments without drug levels. Thus, the ILAE 2008 best practice guidelines generally recommend monitoring drug concentrations during pregnancy and conclude that the timing and frequency of drug concentration monitoring need to be individualised based on the type of AED used and the patient's characteristics.

Pharmacokinetics of Older AEDs in Pregnancy

For older AEDs (see chapter 4 for additional information), a helpful summary is provided by the best practice ILAE guidelines (99): Total and unbound concentrations of phenobarbital decline by up to 50% to 55%; primidone concentrations decline by 10% to 30%, but with a pronounced decrease (70% or more) in its phenobarbital derivative; CBZ concentrations decline by 0% to 40% with 'insignificant' changes in unbound CBZ; total phenytoin concentrations decrease markedly to about 40% of pre-pregnancy concentrations, but with free concentrations decreasing to a lesser extent (20–30%); no significant change is noted in unbound concentrations of valproate despite a fairly marked decrease in total concentrations.

Thus, one may expect that observed decreases in levels may have clinical significance with phenobarbital, to a lesser extent primidone, through its phenobarbital metabolite. Monitoring levels would thus be reasonable. With phenytoin, monitoring is generally recommended, although the drop in total

levels will overestimate the smaller drop in free levels. Because of its non-linear pharmacokinetics and narrow therapeutic window, monitoring maternal free phenytoin levels would be of benefit, where available, to guide dose adjustments. In the non-pregnant state, free phenytoin levels are approximately 10% of total levels. This is affected by displaced binding and albumin levels. The Sheiner–Tozer equation, a correction formula for phenytoin levels, based on albumin concentrations, the principal but not unique protein with which phenytoin binds, has not been tested in the pregnant state. Its applicability is thus uncertain, particularly that it has not been found to accurately predict active free levels in some situations (101). With valproate (which is 90% protein bound), the drop in total levels is generally not associated with a drop in free levels, and hence an observed drop is unlikely to be clinically significant, and automatic dose adjustments are not advised without a clinical indication. With CBZ, the drop in free levels is small and advice on dose changes will be guided by the clinical context.

Pharmacokinetics of Newer AEDs
Data are only available for some of the newer AEDS (see chapter 4 for additional information).

Lamotrigine
Lamotrigine is only 55% protein bound with no significant differences expected in the ratio between free and total serum levels in pregnancy. The clearance of lamotrigine, however, is markedly increased in pregnancy due to increased renal clearance, which occurs earlier in pregnancy, and oestrogenic induction of the hepatic enzyme UGT1A4 catalysing lamotrigine glucuronidation, with resultant falls in serum levels of lamotrigine as reported by many studies, with some showing an associated increase in seizures (102–114). In the last study, median lamotrigine clearance rose by 197% during the first trimester, 236% the second and 248% the third with a maximum of 264% at delivery. According to Patsalos (99), clearance may be increased by up to 300% during pregnancy. The increase is significantly attenuated by co-medication with valproate (115). Of note is the large individual variation observed between patients. After delivery the increased clearance returns to baseline levels by the end of 2 weeks (Fig. 12.1). The available evidence suggests that it is advisable to maintain serum levels of lamotrigine during pregnancy by increasing the dose, however, given the well-documented inter-individual variation, dose changes would need to be tailored to the individual woman. To avoid toxicity post-partum, a reduction in dose may be indicated where a significant dose increase has been made as discussed further below.

Assuming adherence to treatment can be maintained, if the dose is moderate or high, we suggest splitting the total daily lamotrigine dose to avoid high peak levels and to counteract potential loss of efficacy due to fluctuating levels with increased clearance and half-life. Our current practice is to monitor pre-dose lamotrigine levels regularly during pregnancy. Preconception levels, taken when dose and control are optimal, are advised, as well as a when the woman first presents with the pregnancy. Levels are then performed monthly during pregnancy, more often if there is clinical concern or changes made. Dose increases (increments depending on baseline dose – see below) are made in the majority of women on lamotrigine in any of the following circumstances:

a.   Prophylactically, when there is a drop in levels at any stage with the aim of maintaining pre-pregnancy levels and preventing deterioration in seizure control

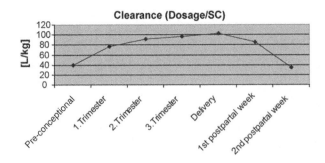

[L/kg]	Pre-conceptional	1.trimester	2.trimester	3.trimester	Delivery	1st postpartal week	2nd postpartal week
Median LTG-clearance	39	77	92	97	103	85	35
25% Percentile	39	68	76	74	71	71	35
75% Percentile	41	154	167	110	179	159	36

Figure 12.1 Median changes in lamotrigine clearance at different stages of pregnancy and puerperium in nine women on lamotrigine monotherapy. *Abbreviation*: SC, lamotrigine-serum concentration. *Source*: From Ref. 113.

b. Prophylactically, if there were significant falls in serum level in previous pregnancies or clinical deterioration

c. In the event of any increase in seizures, the dose is increased on clinical grounds without waiting for serum levels

Interestingly, a similar approach to managing lamotrigine in pregnancy appears successful based on a single practice from Denmark (116), where regular (minimum monthly) assessment and monitoring of lamotrigine levels were carried out. If levels dropped below baseline, a prophylactic increase in dose by 20% to 25% was advised within 1 week of the levels being taken. An increase in seizures occurred in 19% (half of whom had an increase in frequency while half relapsed having been controlled) compared to 45% from the same centre when monitoring was less frequent. This study shows a clear advantage to this approach, although more than one possible explanation for improvement may be postulated.

Post-partum lamotrigine dose, if increased significantly during pregnancy, will need to be decreased to avoid a rise in level and concomitant toxicity to the mother or infant. The aim is to avoid major fluctuations in levels. Figure 12.2 (112) shows the rise in lamotrigine levels post-partum in patients who, all but one, had not had dose alterations. A decision needs to be made, depending on the individual case, whether to aim for pre-pregnancy doses/levels or aim higher to provide more protection during a vulnerable period. Pennell et al. (116) began prescribing an 'empiric postpartum taper schedules to decrease the dose by steady increments at postpartum days 3, 7, and 10, with return to preconception dose or preconception dose plus 50 mg to help counteract the effects of sleep deprivation'. Those without this taper were more likely to experience symptoms of toxicity (117). We also follow an empiric taper in those where the dose has been increased significantly. We recommend deciding on the intended dose in consultation with the woman before delivery, then, if appropriate, planning a gradual reduction over the first 2 weeks post-partum until this is achieved, with the advice that side effects or seizures would modify the regime. Some authors advise regular post-partum levels, for example, weekly (113) or consider that levels every second day for 1 week after delivery could be justified (99). While prompt results of levels, if available, would be helpful, this is unlikely to be practical in many settings.

Oxcarbazepine

In the EURAP study there was an association between being on oxcarbazepine monotherapy and the occurrence of GTCS in pregnancy. Oxcarbazepine is only 40% protein bound and the ratio between free and total serum levels is not altered by pregnancy. The active metabolite of oxcarbazepine, like lamotrigine, is metabolised via glucuronidation with a significant drop in levels of its active metabolite observed in pregnancy, with inter-individual variation observed. In a study of five women taking oxcarbazepine as monotherapy, the level of the active moiety [10-hydroxycarbazepine (MHD)] decreased markedly during gestation and, in four of the five patients, increased strikingly after delivery (118). Similar changes were noted in another study of nine pregnancies in seven women (119). Although conclusions were limited regarding the relationship between decrease in levels and seizures, in one of the studies (118), in at least 2/5 patients lower plasma concentrations were associated with emergence of seizures and improvement following dose increase. In a retrospective Danish study looking at 13 pregnancies in 10 women on oxcarbazepine monotherapy, and 1 on polytherapy (with topiramate), significant decreases of the mean of the ratio of plasma concentration of MHD to dosage was observed (by 26.2%, 36.5% and 38.2% during the first, second and third trimester, respectively) compared to non-pregnant levels. Eight had seizure deterioration during pregnancy, five of whom had been seizure-free before (120). While awaiting more data, we advocate close monitoring of women on oxcarbazepine during pregnancy with monthly TDM and dose adjustments aiming to maintain levels stable in pregnancy and post-partum. The dose would need to be increased if there is any clinical deterioration on a drop in levels.

Levetiracetam

Levetiracetam has minimal protein binding and is mostly excreted unchanged by the kidneys with about one-quarter of a dose undergoing extrahepatic hydrolysis. In a prospective study, Tomson et al. (121) studied levetiracetam disposition in up to 15 pregnancies (14 women). A trend towards a decline in concentrations in the first two trimesters was observed with a significant drop in levels in the third trimester to 40% of baseline concentrations outside pregnancy (n = 7). Five of

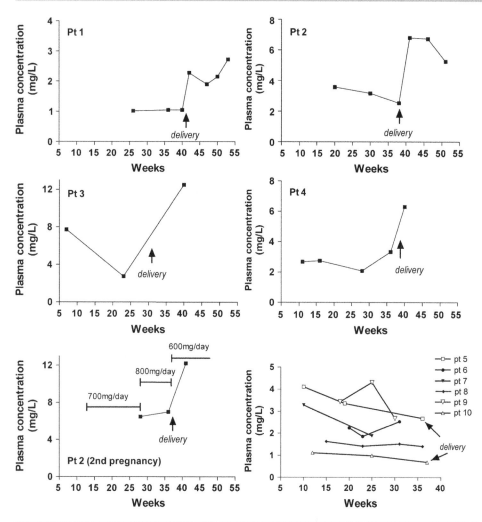

Figure 12.2 Individual plasma concentrations of lamotrigine in five pregnancies assessed before and after delivery (patients 1–4) and in six additional pregnancies assessed at different gestational periods. In second pregnancy from patient 2, reported concentrations are normalised to a 600 mg daily dose (actual dosages taken are also specified). *Source*: From Ref. 112.

seven patients remained controlled, despite a drop in levels and no change in treatment dose. A drop in levetiracetam levels was also reported by Westin et al. (122) in a retrospective study of 21 consecutive pregnancies in 20 women. Mean C/D ratio in the third trimester was 50% of the mean C/D ratio at baseline ($p < 0.001$, $n = 11$). Baseline levels were reached within the first weeks after pregnancy. Reduced seizure frequency was observed in 5/19 completed pregnancies and increased seizure frequency in 7/19 necessitating AED dose increases. However, the observed decline in C/D ratio was not more pronounced in those with increased seizures. Inter-individual variability was pronounced as shown in Figure 12.3. A third study showed similar findings with a drop in levels in 4/5 cases with unchanged dosages of levetiracetam with mean (SD) levetiracetam plasma concentrations as follows: 13.5 (2.4) mg/L in the first trimester; 11.4 (4.4) mg/L in the second trimester; 11.2 (3.5) mg/L in the third trimester; and 23.8 (10.7) and 18.1 (4.1) mg/L at 2 and 12 months post-delivery, respectively. The reason for the difference between the second month and 12 months after delivery is not clear (123). Thus, pregnancy is associated with declines (30–50%) in serum drug concentrations of levetiracetam (124). The clinical implication of this requires more data to be established and it is not possible to give firm recommendations at this stage.

Topiramate
Topiramate is only 15% protein bound. Two studies show significant changes in topiramate pharmacokinetics in

pregnancy. Westin et al. (125) showed average C/D ratios in the second and third trimester at 30% and 34% lower than baseline values, respectively, with pronounced inter-individual variability. Although increased seizure frequency was common, correlation to the decline in C/D ratio could not be established (125). In another study from Sweden, higher topiramate dose/concentration ratios (D/C ratio) in pregnancy were reported indicating a drop in levels in pregnancy (126). Again, a clear correlation between the extent of the increase in D/C ratio in the third trimester and increase in seizures during pregnancy was not demonstrated, but topiramate dose was increased as a response to seizures or a decline in levels. A study in pregnant rabbits was reported as showing a rise rather than a fall in levels (127), with an increase in half-life and decease in clearance. As with levetiracetam, the clinical impact of the decrease in topiramate levels in pregnancy remains to be established.

MANAGEMENT OF EPILEPSY IN WOMEN OF CHILDBEARING AGE: PRACTICAL CONSIDERATIONS

The key to optimising treatment regimens and minimising risk in pregnancy is through prior planning and providing information to WWE. The latter is a long process which begins with the diagnosis of epilepsy and develops over many consultations with different health providers. Despite guidelines, evidence suggests that there is considerable scope for

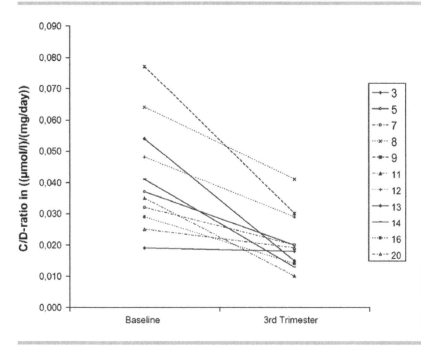

Figure 12.3 Individual serum concentration/dose ratios [(mmol/L)/(mg/day)] at baseline and during the third trimester, in 11 women on levetiracetam. *Abbreviation*: C/D, concentration/dose. *Source*: From Ref. 122.

improvement. As structural teratogenesis occurs during organogenesis which occupies the first trimester, the patient most needs to be on the optimum AED medication and folic acid supplementation at the time of conception and through the first trimester to avoid MCM. For these reasons, the ideal is to achieve the optimisation of medication through preconceptual counselling, although a Cochrane review concluded that there is no evidence to inform the content, methods of delivery or effectiveness of preconception counselling to improve pregnancy outcomes (128). The major issues in this respect are listed here and discussed in more detail below.

- Preconceptual counselling is aimed at optimising outcome and the great majority of children born to WWE do not have congenital malformations.
- Consideration of minimising teratogenesis should begin early. It should be considered in all females of childbearing age *and below including any female child with epilepsy.*
- In females of appropriate age, the topic should be fully discussed and backed-up with supportive literature.
- There may be insufficient time to fully address all the issues in a busy clinic and additional appointments are often needed, including, if available, with a specialist epilepsy nurse.
- A central aim, where possible, is for monotherapy at the minimum effective dose.
- Folic acid is recommended to all women who might conceive with the aim of reducing NTD.
- Additional teratogens should be avoided: other medications, alcohol, tobacco, illicit drugs.
- Pregnant WWE should have fetal ultrasound scans (see below and chapter 3).
- An important aim is to avoid GTCS in pregnancy. It has to be acknowledged that this is not always possible. Although GTCS can lead to an adverse outcome, their occurrence is compatible with the delivery of a healthy child.
- There are no absolutes in AED prescribing for WWE. Given the many uncertainties in this area, input from a clinician with a good level of expertise in epilepsy is recommended.

CONSIDERATIONS REGARDING CONTRACEPTION AND THE MORNING-AFTER PILL

A detailed discussion of contraception is outside the scope of this chapter. However, the following is relevant.

- Enzyme-inducing AEDs reduce the efficacy of contraceptive implants, the oral contraceptive pill and the morning-after pill. It is recommended that the dose of the latter is increased in this situation. The dose of the pill, if the woman does not wish to consider other contraception, needs to be increased sufficiently to abolish mid-cycle bleeding. Barrier methods should be used until the dose is sufficient. The woman would still need to be informed that protection is nevertheless reduced and encouraged to consider other methods of contraception. Folic acid should be recommended whenever protection is deemed suboptimal.
- The oestrogen component of the oral contraceptive pill reduces the level and clinical effect of lamotrigine (102).
- There is no specific contraindication in epilepsy to the use of the intrauterine device (including those which are progesterone coated).
- Depot progesterone injections are suitable and there is no good evidence to reduce the frequency of administration in WWE on enzyme-inducing AEDs. There is, however, an association with osteoporosis and depot progesterone, and this form of contraception is therefore generally not recommended in very young women.

CONSIDERATIONS REGARDING ATTEMPTED AED WITHDRAWAL BEFORE CONCEPTION

In general, AED withdrawal is usually only considered if the epilepsy has been fully controlled for a few years or if the seizure type has always been very mild. The decision will depend on whether the woman is willing to take the risk of relapse on slow withdrawal, a risk which varies between cases. The individual woman's risk of relapse over the next year can be estimated from the MRC AED withdrawal study (129) and is often significant. The outcome of any previous attempts at withdrawal, whether undertaken after consultation or independently by the patient, should be sought. Furthermore, a careful history concerning minor seizures is needed. Women in whom the epilepsy is supposedly controlled are sometimes referred for consideration of withdrawal, but a more detailed history may reveal that they are experiencing infrequent auras, partial seizures, absences or myoclonus. Whilst these may be mild and need not necessarily pose a risk during pregnancy, they indicate that the epilepsy is active and that withdrawal of AEDs is unlikely to be appropriate where there is a previous history of more severe seizures. However, women who have only ever had mild seizures (myoclonus, brief absences, auras) with no history of GTCS or other more severe seizures may wish to come off medication before conception. This is reasonable so long as the woman is aware that while the risk of GTCS or more severe seizures may be low in her case, the occurrence of such seizures cannot be excluded. This possibility and its potential consequences would need to be discussed.

Before a woman whose epilepsy is fully controlled undertakes AED withdrawal, she would need to consider the potential consequences of seizures to herself and to the fetus or infant, including the increased risk of seizures with sleep deprivation later in pregnancy and post-partum, and balance this against the risk of AED-induced structural or cognitive teratogenicity, discussed above. Whenever AED withdrawal is advised, physical risks related to seizures need to be discussed and precautions, where possible, taken. Seizures, particularly GTCS, carry a small risk of serious physical injury and of drowning as well as a small risk of sudden death. Relevant local driving regulations also need to be imparted. For those dependent on driving, this can prove to be an important deciding factor. In the United Kingdom, for example, the advice is to refrain from driving for the period of withdrawal and for 6 months after. Regulations vary in different countries and local advice needs to be communicated.

A woman who is fully controlled may opt to (a) continue AED treatment before and during pregnancy while optimising her treatment regime or (b) gradually attempt drug withdrawal before conception. Those who opt for the latter have the option of restarting medication at any time, not only if seizures recur, but also prophylactically for protection later in pregnancy, during delivery and while looking after the infant. Of relevance in this context is that many AEDs need to be reintroduced gradually. Time to conception is very variable and age has an important effect of the chance of spontaneous conception. Thus, the woman may be left without AED cover for some time. Where medication is withdrawn, and to avoid later delay, discussion is advised regarding the AED regime recommended if seizures recur. Often, but by no means always, this will be the same previously successful regime.

Where appropriate to withdraw AEDs, this is usually carried out slowly and gradually. The rate at which this is recommended varies per case and the habituating potential of the AED(s) taken. Long-term phenobarbital, primidone and benzodiazepines, for example, must be withdrawn extremely slowly and early planning is vital. Where time allows, the case can be made for very slow withdrawal with all AEDs. If control is maintained at a given dose for a reasonable period, but a seizure occurs when the dose is reduced further, this allows for an estimate of the minimum effective dose. An older woman, however, may not wish to delay the process unduly.

The above are considerations and recommendations are for changes in AEDs before conception and it should be remembered that considerable time is usually needed to complete withdrawal and assess if this is successful.

AED IN MONOTHERAPY, WHICH DRUG AND WHAT DOSE?

Monotherapy is considered safer than polytherapy in pregnancy with more than 95% of women on monotherapy with most AEDS having children within normal. Nevertheless, children with malformations are born to women on monotherapy, as indeed to women without epilepsy and AEDs. It is therefore important to minimise the risk, wherever possible, for all women including the 'low-risk' monotherapy group. On the basis of current knowledge, this is done by the choice of AED, minimum effective doses and more frequent dosing schedules to avoid high peak levels, although there are no clinical data to support the latter recommendation. In addition, general measures to reduce malformations are advised including giving supplements and reducing other unrelated risk factors, such as excess alcohol and other medication.

Whichever medication is taken needs to be effective in the woman's case in preventing seizures, particularly GTCS. An ineffective AED in an individual case, even if considered to carry a lower risk in pregnancy, means that the woman is exposed to both potential teratogenicity and to risks associated with uncontrolled seizures. Potential future pregnancies need to be considered right at the outset of epilepsy treatment even in girls not yet of childbearing age or women who are not yet sexually active. Where possible, AEDs known to be safer in pregnancy are offered first, so that by the time the woman is contemplating pregnancy, she has already established the optimal medication for her. Given sufficient time, a woman contemplating pregnancy who has never tried other AEDs and who is on medications considered less safe, such as valproate, is offered the option of changing AED prior to conception to an AED associated with better pregnancy outcomes. The woman needs to know that the next medication may not suit her and success is not guaranteed. It is important that contraception is continued during the changeover period to avoid conception on two AEDs. Safety advice needs to be given during any change in addition to guidance regarding driving. If AEDs associated with lower teratogenicity are not successful, the woman may consider changing from a medication considered unsafe to another which is relatively unknown in pregnancy. Given the lack of evidence, such a decision is based on the individual case, incomplete data, the woman's preference and outcome of any previous pregnancies.

As discussed above, ongoing pregnancy registers will continue to improve the scope and quality of data in relation to structural teratogenicity with both established and new AEDs. Currently, CBZ and lamotrigine have been shown to carry a lower associated risk of major malformations. Valproate, particularly with higher doses, is associated with a greater risk of structural and cognitive teratogenicity. The risk with many other drugs remains unknown. Levetiracetam appears promising, although more data are needed. Thus, in someone with focal epilepsy, CBZ or lamotrigine is reasonable first-choice option as they are associated with a relatively low risk. The much greater drop in lamotrigine levels compared to CBZ during pregnancy, however, necessitates more active management. On the other hand, lamotrigine is not associated with any adverse developmental outcome while a small effect from CBZ is not excluded. In generalised epilepsy, and although sodium valproate is more effective, it should not be offered as first line to a woman of childbearing age (98). Here, lamotrigine is a reasonable choice, although not as effective as valproate. Where lamotrigine is ineffective, other options are offered and levetiracetam appears a reasonable choice at this time. Information on zonisamide is limited, and breastfeeding is not advised with it. Teratogenicity has also been reported with topiramate, but there is no comparative data between it and valproate. CBZ, while not first choice in those with generalised epilepsy syndromes, may be effective in treating GTCS in this context, although exacerbations, particularly but not exclusively of absences and myoclonus, may occur. If after trying other suitable AEDs, valproate is deemed the most effective in a given case, and with the woman's informed consent, the dose advised needs to (a) be the minimum that controls GTCS, (b) be kept below 800 to 1000 mg for as much of the pregnancy as possible and (c) although there is no direct clinical evidence to support this, be taken in divided doses in a long-acting formulation to reduce peak levels. Of note is that maximum benefit from valproate is not always immediate and fast titration may miss the minimum effective dose. Throughout, a priority is to maximise the safety of the woman.

With all drugs it is sensible to maintain the woman on the lowest dose that will control attacks. To guide this, a detailed previous medication history is needed. How was the AED first titrated? Was the dose the woman is on when contemplating pregnancy one she was advised to reach automatically or was it needed to achieve control? Will it be possible to reduce the dose with reasonable expectation of maintaining control of convulsive or other potentially dangerous seizures?

AED IN POLYTHERAPY, WHAT ARE THE OPTIONS?

As already discussed, teratogenicity risk is higher with polytherapy than monotherapy. In each individual case, whether the epilepsy is controlled or not, consideration should be given to simplifying medication, although this is not possible in all cases. In some women, the risk from the epilepsy is such that despite less than ideal AED regimens, no change is made. An example might be someone with a history of status epilepticus with previous attempts to withdraw AEDs. Some women may also chose not to make any change in their AED treatment if the epilepsy had been severe and required many attempts to become stable.

In those on polytherapy who wish to attempt rationalisation of treatment, even if the epilepsy is not fully controlled, and in whom this is judged to be a reasonable course of action, an attempt is made to withdraw one, or more if appropriate, of the AEDs. Which AED reduction is attempted first varies depending on the individual case. The following information may help guide this process: Which of the AEDs taken has a better profile in pregnancy? How were AEDs introduced and which appeared the more effective for more severe seizure types? Which AED controlled convulsions? Were any of the medications added to control auras or brief absences, and could they be safely withdrawn? Which AED may cause neonatal drowsiness at birth or is more likely to cause problems with breastfeeding? With which AED was reduction attempted before and how successful was the reduction? Which AED is habituating and how much time does the woman have for making changes? What interactions need to be considered between the concomitant AEDs? If an enzyme-inducing drug is withdrawn, side effects may emerge, for example, due to a rise in blood level of the remaining AED, if hepatically metabolised. Conversely, if valproate is withdrawn, the loss of enzyme inhibition would result in, for example, decrease in lamotrigine level and may result in loss of seizure control. Dose adjustments in the remaining drugs may be needed.

If withdrawing one AED is unsuccessful, it may then be worth trying to reduce or withdraw another AED so long as

the woman's safety is not compromised. Even if withdrawing an AED proves unsuccessful, the process, if carried out slowly, would have helped establish the minimum effective dose. It is usually important for the woman to go forward with planning a pregnancy knowing that she has optimised her treatment as much as she is safely able to.

EARLY MANAGEMENT OF AN UNPLANNED PREGNANCY

Even if the main time period during which organogenesis takes place (see Table 3.1 in chapter 3) has already passed by the time the woman presents, if still relatively early in pregnancy, it is still worth considering developmental outcome, for example, in someone on valproate. Thus, without recommending abrupt changes, reviewing AEDS as well as doses given, as discussed above, may be appropriate. If it is possible to minimise AED exposure, for example, by reducing valproate dose, *if this can be safely achieved*, this can be considered. Addressing unrelated risk factors and ensuring a good diet with adequate supplementation are also needed.

DURING PREGNANCY

While many pregnancies in WWE proceed without difficulty, expert advice and support may be needed. Drug levels and doses have been discussed above. The woman is encouraged to take responsibility for aiding the monitoring process, where indicated, and for reporting promptly any change in seizures. Review can be provided by midwife, obstetrician, family physician, neurologist and epilepsy nurse. Routine scans are carried out (see below and chapter 3). Information provision is important with advice on adherence to treatment, breastfeeding, lifestyle and safety issues in relation to looking after the infant is needed (see specimen clinical form and specimen clinical checklist in text boxes 2a and 2b below) along with discussion with the obstetrician regarding delivery options. Because of the association of epilepsy with fetal growth restriction in some reports, consideration should be given to performing scans for fetal growth in the third trimester of pregnancy, especially in those women who have poorly controlled epilepsy or who are taking multiple AEDs.

Hospital delivery is recommended in case seizures occur, although some women who have been seizure-free for several years and who remain seizure-free in pregnancy consider homebirth. Although an increased rate of caesarean section is observed in some studies, vaginal delivery is the most likely expectation for WWE.

VITAMIN SUPPLEMENTATION: FOLIC ACID AND VITAMIN K₁
Folic Acid Supplementation

It is accepted, on the basis of high-quality evidence, that folic acid supplementation to women in general at and around the time of conception reduces the risk of NTD such as spina bifida. This applies to both primary (4 mg dose used) (130) and secondary prevention with lower doses used (previous child with NTD or first-degree relative with a child with NTD). In the United Kingdom, it is recommended that all women who may fall pregnant should take folic acid 400 mcg/day and this should be continued to the end of the 12th week of pregnancy. There is a question as to whether supplementation should be continued for longer in the hope that this may reduce the risk of other later occurring malformations such as cleft lip and palate, although this has not been demonstrated in the general population (131). The role of folate in reducing malformations specifically associated with AEDs has not been established and evidence is still inconclusive. An evidence evaluation (22) concluded that the risk of MCMs in the offspring of WWE is possibly decreased by folic acid supplementation on the basis of two adequately sensitive class III studies. In pregnancy, and although folic acid supplementation is advised, recommendations vary and doses to some extent depend on available formulations. Some AEDs interfere with folic acid metabolism. In the United Kingdom, the recommendation in reference guidelines followed by many practitioners is for 5 mg/day, a dose which cannot be obtained without a prescription. Despite this recommendation, Morrow found that in only 41% of cases was the vitamin commenced before conception and 21% of those who commenced it at any stage had the lower 400 mcg dose. Overall, only 32% had the higher dose at the appropriate time (132). The glib condition: *'woman who may fall pregnant'* glosses over a sea of uncertainty. The appropriateness of folic acid supplementation for any individual depends on clinical judgement (and common sense). In general, the tendency has been to be very liberal in recommending the vitamin on the basis that it is harmless and *'just in case'*, although lack of harm cannot be assumed. High-dose folic acid may be detrimental in pernicious anaemia.

In conclusion, it is recommended that folic acid supplementation be given before conception and during pregnancy for at least the first 12 weeks (131). As some AEDs may reduce maternal folate levels there may be an argument for continuing folate throughout pregnancy in women taking these drugs. As the optimal duration and dose of supplementation have not been established, clinicians are advised to follow national guidelines.

Vitamin K$_1$

For many years, (soluble) Vitamin K$_1$ was recommended at 10 to 20 mg/day for the last 4 weeks of pregnancy in those on enzyme-inducing AEDs, in addition to being given routinely to neonates at delivery at 1 mg intramuscularly (IM) to reduce risk of haemorrhagic disease of the newborn. The advice regarding oral supplementation to the mother, however, has been questioned given lack of evidence. The 2009 Report of the Quality Standards Subcommittee and Therapeutics and Technology Assessment Subcommittee of the American Academy of Neurology and the American Epilepsy Society reviewed published studies on incidence of haemorrhagic complications in the newborn (any haemorrhage within 24 hours of birth), excluding studies which only looked at surrogate markers of risk (100). Eight articles were rated class IV, one class III (133) and one II (134). Neither of the latter two studies showed an increased risk of neonatal haemorrhagic complications in newborns of WWE taking AEDs (and not receiving oral Vitamin K$_1$) compared to newborns of women without epilepsy, with the Kaaja study looking specifically at enzyme-inducing AEDs. However, in this study, the high upper limit of the CI (OR, 1.1; 95% CI, 0.3–4.6; $p = 0.8$) 'indicates that the possibility of a substantial risk cannot be excluded'. The majority of haemorrhages in AED-exposed newborns were accounted for by premature birth (<34 weeks). A Cochrane review looked at evidence in relation to the use of Vitamin K before preterm birth and concluded that 'Vitamin K administered to women prior to very preterm birth has not been shown to significantly prevent periventricular haemorrhages in preterm infants or improve neurodevelopmental outcomes in childhood' (135).

The conclusion of the 2009 report (100) was that there is insufficient evidence to determine if the risk of neonatal haemorrhagic complications in the newborns of WWE taking AEDs is substantially increased based on one inadequately sensitive class

II study, with the recommendation that counselling of pregnant WWE pregnancy should reflect this. Furthermore, they found no evidence, higher than class IV, that prenatal vitamin K supplementation reduces the risk of haemorrhagic complications in the newborns of WWE taking AEDs, with the recommendation that there is insufficient evidence to support or refute a benefit of *prenatal* vitamin K supplementation for reducing the risk of haemorrhagic complications in the newborns of WWE. Prophylactic administration of Vitamin K to all newborns is standard. In the United Kingdom, NICE guidelines (2006) state that all parents should be offered vitamin K prophylaxis for their babies, that Vitamin K should be administered as a single dose of 1 mg IM and that, if parents decline IM vitamin K for their baby, oral vitamin K should be offered as a second-line option (http://www.nice.org.uk/nicemedia/pdf/CG37NICEguideline.pdf).

FETAL SONOGRAPHY – AND MAJOR MALFORMATIONS

In the United Kingdom, fetal ultrasonography for the detection of anatomical anomalies is routinely offered at 12 weeks and/or between 18 and 23 weeks. Ultrasound examination has its intrinsic limitations and its efficacy is reduced by body mass index, fetal position, operator experience and inadequate machinery. High-resolution scanning with four-chamber view of the heart and outflow tracts should be offered. Where the risk of an anomaly is particularly high, an anomaly scan at 12 weeks could be offered. The early identification of a major anomaly at 12 weeks allows for the possibility of vaginal termination of pregnancy. If this is not chosen then the recognition of the problem may allow appropriate material and emotional preparation for the child's arrival and the identification of the optimum birth management and specialist centre. In a minority of cases, intrauterine treatment may be possible. The woman and her partner need to be supported through a very difficult time and a difficult decision-making process often with an uncertain outcome. Expert advice and counselling should be offered. Ethical considerations are discussed in more detail in chapter 9. The implications to future pregnancies of the woman's AED treatment would need to be later reviewed and AED treatment reconsidered.

MANAGEMENT OF WORSENING SEIZURE CONTROL IN PREGNANCY

If there is a significant change in seizure frequency, severity or pattern, particularly if this is not responsive to an increase in AED dose, a review of the diagnosis or underlying pathology is indicated. Sometimes a diagnosis of psychogenic seizures is made following EEG video telemetry or new or progressive pathology identified. Indeed, if there is any diagnostic doubt, wherever possible, this is better resolved before pregnancy (see chapter 11). In a small proportion of patients, epilepsy control appears to deteriorate significantly in pregnancy without this being due to new pathology, AED-related factors or sleep deprivation. Where a new AED is started in pregnancy consideration should be given to teratogenicity as well as the potential effect on the neonate depending on the stage in pregnancy. In late pregnancy, medications that take a long time to be titrated safely are best voided as are medication more likely to sedate the infant. Additional treatment goals in this setting include preventing severe seizures, clusters or serial seizures or status epilepticus, as well as maintaining some measure of stability until such a time in pregnancy when planned delivery may be contemplated. Rescue medication with benzodiazepine can be used but are kept to a minimum near delivery to minimise neonatal drowsiness.

MANAGEMENT DURING DELIVERY

Management during delivery consists of making sure medication is taken promptly, that the woman does not get too tired and that appropriate obstetric and medical support for the mother and baby is in place should seizures occur. In the EURAP study, seizures occurred during delivery in 60/1956 pregnancies (3.5%), more commonly in women with seizures during pregnancy (OR, 4.8; 2.3–10.0). Local labour ward protocols in maternity units for the management of WWE in labour should emphasise the importance of continuous electronic fetal monitoring if the fetus is thought to be growth restricted, contain details of drugs that should be used to terminate a grand mal seizure and the protocol for the management of a pregnant woman during a seizure. Protocols should emphasise that seizures during labour that do not cause fetal distress (e.g. one brief partial seizure) may be self-limiting and do not in themselves imply that delivery of the fetus should be immediate. The protocol should also indicate which medical staff should be contacted in the event of a seizure. It should be ensured that drugs used for the termination of a seizure are kept on the labour ward as ward stock.

MANAGEMENT POST-PARTUM

Medication reduction may be needed to avoid toxicity with certain AEDs, notably lamotrigine, if the dose was increased by a significant amount during pregnancy to maintain blood levels, as discussed above. For the mother, minimising sleep deprivation, regular adherence to treatment, encouraging and accepting support from family members and adopting safe practice in looking after the infant are key considerations discussed further below.

BREASTFEEDING

This is also discussed in chapters 4 and 5. WWE often have concerns about AEDs and breastfeeding. In general, breast-feeding is recommended where possible. Furthermore, given that all AEDs cross the placenta in significant quantities, the baby would have been exposed to the medication in the womb and withholding breastfeeding may give rise to withdrawal symptoms. The amount of AED which passes into breast milk is often very small although this is not always the case depending on the medication (Table 12.6).

Drug clearance in the infant is different from that of the mother and accumulation may occur, this being more of a concern if the infant is premature. Other considerations include the physical safety of the infant if the mother has uncontrolled epilepsy and exacerbation of sleep deprivation with nocturnal breastfeeding. Breastfeeding at ground level with the mother's back supported, with help present, may

Table 12.6 Relative Infant Doses for Some AEDS

Carbamazepine	4.35
Diazepam	8.1
Gabapentin	6.5
Lamotrigine	22.8
Levetiracetam	5.4
Lorazepam	2.5
Phenobarbital	23.9
Phenytoin	7.7
Sodium valproate	0.68
Topiramate	24.4
Zonisamide	*33*

Source: Adapted from Ref. 136.

reduce risk, and the mother can avoid getting up at night by expressing her milk beforehand. In practice, breastfeeding is generally recommended with most AEDs (see chapter 5 for exceptions), with the proviso that if the baby is drowsy or not feeding well, breastfeeding should be avoided or supplemented by formula milk to reduce the daily dose of AED the infant receives. This advice applies to term infants. More caution is required in premature infants.

The amount of drug excreted into breast milk depends on concentrations in maternal plasma, molecular weight, protein binding and lipid solubility. Drugs more likely to transfer into human milk attain high concentrations in maternal plasma, are low in Molecular Weight (MW), have low protein binding and high lipid solubility. A method of measuring risk is the relative infant dose (RID) calculated by dividing the infant's dose via milk (mg/kg/day) by the mother's dose (mg/kg/day). The RID indicates how much medication the infant is exposed to on a weight-normalised basis (Table 12.6).

EPILEPSY AND PREGNANCY: THE ROLE OF THE EPILEPSY NURSE

In some countries, the epilepsy specialist nurse (ESN) has become an integral part of the team. In the United Kingdom, this is supported by national guidelines (137) which advocate that people with epilepsy should have access to ESNs at the time of diagnosis and when they are reviewed. These guidelines also state that 'WWE and their partners, as appropriate, must be given accurate information and counselling about contraception, conception, pregnancy, caring for young children, breast feeding and menopause'. The ENS has a pivotal role in ensuring that this guidance is met. In one survey carried out by the U.K. national charity, Epilepsy Action, in 2002, the majority of women (87%) considering having children would have liked more information about epilepsy treatment and the possible risk to the unborn child. More than half (57%) wanted the latest information on epilepsy treatment and the risk of birth defects on an ongoing basis, even if data was incomplete. Many WWE said they were not receiving vital preconception counselling, or specialist antenatal care during pregnancy (138). One possible reason for this might be the variation in the provision of epilepsy services in the United Kingdom. Bell et al. (139) point out that women do not always recall being given relevant information, hence the need to repeat this regularly.

In addition to providing expert information, advice and support to people with epilepsy and their families on all aspects concerning living with epilepsy, the ESN is ideally placed to act as the first point of contact for patients, General Practitioners (GPs) and other health care professionals, liaising between agencies to ensure continuity of care. Telephone consultations may take place in addition to, or in place of, nurse-led clinics, depending on individual need and preference. Patients are generally encouraged to telephone the ESN if they run into difficulties or if there are any concerns between scheduled appointments. Some nurses hold dedicated preconception clinics where all the issues concerning pregnancy planning are addressed with the aid of a checklist (see text box 2b). A letter to the woman's general practitioner/family doctor outlining what was discussed is copied to the patient, thus reinforcing advice given, and literature, in the form of leaflets produced by voluntary bodies, is provided along with the contact details for the nurse. Some specialist centres provide joint adolescent or transition clinics where, as appropriate, issues concerning women and epilepsy are raised. Information needs to imparted early depending on the individual case, with only 44% of pregnancies in WWE planned in a U.K.

Text box 2a: Specimen clinical form
Women with Epilepsy: Preparing for Pregnancy

Patient's surname		Title	First name(s)	
Date of birth ____/____/____		Hospital number		
Named GP		Epilepsy Specialist		Epilepsy Nurse
Date of first visit to clinic ____/____/____		Obstetrician		
Date of return visit to clinic ____/____/____		Midwife		

Confirm
Security of diagnosis of epilepsy   _____

Seizure type(s) (e.g., tonic-clonic, absence e.t.c.)   _____

Current seizure frequency   _____

Epilepsy syndrome (if known, e.g., idiopathic generalised)   _____

Cause (if known; consider genetic causes e.g., T.S.)   _____

Precipitating factors (e.g., photosensitivity, catamenial)   _____

History of accidents / injuries   _____

Prolonged/serial seizures/status   _____

Non-epileptic seizures   _____

Previous antiepileptic medication

Brand name	Date initiated	Date stopped	Maximum dose reached	Reason for withdrawal

Current antiepileptic medication

Brand name	Dose	Time(s)	Date initiated

Is there an issue regarding compliance?   _____

Are there side effects?   _____

study (14). Pregnant WWE need regular follow-up and a delivery plan with liaison between the obstetrician, midwife and specialist or epilepsy team. This can be facilitated by the ESN who can ensure that systems are in place to prevent WWE who are pregnant from being lost to follow-up. This also applies to the first few weeks following the birth. Other areas where the nurse may help include providing supporting letters to their partner's employers requesting that they be allowed additional time off work to help care for the new infant. This can help to prevent the mother from becoming too exhausted which can trigger attacks. If she is a single mother without family nearby, it might be appropriate to discuss the possibility of referring her for outside help. Many women with poorly controlled seizures are fearful that social services will intervene; this needs to be addressed and the necessary reassurance and support given. Advice about safety

issues in relation to caring for the new infant should be given before the birth so that there is adequate time to prepare and for the woman to absorb the information. In rare circumstances when a woman miscarries, the ESN can also offer support and counselling and guide the woman to where further support is available.

To maximise safety, the mother is encouraged to look after herself and to do her best to avoid common trigger factors for her seizures. Having a supportive family and friends can be invaluable but this should not be at the expense of affecting the mother's confidence and interfere with bonding between mother and baby through overprotection. It is important that she eats regularly. Remembering to take medication at the correct times is important and can be more difficult with a new baby in the house disrupting everyone's routine. Ensuring

Text box 2b: Specimen clinical checklist

Date and initials

Reassurance that the majority of WWE have unproblematic ☐ __/__/__ _____
pregnancies and deliver healthy babies
Importance of planned pregnancies ☐ __/__/__ _____
Menstrual cycle ☐ __/__/__ _____
Potential effect of menstrual cycle on seizure frequency ☐ __/__/__ _____
Potential effect of AEDs on monthly cycle ☐ __/__/__ _____
Cosmetic side effects of AEDs ☐ __/__/__ _____
Sexual activity ☐ __/__/__ _____
Appropriate (reliable) method of contraception ☐ __/__/__ _____
AED interaction with OCP ☐ __/__/__ _____
Fertility ☐ __/__/_ _____
Experience in previous pregnancies ☐ __/__/_ _____
Importance of achieving optimum seizure control (compliance) ☐ __/__/_ _____
Baseline AED serum levels ☐ __/__/_ _____
AED regime (e.g., reduction in dose/withdrawal/switching)
- increased risk of seizures/teratogenicity ☐ __/__/_ _____
Teratogenic effect of AEDs on fetus (include alcohol, cigarettes) ☐ __/__/_ _____
Previous family history of malformations ☐ __/__/_ _____

The availability of prenatal testing ☐ __/__/_ _____
Folic acid supplementation ☐ __/__/__ _____
Potential effect of epilepsy (seizures) on *mother* and fetus ☐ __/__/__ _____
Risk of child developing epilepsy (role of genetic counseling) ☐ __/__/_ _____
Vitamin K supplementation if on enzyme-inducing AEDs if considered appropriate ☐ __/__/_ _____
Importance of taking medication into hospital ☐ __/__/_ _____
Risk of seizures during labor and post partum ☐ __/__/_ _____
Pain control during labor
Post natal fatigue and seizure frequency ☐ __/__/_ _____
Appropriateness of breast feeding ☐ __/__/_ _____
Childcare (e.g., handling, feeding and bathing) ☐ __/__/_ _____
- minimize risk yet maximize opportunities for bonding ☐ __/__/_ _____

Further help and support
Statutory and voluntary organizations ☐ __/__/__ _____
The Pregnancy Registers ☐ __/__/__ _____

sufficient rest and sleep is paramount. A partner can share the responsibilities, especially during the night by giving the baby either formula or expressed milk. Specific examples of practical advice are listed in text box 3.

Text box 3: Practical advice for activities

Feeding	Supervised if seizures
	At floor level on a rug or blanket, leaning against the wall and supported by pillows
	Lower 'high' chair when child is older.
Changing and dressing	At floor level using changing mat.
	Changing units not advised.
Bathing	Only when another adult present; otherwise sponge bath on the floor.
Carrying	Avoid unnecessary use of stairs whenever possible.
	Use of a padded carrycot or car seat.
Around the home	Playpens
	Safety gates to block all exits and stairways.
Outdoors	Deadlocks on pram/pushchair to prevent from rolling away if the mother lets go.
	Reins when the child is older.

Text box 4: Relevant websites
Epilepsy Action: http://www.epilepsy.org.uk/
Epilepsy Society: http://www.epilepsysociety.org.uk/
The American Epilepsy Society: http://www.aesnet.org/
Epilepsy Foundation: http://www.epilepsyfoundation.org/

The U.K. Epilepsy and Pregnancy Register: http://www.epilepsyandpregnancy.co.uk/
An International Registry of Antiepileptic Drugs and Pregnancy (EURAP): http://www.eurapinternational.org
North American Antiepileptic Drug Pregnancy Registry: http://www.aedpregnancyregistry.org/
The Australian Pregnancy Register for Women on Antiepileptic Medication: http://www.apr.org.au

REFERENCES

1. Herzog A. Disorders of reproduction in patients with epilepsy: primary neurological mechanisms. Seizure 2008; 17(2):101–110.
2. Isojärvi J. Disorders of reproduction in patients with epilepsy: antiepileptic drug related mechanisms. Seizure 2008; 17(2): 111–119.

3. Taubøll E, Røste LS, Svalheim S, et al. Disorders of reproduction in epilepsy—what can we learn from animal studies? Seizure 2008; 17(2):120–126.

4. Sukumaran SC, Sarma PS, Thomas SV. Polytherapy increases the risk of infertility in women with epilepsy. Neurology 2010; 75(15):1351–1355.

5. Kariuki JG, Joshi MD, Adam AM, et al. Fertility rate of epileptic women at Kenyatta National Hospital. East Afr Med J 2008; 85 (7):341–346.

6. Löfgren E, Pouta A, von Wendt L, et al. Epilepsy in the northern Finland birth cohort 1966 with special reference to fertility. Epilepsy Behav 2009; 14(1):102–107.

7. Artama M, Isojärvi JI, Raitanen J, et al. Birth rate among patients with epilepsy: a nationwide population-based cohort study in Finland. Am J Epidemiol 2004; 159(11):1057–1063.

8. Wallace H, Shorvon S, Tallis R. Age-specific incidence and prevalence rates of treated epilepsy in an unselected population of 2,052,922 and age-specific fertility rates of women with epilepsy. Lancet 1998; 352(9145):1970–1973.

9. Jalava M, Sillanpaa M. Reproductive activity and offspring health of young adults with childhood-onset epilepsy: a controlled study. Epilepsia 1997; 38(5):532–540.

10. Webber MP, Hauser WA, Ottman R, et al. Fertility in persons with epilepsy. Epilepsia 1986; 27(6):746–752.

11. Schupf N, Ottman R. Reproduction among individuals with idiopathic/cryptogenic epilepsy: risk factors for reduced fertility in marriage. Epilepsia 1996; 9:833–840.

12. Isojärvi J, Laatikainen TJ, Pakarinen AJ, et al. Polycystic ovaries and hyperandrogenism in women taking valproate for epilepsy. N Engl J Med 1993; 329:1383–1388.

13. Morrell MJ, Guldner GT. Hyperandrogenism, ovulatory dysfunction, and polycystic ovary syndrome with valproate versus lamotrigine. Ann Neurol 2008; 64(2):200–211.

14. Fairgrieve SD, Jackson M, Jonas P. Population based, prospective study of the care of women with epilepsy in pregnancy. BMJ 2000; 321(7262):674–675.

15. Olafsson E, Hallgrimsson JT, Hauser WA, et al. Pregnancies of women with epilepsy: a population-based study in Iceland. Epilepsia 1998; 39(8):887–892.

16. Seale CG, Morrell MJ, Nelson L, et al. Analysis of prenatal and gestational care given to women with epilepsy. Neurology 1998; 51(4):1039–1045.

17. Viinikainen K, Eriksson K, Mönkkönen A, et al. The effects of valproate exposure in utero on behavior and the need for educational support in school-aged children. Epilepsy Behav 2006; 9(4):636–640.

18. The Eurap Study Group. Seizure control and treatment in pregnancy: observations from the EURAP epilepsy pregnancy registry. Neurology 2006; 66(3):354–360.

19. Knight AH, Rhind EG, Epilepsy and pregnancy: a study of 153 pregnancies in 59 patients. Epilepsia 1975; 16(1):99–110.

20. Richmond JR, Krishnamoorthy P, Andermann E, et al. Epilepsy and pregnancy: an obstetric perspective. Am J Obstet Gynecol 2004; 190(2):371–379.

21. Vajda FJ, Hitchcock A, Graham J, et al. Seizure control in antiepileptic drug-treated pregnancy. Epilepsia 2008; 49(1):172–176.

22. Harden CL, Hopp J, Ting TY, et al. Practice Parameter update: Management issues for women with epilepsy—Focus on pregnancy (an evidence-based review): Vitamin K, folic acid, blood levels, and breastfeeding. Neurology 2009; 73:142–149.

23. Viinikainen K, Heinonen S, Eriksson K, et al. Community-based, prospective, controlled study of obstetric and neonatal outcome of 179 pregnancies in women with epilepsy. Epilepsia 2006; 47 (1):186–192.

24. Borthen I, Eide M, Daltveit AK, et al. Delivery outcome of women with epilepsy: a population-based cohort study. BJOG 2010; 117(12):1537–1543.

25. Borthen I, Eide M, Daltveit AK, et al. Obstetric outcome in women with epilepsy: a hospital-based, retrospective study. BJOG 2011; 118(8):956–965.

26. The Eighth Report on Confidential Enquiries into Maternal Deaths in the United Kingdom. Saving mothers' lives: reviewing maternal deaths to make motherhood safer: 2006–08. BJOG 2011; 118(suppl 1):1–203.

27. Ottman R, Hirose S, Jain S, et al. Genetic testing in the epilepsies—report of the ILAE Genetics Commission. Epilepsia 2010; 51(4):655–670.

28. Berg AT, Berkovic S, Brodie MJ, et al. Revised terminology and concepts for organization of seizures and epilepsies: report of the ILAE Commission on Classification and Terminology, 2005–2009. Epilepsia 2010; 51(4):676–685.

29. Sisodiya SM, Mefford, HC. Genetic contribution to common epilepsies. Curr Opin Neurol 2011; 24(2):140–145.

30. Winawar MR, Shinnar SGH. Epidemiology of epilepsy or what do we tell families? Epilepsia 2005; 46(suppl 10):24–30.

31. Doose H, Waltz S. Photosensitivity – genetics and clinical significance. Neuropediatrics 1993; 24(5):249–255.

32. Waltz S, Stephani U. Inheritance of photosensitivity. Neuropediatrics 2000; 31(2):82–85.

33. Tauer U, Lorenz, S, Lenzen, K, et al. Genetic dissection of photosensitivity and its relation to idiopathic generalized epilepsy. Ann Neurol 2005; 57(6):866–873.

34. Vadlamudi L, Andermann E, Lombroso CT, et al. Epilepsy in twins: insights from unique historical data of William Lennox. Neurology 2004; 62:1127–1133.

35. Berkovic SF, Howell RA, Hay DA, et al. Epilepsies in twins: genetics of the major epilepsy syndromes. Ann Neurol 1998; 43:435–445.

36. Winawer MR, Marini C, Grinton BE, et al. Evidence for distinct genetic influences on generalized and localization related epilepsy. Epilepsia 2003; 44:1176–1182.

37. Winawer MR, Rabinowitz D, Pedley TA, et al. Genetic influences on myoclonic and absence seizures. Neurology 2003; 61:1576–1581.

38. Ottman R, Lee JH, Hauser WA, et al. Are generalized and localization-related epilepsies genetically distinct? Arch Neurol 1998; 55(3):339–344.

39. Marini C, Scheffer IE, Crossland KM, et al. Genetic architecture of idiopathic generalized epilepsy: clinical genetic analysis of 55 multiplex families. Epilepsia 2004; 45:467–s78.

40. Italian League Against Epilepsy Group. Concordance of clinical forms of epilepsy in families with several affected members. Epilepsia 1993; 34(5):819–826.

41. Marini C, Harvey AS, Pelekanos JT, et al. Epilepsy in offspring of whom both parents have idiopathic generalized epilepsy: biparental inheritance. Epilepsia 2003; 44(9):1250–1254.

42. Jansen AC, Andermann E, and Andermann F. Biparental inheritance in idiopathic generalized epilepsy. Epilepsia 45(10):1294–1295.

43. Doose H, Maurer A. Seizure risk in offspring of individuals with a history of febrile convulsions. Eur J Pediatr 1997; 156(6):476–481.

44. Helbig KL, Bernhardt BA, Conway LJ, et al. Genetic risk perception and reproductive decision making among people with epilepsy. Epilepsia 2010; 51(9):1874–1877.

45. Harden CL, Pennell PB, Koppel BS. Management issues for women with epilepsy – focus on pregnancy (an evidence-based review): II. Teratogenesis and perinatal outcomes. Epilepsia 2009; 50(5):1237–1246.

46. Adab N, Kini U, Vinten J, et al. The longer term outcome of children born to mothers with epilepsy. J Neurol Neurosurg Psychiatry 2004; 75(11):1575–1583.

47. Nashef L, Walker W, Allen P, et al. Apnoea and bradycardia during epileptic seizures: relation to sudden death in epilepsy. J Neurol Neurosurg Psychiatry 1996; 60(3):297–300.

48. Seyal M, Bateman LM, Albertson TE, et al. Respiratory changes with seizures in localization-related epilepsy: analysis of periictal hypercapnia and airflow patterns. Epilepsia 2010; 51(8):1359–1364.

49. Sahoo S, Klein P. Maternal complex partial seizure associated with fetal distress. Arch Neurol 2005; 62(8):1304–1305.

50. Delgado-Escueta AV, Janz D. Consensus guidelines: preconception counselling, management, and care of the pregnant woman with epilepsy. Neurology 1992; 42(4):149–160.

51. Tomson T, Battino D. Teratogenicity of antiepileptic drugs: state of the art. Curr Opin Neurol 2005; 18(2):135–140.

52. Holmes LB, Wyszynski DF, Lieberman ES. The AED (antiepileptic drug) pregnancy registry: a 6-year experience. Arch Neurol 2004; 61(5):673–678.

53. Vajda FJ, O'Brien TJ, Hitchcock A, et al. Critical relationship between sodium valproate dose and human teratogenicity: results of the Australian register of anti-epileptic drugs in pregnancy. J Clin Neurosci 2004; 11(8):854–858.

54. Morrow J, Russell A, Gutherie E, et al. Malformation risks of antiepileptic drugs in pregnancy: a prospective study from the UK Epilepsy and Pregnancy Register. Neurol Neurosurg Psychiatry 2006; 77(2):193–198.

55. Thomas SV, Ajaykuma B, Indhu K, et al. Motor and mental development of infants exposed to antiepileptic drugs in utero. Epilepsy Behav 2008; 13(1):229–236.

56. Cunnington MC, Weil JG, Messenheimer JA, et al. Final results from 18 years of the International Lamotrigine Pregnancy Registry. Neurology 2011;,76(21):1817–1823.

57. Tomson T, Battino D, Craig J, et al; ILAE Commission on Therapeutic Strategies. Pregnancy registries: differences, similarities, and possible harmonization. Epilepsia 2010; 51(5):909–915.

58. Vajda FJ, Graham J, Hitchcock AA, et al. Foetal malformations after exposure to antiepileptic drugs in utero assessed at birth and 12 months later: observations from the Australian pregnancy register. Acta Neurol Scand 2011; 124(1):9–12.

59. Wyszynski DF, Nambisan M, Surve T, et al. Antiepileptic drug pregnancy registry. Increased rate of major malformations in offspring exposed to valproate during pregnancy. Neurology 2005; 64(6):961–965.

60. Samrén EB, van Duijn CM, Koch S, et al. Maternal use of antiepileptic drugs and the risk of major congenital malformations: a joint European prospective study of human teratogenesis. Epilepsia 1997; 38(9):981–990.

61. Tomson T, Battino D, Bonizzoni E, et al. Dose-dependent risk of malformations with antiepileptic drugs: an analysis of data from the EURAP epilepsy and pregnancy registry. Lancet Neurol 2011; 10(7):609–617; [Epub5 June 2011].

62. Holmes LB, Mittendorf R, Shen A, et al. Fetal effects of anticonvulsant polytherapies: different risks from different drug combinations. Arch Neurol 2011; 68(10):1275–1281; [Epub 13 Jun 2011].

63. Holmes LB, Baldwin EJ, Smith CR, et al. Increased frequency of isolated cleft palate in infants exposed to lamotrigine during pregnancy. Neurology 2008; 70(22 pt 2):2152–2158. Erratum in: Neurology 2009; 72(16):1449.

64. Holmes LB, Wyszynski DF. North American antiepileptic drug pregnancy registry. Epilepsia 2004; 45(11):1465.

65. Mølgaard-Nielsen D, Hviid A. Newer-generation antiepileptic drugs and the risk of major birth defects. JAMA 2011; 305 (19):1996–2002.

66. ten Berg K, Samren EB, van Oppen AC, et al. Levetiracetam use and pregnancy outcome. Reprod Toxicol 2005; 20(1):175–178.

67. Shallcross R, Bromley RL, Irwin B, et al. Child development following in utero exposure: levetiracetam vs sodium valproate. Neurology 76(4):383–389.

68. Hunt S, Russell A, Smithson WH, et al. UK Epilepsy and Pregnancy Register. Topiramate in pregnancy: preliminary experience from the UK Epilepsy and Pregnancy Register. Neurology 2008; 71(4):272–276.

69. Ornoy A, Zvi N, Arnon J, et al. The outcome of pregnancy following topiramate treatment: a study on 52 pregnancies. Reprod Toxicol 2008; 25(3):388–389.

70. Oyen N, Vollset SE, Eide MG, et al. Maternal epilepsy and offsprings' adult intelligence: a population based study from Norway. Epilepsia 2007; 48(9):1731–1738.

71. Finnell RH, Dansky LV. Parental epilepsy, anticonvulsant drugs, and reproductive outcome: epidemiologic and experimental findings spanning three decades; 1: animal studies. Reprod Toxicol 1991; 5(4):281–299.

72. Meador KJ, Zupanc ML. Neurodevelopmental outcomes of children born to mothers with epilepsy. Cleve Clin J Med 2004; 71(suppl 2):S38–S41.

73. Dean JC, Hailey H, Moore SJ, et al. Long term health and neurodevelopment in children exposed to antiepileptic drugs before birth. J Med Genet 2002; 39(4):251–259.

74. Eriksson K, Viinikainen K, Monkkonen A, Aikia M, et al. Children exposed to valproate in utero–population based evaluation of risks and confounding factors for long-term neurocognitive development. Epilepsy Res 2005; 65(3):189–200.

75. Titze K, Koch S, Helge H, et al. Prenatal and family risks of children born to mothers with epilepsy: effects on cognitive development. Dev Med Child Neurol 2008; 50(2):117–122.

76. Koch S, Tize K, Zimmerman RB, et al. Long-term neuropsychological consequences of maternal epilepsy and anticonvulsant treatment during pregnancy for school-age children and adolescents. Epilepsia 1999; 40(9):1237–1243.

77. Speidel BD, Meadow SR. Maternal epilepsy and abnormalities of the fetus and newborn. Lancet 1972; 2(7782):839–843.

78. Gaily E, Kantola-Sorsa E, Granström ML. Specific cognitive dysfunction in children with epileptic mothers. Med Child Neurol 1990; 32(5):403–414.

79. Reinisch JM, Sanders SA, Mortensen EL, et al. In utero exposure to phenobarbital and intelligence deficits in adult men. JAMA 1995; 274(19):1518–1525.

80. Jones KL, Lacro RV, Johnson KA, et al. Pattern of malformations in the children of women treated with carbamazepine during pregnancy. N Engl J Med 320(25):1661–1666.

81. Skolnik D, Nulman I, Rovet J, et al. Neurodevelopment of children exposed in utero to phenytoin and carbamazepine monotherapy. JAMA 1994; 271(10):767–770.

82. Wide K, Winbladh B, Tomson T, et al. Psychomotor development and minor anomalies in children exposed to antiepileptic drugs in utero: a prospective population-based study. Dev Med Child Neurol 2000; 42(2):87–92.

83. Ornoy A, Cohen E. Outcome of children born to epileptic mothers treated with carbamazepine during pregnancy. Arch Dis Childhood 1996; 75:517–520.

84. Gaily E, Kantola-Sorsa E, Hiilesmaa V, et al. Normal intelligence in children with prenatal exposure to carbamazepine. Neurology 2004; 62(1):28–32.

85. Kantola-Sorsa E, Gaily E, Isoaho M, et al. Neuropsychological outcomes in children of mothers with epilepsy. J Int Neuropsychol Soc 2007; 13(4):642–652.

86. Vanoverloop D, Schnell RR, Harvey EA, et al. The effects of prenatal exposure to phenytoin and other anticonvulsants on intellectual function at 4 to 8 years of age. Neurotoxicol Teratol 1992; 14(5):329–335.

87. Holmes LB, Rosenberger PB, Harvey EA, et al. Intelligence and physical features of children of women with epilepsy. Teratology 2000; 61(3):196–202.

88. Lösche G, Steinhausen H-C, Koch S, et al. The psychological development of children of epileptic parents. II. The differential impact of intrauterine exposure to anticonvulsant drugs and further influential factors. Acta Paediat 1994; 83(9):961–966.

89. Steinhausen HC, Lösche G, Koch S, et al. The psychological development of children of epileptic parents. I. Study design and comparative findings. Acta Paediatr 1994; 83(9): 955–960.

90. Hirano T, Fujioka K, Okada M, et al. Physical and psychomotor development in the offspring born to mothers with epilepsy. Epilepsia 2004; 45(suppl 8):53–57.

91. Parisi P, Francia A, Vanacore N, et al. Psychomotor development and general movements in offspring of women with epilepsy and anticonvulsant therapy. Early Hum Dev 2003; 74(2):97–108.

92. Hill RM, Verniaud WM, Horning MG, et al. Infant exposed in utero to antiepileptic drugs. A prospective study. Am J Dis Child 1974; 127:645–653.

93. Nadebaum C, Anderson V, Vajda F, et al. Language skills of school-aged children prenatally exposed to antiepileptic drugs. Neurology 2011; 76(8):719–726.

94. Nadebaum C, Anderson VA, Vajda F, et al. The Australian brain and cognition and antiepileptic drugs study: IQ in school-aged children exposed to sodium valproate and polytherapy. J Int Neuropsychol Soc 2011; 17(1):133–142.

95. Cummings C, Stewart M, Stevenson M, et al. Neurodevelopment of children exposed in utero to lamotrigine, sodium valproate and carbamazepine. Arch Dis Child. 2011; 96(7):643-647. [Epub 2011, Mar 17].

96. Meador KJ, Baker GA, Browning N, et al., NEAD Study Group. Foetal antiepileptic drug exposure and verbal versus non-verbal abilities atthree years of age. Brain. 2011;134(Pt 2):396-3404. [Epub 2011, Jan 11].

97. Meador KJ, Baker GA, Browning N, et al. Loring Cognitive function at 3 years of age after fetal exposure to antiepileptic drugs. N Engl J Med 2009; 360(16):1597–1605.

98. Tomson T, Battino D. Teratogenic effects of antiepileptic medications. Neurol Clin 2009; 27(4):993–1002.

99. Patsalos PN, Berry DJ, Bourgeois BF, et al. Antiepileptic drugs—best practice guidelines fortherapeutic drug monitoring: a position paper by the subcommission on therapeutic drug monitoring, ILAE Commission on Therapeutic Strategies. Epilepsia 2008; 49(7):1239–1276.

100. Harden CL, Hopp J, Ting TY, et al. American Academy of Neurology; American Epilepsy Society. Management issues for women with epilepsy-Focus on pregnancy (an evidence-based review): I. Obstetrical complications and change in seizure frequency. Epilepsia 2009; 50(5):1229–1236.

101. Hong JM, Choi YC, Kim WJ.. Differences between the measured and calculated free serum phenytoin concentrations in epileptic patients. Yonsei Med J 2009; 50(4):517–520.

102. Reimers A, Helde G, Brodtkorb E. Ethinyl estradiol, not progestogens, reduces lamotrigine serum concentrations. Epilepsia 2005; 46(9):1414–1417.

103. Tomson, T. Gender aspects of pharmacokinetics therapeutic drug monitoring. Epilepsia 2005; 27:718–721.

104. Tomson T, Ohman I, Vitols S. Lamotrigine in pregnancy and lactation: a casereport. Epilepsia. 1997; 38(9):1039-1041.

105. Ohman I, Vitols S, Tomson T. Lamotrigine in pregnancy: pharmacokinetics during delivery, in the neonate, and during lactation. Epilepsia. 2000; 41(6):709-713.

106. Pennell PB, Newport DJ, Stowe ZN, et al. Theimpact of pregnancy and childbirth on the metabolism of lamotrigine. Neurology 2004; 62(2):292-295. Erratum in: Neurology 2010; 74(24):2028.

107. Tran TA, Leppik IE, Blesi K, et al. Lamotrigine clearance during pregnancy. Neurology 2002; 59(2):251–255.

108. de Haan GJ, Edelbroek P, Segers J, et al. Gestation-induced changes in lamotrigine pharmacokinetics: amonotherapy study. Neurology 2004; 63(3):571-573.

109. Petrenaite V, Sabers A, Hansen-Schwartz J. Individual changes in lamotrigine plasma concentrations during pregnancy. Epilepsy Res 2005; 65(3):185–188.

110. Pennell PB, Peng L, Newport DJ, et al. Lamotrigine in pregnancy: clearance, therapeutic drug monitoring, and seizure frequency. Neurology 2008; 70(22 Pt 2):2130-2136. [Epub 2007, Nov 28].

111. Ohman I, Beck O, Vitols S, et al. Plasma concentrations of lamotrigine and its 2-N-glucuronide metabolite during pregnancy in women with epilepsy. Epilepsia 2008; 49(6):1075–1080.

112. Franco V, Mazzucchelli I, Gatti G, et al. Changes in lamotrigine pharmacokinetics during pregnancy and the puerperium. Ther Drug Monit 2008; 30(4):544–547.

113. Fotopoulou C, Kretz R, Bauer S, et al. Prospectively assessed changes in lamotrigine-concentration in women with epilepsy during pregnancy, lactation and the neonatal period. Epilepsy Res 2009; 85(1):60–64.

114. Reimers A, Helde G, Bråthen G, et al. Lamotrigine and its N2-glucuronide during pregnancy: The significance of renal clearance and estradiol. Epilepsy Res 94(3):198–205.

115. Tomson T, Luef G, Sabers A, et al. Valproate effects on kinetics of lamotrigine in pregnancy and treatment with oral contraceptives. Neurology 2006; 67(7):1297–1299.

116. Sabers A, Petrenaite V. Seizure frequency in pregnant women treated with lamotrigine monotherapy. Epilepsia 2009; 50 (9):2163–2166.

117. Pennell PB, Peng L, Newport DJ. Lamotrigine in pregnancy: clearance, therapeutic drug monitoring, and seizure frequency. Neurology 2008; 70(22 pt 2):2130–2136.

118. Mazzucchelli I, Mazzucchelli I, Onat FY, et al. Changes in the disposition of oxcarbazepine and its metabolites during pregnancy and the puerperium. Epilepsia 2006; 47(3):504–509.

119. Christensen J, Sabers A, Sidenius P. Oxcarbazepine concentrations during pregnancy: a retrospective study in patients with epilepsy. Neurology 2006; 67(8):1497–1499.

120. Petrenaite V, Sabers A, Hansen-Schwartz J. Seizure deterioration in women treated with oxcarbazepine during pregnancy. Epilepsy Res 2009; 84(2–3):245–249.

121. Tomson T, Palm R, Kallen K, et al. Pharmacokinetics of levetiracetam during pregnancy, delivery, in the neonatal period, and lactation. Epilepsia 2007; 48(6):1111–1116.

122. Westin AA, Reimers A, Helde G, et al. Serum concentration/dose ratio of levetiracetam before, during and after pregnancy. Seizure 2008; 17(2):192–198.

123. López-Fraile IP, Cid AO, Juste AO, et al. Levetiracetam plasma level monitoring during pregnancy, delivery, and postpartum: clinical and outcome implications. Epilepsy Behav 2009; 15 (3):372–375.

124. Tomson T, Palm R, Källén K, et al. Pharmacokinetics of levetiracetam during pregnancy, delivery, in the neonatal period, and lactation. Epilepsia 2007; 48(6):1111-1116. [Epub 2007, Mar 22].

125. Westin AA, Nakken, KO, Johannessen S, et al. Serum concentration/dose ratio of topiramate during pregnancy. Epilepsia 2009; 50(3):480–485.

126. Ohman I, Sabers A, de Flon P, et al. Pharmacokinetics of topiramate during pregnancy. Epilepsy Res 2009; 87(2–3): 124–129.

127. Matar KM, Marafie NA. Effect of pregnancy on topiramate pharmacokinetics in rabbits. Xenobiotica 2011; 41(5):416–421.

128. Winterbottom JB, Smyth RM, Jacoby A, et al. Preconception counselling for women with epilepsy to reduce adverse pregnancy outcome. Cochrane Database Syst Rev 2008; (3): CD006645.

129. Medical Research Council Antiepileptic Drug Withdrawal Study Group. Prognostic index for recurrence of seizures after remission of epilepsy. BMJ 1993; 306:1374–1378.

130. MRC Vitamin Study Research Group. Prevention of neural tube defects: results of the Medical Research Council Vitamin Study. Lancet 1991; 338(8760):131–137.

131. De-Regil LM, Fernández-Gaxiola AC, Dowswell T, et al. Effects and safety of periconceptional folate supplementation for preventing birth defects. Cochrane Database Syst Rev 2010; (10): CD007950.

132. Morrow JI, Hunt SJ, Russell AJ, et al. Folic acid use and major congenital malformations in offspring of women with epilepsy: a prospective study from the UK Epilepsy and Pregnancy Register. J Neurol Neurosurg Psychiatry 2009; 80(5):506–511.

133. Choulika S, Grabowski E, Holmes LB. Is antenatal vitamin K prophylaxis needed for pregnant women taking anticonvulsants? Am J Obstet Gynecol 2004; 190(4):882–883.

134. Kaaja E, Kaaja R, Matila R, et al. Enzyme-inducing antiepileptic drugsin pregnancy and the risk of bleeding in the neonate. Neurology 2002; 58(4):549–553.

135. Crowther CA, Crosby DD, Henderson-Smart DJ. Vitamin K prior to preterm birth for preventing neonatal periventricular haemorrhage. Cochrane Database Syst Rev 2010; (1):CD000229.

136. Alarcon G, Nashef L, Cross H, et al. Oxford specialist handbooks in neurology: epilepsy. Oxford: Oxford University Press, 2009.

137. NICE, Department of Health, 2004. Available at: http://www.nice.org.uk.

138. Crawford P, Hudson S. Understanding the information needs of women with epilepsy at different lifestages: results of the 'Ideal World' survey. Seizure 2003; 12(7):502–507.

139. BELL GS, Nashcf L, Kendall S, et al. Information recalled by women taking anti-epileptic drugs for epilepsy: a questionnaire study. Epilepsy Res 2002; 52:139–146.

13

Headache in pregnancy

Anish Bahra

INTRODUCTION

The majority of women who present with headache during pregnancy and post-partum will have a primary headache disorder. Therefore, this chapter largely concentrates on the diagnosis and management of primary headache. These disorders have been clinically classified by the International Headache Society (IHS) and are detailed in the Appendix. All causes of secondary headache can occur in pregnancy as in the non-pregnant state. However, management is restricted to the investigative procedures and drug treatments which are deemed safe in pregnancy. There are some important secondary causes of headache which are particularly common in pregnancy and the peri-partum period.

MIGRAINE AND TENSION-TYPE HEADACHE

Migraine and tension-type headache are the most common headache disorders, and the most common encountered during pregnancy (1). The 1-year prevalence of frequent tension-type headache (more than once a month) in adult women is 30% to 40% (2,3). The 1-year prevalence of migraine in adult women is 15% to 18% (4,5). Between 20% and 25% of women have frequent migraine attacks, more than once in a month (6). Although tension-type headache is more prevalent than migraine, disabling tension-type headache is rare (7), whereas disabling migraine is common (8,9). The highest prevalence of migraine and tension-type headache occurs during childbearing years (10,11). During pregnancy, the pattern of attacks in those suffering from tension-type headache is similar to that in migraine sufferers (12).

There remains a dearth of evidence-based treatments for tension-type headache. However, many patients diagnosed with tension-type headache respond to treatments effective in migraine (13–15). Thus, any patient presenting with a diagnosis of disabling tension-type headache ultimately is likely to be treated as for a migraine headache disorder. This adds further weight to the concept that tension-type headache and migraine fall within a spectrum of the same biological disorder (16). Therefore, the management of tension-type headache requiring treatment in pregnancy is similar to the treatment for migraine.

MIGRAINE AND FEMALE SEXUAL HORMONES

Migraine both with and without aura show a relationship to menarche, menstruation and pregnancy; these relationships appear to be stronger for migraine without aura (17–19).

The female:male ratio for migraine during childhood is 1:1 (20). About 4% of school children suffer from migraine (21). Ten percent to 20% of women report onset of migraine at menarche. From puberty the gender ratio gradually changes to 3:1, peaking during the 4th to 5th decade (22). At least 50% of women report an association between menstruation and

migraine (22). Migraine without aura is more commonly associated with menstruation (19). Pure menstrual migraine is less common (23). This is defined by attacks which occur exclusively on day 1 ± 2 of menstruation in at least 2 of 3 menstrual cycles, and at no other times of the cycle.

It has been observed that menstrual attacks of migraine have been associated with falling levels of oestrogen, seen in the late luteal and early follicular phase of the menstrual cycle. The absolute levels to which oestrogen falls seem less relevant than the actual decline in levels. Oestrogen given pre-menstrually delays the onset of migraine but not menstruation. Progesterone administration delays menstruation but does not prevent migraine. Moreover, several days of high levels of oestrogen are required to precipitate oestrogen-withdrawal migraine. In early studies erratic pre-emptive therapeutic oestrogen delivery resulted in irregular bleeding and headache (24–27). More recent studies with oestrogen gels or patches have reported conflicting results (28,29).

The combined oral contraceptive pill, menopause and hormone replacement therapy (HRT) can be associated with no change, improvement or worsening of migraine with and without aura, and new-onset migraine (30–32).

There is increasing support for a genetic predisposition to migraine (33,34). Functional consequences of known pathological mutations in a rare form of migraine with aura, familial hemiplegic migraine, suggest a dysfunction of ion channel transport. Genetic models have and are likely to continue to facilitate research into an increased sensitivity to migraine triggers and metabolic homeostasis (35).

COURSE OF MIGRAINE DURING PREGNANCY

Migraine appears to have no adverse impact on fertility or pregnancy (12,36). Table 13.1 summarises the course of migraine during pregnancy. The majority of women improve, most commonly during the second and third trimester with worsening, in some individuals peri-partum (43,44). Up to 20% can attain complete remission from attacks during pregnancy. Improvement of migraine during pregnancy is more commonly reported by those who experience migraine in association with menstruation (19). Although greater parity has been reported to be associated with less consistent improvement of headache during pregnancy, this has not been confirmed and the observation attributed to reporting bias (45).

A small but noteworthy proportion of individuals experience worsening or new-onset migraine during pregnancy. It is this group which generates the greatest concern about potential secondary headache and drug management. This is particularly so in new-onset migraine with aura.

Table 13.1 Course of Headache During Pregnancy

	N	Age Range	Past headache	Headache type %	Improvement %	Worse %	No change %	New-onset headache %
(1)	1101	12–15 5.3% 16–19 27.7% 20–34 2.31% >35 4.63%	93.5	Probable MO 34.6 MOH 0.8 Oestrogen-withdrawal 0.9 Cold-stimulus 0.5 Primary stabbing 0.8 TTH 10.2 MA 8.8 MO+MA 4.9 Chronic migraine 0.7 MO 33.9 Probable TTH 1.1 Probable MA 2.2 Basilar-type migraine 0.2 Other 0.3	First trimester 55 Second trimester 60 Third trimester 65	18.1 11.5 8.9	Variable 1.0 0.9 1.1	7.2 – Total 3.4 – New-onset 3.8 – Different headache to pre-gestational headache Of the above 3.9 % had secondary headache
(12)	149	–	–	MO 54.4 MA 8.1 TTH 22.1 Non-IHS 8.7 Secondary 6.7	First trimester[a] 71.4 Second trimester 77.8 Third trimester 84.1	6.3 0.8 1.6	30.2 13.5 14.3	New-onset primary headache (MO) 0.8
(37)[b]	703	–	–	MO 77.7 MA 22.3	69.4 – Unrelated to trimester	6.8	7.5	10.9
(19)[b]	151	–	88.7	MO 76.8 MA 23.2	42.5	4.5	5.3	11.3
(38)[b]	484	<20 24% 21–30 56.8% >31 19.2%	All had pre-existing headache	MO and MA	43.6 – Remission/improved 35.3 – Probably improved	21.1 – Unimproved		Not addressed
(39)[b]	571	–	All had pre-existing active headache	MO and MA	17.4 – Remission 49.9 – Improvement	3.5	29.2	Not addressed
(40)[b]	49	29.3 ± 3.2 (mean)	All had pre-existing active headache	MO 96 MA 4	66.6 – Remission/improved First trimester 57.4 Second trimester 83 Third trimester 87.2	0	16.7	4

Headache diagnoses have used IHS Criteria (8, 41) or prior to 1988 the Ad Hoc Committee Classification of Headache (42).
[a]Total for MO+MA+TTH.
[b]Migraine only studied.
Abbreviations: MO, migraine without aura; MA, migraine with aura; MOH, medication overuse headache; TTH, tension-type headache.

HEADACHE AND NEUROLOGICAL SYMPTOMS IN PREGNANCY

In a prospective study of 1631 pregnant women attending Trondhein Hospital from May 1997 to June 1998, 410 women suffered from migraine and, 856 from non-migrainous headache, of which 80% were diagnosed as tension-type headache (46). Eighty-six patients who had a diagnosis of non-migrainous headache prior to pregnancy fulfilled the criteria for migraine during pregnancy. A total of 41 patients, from this cohort, were investigated for transient focal neurological deficits. This included magnetic resonance imaging (MRI), cardiac investigations and blood screen for a prothrombotic tendency either during pregnancy or after delivery (all MRIs were done after delivery). A control group of 41 women from the 1631 patient cohort had similar investigations except MRI. Patients and controls were contacted yearly for 5 years by mailed questionnaire asking whether they had developed any medical disorder during the past year. Data on headache, aura and medication use over each year were also collated.

Results are shown in Tables 13.2–13.4. Focal transient neurological symptoms increased throughout pregnancy, with highest occurrence in the third trimester. Migraine aura, as defined by IHS criteria, was the most common transient neurological symptom presenting during pregnancy. Migraine attacks prior to pregnancy were reported by 18 patients, 12 of whom had migraine with aura and all of whom had experienced visual symptoms as part of their migraine aura. During pregnancy, visual symptoms were reported by 20 of the 41 patients. Furthermore, four patients reported paraesthesia before pregnancy, compared with 26 patients during pregnancy, and speech disturbance was not reported by any patients before pregnancy, but seven patients experienced this during pregnancy. The authors concluded that transient

Table 13.2 Transient Neurological Presentations in 41 Pregnant Women

Diagnosis	N	Pathological findings and investigations
Migraine with aura	34	MRI: one had signs of a previous stroke (incidental), two had non-specific white matter lesions. ECG: three had right bundle branch block. Ultrasound: one had a false-positive finding.
Stroke	2	MRI: two had changes compatible with recent stroke blood chemistry: one had positive antiphospholipid antibodies (IgG and IgM), positive antinuclear factor and lupus anticoagulant and luetic antibodies; one had elevated fibrinogen, AT3, protein C, and low protein S and APC resistance, and was heterozygous for the factor V Leiden on gene testing.
Presyncope	1	Blood chemistry: anaemia
MS	1	MRI and cerebrospinal fluid: typical findings for MS
Epilepsy	1	EEG: negative first year, later developed focal epilepsy
CTS	2	Symptomatic CTS confirmed by neurophysiology

Abbreviations: APC, activated protein C; AT3, antithrombin III; CTS, carpel tunnel syndrome; ECG, electrocardiography; EEG, electroencephalography; MRI, magnetic resonance imaging; MS, multiple sclerosis.
Source: Adapted from data in Ref. 46.

Table 13.3 Migraine Subtype in Patients with Transient Neurological Deficit During Pregnancy

ICHD-II diagnosis	N
1.2.1 Typical aura with migraine headache	9
1.2.2 Typical aura with non-migraine headache	12
1.2.3 Typical aura without headache	5
1.2.5 Sporadic hemiplegic migraine	1
1.6.2 Probable MA	6
1.6.6 Probable basilar-type migraine	1

Based on Examination and Interview by Neurologist.
Abbreviations: ICHD, International Classification of Headache Disorders; MA, migraine with aura.
Source: Adapted from data in Ref. 46.

Table 13.4 Symptoms in Patients with Typical Aura

Nature of aura symptoms	N
Visual aura only	4
Sensory only	12
Dysphasic only	0
Visual and sensory	10
Visual and dysphasic	2
Sensory and dysphasic	1
Visual, sensory and dysphasic	4

Source: Adapted from data in Ref. 47.

neurological symptoms were less common in individuals without or with non-migrainous headache; those with migraine had an increased susceptibility to experience these symptoms during pregnancy.

MIGRAINE IN THE POST-PARTUM PERIOD

Headache post-partum occurs in 30% to 40% of women, most commonly on days 3 to 6 post-partum (43). Post-partum headache is commonly associated with a past or family history of migraine. About 60% of migraineurs will experience post-partum headache (44,48); new-onset headache post-partum can also occur, with or without a past or family history of headache. As for antenatal new-onset headache, secondary headache remains the main concern and a diagnosis of new-onset primary headache is usually that of exclusion.

TREATMENT OF MIGRAINE DURING PREGNANCY AND LACTATION

The principles of drug treatment in pregnancy and lactation are the same as in the non-parous state, but with restriction of type of drug use. Tables 13.5 and 13.6 provide guidelines on available effective acute and preventative treatments and their associated risks in pregnancy. The information is sourced from the British National Formulary, the UK Teratology Information Service: http://www.nyrdtc.nhs.uk/Services/teratology/teratology.html. and National electronic Library for Medicines (www.nelm.nhs/uk/NeLM).

Acute Treatment

There have been two approaches to use of acute attack treatment: step care and stratified care (49). The *step care* approach escalates treatment according to safety, cost and efficacy, both within and across attacks. Thus, this may start with a simple analgesic, with or without an anti-emetic, and if this approach fails, a triptan is used. This same approach is used within and across attacks. Thus, within an attack if at 2 hours a simple analgesic has failed then a migraine-specific drug is used.

Table 13.5 Drug Safety in Pregnancy and Lactation: Acute-Relief Medication

Drug	Pregnancy	Lactation
Paracetamol	Not known to be harmful	Amount too small to be harmful
NSAIDs	Most manufacturers advise avoiding the use of NSAIDs during pregnancy or avoiding them unless the potential benefit outweighs the risk. NSAIDs should be avoided during the third trimester because use is associated with a risk of closure of fetal ductus arteriosus in utero and possibly persistent pulmonary hypertension of the newborn. In addition, the onset of labour may be delayed and its duration may be increased.	NSAIDs should be used with caution during breastfeeding; see also individual drugs.
i Aspirin	Use with caution during third trimester; impaired platelet function and risk of haemorrhage; delayed onset and increased duration of labour with increased blood loss; avoid analgesic doses if possible in last few weeks (low doses probably not harmful); with high doses, closure of fetal ductus arteriosus in utero and possibly persistent pulmonary hypertension of newborn; kernicterus in jaundiced neonates	i Avoid – possible risk of Reye syndrome; regular use of high doses could impair platelet function and produce hypoprothrombinaemia in infant if neonatal vitamin K stores low
ii Ibuprofen		ii Amount too small to be harmful but some manufacturers advise to avoid (including topical use)
iii Naproxen		iii Amount too small to be harmful but manufacturer advises to avoid
iv Diclofenac		iv Amount in milk too small to be harmful
v Indomethacin		v Amount probably too small to be harmful – manufacturers advise to avoid
Triptans Almotriptan, eletriptan, frovatriptan, naratriptan, rizatriptan, zolmitriptan	There is limited experience of using $5HT_1$-receptor agonists during pregnancy; manufacturers advise that they should be avoided unless the potential benefit outweighs the risk.	Present in milk in *animal* studies – withhold breastfeeding for 24 hours
Sumatriptan	Limited first-trimester data: no significant differences in congenital malformations or poor pregnancy outcomes compared with expected rates in the general population or with the observed rates in control subjects. Little information on exposure in middle and late pregnancy.	Present in milk but amount probably too small to be harmful; withhold breastfeeding for 12 hours
Ergotamine tartrate	Avoid; oxytocic effect on the uterus	Avoid; oxytocic effect on the uterus
Opioids Codeine phosphate	Respiratory depression and withdrawal symptoms can occur in the neonate if opioid analgesics are used during delivery; also gastric stasis and inhalation pneumonia has been reported in the mother if opioid analgesics are used during labour.	Amount usually too small to be harmful; however, mothers vary considerably in their capacity to metabolise codeine – risk of morphine overdose in infant
Pethidine		Present in milk but not known to be harmful
Morphine salts		Therapeutic doses unlikely to affect infant; withdrawal symptoms in infants of dependent mothers; breastfeeding not best method of treating dependence in offspring
Domperidone	Use only if potential benefit outweighs risk.	Amount too small to be harmful
Metoclopramide	Not known to be harmful	Small amount present in milk; avoid
Prochlorperazine	Extrapyramidal effects have been reported occasionally in the neonate when antipsychotic drugs are taken during the third trimester of pregnancy.	There is limited information available on the short- and long-term effects of antipsychotics on the breastfed infant. *Animal* studies indicate possible adverse effects of antipsychotic medicines on the developing nervous system. Chronic treatment with antipsychotics whilst breastfeeding should be avoided unless absolutely necessary.

Stratified care is based on selecting the most appropriate treatment following initial assessment of disease severity; this includes attack severity, frequency and associated disability, co-morbidity and previous ineffective/tolerated treatments. Although the direct costs of the latter approach may seem high, this approach has lower indirect costs (e.g., general practitioner and hospital visits, less disability and thus improved attendance at work) and improved health-related quality of life (49,50).

The ideal end point is rapid achievement of a pain-free state. Realistically a reduction of pain from moderate or severe to mild or none at 2 hours is the end point adopted by most recent acute treatment trials. If no response is obtained at 2 hours, repeat dosing with the same drug and/or dose that

Table 13.6 Drug Safety in Pregnancy and Lactation: Preventative Treatment

Drug	Pregnancy	Lactation
Beta-blockers		
Propranolol Atenolol Metoprolol	Beta-blockers may cause intra-uterine growth restriction, neonatal hypoglycaemia and bradycardia; the risk is greater in severe hypertension. If beta-blockers are used close to delivery, infants should be monitored for signs of beta-blockade.	Infants should be monitored as there is a risk of possible toxicity due to beta-blockade, but the amount of most beta-blockers present in milk is too small to affect infants. Atenolol is present in milk in greater amounts than other beta-blockers.
Anticonvulsants		
i Topiramate ii Sodium valproate iii Gabapentin iv Lamotrigine v Carbamazepine	There is an increased risk of teratogenicity associated with the use of anti-epileptic drugs (especially if used during the first trimester and if the patient takes two or more anti-epileptic drugs). Valproate is associated with the highest risk of major and minor congenital malformations, and with developmental delay; doses greater than 1 g daily are associated with an increased risk of teratogenicity. Neonatal bleeding (related to hypofibrinaemia) and neonatal hepatotoxicity also reported with valproic acid. There is also an increased risk of teratogenicity with lamotrigine and carbamazepine. There is not enough evidence to establish the risk of teratogenicity with other anti-epileptic drugs. Women of childbearing potential who take anti-epileptic drugs should be given contraceptive advice. The effectiveness of *combined* oral contraceptives, *progestogen-only* oral contraceptives contraceptive patches, and vaginal rings can be considerably reduced by interaction with drugs that induce hepatic enzyme activity – carbamazepine, oxcarbazepine and topiramate. Alternative contraception should be considered or the dose of combined oral contraceptives should be adjusted to provide ethinylestradiol 50 μg or more daily (unlicensed use); furthermore, additional contraceptive precautions should be taken whilst taking the enzyme-inducing drug and for 4 weeks after stopping it.	i Manufacturer advises to avoid – present in milk ii Amount too small to be harmful iii Present in milk – manufacturer advises use only if potential benefit outweighs risk. iv Present in milk but limited data suggest no harmful effects on infants v Amount probably too small to be harmful but monitor infant for possible adverse reactions
Tricyclics		
Amitriptyline Imipramine	Use only if potential benefit outweighs risk. Colic, tachycardia, dyspnoea, irritability and muscle spasms reported in neonates when used in the third trimester.	The amount of tricyclic antidepressants secreted into breast milk is too small to be harmful.
Nortriptyline Dosulepin	Use only if potential benefit outweighs risk. Use only if potential benefit outweighs risk.	
Calcium channel blockers		
Flunarizine Verapamil	Avoid May reduce uterine blood flow with fetal hypoxia; manufacturer advises to avoid in first trimester unless absolutely necessary; may inhibit labour	Avoid Amount too small to be harmful
Other		
Pizotifen	Avoid unless potential benefit outweighs risk.	Amount probably too small to be harmful, but manufacturer advises to avoid.
Methysergide	Avoid	Avoid

have not shown to be effective (51,52) Thus, treatment should be escalated to a higher dose of the same drug or a different treatment. The response across three attacks has been taken to give a measure of consistency. Two from three failed responses to the maximum tolerated dose of a treatment should prompt progression to an alternative drug.

Table 13.5 gives a list of acute-relief treatments for migraine headache. Paracetamol carries the best safety data.

The use of triptans in pregnancy warrants a special note. Triptans are selective 5-HT1B and 5-HT1D agonists with putative vascular, peripheral and central neural sites of action. In 2008, all retrospective and prospective studies reporting on pregnancy outcomes after the use of a triptan were critically evaluated (53). Data from all available manufacturer-sponsored pregnancy registries were also included. The data exist primarily for exposure in the first trimester and are available in larger numbers only for sumatriptan, with smaller numbers of women treated with naratriptan and rizatriptan. The data show no significant differences in congenital malformations or poor pregnancy outcomes when compared with expected rates in the general population or with the observed rates in control subjects. There was little information on exposure in middle and late pregnancy. It was concluded that sumatriptan appears to be a safe acute treatment for pregnant women who experience new-onset or worse migraines in the first trimester. There is, as yet, inadequate information about sumatriptan use in later trimesters and/or other agents within this class throughout pregnancy (53).

Sumatriptan is the first and most widely used triptan. It is also the only triptan available in oral, rectal, intranasal and subcutaneous preparations. The efficacy of the rectal (54) and intranasal preparations (55) is similar to the oral preparation. The rectal preparation is not available in the United Kingdom. Subcutaneous sumatriptan provides the most effective acute attack treatment (51). However, oral preparations tend to be preferred and the adverse effect profile is greater with subcutaneous than with oral sumatriptan. The most typical adverse effects include tingling, paraesthesias and warm sensations in the head, neck, chest and limbs. Less frequently experienced side effects are dizziness, flushing, neck pain or stiffness. Patients may experience chest tightness. However, such patients can also experience tightness in other parts of the body. There is currently no evidence to support that the origin of this chest tightness is due to cardiac ischaemia. While triptans can cause coronary artery vasoconstriction, cardiac adverse events are rare (56). In most, but not all, patients with serious cardiac events, cardiac risk factors and underlying cardiac disease have been found. Therefore, the current recommendation is that a triptan should not be used in patients with ischaemic heart disease, uncontrolled hypertension, cerebrovascular and peripheral vascular disease.

Triptans taken pre-emptively during the aura phase are safe but do not prevent the headache phase of the attack (57,58).

Nausea and vomiting are common in migraine attacks. During migraine there is gastric stasis which delays oral drugs absorption (59). Metoclopramide 10 mg orally or intramuscularly has been shown to reverse the delayed gastric emptying (60). It can also be used as a 20 mg suppository. In placebo-controlled studies, metoclopramide appears to improve outcome *with* an acute-relief medication but not alone (61,62). Caution should be maintained in individuals below the age of 20 years due to the increased risk of dystonic adverse effects. Domperidone, 10 to 20 mg orally or 60 mg rectally, is an alternative compared to placebo. Domperidone has been shown to be effective in the pre-emptive treatment of migraine attacks.

Prochlorperazine 10 mg parenterally has been shown to be effective for pain and nausea compared to placebo and metoclopramide (62,63). These studies addressed a reduction in pain scores at 30 minutes for intravenous prochlorperazine and 60 minutes for intramuscular prochlorperazine.

About 70% of migraine attacks last between 4 and 72 hours, hence the IHS definition. Attacks lasting more than 72 hours occur in less than 5% of cases; in one study, well-documented duration greater than 72 hours occurred in about 1% of patients (64–66). A prolonged attack of migraine lasting more than 72 hours is termed *status migrainosus*. This is an arbitrary definition and much of the original observation was compounded by patients with acute-relief medication overuse (67) Furthermore, this definition does not give an upper limit.

The frequent use of acute-relief medication can lead to chronic daily headache in predisposed individuals (68,69). The current definition for medication overuse headache is headache on more than 15 days/mo associated with the use of analgesics on more than 15 days a month or a triptan, ergotamine or opioid use on more than 10 days a month for at least 3 months. The headache resolves or reverts to its previous pattern within 2 months after discontinuation of the acute-relief medication (8). However, historical data suggest that medication overuse headache can be associated with acute-relief medication use on 2 to 3 days a week (70). Development of medication overuse headache is associated with lower frequency of use and dosing with triptans (69). Thus, the 10 days a month may in fact be too lenient and a lower frequency of dosing warranted to truly avoid medication overuse headache, particularly in this drug group.

Preventative Treatment

Individuals experiencing 4 to 5 disabling headache days each month which require treatment should be considered for preventative therapy. The number of headache days is somewhat arbitrary but serves to prompt a re-evaluation in management strategy in an individual who may otherwise begin to venture into the realm of medication overuse headache. This is based on the above data that, at least for ergotamine and triptans, medication overuse headache can result with acute-relief medication use as little as 2 days/wk. Moreover, preventative treatment is rendered less effective in the presence of medication overuse (71,72). On the basis that most women experience improvement of their headache disorder during pregnancy preventative treatment is usually not required.

Table 13.6 gives a list of preventive medication in the treatment of migraine headache. The tricyclics are likely to be the safest preventative drug treatment that can be used in pregnancy. In women with chronic migraine, preventative treatments with drugs other than tricyclics should be reviewed carefully in women who wish to become pregnant or who become pregnant. Post-partum reintroduction can be considered depending upon whether the mother chooses to breastfeed.

Probably the safest preventative treatment in pregnancy for intractable headache of any phenotype is the use of local nerve blocks. The most commonly used is the greater occipital nerve block. This is based on the physiological functional connections between primarily first division trigeminal (V1) and upper cervical nociceptive pathways. Thus, targeting C2 will modulate sensory (including nociceptive) perception in V1, and the converse (73,74). An audit of greater occipital nerve blockade showed that 46% of injections in 54 migraineurs resulted in complete or partial improvement in pain for a median of 30 days (75). There was a significant association between response and tenderness at the most proximal superficial site of the nerve. However, there was no association between response and paraesthesia produced by the block, nor with medication overuse.

Management of *chronic daily headache* is based on minimisation of medication overuse and if required establishment of preventative treatment. Following analgesic withdrawal it may take more than 2 months to be able to establish an individual's underlying pattern of attacks and hence to determine which patients have chronic migraine or tension-type headache, defined as 15 headache days a month in the absence of acute-relief medication overuse (76). The data for headache improvement during pregnancy (Table 13.1) have included patients with chronic headache. However, the numbers are small, thus there are no subgroup analyses nor details about associated medication overuse (1). Most women, even those who experience no change or worsening of their headache disorder during pregnancy, prefer to avoid drug treatment during this time. In the event of significant disability the safest preventative treatment options in early pregnancy are the tricyclic group. The greater occipital nerve block can provide a safer option with the main caution being transient worsening of pain in some individuals (personal experience and communication).

New daily persistent headache (NDPH) is defined as headache which is daily and unremitting from onset (within 3 days) and has the clinical syndrome of tension-type headache (8). However, it is clear from the reported patient cohorts that more than half experienced typically migrainous symptoms (77). It is assumed that if an 'attack' persisted daily for at least 3 months, that is, in descriptive terms, the headache is 'new onset', 'daily' and 'persistent'. In this situation it is prudent to ensure there is no secondary precipitant such as a cerebral venous sinus thrombosis, low cerebrospinal fluid pressure due to an indolent leak or other cause. If the attack remits but henceforth the individual experiences more than 15 headache days a month for at least 3 months, then the diagnosis is chronic migraine. It must also be borne in mind that, otherwise episodic headache may manifest as NDPH or chronic migraine in the presence of frequent acute-relief medication overuse.

Particularly in pregnancy, the likelihood is that women will tend to treat pain with acute-relief medication. In both NDPH and chronic migraine management remains minimisation of analgesics and if required establishment of preventative treatment. The question of when should acute treatment be restricted and a preventative considered is more difficult. There are no prospective data on time to development of medication overuse headache in adequately sized patient groups. Retrospective data suggest this is most rapid and with the lowest frequency of medication use, for triptans, followed by opioids and then simple analgesics (69). The lowest monthly frequency of triptan use was 10 days and duration of use 4 months. Thus, clinical judgement will need to be made based on trimester, disability and social support.

CLUSTER HEADACHE AND PREGNANCY

The population prevalence of cluster headache is about 0.1% with a male-to-female ratio about 3:1. Although uncommon, cluster headache is one of the most phenotypically stereotyped headache disorders. Although the term 'Cluster' is a characteristic, it is not necessarily this aspect of the syndrome which is so distinctive. The pain of the attack is strictly unilateral, and predominantly in the distribution of the first and second division of the trigeminal nerve and C2. The pain is accompanied by prominent ipsilateral autonomic features, such as lacrimation, conjunctival injection, nasal congestion, rhinorrhoea, ptosis, partial Horner's and eyelid swelling. Individuals are typically restless during the pain, in marked contrast to migraine during which individuals are particularly sensitive to movement. Attacks are short-lived, 15 to 180 minutes, and recurrent up to 8 times throughout the day with regularity. Patients typically are awoken from sleep (usually REM sleep). During an active period, alcohol can precipitate an attack, usually within the hour. The majority experience attacks daily for periods of several weeks at a time, typically 2 to 12 weeks, interspersed by months or

years of complete remission from pain before experiencing a further 'Cluster' period. The latter often occurs each time at similar times of the year (78–80). The current IHS definition for chronicity is 1 year without remission periods greater than 1 month.

The lower prevalence, male predominance and periodicity of the disorder preclude the study of the effects of pregnancy in adequately sized patient populations. However, the limited data which exist suggest that menstruation, the oral contraceptive pill, pregnancy, menopause and HRT have little impact on the course of cluster headache (78,81). However, there does seem to be a tendency in women who are due to come into their bout for the bout to be missed or delayed to the post-partum period. In a recent observational study, 26 of 111 (23%) episodic cluster headache patients who had been pregnant reported that an 'expected' cluster period did not occur during pregnancy. In eight of these a cluster period started within 1 month after delivery (81).

Treatment of Cluster Headache During Pregnancy and Lactation

High-flow oxygen is the safest acute treatment of cluster headache attacks. The use of 100% oxygen at 7 to 12 L/min for at least 15 minutes has been shown to be effective (82,83). Subcutaneous sumatriptan 6 mg has been shown to be the most effective acute treatment (84). An early observational study of subcutaneous sumatriptan 6 mg (maximum 2/day) enrolled 3604 women of childbearing potential. During the study, 173 (4.8%) became pregnant with well-documented data in 168. Sumatriptan was used at least once in the first trimester in 76 women; one woman also used the drug in the second trimester. There was no significant difference in spontaneous abortion nor congenital fetal abnormalities; preterm delivery and birth weight were not addressed (85). However, there is currently inadequate data addressing frequent use of subcutaneous sumatriptan to recommend the drug for regular use in pregnancy. There is support for the efficacy of intranasal sumatriptan 20 mg (86) and zolmitriptan 5 and 10 mg (87) and oral zolmitriptan 5 and 10 mg (88) at 30 minutes. Again extrapolation of safety data in pregnancy from existing data for oral sumatriptan and naratriptan remains presumptive. Intranasal lidocaine can provide modest benefit (89). The preparation is not packaged as a nasal spray; therefore, the practicalities of self-administration can limit use.

Prednisolone is safe and effective in the preventative treatment of cluster headache (90). However, whilst still in a cluster headache bout, once doses fall below 30 to 40 mg attacks begin to recur. Prednisolone is usually given as a short-term measure in patients with frequent daily attacks while an alternative preventative is introduced. Unfortunately most preventive treatments effective in cluster headache are not recommended in pregnancy. These include verapamil, methysergide, lithium and topiramate (91). Greater occipital nerve blockade is the safest option in this circumstance (75).

OTHER TRIGEMINAL AUTONOMIC CEPHALALGIAS

Paroxysmal hemicrania (PH) and the syndrome of SUNCT (short-lasting unilateral neuralgiform headache attacks with conjunctival injection and tearing) share with cluster headache site and strict unilaterality of pain, and the ipsilateral autonomic features (8). Hence, the IHS has categorised these disorders as the trigeminal autonomic cephalalgias (TACs). In comparison to cluster headache, in PH and SUNCT attacks are shorter and more frequent. Traits of cluster headache such as periodicity, restlessness and alcohol triggering are less consistent. Both disorders have a propensity towards chronicity and each disorder responds to different drug treatments.

PH is defined by an absolute response to indomethacin (8). Attacks tend to last 2 to 30 minutes, and can occur up to 20 times a day (92). Animal studies have suggested that early in pregnancy, transplacental passage of indomethacin is minimal. Indomethacin has been found to cross the placenta freely during the second half of human gestation (93). In accordance with this, data available on first-trimester exposure during human pregnancy suggest that the drug does not produce malformations. However, as with other non-steroidal anti-inflammatory drugs (NSAIDs), at >32 weeks' gestation, indomethacin can cause in utero fetal pulmonary hypertension due to constriction of the ductus arteriosus. Other complications include decreased renal output in the fetus, oligohydramnois and delayed labour. Therefore, the recommendation is to avoid the drug during pregnancy. There has been a report of convulsions in one breastfed infant associated with indomethacin use. Cyclo-oxygenase-II inhibitors (94,95) have reported efficacy in PH but are not recommended for use during pregnancy and lactation. Anecdotal responses to topiramate, piroxicam and verapamil are reported (Table 13.7b).

The syndrome of SUNCT is characterised by even shorter and more frequent attacks of pain. Attacks last 5 to 240 seconds and can occur from 3 to 200 times a day (108). Attacks can be spontaneous, or triggered by trigeminal and extra-trigeminal region manoeuvres. Patients are often misdiagnosed with trigeminal neuralgia. However, the pain in SUNCT is predominantly first division trigeminal in distribution, while that in trigeminal neuralgia is second and third division. The duration of attacks is usually longer in SUNCT and autonomic features are prominent. Trigeminal neuralgia is characterised by a refractory period after a run of attacks, which is not seen in SUNCT. Most importantly treatment responses differ. While trigeminal neuralgia has a good response to carbamazepine and surgical intervention (109), SUNCT responds only partially to carbamazepine and has a poor response to similar surgical procedures (110). The best reported treatment response in SUNCT is with lamotrigine (111).

Where the disability associated with cluster headache, PH and SUNCT is considered by the mother to outweigh the risks associated with effective drug treatment, her informed decision should be well documented.

OTHER PRIMARY HEADACHE DISORDERS

Other primary headache disorders are less common than cluster headache; therefore, activity of the disorders in relation to pregnancy is less well described. Table 13.8 summarises treatments effective in other IHS-defined primary headache disorders.

Hemicrania continua is a strictly unilateral predominantly first division trigeminal head pain, which is continuous, unremitting and varies in intensity. Exacerbations may be accompanied by ipsilateral autonomic features. It is defined by an absolute response to indomethacin. The disorder seems to straddle migraine and the TACs phenotypically and biologically (115,116). Individuals with the TACs do not seem to report medication overuse headache. In patients with cluster headache who developed medication overuse headache the patients had a migrainous predisposition, thus a past or family history of migraine (117). The clinical syndrome of the medication overuse headache was consistent with either tension-type headache or migraine and responded similarly to drug withdrawal. Medication overuse in patients with migraine tends to render prophylaxis inadequately efficacious (71). This is similarly reported in hemicrania continua; patients overusing analgesics do not respond to indomethacin until the acute-relief medication has been withdrawn (118). Anecdotal responses to topiramate, piroxicam and verapamil are reported (Table 13.7b).

Most preventative treatments for the TACs and hemicrania continua are not advised during pregnancy. Local nerve blockade has reported benefit in the both groups and has no known adverse consequences in pregnancy.

Short-lived recurrent paroxysmal primary headache disorders seem to most consistently respond to indomethacin. Anecdotal reports exist for a number of other treatments (Tables 13.7 and 13.8) most of which, as is the case with indomethacin, are not recommended in pregnancy. Cough headache has been reported to respond to withdrawal of cerebrospinal fluid by lumbar puncture. Limited data exist for safety of naratriptan (53). Whether these disorders respond to local nerve blocks remains unknown due to the rare occurrence of the disorders.

SECONDARY HEADACHE

Primary headache syndromes can be precipitated by other pathologies in the brain (secondary headache) (8). Although pathologies in specific brain regions have been associated with particular headache syndromes (119–121), this is likely to reflect publication bias. Indeed as reports of secondary headache increase it has become evident that diverse pathologies affecting many different brain regions can precipitate the same headache phenotype (122). Moreover, secondary headaches can respond to the same treatments used for the corresponding primary headache phenotypes (123,124). This is not altogether surprising given the widespread functional connectivity of the peripheral and central nociceptive–anti-nociceptive network. The most consistent indicators of secondary headache are age over 50 years, sudden onset headache, abnormal neurological examination and additional features (125,126). Any patient presenting with thunderclap headache should be investigated as primary and secondary thunderclap headache cannot be clinically differentiated (127). Table 13.9 gives causes of secondary thunderclap headache. Particular to pregnancy, subarachnoid haemorrhage, cerebral venous sinus thrombosis and pituitary apoplexy should be considered. A diagnosis of primary thunderclap headache remains that of exclusion. In line with prevalence of primary headache syndromes, the most common disabling secondary headache syndrome is consistent with migraine (125,128). The data for imaging isolated migraine with and without typical aura, episodic and chronic, show that the yield of relevant associated pathology does not warrant neuroimaging (129,130). Adequate data do not exist for the more uncommon primary headache disorders outside of pregnancy, let alone during pregnancy. Therefore, the difficulty arises as to whether new onset during pregnancy of these less common headache syndromes should be imaged. It is likely that neurologists would image, but wait until after the first trimester, unless indicated by development of abnormal neurology and/or additional features, as supported by data from studies of secondary headache cited.

Table 13.7 Treatment of Other Primary Headache Disorders in Pregnancy and Lactation

7a.

Primary headache	Acute treatment	Pregnancy	Lactation
Cluster headache (91)	Triptans	As above	As above
	High-flow oxygen	No harm reported	No harm reported
	Intranasal lidocaine	No harm reported	No harm reported
	Ergotamine tartrate	As above	As above
Paroxysmal hemicrania (91)	None	NA	NA
SUNCT[a] (91)	IV Lidocaine (Data from doses used to treat cardiac arrhythmia)	Large doses can cause fetal bradycardia	Present in milk but amount too small to be harmful
Idiopathic stabbing headache	None	NA	NA
Cough headache	None	NA	NA
Exertional headache	None	NA	NA
Sexual headache	None	NA	NA
Thunderclap headache	None	NA	NA
Hemicrania continua	None	NA	NA

7b.

Primary headache	Preventative treatment	Pregnancy	Lactation
Cluster headache (91)	Verapamil	As above	As above
	Lithium	Avoid if possible in the first trimester (risk of teratogenicity, including cardiac abnormalities); dose requirements increased during the second and third trimesters (but on delivery return abruptly to normal); close monitoring of serum-lithium concentration advised (risk of toxicity in neonate)	Present in milk and risk of toxicity in infant – avoid
	Methysergide	As above	As above
	Corticosteroids	Corticosteroids vary in their ability to cross the placenta; dexamethasone cross the placenta readily while 88% of prednisolone is inactivated as it crosses the placenta; there is no convincing evidence that systemic corticosteroids increase the incidence of congenital abnormalities such as cleft palate or lip; when administration is prolonged or repeated during pregnancy, systemic corticosteroids increase the risk of intrauterine growth restriction; there is no evidence of intrauterine growth restriction following short-term treatment (e.g., prophylactic treatment for neonatal respiratory distress syndrome); any adrenal suppression in the neonate following pre-natal exposure usually resolves spontaneously after birth and is rarely clinically important.	Prednisolone appears in small amounts in breast milk but maternal doses of up to 40 mg daily are unlikely to cause systemic effects in the infant; infants should be monitored for adrenal suppression if the mothers are taking a higher dose.
	Anticonvulsant group[b]	As above	As above
	Melatonin	No information available – avoid	Present in milk – avoid
Paroxysmal hemicrania and hemicrania continua (91, 96–100)	Indomethacin	As above	As above
	Topiramate	As above	As above
	Verapamil	As above	As above
	Piroxicam	As for other NSAIDs	Amount too small to be harmful
SUNCT[a] (91)	Lamotrigine	As above	As above
	Topiramate	As above	As above
	Gabapentin	As above	As above
All TACs[c] and hemicrania continua (75, 101)	Greater occipital nerve block	No harm reported	No harm reported

(Continued)

Table 13.7 Treatment of Other Primary Headache Disorders in Pregnancy and Lactation (*Continued*)

Primary headache	Acute treatment	Pregnancy	Lactation
Idiopathic stabbing headache (102)	Indomethacin	As above	As above
Cough headache (103, 104)	Indomethacin		
Exertional headache (103, 105)	Indomethacin		
Sexual headache (106, 107)	Indomethacin		

NA – Not applicable.
[a]SUNCT – short-lasting unilateral neuralgiform attacks with conjunctival injection and tearing.
[b]Topiramate, sodium valproate, gabapentin, lamotrigine.
[c]TAC – Trigeminal autonomic cephalalgia.

Table 13.8 Diagnosis and Treatment of Other Primary Headache Disorders

	Cough headache	Exertional headache	Sexual headache	Stabbing headache
Site of pain	Usually bilateral	Bilateral	Bilateral	Varying site – mainly V1 trigeminal
Character of pain	Sharp, stabbing	Throbbing	Thunderclap – before/at orgasm or bilateral pressure headache gradually increasing in severity towards orgasm	Single jabs or series of jabs
Additional features	Nausea, photophobia and phonophobia uncommon	With or without nausea, photophobia and phonophobia	None	None
Duration	Seconds to 30 min	5 min to 48 hr	1 min to 3 hr	Seconds
Frequency	Sudden and precipitated by coughing, straining or Valsalva	Pain precipitated by and occurs during or after physical exertion	Associated with orgasm	Irregular frequency
Preventative treatment	Indomethacin Acetazolamide Methysergide Parenteral dihydroergotamine Naproxen (112, 113) Propranolol Lumbar puncture	Indomethacin Propranolol Naproxen Ergotamine derivatives	Indomethacin Propranolol Pre-emptive Naratriptan	Indomethacin

Source: Adapted from data in Ref. 114.

Table 13.9 Secondary Thunderclap Headache

- Subarachnoid haemorrhage
- Cerebral venous sinus thrombosis
- Intra- and extracranial arterial dissection
- Pituitary apoplexy
- Intracerebral haemorrhage
- Spontaneous intracranial hypotension
- Colloid cyst of third ventricle
- Hypertensive encephalopathy with posterior leukoencephalopathy

SUMMARY

The most common disabling headache presenting in pregnancy is migraine. Individuals diagnosed with tension-type headache which is disabling are likely to have an underlying migraine disorder, and respond to treatments effective in migraine. The natural history is to improve during the sec-

ond and third trimesters. There can be worsening towards the end of the third trimester, and up to 40% of women experience post-partum headache. The safest acute treatment is paracetamol. Sumatriptan appears to be safe from first-trimester data. Acute-relief medication overuse should be avoided as this can potentiate the headache disorder and render preventative treatment less adequately efficacious. The safest preventative treatment is the tricyclic group of drugs.

A small proportion of individuals present with new-onset headache during pregnancy. This is most concerning if associated with neurological features. However, migraine aura is the most common transient neurological symptom presenting during pregnancy. Secondary headache in pregnancy is uncommon but further investigation should be prompted by any headache which is thunderclap in onset or associated with additional neurological features which are not typical for migraine aura.

REFERENCES

1. Melhado EM, Maciel JAJ, Guerreiro CA. Headache during gestation: evaluation of 1101 women. Can J Neurol Sci 2007; 34 (2):187–192.
2. Jensen R, Symond D. Epidemiology of tension-type headaches. In: Olesen J, Goadbsy PJ, Ramadan NM, et al. eds. The Headaches. 3rd ed. Philadelphia: Lippincott Williams and Wilkins, 2006:621–624.
3. Lyngberg AC, Rasmussen BK, Jørgensen T, et al. Has the prevalence of migraine and tension-type headache changed over a 12-year period? A Danish population survey. Eur J Epidemiol 2005; 20(3):243–249.
4. Steiner TJ, Scher AI, Stewart WF, et al. The prevalence and disability burden of adult migraine in England and their relationship to age, gender and ethnicity. Cephalalgia 2003; 23 (7):519–527.
5. Rasmussen BK, Jensen R, Olesen J. A population-based analysis of the diagnostic criteria of the International Headache Society. Cephalalgia 1991; 11(3):129–134.
6. Rasmussen BK. Epidemiology of migraine. In: Olesen J, Goadbsy PJ, Ramadan NM, et al. eds. The Headaches. 3rd ed. Philadelphia: Lippincott Williams and Wilkins, 2006:235–242.
7. Lipton RB, Cady RK, Stewart WF, et al. Diagnostic lessons from the Spectrum Study. Neurology 2002; 58(suppl 6):S27–S31.
8. Headache Classification Subcommittee of the International Headache Society. The International Classification of Headache Disorders (II). Cephalalgia 2004; 24(suppl 1):1–160.
9. Leonardi M, Steiner TJ, Scher AI, et al. The global burden of migraine: measuring disability in headache disorders with WHO's Classification of Functioning, Disability and Health (ICF). J Headache Pain 2005; 6:429–440.
10. Lipton RB, Scher AI, Steiner TJ, et al. Patterns of health care utilization for migraine in England and in the United States. Neurology 2003; 60(3):441–448.
11. Schwartz BS, Stewart WF, Simon D, et al. Epidemiology of tension-type headache. JAMA 1998; 279(5):381–383.
12. Maggioni F, Alessi C, Maggino T, et al. Headache during pregnancy. Cephalalgia 1997; 17(7):765–769.
13. Lipton RB, Stewart WF, Cady R, et al. Wolfe award. Sumatriptan for the range of headaches in migraine sufferers: results of the Spectrum Study. Headache 2000; 40(10):783–791.
14. Lampl C, Marecek S, May A, et al. A prospective, open-label, long-term study of the efficacy and tolerability of topiramate in the prophylaxis of chronic tension-type headache. Cephalalgia 2006; 26(10):1203–1208.
15. Yurekli VA, Akhan G, Kutluhan S, et al. The effect of sodium valproate on chronic daily headache and its subgroups. J Headache Pain 2008; 9(1):37–41.
16. Cady R, Schreiber C, Farmer K, et al. Primary headaches: a convergence hypothesis. Headache 2002; 42(3):204–216.
17. Rasmussen BK, Olesen J. Migraine with and without aura: an epidemiological study. Cephalalgia 1992; 12(4):221–228.
18. Mattsson P. Hormonal factors in migraine: a population-based study of women aged 40 to 74 years. Headache 2003; 43(1):27–35.
19. Cupini LM, Matteis M, Troisi E, et al. Sex-hormone-related events in migrainous females. A clinical comparative study between migraine with aura and migraine without aura. Cephalalgia 1995; 15(2):140–144.
20. Rasmussen BK. Epidemiology of headache. Cephalalgia 1995; 15 (1):48–68.
21. Bille B. A 40-year follow-up of school children with migraine. Cephalalgia 1997; 17(4):488–491.
22. Stewart WF, Lipton RB, Celentano DD, et al. Prevalence of migraine headache in the United States: relation to age, income, race and other sociodemographic factors. JAMA 1992; 267(1): 64–69.
23. MacGregor EA, Chia H, Vohrah RC, et al. Migraine and menstruation: a pilot study. Cephalalgia 1990; 10(6):305–310.
24. Somerville BW. Estrogen-withdrawal migraine. I. Duration of exposure required and attempted prophylaxis by premenstrual estrogen administration. Neurology 1975; 25(3):239–244.
25. Somerville BW. Estrogen-withdrawal migraine. II. Attempted prophylaxis by continuous estradiol administration. Neurology 1975; 25(3):245–250.
26. Somerville BW. The role of estradiol withdrawal in the etiology of menstrual migraine. Neurology 1972; 22(4):355–365.
27. Somerville BW. The role of progesterone in menstrual migraine. Neurology 1971; 21(8):853–859.
28. MacGregor EA, Frith A, Ellis J, et al. Prevention of menstrual attacks of migraine: a double-blind placebo-controlled crossover study. Neurology 2006; 67(12):2159–2163.
29. Dennerstein L, Morse C, Burrows G, et al. Menstrual migraine: a double-blind trial of percutaneous estradiol. Gynecol Endocrinol 1988; 2(2):113–120.
30. Silberstein SD, de Lignières B. Migraine, menopause and hormonal replacement therapy. Cephalalgia 2000; 20(3):214–221.
31. Massiou H, MacGregor EA. Evolution and treatment of migraine with oral contraceptives. Cephalalgia 2000; 20(3):170–174.
32. Loder E, Rizzoli P, Golub J. Hormonal management of migraine associated with menses and the menopause: a clinical review. Headache 2007; 47(2):329–340.
33. Lichten EM, Lichten JB, Whitty A, et al. The confirmation of a biochemical marker for women's hormonal migraine: the depo-estradiol challenge test. Headache 1996; 36(6):367–371.
34. Sicuteri F, Del Bene E, Poggioni M, et al. Unmasking latent dysnociception in healthy subjects. Headache 1987; 27(4):180–185.
35. van den Maagdenberg AM, Haan J, Terwindt GM, et al. Migraine: gene mutations and functional consequences. Curr Opin Neurol 2007; 20(3):299–305.
36. Wainscott G, Volans GN. The outcome of pregnancy in women suffering from migraine. Postgrad Med J 1978; 54(628):98–102.
37. Ratinahirana H, Darbois Y, Bousser M-G. Migraine and pregnancy: a prospective study in 703 women after delivery. Neurology 1990; 40(suppl 1):437.
38. Chen TC, Leviton A. Headache recurrence in pregnant women with migraine. Headache 1994; 34(2):107–110.
39. Granella F, Sances G, Zanferrari C, et al. Migraine without aura and reproductive life events: a clinical epidemiological study in 1300 women. Headache 1993; 33(7):385–389.
40. Sances G, Granella F, Nappi RE, et al. Course of migraine during pregnancy and postpartum: a prospective study. Cephalalgia 2003; 23(3):197–205.
41. Headache Classification Committee of the International Headache Society. Classification and diagnostic criteria for headache disorders, cranial neuralgias and facial pain. Cephalalgia 1988; 8 (7):1–96.
42. Ad Hoc Committee on the Classification of Headache. Classification of headache. J Am Med Assoc 1962; 179:717–718.
43. Stein GS. Headaches in the first post partum week and their relationship to migraine. Headache 1981; 12(5):201–205.
44. Scharff L, Marcus DA, Turk DC. Headache during pregnancy and in the postpartum: a prospective study. Headache 1997; 37 (4):203–210.
45. Marcus DA, Scharff L, Turk D. Longitudinal prospective study of headache during pregnancy and postpartum. Headache 1999; 39(9):625–632.
46. Ertresvåg JM, Zwart JA, Helde G, et al. Headache and transient focal neurological symptoms during pregnancy, a prospective cohort. Acta Neurol Scand 2005; 111(4):233–237.
47. Ertresvg JM, Stovner LJ, Kvavik LE, et al. Migraine aura or transient ischemic attacks? A five-year follow-up case-control study of women with transient central nervous system disorders in pregnancy. BMC Med 2007; 5:19.
48. Wright GD, Patel MK. Focal migraine and pregnancy. Br Med J (Clin Res Ed) 1986; 293(6561):1557–1558.
49. Lipton RB, Stewart WF, Stone AM. Stratified care vs step care strategies for migraine: results of the Disability in Strategies of Care (DISC) Study. JAMA 2000; 284(20):754–763.
50. Sculpher M, Millson D, Meddis D, et al. Cost-effectiveness analysis of stratified versus stepped care strategies for acute

treatment of migraine: The Disability in Strategies for Care (DISC) Study. Pharmacoeconomics 2002; 20(2):91–100.

51. Treatment of acute migraine with sumatriptan: The Subcutaneous Sumatriptan International Study Group. N Engl J Med 1991; 325(5):316–321.

52. Tfelt-Hansen P, Rolan P. Non-steroidal anti-Inflammatory drugs in the acute treatment of migraines. In: Olesen J, Goadsby PJ, Ramadan NM, et al. eds. The Headaches. 3rd ed. Philadelphia: Lippincott Williams and Wilkins, 2006:449–457.

53. Evans EW, Lorber KC. Use of 5-HT1 agonists in pregnancy. Ann Pharmacother 2008; 42(2):543–549.

54. Dahlof C. Clinical efficacy and tolerability of sumatriptan tablet and suppository in the acute treatment of migraine: a review of data from clinical trials. Cephalalgia 2001; 21(S1):9–12.

55. Dahlof C. Sumatriptan nasal spray in the acute treatment of migraine: a review of clinical studies. Cephalalgia 1999; 19 (9):769–778.

56. Welch KMA, Mathew NT, Stone P, et al. Tolerability of sumatriptan: clinical trials and post-marketing experience. Cephalalgia 2000; 20(8):687–695.

57. Olesen J, Diener HC, Schoenen J, et al. No effect of eletriptan administration during the aura phase of migraine. Eur J Neurol 2004; 11(10):671–677.

58. Bates D, Ashford E, Dawson R, et al. Subcutaneous sumatriptan during migraine aura. Neurology 1994; 44(9):1587–1592.

59. Thomsen LL, Dixon R, Lassen LH, et al. 311C90(Zolmitriptan), a novel centrally and peripheral acting oral 5-hydroxytryptamine-1D agonist: a comparison of its absorption during a migraine attacks and in a migraine-free period. Cephalalgia 1996; 16 (4):270–275.

60. Ross-Lee LM, Eadie MJ, Heazlewood V, et al. Aspirin pharmacokinetics in migraine. The effect of metoclopramide. Eur J Clin Pharmacol 1983; 24(6):777–785.

61. Tokola RA, Kangasniemi P, Neuvonen PJ, et al. Tolfenamic acid, metoclopramide, caffeine and their combinations in the treatment of migraine attacks. Cephalalgia 1983; 4(4):253–263.

62. Coppola M, Yealy DM, Leibold RA. Randomized, placebo-controlled evaluation of prochlorperazine versus metoclopramide for emergency department treatment of migraine headache. Ann Emerg Med 1995; 26(5):541–546.

63. Jones J, Pack S, Chun E. Intramuscular prochlorperazine versus metoclopramide as single-agent therapy for the treatment of acute migraine headache. Am J Emerg Med 1996; 14(3):262–264.

64. Russell MB, Andersson PG, Iselius L. Cluster headache is an inherited disorder in some families. Headache 1996; 36(10):608–612.

65. Davies PTG, Peatfield RC, Steiner TJ, et al. Some clinical comparisons between common and classical migraine. Cephalalgia 1991; 11(5):223–227.

66. Henry P, Michel P, Brichet B, et al. A nationwide survey of migraine in France: prevalence and clinical features in adults. Cephalalgia 1992; 12(4):229–237.

67. Couch JR, Diamond S. Status migrainosus: causative and therapeutic aspects. Headache 1983; 23(3):94–101.

68. Bahra A, Walsh M, Menon S, et al. Does chronic daily headache arise de novo in association with regular analgesic use? Headache 2003; 43(3):179–190.

69. Limmroth V, Katsarava Z, Fritsche G, et al. Features of medication overuse headache following overuse of different acute headache drugs. Neurology 2002; 59(7):1011–1014.

70. Saper JR. Ergotamine dependency – a review. Headache 1987; 27 (8):435–438.

71. Zeeberg P, Olesen J, Jensen R. Discontinuation of medication overuse in headache patients: recovery of therapeutic responsiveness. Cephalalgia 2006; 26(10):1192–1198.

72. Kudrow L. Paradoxical effects of frequent analgesic use. Adv Neurol 1982; 33:335–341.

73. Goadsby PJ, Knight YE, Hoskin KL. Stimulation of the greater occipital nerve increases metabolic activity in the trigeminal nucleus caudalis and cervical dorsal horn of the cat. Pain 1997; 73(1):23–28.

74. Busch V, Jakob W, Juergens T, et al. Occipital nerve blockade in chronic cluster headache patients and functional connectivity between trigeminal and occipital nerves. Cephalalgia 2007; 27 (11):1206–1214.

75. Afridi SK, Shields KG, Bhola R, et al. Greater occipital nerve injections in primary headache syndromes – prolonged effects from a single injection. Pain 2006; 122(1–2):126–129.

76. Rapoport AM, Weeks RE, Sheftell FD, et al. Analgesic rebound headache: theoretical and practical implications. Cephalalgia 1985; 5(suppl 3):448.

77. Li D, Rozen TD. The clinical characteristics of new persistent daily headache. Cephalalgia 2002; 22(1):66–69.

78. Bahra A, May A, Goadsby PJ. Cluster headache: a prospective clinical study with diagnostic implications. Neurology 2002; 58 (3):354–361.

79. Schurks M, Kurth T, de Jesus J, et al. Cluster headache: clinical presentation, lifestyle features, and medical treatment. 2006; 46 (8):1246–1254.

80. Torelli P, Cologno D, Cademartiri C, et al. Application of the International Headache Society classification criteria in 652 cluster headache patients. Cephalalgia 2001; 21(2):145–150.

81. van Vliet JA, Favier I, Helmerhorst FM, et al. Cluster headache in women: relation with menstruation, use of oral contraceptives, pregnancy, and menopause. J Neurol Neurosurg Psychiatry 2006; 77(5):690–692.

82. Cohen AS, Burns B, Goadsby PJ. High-flow oxygen for treatment of cluster headache: a randomized trial. JAMA 2009; 302 (22):2451–2457.

83. Fogan L. Treatment of cluster headache. Arch Neurol 1985; 42 (4):362–363.

84. Ekbom K. The Sumatriptan Cluster Headache Study Group. Treatment of acute cluster headache with sumatriptan. N Engl J Med 1991; 325(5):322–326.

85. O'Quinn S, Ephross SA, Williams V, et al. Pregnancy and perinatal outcomes in migraineurs using sumatriptan: a prospective study. Arch Gynaecol Obstet 1999; 263(1–2):7–12.

86. van Vliet JA, Bahra A, Martin V, et al. Intranasal sumatriptan is effective in the treatment of acute cluster headache – a double-blind placebo-controlled crossover study. Cephalalgia 2001; 21 (4):270–271.

87. Cittadini E, May A, Straube A, et al. Effectiveness of intranasal zolmitriptan in acute cluster headache: a randomised placebo-controlled crossover study. Arch Neurol 2006; 63(11):1537–1542.

88. Bahra A, Gawel MJ, Hardebo J-E, et al. Oral zolmitriptan is effective in the acute treatment of cluster headache. Neurology 2000; 54(9):1832–1839.

89. Costa A, Pucci E, Antonaci F, et al. The effect of intranasal cocaine and lidocaine on nitroglycerin-induced attacks in cluster headache. Cephalalgia 2000; 20(2):85–91.

90. Jammes JL. The treatment of cluster headaches with prednisone. Dis Nerv Syst 1975; 36(7):375–376.

91. May A, Leone M, Afra J, et al. EFNS guidelines on the treatment of cluster headache and other trigeminal – autonomic cephalalgias. Eur J Neurol 2006; 13(10):1066–1077.

92. Cittadini E, Matharu MS, Goadsby PJ. Paroxysmal hemicrania: a prospective clinical study of thirty-one cases. Brain 2008; 131(pt 4):1142–1155.

93. Norton ME. Teratogen update: fetal effects of indomethacin administration during pregnancy. Teratology 1997; 56:282–292.

94. Mathew NT, Kailasam J, Fischer A. Responsiveness to celecoxib in chronic paroxysmal hemicrania. Neurology 2000; 55(2):316.

95. Siow HCC. Seasonal episodic paroxysmal hemicrania responding to cyclooxygenase-2 inhibitors. Cephalalgia 2004; 24(5):414–415.

96. Sjaastad O, Antonaci F. A piroxicam derivative partly effective in chronic paroxysmal hemicrania and hemicrania continua. Headache 1995; 35(9):549–550.

97. Trucco M, Antonaci F, Sandrini G. Hemicrania continua: a case responsive to piroxicam-beta-cyclodextrin. Headache 1992; 32 (1):39–40.

98. Rajabally YA, Jacob S. Hemicrania continua responsive to verapamil. Headache 2005; 45(8):1082–1083.

99. Cohen AS, Goadbsy PJ. Paroxysmal hemicrania responding to topiramate. J Neurol Neurosurg Psychiatry 2007; 78(1):96–97.

100. Camarda C, Camarda R, Monastero R. Chronic paroxysmal hemicrania and hemicrania continua responding to topiramate: two case reports. Clin Neurol Neurosurg 2008; 110(1):88–91.

101. Antonaci F, Pareja JA, Caminero AB, et al. Chronic paroxysmal hemicrania and hemicrania continua: anaesthetic blockades of pericranial nerves. Functional Neurology 1997; 12(1):11–15.

102. Pareja JA, Rutz J, de Isla C. Idiopathic stabbing headache. Cephalalgia 1996; 16(2):93–96.

103. Mathew NT. Indomethacin responsive headache syndromes. Headache 1981; 21(4):147–150.

104. Raskin N. The cough headache syndrome: treatment. Neurology 1995; 45(9):1784.

105. Diamond S, Medina JL. Benign exertional headache: successful treatment with indomethacin. Headache 1979; 19:249.

106. Pascual J, Iglesias F, Oterino A, et al. Cough, exertional, and sexual headaches: an analysis of 72 benign and symptomatic cases. Neurology 1996; 46(6):1520–1524.

107. Raskin NH. Short-lived head pains. Neurol Clin 1997; 15:143–145.

108. Cohen AS, Matharu MS, Goadbsy PJ. Short-lasting unilateral neuralgiform headache attacks with conjunctival injection and tearing (SUNCT) or cranial autonomic features (SUNA)—a prospective clinical study of SUNCT and SUNA. Brain 2006; 129 (10):2746–2760.

109. Cruccu G, Gronseth G, Alksne J, et al. AAN-EFNS guidelines on trigeminal neuralgia management. Eur J Neurol 2008; 15 (10):1013–1028.

110. Pareja JA, Kruszewski P, Sjaastad O. SUNCT syndrome: trials of drugs and anaesthetic blockades. Headache 1995; 35(3):138–142.

111. Pareja JA, Caminero AB, Sjaastad O. SUNCT Syndrome: diagnosis and treatment. CNS Drugs 2002; 16(6):373–383.

112. Mateo I, Pascual J. Coexistence of chronic paroxysmal hemicrania and benign cough headache. Headache 1999; 39(6):437–438.

113. Raskin NH. The indomethacin-responsive syndromes. In: Raskin NH, ed. Headache. New York: Churchill Livingstone, 1988:255–268.

114. Bahra A. Unusual headache disorders. Adv Clin Neurosci Rehabilitation 2006; 6(6):12–13.

115. Newman HC, Lipton RB, Solomon S. Hemicrania continua: ten new cases and a review of the literature. Neurology 1994; 44 (11):2111–2114.

116. Matharu MS, Cohen AS, McGonigle DJ, et al. Posterior hypothalamic and brainstem activation in hemicrania continua. Headache 2004; 44(8):747–761.

117. Paemeleire K, Bahra A, Evers S, et al. Medication-overuse headache in patients with cluster headache. Neurology 2006; 67(1):109–113.

118. Young WB, Silberstein SD. Hemicrania continua and symptomatic medication overuse. Headache 1993; 33(9):485–487.

119. Palmieri A, Mainardi F, Maggioni F, et al. Cluster-like headache secondary to cavernous sinus metastasis. Cephalalgia 2005; 25 (9):743–745.

120. Todo T, Inoya H. Sudden appearance of a mycotic aneurysm of the intracavernous carotid artery after symptoms resembling cluster headache: case report. Neurosurgery 1991; 29 (4):594–598.

121. Haas DC, Kent PF, Friedman DI. Headache caused by a single lesion of multiple sclerosis in the periaqueductal gray area. Headache 1993; 33(8):452–455.

122. Trucco M, Mainardi F, Maggioni F, et al. Chronic paroxysmal hemicrania, hemicrania continua and SUNCT syndrome in association with other pathologies: a review. Cephalalgia 2004; 24(3):173–184.

123. Tfelt-Hansen P, Paulson OB, Krabbe A. Invasive adenoma of the pituitary gland and chronic migrainous neuralgia: a rare coincidence or a causal relationship? Cephalalgia 1982; 2(1):25–28.

124. Rosenberg JH, Silberstein SD. The headache of SAH responds to sumatriptan. Headache 2005; 45(5):597–598.

125. Locker T, Mason S, Rigby A. Headache management – are we doing enough? An observational study of patients presenting with headache to the emergency department. Emerg Med J 2004; 21(3):327–332.

126. Ramirez-Lassepas M, Espinosa CE, Cicero JJ, et al. Predictors of intracranial pathologic findings in patients who seek emergency care because of headache. Arch Neurol 1997; 54 (12):1506–1509.

127. Linn FHH, Rinkel GJE, Algra A, et al. Headache characteristics in subarachnoid haemorrhage and benign thunderclap headache. J Neurol Neurosurg Psychiatry 1998; 65(5):791–793.

128. Barton CW. Evaluation and treatment of headache in the emergency department: a survey. Headache 1994; 34(2):91–94.

129. Detsky ME, McDonald DR, Baerlocher MO, et al. Does this patient with headache have a migraine or need neuroimaging? JAMA 2006; 13(296):1274–1283.

130. Alter M, Daube JR, Franklin G, et al. Practice parameter: the utility of neuroimaging in the evaluation of headache in patients with normal neurologic examinations (summary statement). Report of the Quality Standards Subcommittee of the American Academy of Neurology. Neurology 1994; 44(7):1353–1354.

14

Infections in pregnancy

Iskandar Azwa, Michael S. Marsh, and David A. Hawkins

INTRODUCTION

Despite the advent of antibiotics and improved diagnostic facilities, infectious diseases in pregnancy continue to contribute significantly to maternal and neonatal morbidity and mortality (1). These are most common in the developing world. About 99% of maternal deaths in the world in 2005 occurred in developing countries and 25% of maternal deaths in the developing world are due to infections in pregnancy mainly due to puerperal sepsis and septic abortion.

Obstetric sepsis was the leading cause of maternal mortality in the United Kingdom until the introduction of antibiotics into clinical practice in the late 1930s. The incidence has now declined rapidly but there were still 18 direct deaths from genital tract sepsis (0.06% of maternal deaths) reported in the 2003 to 2005 triennium in the Confidential Enquiry into Maternal Deaths (CEMD), the majority associated with beta-haemolytic streptococcus Lancefield group A and *Escherichia coli* infection (2). Eight out of the 18 deaths occurred during labour or before delivery. The CEMD identified risk factors for maternal sepsis which included diabetes, anaemia, history of pelvic infection, impaired immunity, history of group B streptococcal infection, amniocentesis and other invasive intrauterine procedures, cervical cerclage, prolonged spontaneous rupture of membranes, caesarean section and retained products of conception post-miscarriage or -delivery. Obesity was also identified as a risk factor for infection and led to practical difficulties in managing care. The CEMD highlighted the need to avoid complacency in maternal infection and made a number of key specific recommendations. It emphasised the importance of increased awareness by health care professionals of symptoms and signs of sepsis and septic shock and the importance of regular frequent observations if pelvic sepsis was suspected. It also stressed the importance of implementation of guidelines within individual maternity units for the management of genital tract sepsis. Prompt treatment with high-dose broad-spectrum antibiotics should be started prior to obtaining microbiology results.

Maternal infections also have a major impact in the transmission of infections to the fetus, with a risk of adverse outcomes such as preterm deliveries, stillbirth, intrauterine growth restriction, congenital anomalies and neonatal infection. In addition, increased foreign travel of pregnant women and the increase in immigrants from developing countries pose challenges to obstetricians and neonatologists in the overall management of infectious diseases in the United Kingdom. Early involvement of a multidisciplinary team involving microbiologists, maternal-fetal medicine specialists, pharmacists and the critical care team is essential. With evidence of sexually transmitted infections (STIs), genitourinary medicine specialists should be involved, and screening for other STIs should be undertaken.

In contrast to the common infections found in pregnancy, central nervous system (CNS) infections rarely complicate pregnancy, although when they do the effects can be severe.

This chapter is divided into two sections. The first discusses the screening and prevention of maternal infections and outlines some of the more common infections in pregnancy encountered in the developed world and their consequences. Investigations and management to improve fetal and maternal outcomes are also discussed. The second section deals with the CNS infections that can complicate pregnancy, including acute and chronic meningitis, encephalitis, brain abscess and spinal cord infection.

Management recommendations and guidelines have been based on the most recently revised guidelines from the U.K. Royal College of Obstetricians and Gynaecologists (RCOG), Health Protection Agency (HPA), Department of Health (DOH), British Association for Sexual Health and HIV (BASHH), British HIV Association (BHIVA), U.S. Centers for Disease Control and Prevention (CDC) and World Health Organization (WHO), when available.

GENERAL INFECTION IN PREGNANCY
The U.K. Antenatal Screening Programme
Since 2003, the U.K. DOH has recommended screening all pregnant women with a single blood sample for human immunodeficiency virus (HIV), hepatitis B, rubella and syphilis during their first and all subsequent pregnancies (3). Other infections, not routinely investigated as part of the U.K. antenatal screening programme, may be appropriate in other countries depending on the prevalence and risk of exposure. These include cytomegalovirus (CMV), *Chlamydia trachomatis*, bacterial vaginosis, hepatitis C, group B streptococcus, toxoplasma, genital herpes simplex and human T-lymphotropic virus type-1. The important factors to consider when deciding to undertake screening of any infectious agent during pregnancy are the incidence of maternal infection, the risk of transmission to the fetus, the fetal damage if infection occurs, the availability of a reliable screening test and the availability of a safe and effective intervention to prevent fetal infection and reduce damage.

Prevention of Infection in Pregnant Women
Pregnant women should be advised about preventive measures to reduce the risk of toxoplasma infection such as avoiding eating unwashed fruits, vegetables and inadequately cooked meat and avoiding contact with cat litter (4). To reduce the risk of listeriosis, pregnant women should avoid eating unpasteurised dairy products. Pregnant women should also avoid unprotected intercourse if their partners are known to have HIV, hepatitis B, herpes simplex virus (HSV) or other STIs. Women from non-endemic areas should be advised against travel to a malaria-endemic area (5). If travel is unavoidable, advice should be given about personal protection

and chemoprophylaxis. This advice also applies to previously immune women from malaria-endemic areas who have lived in the United Kingdom for more than 2 years and who will therefore have lost much of their pre-existing immunity.

Protection against infection may be achieved by active and passive immunisation and all health care providers should obtain an immunisation history from women accessing prenatal care. Live and/or live-attenuated vaccines are contra-indicated in pregnancy due to theoretical concerns of terato-genicity. If immunisation is to be given in anticipation of later risks, it is preferable for administration after the first trimester. Immunisation programmes for rubella in childhood should provide protection throughout the childbearing years. Following the mumps, measles and rubella (MMR) vaccine controversy, first reported in 1998, immunisation rates in the United Kingdom fell to 80% in 2003. However, the uptake of the vaccine is beginning to increase again, attaining 85% coverage in 2008. Women without a previous history of varicella should be screened for varicella zoster virus (VZV) antibodies at booking or rapidly after exposure, that is, within 48 hours after contact (5). Following exposure of a pregnant woman to varicella, non-immune women should be offered passive immunisation with varicella zoster immune globulin up to 10 days after contact. Pregnant women are at increased risk of complications of influenza and all pregnant women should be offered the inactivated vaccine during the influenza season. Women who are breastfeeding can still be immunised.

Immunology of Pregnancy

The 'paradox of pregnancy', in which immunological tolerance to paternally derived fetal antigens is achieved despite an apparently adequate maternal defence against infection, continues to intrigue immunologists. Evidence indicates that immunological tolerance of the fetus may occur by suppression of maternal cell-mediated immunity while retaining normal humoral (antibody-mediated) immunity. This occurs as a result of decreased T-helper type 1(Th-1) lymphocyte responses (which stimulate cell-mediated immunity) with a shift to T-helper type 2 (Th-2) dominance (which augment the humoral immune response) (6). The cell-mediated immunity is responsible for controlling intracellular pathogens and the immunological changes that occur in pregnancy may lead to increased severity and susceptibility to intracellular pathogens, including viruses, intracellular bacteria and parasites.

Effect of Infections on the Fetus

Infections that affect the fetus and neonate are predominantly viral infections with a smaller number due to bacterial and protozoal infections. Infections can develop in the neonate transplacentally, perinatally (from vaginal secretions or blood), or post-natally (from breast milk). Blood-borne viruses such as HIV, hepatitis B and C are mainly associated with perinatal infections, whereas rubella, CMV, parvovirus B19 and VZV are associated with in utero infection and placental transmission.

Infections traditionally known to produce congenital defects have been described with the acronym TORCH (toxoplasma, others, rubella, CMV, herpes). The 'others' category has now rapidly expanded to include parvovirus B19, VZV, West Nile virus, measles virus, enteroviruses, adenovirus and HIV.

The effect of infection in the fetus is determined by the virulence of microbes, the size of the inoculum, the immune response of the fetus at different gestational ages

and passively derived maternal antibodies. Infection in pregnancy can lead to miscarriage, stillbirth, prematurity, structural defects and intrauterine growth restriction.

Investigation of Suspected Infection in Pregnancy

Serological methods are often used for diagnosing viral infections in pregnancy and look for changes in immunoglobulin G (IgG) antibody titres with serial samples and the presence of immunoglobulin M (IgM) in order to determine if recent infection has occurred. It is often helpful to compare a current sample with any previous samples taken earlier in the pregnancy, for example, samples taken at the time of booking, which are often stored in the laboratory for a period of time. Absence of IgG antibodies in early pregnancy identifies susceptible women. The presence of IgG antibodies suggests previous infection or vaccination. Measurement of IgG avidity when available is useful. Low IgG avidity indicates primary infection. This is based on the fact that antibody binds less avidly to antigens during the early phases than in the later or chronic phase of infection. In order to aid interpretation of serological tests, it is important to give as much clinical information as possible to the laboratory such as date and type of exposure, time of symptom onset, history of previous vaccination or infection and gestation of pregnancy.

It is important to remember that only some cases of maternal infection will result in fetal infection and not all cases of fetal infection will result in the fetus being affected or damaged by infection. Referral to a fetal medicine unit for prenatal diagnostic testing such as amniotic fluid culture and polymerase chain reaction (PCR) may establish whether a fetus has been infected, but it cannot confirm or refute the possibility that the fetus has been affected.

Uterine Infections

Chorioamnionitis

Chorioamnionitis is infection or inflammation of the amniotic fluid and/or the fetal membranes, the chorion and amnion. It can be either a histological or clinical diagnosis. Clinical chorioamnionitis is present in up to 5% of term deliveries and in 10% to 25% of preterm deliveries, with the highest risk in those with preterm premature rupture of membranes (PPROM) (6). Other risk factors of chorioamnionitis include prolonged labour, repeated vaginal examinations, internal fetal monitoring, bacterial vaginosis and group B streptococcal colonisation. Most cases are secondary to ascending infection from the vagina and cervix.

The diagnosis of chorioamnionitis is suggested by maternal fever, uterine tenderness, offensive liquor, maternal and fetal tachycardia. Management involves expediting delivery and treatment with broad-spectrum intravenous antibiotics such as ampicillin, gentamicin and metronidazole (or clindamycin for anaerobic cover) after taking blood cultures. Consequences of chorioamnionitis include premature rupture of membranes, premature labour, increased risk of neonatal pneumonia, bacteraemia and meningitis. Severe chorioamnionitis may be accompanied by a fetal inflammatory response leading to vasculitis of the umbilical vessels and funisitis (inflammation of the umbilical cord's connective tissue).

There is a causal link between chorioamnionitis and brain injury in preterm and term infants. It has been shown that there is a significant association between intrauterine infection and brain injury in the form of cerebral white matter lesions and periventricular leucomalacia in preterm neonates. This association also applies to term infants, but with a much stronger association. It is uncertain whether the resulting brain injury is directly the result of maternal infection or indirectly via the fetus' inflammatory response.

Puerperal Sepsis

Ninety percent of infections arising in the first 14 days after delivery are of genital or urinary tract in origin. Other causes include mastitis, wound infections (following caesarean section, episiotomy or perineal tears), venous thrombophlebitis and post general anaesthesia pneumonia; pneumonia is very rare after epidural anaesthesia during labour.

Puerperal infection of the uterus is a common cause of post-natal pyrexia (7). There is an increased risk of endometritis following prolonged rupture of membranes and instrumental delivery. Infections are often polymicrobial, caused by a variety of organisms ascending from the vagina such as *E. coli*, *Streptococcus* A or B, anaerobes, *Bacteroides* spp., *Mycoplasma hominis* and *Ureaplasma urealyticum*. Post-partum endometritis should be suspected in women presenting with high-grade fever, lower abdominal pain, uterine tenderness and leucocytosis. An antibiotic regimen consisting of clindamycin and an aminoglycoside is recommended. Routine use of prophylactic antibiotics for elective and emergency caesarean sections is recommended by the U.K. RCOG national guidelines. The antibiotic used should be limited to one dose to reduce the possibility of resistance.

Viral Infections

Rubella (German Measles)

This is caused by an RNA togavirus and is acquired by respiratory droplet exposure. After an incubation period of 2 to 3 weeks, a mild febrile illness with a macular rash, suboccipital and posterior auricular lymphadenopathy and arthralgia occur. The affected individual is infectious for 1 week before the onset of the rash until 4 days afterwards. The incidence of rubella infection has considerably reduced since the introduction of the rubella vaccine programme in most developed countries. About 2% to 3% of women do not respond to the rubella vaccine and therefore remain susceptible to the infection.

Rubella infection in pregnancy has marked embryopathic consequences to the fetus when acquired by the fetus in utero (8). Risk of transmission to the fetus with resultant congenital anomalies occurs is over 90% in the first trimester, dropping to about 35% by weeks 13 to 16. The range of congenital defects seen maybe permanent and includes cardiac anomalies (commonly patent ductus arteriosus or peripheral pulmonary artery stenosis), ocular defects (cataracts, glaucoma), microcephaly, developmental delay, sensorineural deafness, hepatosplenomegaly and thrombocytopaenic purpura. The severity of these anomalies merits the offer of termination of pregnancy to the mother in cases where the fetus may be affected. The predominant defects in first-trimester infection are cardiac disease and deafness whilst deafness alone is the main defect seen in second-trimester infection. Congenital defects are rare with maternal infection after 16 weeks. Maternal re-infection in immune women is usually subclinical and the risk to the fetus is thought to be relatively low (<5%).

Clinical diagnosis is difficult because of its atypical presentation and a similar rash may be caused by other viral infections such as parvovirus B19, varicella, measles, enteroviruses and infectious mononucleosis. Suspected cases should be investigated promptly with serology testing for rising antibody titre and rubella-specific IgM which confirms recent infection. IgM may be present on day 4 or 5 of the clinical illness and persist for 6 weeks. IgG can be detected within 6 weeks of infection. Prenatal diagnostic tests such as amniocentesis and amniotic fluid viral culture, PCR or fetal blood IgM may be used to establish infection of the fetus, but have low positive predictive value and does not prove damage of the fetus by infection. If maternal seroconversion occurs within the first 12 weeks where the risk of congenital infection is greatest, then a termination of pregnancy may be offered without invasive prenatal diagnosis.

All pregnant women should be tested in early pregnancy to confirm immunity. Prevention is through childhood vaccination as well as assessment of rubella immunity pre-pregnancy in women seeking pre-conceptual counselling or advice on sub-fertility. All women found to be non-immune during pregnancy should be offered post-natal vaccination. The vaccine is a live-attenuated vaccine and contraindicated in pregnancy. There is no evidence that inadvertent use in pregnancy is associated with congenital infection and not considered in itself an indication for termination of pregnancy.

Cytomegalovirus

CMV is a member of the herpes virus family and represents the most frequent congenital infection. Approximately 1% (range 0.5–2.5%) of all newborns are congenitally infected with CMV. Infection of the fetus is the second most common cause of mental retardation after Down syndrome (7). The virus is transmitted by contact with infected body fluids: saliva, urine, blood, semen and cervical secretions. Vertical infection can occur antenatally through the placenta, during delivery through contact with cervical secretions and blood and post-natally through breastfeeding. Adult seroprevalence in developed countries is around 50%, but in developing countries where most infections are acquired during childhood, it may be as high as 90% to 100%. Women of child-bearing age who are CMV seronegative are at major risk of giving birth to infants with symptomatic congenital infection if primary infection is acquired during pregnancy. Primary maternal CMV infection in adults may be asymptomatic or lead to an infectious mononucleosis-like syndrome. Viral shedding after primary infection continues for some months before it establishes latency. Children represent an important infectious source to pregnant mothers as viral shedding can persist for years after a primary infection. Secondary infection can occur due to reactivation of latent virus or due to re-infection with a different strain. Most maternal CMV infections are most likely due to reactivation of latent virus.

Vertical transmission of CMV can occur at any stage of pregnancy; however, severe sequelae are more common with infection in the first trimester, while overall risk of transmission is greatest in the third trimester. Primary CMV infection during pregnancy leads to transplacental fetal infection in 40% of cases, whereas secondary infection carries a significantly smaller risk of vertical transmission of 1%. Seven to ten percent of infected fetuses will present at birth with defects, the most common being petechiae, hepatosplenomegaly, microcephaly, jaundice, chorioretinitis and intrauterine growth restriction. There is a mortality rate of up to 20% in this group. Of those asymptomatic at birth, a further 10% to 15% will develop long-term neurological sequelae such as sensorineural deafness and psychomotor delay during the first 2 years of life.

The diagnosis of primary maternal infection is made by demonstration of seroconversion of CMV-specific IgG antibodies from negative to positive. A rise in IgG titre is not indicative of primary infection as it can occur with reactivation. CMV-specific IgM is not a reliable marker of primary infection as circulating IgM may persist for up to 12 months after primary infection and may cause uncertainty as to whether infection has occurred during or shortly before pregnancy. IgG avidity testing can be very helpful in differentiating between acute and chronic infection. Low-avidity IgG is suggestive of primary infection. The diagnosis can also be made by PCR testing of serum or urine during acute illness.

Following confirmation of primary maternal infection, fetal infection may be diagnosed by detection of the virus in the amniotic fluid by culture and PCR. The sensitivity of amniotic fluid testing before 21 weeks of gestation is low as it is only after this time that the infected fetus sheds virus in its urine and into the amniotic fluid. Higher viral loads on quantitative PCR are associated with a higher likelihood of fetal infection and termination may be offered. Serial ultrasound scanning may be undertaken to look for features of CMV infection such as ventriculomegaly, periventricular, intracranial and intra-abdominal calcification and echogenic bowel, although none of these features are specific to CMV.

At present, the treatment options to prevent congenital infection are limited but a vaccine is in development and remains a high priority. Screening for maternal immunity is therefore not currently routine in the United Kingdom. There is some evidence that ganciclovir can stop the progression of hearing loss in affected infants and the RCOG guidelines recommend treatment of neonates with congenital CMV infection and neurological signs at birth with ganciclovir.

Parvovirus B19

Parvovirus is a small single-stranded DNA virus that has an affinity for erythroid precursor cells leading to inhibition of erythropoiesis. The virus readily crosses the placenta, causing lytic destruction of fetal red blood cells, with resultant anaemia and viral myocarditis (9). If the anaemia is severe it can lead to cardiac failure and non-immune hydrops, which occurs in less than 3% of pregnancies. The infection is usually transmitted by respiratory droplets but can also be transmitted from blood and blood-derived products. It is common worldwide and the seroprevalence increases with age, so that 15% of preschool children, 50% of younger adults and 85% of the elderly show serological evidence of past infection (10). Infection confers lifelong immunity. Most infections occur in children. Mothers, nursery teachers and health workers who come into contact with school-aged children are at highest risk of contracting the infection. A flu-like illness with fever, headache, coryza and myalgia is followed 1 week later by a characteristic facial rash which spreads to the trunk and limbs and is known as erythema infectiosum or slapped cheek syndrome. A quarter of infections are subclinical. Viraemia reaches its peak 1 week after infection when the risk of transmission is at its greatest. Vertical transmission occurs in one-third of cases.

Serological examination for both parvovirus B19-specific IgM and IgG antibodies should be undertaken if infection is suspected in pregnancy. IgM is present 7 to 10 days after infection and persists for about 2 to 3 months. IgG appears shortly after IgM and persists for life with slowly decreasing titres unless boosted by subsequent encounters with the virus. Nucleic acid amplification tests are useful in patients lacking an adequate antibody-mediated immune response or in immune-compromised mothers. A positive PCR test in serum indicates acute maternal infection. PCR testing of amniotic fluid or cord blood for detection of viral DNA helps confirm fetal infection. Where maternal infection is confirmed, monitoring of the fetus by serial ultrasound to look for developing hydrops is recommended. If hydrops and/or anaemia are diagnosed by ultrasound and cordocentesis, intrauterine transfusions should be administered to support the fetus until spontaneous recovery occurs. The treatment of parvovirus infection is limited to the treatment of fetal anaemia, as no vaccine or treatment is currently available to infected mothers.

Varicella Zoster Virus

VZV is a DNA virus and a member of the herpes family. It is highly infectious and transmitted through respiratory droplets and close contact with the vesicular fluid of the skin lesions. Patients with primary VZV infection are infectious from up to 2 days before the appearance of the rash until the vesicles crust over. In developed countries, 85% of women of childbearing age are immune to VZV. Following the primary infection (chickenpox), the virus remains latent in the sensory nerve ganglia and can reactivate to cause the rash of herpes zoster (shingles). Although primary infection is thought to confer lifelong immunity, there have been case reports of clinical reinfections.

Pregnant women exposed to VZV and who do not recall having had chickenpox should be blood tested for VZV IgG antibodies, either at the time of suspected infection or from a stored sample (11). If this confirms past immunity, the woman can be reassured that the fetus is not at risk. Non-immune pregnant women who have been exposed to VZV should be offered passive immunisation with varicella zoster immunoglobulin (VZIG). VZIG is known to be effective in preventing or reducing the severity of maternal infection or congenital varicella syndrome (CVS) if given within 72 hours with some residual benefit if administered within 10 days. The varicella vaccine is a live-attenuated vaccine and therefore contraindicated in pregnancy. It can be given as post-exposure prophylaxis in non-pregnant women.

In pregnancy, VZV infection can have both maternal and fetal consequences. Disseminated primary maternal varicella infection, particularly in the third trimester has been associated with maternal complications that include pneumonia (in up to 10% of pregnant women with a higher mortality risk from respiratory failure than in non-pregnant adults), encephalitis (up to 1% of pregnant patients, see below), hepatitis and secondary bacterial infections.

Uncomplicated maternal varicella can be treated orally with aciclovir or valaciclovir if the patient presents within 24 hours of the onset of the rash. Oral aciclovir reduces the duration and severity of symptoms. Treatment should be considered particularly in the latter half of pregnancy when risks of maternal complications are increased and the risk of acyclovir affecting the fetus are minimal. Although no adverse fetal effects have been reported with the use of aciclovir in pregnancy, there is a slight theoretical risk of teratogenesis in the first trimester and its use in pregnancy and relative risks and benefits should be discussed with the mother. Intravenous aciclovir is indicated for pregnant women who develop any signs of pneumonia.

Primary VZV infection in the pregnant woman most often results in the birth of a normal newborn. Rarely, the outcome is CVS and/or fetal death. The highest risk for spontaneous abortion or CVS is within the first 20 weeks of gestation, but the overall risk of CVS in the first 20 weeks is only around 2%. The features of CVS are cicatricial skin scarring in a dermatomal distribution, eye defects (chorioretinitis, cataracts, microphthalmia), limb hypoplasia and neurological abnormalities (microcephaly, cortical atrophy and developmental delay). Features may be detected on ultrasound from 5 weeks after infection. Evaluation of fetal infection after primary infection by amniocentesis is not routinely advised because the risk of CVS is low even when the amniotic fluid is positive for VZV DNA. VZV DNA has a high sensitivity but a low specificity for the development of CVS.

Transplacental passage of the virus resulting in neonatal varicella infection increases with gestational age. Up to 50% of fetuses are affected when maternal infection occurs 1 to 4 weeks before delivery, with up to one-third of the newborns developing clinical varicella. Neonatal varicella infection can be life threatening in 20% to 30% of neonates whose mothers become acutely infected from 5 days prior to delivery to 2 days post-delivery. This represents a high-risk window of time as there has not been sufficient time for the development and passage of maternal antibodies to the fetus. The delivery date should be postponed by 5 to 7 days where possible to allow transfer of maternal antibodies to the fetus. This delay may ameliorate the disease. The baby at risk of congenital varicella infection should be given VZIG immediately after birth and should be isolated from the mother if she has a rash and the baby should be monitored for signs of infection. If infection arises in the neonate, it should be treated with aciclovir. It should be noted that babies born to mothers with VZV infection during pregnancy with no clinical evidence of VZV infection at birth may present later in infancy with herpes zoster due to reactivation of the virus after a primary infection in utero.

Human Immunodeficiency Virus

HIV is a retrovirus that targets the cell-mediated immune system, particularly CD4 + cells. The depressed immunodeficiency increases the risk of opportunistic infections and certain malignancies within the host. The estimated seroprevalence of HIV in the antenatal U.K. population is 0.23%; the majority of women testing positive coming from sub-Saharan Africa. Unlike some other viral infections, maternal HIV infection is not associated with a specific pattern of congenital abnormalities. Vertical transmission is the predominant concern. Without specific interventions, the transmission rate ranges from 15% to 40%. There is a close linear correlation between maternal HIV plasma viral load and risk of transmission, the risk being greatest for women with high viral loads (12). Most mother-to-child transmission of HIV occurs during delivery. The main obstetric risk factors are vaginal delivery, long duration of membrane rupture, chorioamnionitis and preterm delivery, although these risk factors may be less important in the presence of an undetectable viral load. The risk of vertical transmission can be reduced to less than 2% by antiretroviral treatment, planned pre-labour caesarean sections and avoidance of breastfeeding. In cases where the viral load is very low these interventions may not be needed. The key to reducing transmission is early detection. Universal screening of HIV has been routinely offered to all pregnant women since 1999.

In developed countries, short-term combination antiretroviral therapy of three or more drugs is offered to pregnant women for prevention of mother-to-child transmission or to women who require it for their own health (13). Combination antiretroviral therapy is more likely than monotherapy to suppress viral loads to undetectable levels with lower risk of development of viral resistance. It is started in the second trimester and continued up to the time of delivery. Zidovudine is currently the only licensed drug specifically indicated for use in pregnancy, although use of other nucleosides/

nucleotides in pregnancy may be better tolerated and have not demonstrated any increase in adverse fetal or maternal outcomes. Zidovudine monotherapy is an alternative to highly active antiretroviral therapy (HAART) in women with low HIV viral loads. HAART combinations use multiple drugs and aim to increase potency and reduce the development of resistance by suppressing HIV replication using multiple mechanisms. Combinations usually comprise two nucleoside-analogue or a nucleotide reverse transcriptase inhibitor (RTI) and one non-nucleoside-analogue RTI or protease inhibitor.

Use of other single-agent prophylactic regimens such as single-dose nevirapine during onset of labour, an intervention used in many resource-limited settings, may lead to the development of resistance which could compromise future treatment options. There appears to be no increased risk of congenital malformations associated with exposure to antiretroviral drugs during pregnancy. Efavirenz has been associated with neural tube defects in animal studies but there has been no reported increased risk in humans following first-trimester exposure to efavirenz. However, use of HAART in pregnancy, especially protease inhibitors, has been associated with an increased risk of premature delivery, impaired glucose tolerance and pre-eclampsia. Case reports of fatal lactic acidosis in pregnant women receiving didanosine and stavudine in combination prompted a clinical alert recommending the avoidance of this combination in pregnancy. Nevirapine should be avoided in women with CD4 + cell counts >250/mm^3 due to increased risk of serious rash or hepatotoxicity.

Elective caesarean section reduces the risk of vertical transmission by 50% when compared with that of planned vaginal delivery. The risk is further reduced by 90% when combined with antiretroviral treatment. It is effective even with low viral loads (1000 copies/mL) but additional benefit is uncertain in women taking HAART with undetectable viral loads. In the United Kingdom, HIV-positive women who are on HAART are given the option of a vaginal delivery provided they have no detectable viraemia (<50 copies/mL).

All infants born to HIV-positive mothers should be treated with a 4-week course of antiretroviral therapy. Zidovudine monotherapy is an option for neonates born to mothers on any combination therapy who deliver with a viral load of <50 copies/mL, provided the mother's virus is not resistant to zidovudine. Combination post-exposure prophylaxis therapy is recommended for neonates when the mother delivered with persistent maternal viraemia or started antiretroviral treatment late in pregnancy. Use of PCR detection of HIV DNA or RNA is used to diagnose infant infection. A positive result within the first 72 hours of birth is indicative of intrauterine transmission. The infant is tested at birth, 6 weeks and 12 weeks of age. A negative test at 3 months indicates that the child has not been infected. Final confirmation is a negative HIV antibody test at 18 months of age following the loss of maternal antibodies. With later-generation HIV antibody assays maternal antibody may occasionally persist for longer than 18 months and in this situation the test should be repeated a few months later.

Breastfeeding is an important route of transmission of HIV from mother to child. In United Kingdom and other settings where formula feeding is safe, affordable and feasible, HIV-infected mothers are still advised not to breastfeed their infants. However, the risk of mother-to-child transmission from a woman who is on HAART and has a consistently undetectable HIV viral load is likely to be low as long as the mother continues to be fully adherent to HAART whilst she is breastfeeding. Furthermore, in resource-poor settings infants of HIV-infected mothers are at a greater risk of illness and death if they are not breastfed. This has led to a change of advice from the WHO that now recommends that mothers should breastfeed for 12 months provided the HIV-positive mother or her baby is taking combination antiretrovirals throughout this period (14,15).

Herpes Simplex Virus
Genital herpes (GH) is the most frequent cause of genital ulceration worldwide. It results in a chronic recurrent viral genital infection. It is caused by HSV, most commonly HSV-2, although an increasing proportion of GH is now caused by HSV-1 (16). The most devastating complication of acquisition of GH during pregnancy is neonatal herpes. In the United Kingdom, it has a reported incidence of 1.65 births/100,000 births annually. Transmission occurs as a result of direct contact with infected maternal secretions at the time of delivery or by ascending infection following rupture of membranes. The greatest risk of neonatal herpes is when a woman acquires a new infection (primary HSV infection) in the third trimester, particularly within 6 weeks of delivery (17). The risk of neonatal infection under these circumstances is around 31% to 40%. Primary infection is associated with higher viral loads and higher rates of viral shedding than recurrent infection, and acquisition late in pregnancy results in lack of protective maternal neutralising antibodies. Other factors influencing transmission include the duration of rupture of membranes before delivery, the use of fetal scalp electrodes and mode of delivery.

Women with a first episode of GH in the first and second trimester should receive a 5-day course of oral aciclovir and anticipate a vaginal delivery. In the United Kingdom, caesarean section is recommended for all women who present with primary infection at the time of delivery or in the last 6 weeks of pregnancy. Type-specific HSV antibody testing can be used to identify those women with true primary infections in these circumstances and decide which women should proceed to having a caesarean section. These women should also receive daily suppressive therapy with aciclovir in the last 4 weeks of pregnancy. Recurrent infection at term is associated with a much smaller risk of neonatal infection (1–3%) (18), according to two studies quoted in reference 17 (17A, 17B), and the risks of the baby developing neonatal herpes need to balanced with the operative risks to the mother. In the United Kingdom, most women with recurrent lesions at the time of delivery will be delivered by caesarean section. Daily suppressive therapy with antiviral agents should be offered if a woman presents with recurrent lesions during the last 4 weeks of pregnancy.

Hepatitis B Virus
Hepatitis B virus (HBV) is a DNA virus. The carriage rate of hepatitis B varies greatly throughout the world with very high rates of up to 20% in South East Asia and Africa compared to less than 1% in Northern Europe and North America. The major routes of transmission in developed countries are through blood and blood products, sexual activity and injecting drug use, whereas vertical transmission accounts for 50% of transmissions in developing countries. Following primary infection, 10% of women become chronic carriers with persistence of hepatitis B surface antigen (HBsAg). Acute hepatitis B infection in pregnancy is associated with increased risk of premature labour and low birth weight infants (19). The usual route of transmission to the baby is perinatal exposure to contaminated maternal cervical secretions and blood at or near the time of birth. Risk of

transmission is related to maternal viraemia and e-antigen status. Hepatitis B e-antigen status is a marker of infectivity. Vertical transmission occurs in 90% of pregnancies where the mother is hepatitis e-antigen positive and in 10% of surface antigen positive, e-antigen negative mothers. Infected infants are usually too immature to mount an adequate immune response and up to 90% become chronic carriers, 25% of whom will develop chronic liver disease. Administration of hepatitis B immunoglobulin (HBIG) and hepatitis B vaccination at birth can prevent 90% of hepatitis B transmissions. Infants born to HBsAg-positive mothers should receive both the HBV vaccine and HBIG within 12 hours of birth. Treatment with lamivudine during the last month of pregnancy may further reduce transmission rates to the fetus in highly infectious mothers who are hepatitis e-antigen positive with high hepatitis B viral DNA loads. Although caesarean section has been proposed as a means of reducing vertical transmission, the evidence to date has not shown the mode of delivery to influence the likelihood of HBV transmission. Infected mothers may continue to breastfeed, as there is no additional risk of transmission. There is no evidence of risk in vaccinating pregnant or breastfeeding women, thus where there is a definite evidence of exposure, vaccination should be given to non-immune pregnant women. Universal screening for HBsAg carriage should be performed on all pregnant women at their first antenatal visit.

Hepatitis C Virus
Screening for hepatitis C virus (HCV) in pregnancy is offered only to those thought to be at higher risk of infection in the United Kingdom. This would include those women with other blood-borne viruses, are injecting drug users or have been exposed to blood or blood products. The antenatal prevalence of HCV infection in the United Kingdom is estimated to be less than 1%. Risk of transmission overall is up to 6% with a higher level of up to 15% in HCV/HIV co-infected patients. This is probably because the risk is related to HCV viral load which tends to be higher in the latter population.

There is no evidence at present that interventions such as caesarean section and avoidance of breastfeeding decrease the risk of transmission although some would recommend a caesarean section in those with HCV viral loads >1 million copies/mL.

2009 Pandemic H1N1 Influenza A Virus (Swine Flu)
On 11th June 2009, the WHO formally confirmed the first pandemic of influenza in more than 40 years. The novel pandemic H1N1 influenza A virus which is antigenically distinct from the pre-existing seasonal H1N1 human influenza A virus, and contains swine, avian and human elements, began to cause illness in the United Kingdom about 1 month after it first emerged in Mexico in March 2009. Pregnant women are not known to be at an increased risk of contracting 2009 H1N1 influenza virus. However, pregnant women infected with H1N1 are at greater risk of developing complications, especially respiratory complications in the second and third trimesters, than the non-pregnant women (20). Pregnant women are also more likely to require admission to high dependency care or intensive care. Observations from the United States, Canada and Australasia showed that pregnant women formed between 7% and 9% of intensive care unit (ICU) admissions. It has also been observed that in 80% of hospital admissions, no antiviral drug had been started. Only 24% of hospitalised women commenced antiviral treatment within 48 hours of symptom onset. The risk of hospital admission and death in pregnant women are strongly influenced by underlying co-morbidities such as asthma, diabetes, heart disease and obesity.

Most patients with pandemic H1N1 in the United Kingdom experienced mild illness, with 50% of patients recovering within 7 days of symptom onset. The most common symptoms reported were fever, fatigue, dry cough, sore throat and headache. Severe gastrointestinal symptoms such as nausea, vomiting and diarrhoea were also present in adults requiring admission. Complications seen are similar to that seen in seasonal influenza. Half of patients with H1N1 influenza admitted to ICU had viral pneumonitis or adult respiratory distress syndrome (ARDS) and 20% had secondary bacterial infections.

The neuraminidase inhibitors, oseltamivir (Tamiflu) and zanamivir (Relenza) are both active against pandemic H1N1 2009 influenza. In contrast to oseltamivir, zanamivir is given by inhalation and, as well as being effective in the respiratory tract, it is associated with lower systemic exposure. Because of this and the lower potential fetal exposure it is the recommended antiviral for pregnant women in the United Kingdom. Initiation of antivirals has been shown to be very effective and reduces the risks of complications if commenced within 48 hours of symptom onset. However, recent experience with hospitalised patients suggests that even if antivirals are given more than 48 hours and up to 7 days after symptom onset they also confer benefit. Treatment should be started on clinical grounds whilst awaiting confirmatory test results. To date, use of antepartum antiviral treatment has not been linked to adverse maternal or neonatal outcomes. Oseltamivir resistance remains rare.

Maternal pyrexia which often accompanies influenza (of whatever cause) is a risk factor for preterm delivery and has been linked to miscarriage and neural tube defects. It is therefore important to control maternal pyrexia with regular paracetamol and hydration.

In most cases, the decision to deliver will be made for obstetric indications. There may be situations where a preterm baby needs to be delivered by caesarean section in order to improve the outcome of ventilation for a critically ill mother with hypoxia. The decision should involve the obstetric, critical care and neonatal teams. Corticosteroids should be administered prior to delivery to promote fetal lung maturity. There is no contraindication to breastfeeding in affected mothers.

Rapid influenza diagnostic tests (RIDT) and direct immunofluorescence assays (DFA) have variable and lower sensitivities (10–70% and 47–93%, respectively) for detection of H1N1 influenza relative to real-time reverse transcriptase polymerase chain reaction (rRT-PCR). A negative test therefore does not rule out influenza virus infection. A positive RIDT or DFA result, however, is informative as the specificity of both these tests is high (>95%). However, they do not provide information on the subtype of influenza A virus. Nucleic acid amplification tests, including rRT-PCR, are the most sensitive and specific influenza diagnostic tests but false negatives can occur and test results may take several days. Not all nucleic acid amplification assays can specifically differentiate 2009 H1N1 influenza virus from other influenza A viruses. If specific testing for 2009 H1N1 influenza virus is required, testing with an rRT-PCR assay specific for 2009 H1N1 influenza or viral culture should be performed.

As pregnant women are at increased risk of complications from H1N1 influenza, the U.K. DOK and HPA recommend vaccination for pregnant women at any stage of pregnancy. Two different types of vaccines have been licensed by the European Medicines Agency for use in the United Kingdom including pregnant women. Pandemrix is preferred as it only requires one dose and gives more rapid protection than the two-dose Celvapan vaccine. It contains inactivated virus components and an adjuvant, which boosts the immune response thereby reducing the dose of vaccine required.

As of the end of April 2010, pandemic influenza H1N1 activity has significantly reduced in the United Kingdom and remains low in much of the temperate zones. The most active areas of transmission currently are parts of West and Central Africa, with some focal areas of activity in South East Asia and Central America (21).

Bacterial Infections

Syphilis

Prevalence of syphilis in women of reproductive age varies from as high as 20% in some African populations to about 0.02% in high-income countries. More than 1 million cases of congenital syphilis occur worldwide every year. The morbidity and mortality associated with congenital syphilis are preventable and antenatal screening and treatment of syphilis are extremely cost-effective interventions even when the prevalence of infection is very low. Congenital syphilis is seen far less in the United Kingdom due to a well-established antenatal screening programme and low rates of syphilis in pregnant women, although rates are increasing.

Syphilis is a systemic chronic granulomatous infection caused by the spirochaete *Treponema pallidum*. Antenatal syphilis poses a significant threat to both pregnancy and fetus. *T. pallidum* readily crosses the placenta, resulting in fetal infection. Fetal infection can occur at any stage of maternal infection but is more common in primary and secondary syphilis (50%) when maternal spirochataemia is at its greatest, compared with early latent (40%) and late latent syphilis (10%) (22). Although infection may occur at any stage of pregnancy, it is most likely to arise after the 18th week of pregnancy when the fetus is able to mount an immune response. Up to 50% of untreated maternal primary and secondary infections result in fetal loss (stillbirths and perinatal deaths) and 50% in preterm labour. Other manifestations of fetal infection on ultrasound include intrauterine growth restriction, hydrops fetalis, polyhydramnios and hepatomegaly.

The majority of infected women are asymptomatic and are diagnosed following routine antenatal serological screening. If non-treponemal antigen tests such as Venereal Diseases Research Laboratory (VDRL) tests are used as the initial screening test, this can be associated with biological false positive results. Treatment of maternal infection should be undertaken in conjunction with obstetricians, midwives, paediatricians and genitourinary medicine specialists to ensure tracing of partners and prevention of re-infection. The antibiotic of choice is high-dose benzathine penicillin G administered as a single intramuscular dose of 2.4 MU for primary, secondary and early latent syphilis and the same dose for three consecutive weeks for late latent syphilis. Aqueous procaine penicillin may also be used but requires a longer course of daily treatment. Penicillin is by far the preferred choice as it offers a cure rate in excess of 98% compared to non-penicillin alternatives, which are associated with failures of prevention of congenital infection in the neonate. Therefore, desensitisation to penicillin in those reporting allergies should be considered. Patents need to be warned that there is a greater risk of the Jarisch–Herxheimer reaction after treatment of early syphilis in pregnancy. This may precipitate premature labour. Erythromycin is associated with a lower cure rate and does not penetrate the placental barrier in adequate doses to treat the fetus. Likewise, azithromycin is not recommended for similar reasons and there are also concerns regarding azithromycin-resistant strains. Treatment of babies at birth with penicillin is recommended following maternal treatment with macrolides. Mothers treated with a macrolide should be considered for retreatment with doxycycline after delivery and when breastfeeding is completed. Tetracyclines should be avoided because of their potential effects on bone and dentition. All neonates born to mothers with syphilis should be evaluated for congenital syphilis.

Diagnosis of congenital syphilis is made by demonstrating the presence of treponemes by dark ground microscopy and/or PCR of exudates from suspicious lesions or body fluids and by serology. Serological tests detecting IgG may be positive due to passive transfer of maternal antibodies whether or not the infant is infected. A positive anti-treponemal immunoglobulin M (IgM) enzyme immunoassay (EIA) test, a fourfold increase or more of the rapid plasma reagin (RPR) or VDRL titre or the *T. pallidum* particle agglutination assay (TPPA) above that of the mother indicates a diagnosis of congenital infection. Early clinical manifestations of congenital syphilis in newborns include rashes, vesiculobullous lesions, condylomata lata, hepatosplenomegaly, generalised lymphadenopathy, osteochondritis and later periostitis (especially of the long bones), which may present as pseudoparalysis, neurological involvement such as meningitis or chorioretinitis and thrombocytopaenia. Late stigmata include interstitial keratitis, deafness, Clutton's joints and gummata of the nasal septum, palate and throat. Craniofacial malformations may be present with frontal bossing and a bulldog-like appearance with hypoplastic maxilla, high-arched palate and prominent mandible, saddle nose deformity and rhagades. Dental deformities may manifest as Hutchinson's incisors and mulberry molars. Treatment of the infected neonate is with intravenous benzylpenicillin.

Group B Streptococcus

Group B streptococcus is the most common cause of severe early-onset neonatal infection in the developed world. It is also a leading cause of maternal chorioamnionitis and puerperal endometritis. Group B streptococcus is found as a normal vaginal commensal in 25% of pregnant women. Forty to seventy percent of infants born to colonised mothers become colonised in the first week of life with about 1% developing acute infection. Neonatal infection can be classified as early onset (<7 days) or late onset (>7 days). The majority of neonatal infections are early onset, presenting with sepsis, pneumonia or meningitis. The mortality is 10% in this group being significantly higher in preterm infants.

The incidence of early-onset group B streptococcus disease in the United Kingdom is 0.5/1000 births (23). Intrapartum antibiotic prophylaxis to high-risk mothers has been shown to significantly reduce the risk of early-onset neonatal disease. High-risk mothers can be identified by universal antenatal screening or a risk-based strategy. Universal screening of pregnant women for group B streptococcus is not currently offered in the United Kingdom. This is in contrast to the United States where the CDC recommends that all pregnant women undergo bacteriological screening, with vaginal and rectal swabs taken for group B streptococcus culture at 35 to 37 weeks' gestation (24). Those found to be colonised with group B streptococcus are offered intrapartum antibiotic prophylaxis, usually in the form of high-dose intravenous benzylpenicillin or ampicillin which is continued until delivery. With a risk-based strategy, management involves selective antibiotic prophylaxis to women deemed at risk. Recognised risk factors for early-onset disease include preterm labour with preterm rupture of membranes, rupture of membranes >18 hours prior to delivery or pyrexia >38° in labour. The U.K. RCOG guidelines argue in favour of prophylaxis in the presence of two or more risk factors, when group B streptococcus is found incidentally in the vagina or in the urine in the current pregnancy and in women with a previous affected child (23).

Protozoal Infections

Toxoplasmosis

Toxoplasmosis is caused by the protozoan parasite *Toxoplasma gondii*. Domestic cats are the definitive hosts in which the parasite may complete its life cycle. Infection is primarily acquired through ingestion of cysts in infected undercooked meat or by ingestion of oocysts in inadequately washed garden produce that has been contaminated with cat litter. The U.K. prevalence of maternal toxoplasma infection is low at around 2/1000. In the neonate, toxoplasmosis infection presents with chorioretinitis, microcephaly, hydrocephalus, intracranial calcification and mental retardation (25). Maternal primary infection is mostly asymptomatic. Five to fifteen percent of infected women present with a glandular fever like illness with flu-like symptoms and lymphadenopathy. The neurological presentation that can rarely result in an affected mother from cerebral toxoplasmosis is discussed later in this chapter. Data from France, where the prevalence of toxoplasmosis is higher than the United Kingdom indicate that the risk of congenital infection increases with gestational age at maternal seroconversion. The risk of transmission is 10% to 15% in the first trimester, 25% to 40% in the second trimester and over 60% in the third trimester. In contrast, the risk of damage to the fetus is higher when infection occurs early in the first trimester.

Serological testing using *T. gondii* IgG/IgM antibodies, a rise in IgG titres in serial samples and IgG avidity testing are used to diagnose maternal infection. Once maternal infection is confirmed, treatment with spiramycin should be commenced to reduce the risk of vertical transmission and consideration should be given to fetal testing and treatment. Fetal infection can be proven by amplification of *T. gondii* DNA by PCR in amniotic fluid ideally at 18 weeks. In cases of confirmed fetal infection or high risk to the fetus, for example, maternal seroconversion after 32 weeks, three weekly cycles of pyrimethamine, sulphadiazine and folinic acid alternating with spiramycin is recommended and continued until delivery. Pyrimethamine is potentially teratogenic and should not be used in the first trimester of pregnancy. Ultrasound surveillance for abnormalities should be undertaken to detect fetuses that have been affected. Ultrasound abnormalities are a late sign and serial scans are needed. The most common abnormality is ventricular dilatation, with other findings of intracranial calcification, hepatomegaly and placental thickening. Absence of abnormality on ultrasound does not reliably predict whether an infected fetus will be unaffected. Termination of pregnancy may be considered by couples before 24 weeks gestation on the basis of a positive result on PCR testing of amniotic fluid.

Parasitic Infections

Malaria

Malaria is the second most common cause of infectious disease-related death in the world after tuberculosis. Although not common in the United Kingdom, malaria is commonly seen in women from developing countries and in immigrant populations of women who have travelled to endemic areas. It is caused by the four species of *Plasmodium* that infect humans: *vivax*, *ovale*, *malariae* and *falciparum*. *P. falciparum* is associated with the worst prognosis. The infection is transmitted by the bite of the female anopheline mosquito.

The effects of malaria in pregnancy on the mother and fetus depend on the mother's immunity derived from previous exposure to infection. Women from non-endemic areas with no pre-existing immunity are more likely to be symptomatic when parasitaemic, and are at greater risk of developing severe disease and death. In areas with moderate to high transmission rates, women have a high level of immunity to malaria that is maintained by continual exposure (26). This immunity is altered by pregnancy, especially in women in their first ongoing pregnancy with high parasite loads, although the risk is reduced with subsequent pregnancies. Pregnant women are more likely to suffer from more severe disease compared with non-pregnant women. In addition, pregnant women have an increased risk of symptomatic hypoglycaemia during *Plasmodium* infection and are more likely to suffer from severe anaemia as a result of placental sequestration of infected erythrocytes. Adverse consequences of malaria in pregnancy include an increased risk of spontaneous abortion, stillbirth, preterm labour and low birth weight.

Malaria in non-immune pregnant women should be treated as an emergency, and these women should be admitted to hospital and monitored closely. Selection of a specific drug for malarial treatment in pregnancy depends on any known regional drug sensitivities or resistance, severity of disease and safety of the drugs in pregnancy. Uncomplicated chloroquine-resistant falciparum malaria in pregnancy should be treated with quinine (27). Close observation including uterine and fetal heart monitoring for development of complications is necessary. Quinine should be combined with a second drug, clindamycin rather than doxycycline, to ensure complete eradication of parasites. Both drugs have a good safety record in pregnancy. The side effects of quinine are tinnitus, dizziness and hypoglycaemia. The RCOG guidelines state that atovaquone-proguanil (Malarone) and arthemeter-lumefantrine (Riamet) can be used as alternatives to quinine. The U.S. CDC guidelines are more cautious owing to concerns of lack of safety data in the first trimester and state that both treatments may be used if other treatment options are not available or if the potential benefit is judged to outweigh the benefits (28). Because of the possible association with mefloquine treatment during pregnancy and an increase in stillbirths, the CDC guidelines restrict its use to situations where there are no other treatments available. Chloroquine is the drug of choice for treatment of the erythrocyte asexual forms for all non-falciparum malaria. Chloroquine resistance to *P. vivax* is an increasing problem since 1992 in the regions of Papua New Guinea and Indonesia. The CDC and RCOG guidelines recommend the use of quinine as first line for suspected chloroquine-resistant vivax infections. Primaquine, which is used for the eradication of liver hypnozoites in *P. vivax* and *P. ovale* infections to prevent relapse, is contraindicated in pregnancy. Pregnant women with these infections should be maintained on weekly chloroquine for the duration of the pregnancy and should be treated after delivery with primaquine. Treatment in pregnancy may have lower efficacy than in non-pregnant patients and these women should be advised about the risk of recurrence.

Pregnant women from non-endemic areas and those originally from those areas but now residing elsewhere should be advised to avoid travelling to endemic areas, if possible for the duration of the pregnancy (29). If travel is unavoidable they should be advised to take antimalarial prophylaxis. The CDC and RCOG guidelines recommend chloroquine or, if travelling to areas where chloroquine resistance is present, mefloquine should be used. Its use at prophylactic doses during the second and third trimester is not associated with adverse fetal or pregnancy outcomes. This should be combined with other preventative strategies such as avoiding mosquito bites by covering exposed skin, using insect repellents and insecticide-treated mosquito bed nets. WHO recommends that pregnant women living in malaria-endemic areas should receive intermittent antimalarial chemoprophylaxis after 20 weeks' gestation.

CNS INFECTIONS IN PREGNANCY
Meningitis
Bacterial Meningitis

Bacterial meningitis has an annual incidence of 5 to 10 cases per 100,000 adults and each year causes about 135,000 deaths worldwide. Acute bacterial meningitis is a life-threatening medical emergency which may evolve rapidly in hours, and requires prompt recognition and treatment. Lumbar puncture can be used to confirm the diagnosis in patients presenting with suspected meningitis but treatment should not be delayed if suspicion is high. Imaging with MRI should be performed first in patients with new-onset seizures, an immunocompromised state, signs concerning for mass lesion or moderate or severe impairment of consciousness.

The clinical features and prognostic factors in adults with bacterial meningitis were recently reported in a study of 696 cases, none of whom were reported to be pregnant (30). The most common pathogens were *Streptococcus pneumoniae* (51%) and *Neisseria meningitidis* (37%). The classic triad of fever, neck stiffness, and a change in mental status was present in only 44% of episodes. However, 95% had at least two of the four symptoms of headache, fever, neck stiffness and altered mental status. Risk factors for an unfavourable outcome that are relevant to pregnancy were the presence of otitis/sinusitis, absence of rash, low score on Glasgow coma score on admission, tachycardia (>120 bpm), a positive blood culture, low CSF white cell count (WCC) (<100/mm^3) and infection with *S. pneumoniae*. An elevated erythrocyte sedimentation rate (>56) and decreased platelet count (<180, 000/mm^3) were also found to be important predictors of poor outcome, but are less relevant for the pregnant women as these changes can be found in normal pregnancy.

In patients that survive the initial insult, neurologic sequelae including seizures, hearing loss, impaired mental status and/or cognition may occur in as many as 30% of all cases (31). Local extension from contiguous extracerebral infection (e.g., otitis media, mastoiditis or sinusitis) is a common cause of sequelae.

The CSF usually shows an elevated opening pressure, a high WCC (up to 10,000), low glucose (<40 mg/dL) and elevated protein (100–500 mg/dL). The gram stain or smear will be positive. Bacterial culture is positive in 70% to 85% of cases (32). CSF glucose should be compared with the maternal serum glucose, the normal CSF/blood ratio is 2:3.

Case reports of pneumococcal meningitis in pregnancy describe cases in each trimester, with variable presentations varying from coma, preterm labour, fever and contractions to the more classical features of fever, neck pain, headache and altered consciousness. Some reports describe successful treatment with full maternal recovery and normal vaginal delivery some weeks later. In contrast, in three cases the neonate was delivered less than 36 hours after the onset of maternal illness. In two reports neonates were infected with *S. pneumoniae* and died. In one case, post-mortem caesarean section delivery of a 2.4-kg live infant was performed around 32 weeks and the infant made good progress and had normal development at 5 years. (33–38). In summary, although reports of pneumococcal pneumonia in pregnancy are scant, it appears that in cases in which preterm labour does not occur, when there is a good maternal response to treatment and near continuous fetal monitoring indicates fetal health then iatrogenic premature delivery is not needed to aid maternal recovery.

Dissemination of *Neisseria gonorrhoeae* in women usually occurs during the third trimester of pregnancy. The most common manifestation of gonococcal bacteraemia is arthritis affecting the medium-sized joints or a sparse centrifugal pustular skin rash. Cases of *N. gonorrhoeae* meningitis in pregnancy have been reported. A recent report from South Carolina described a woman with disseminated *N. gonorrhoeae* presenting in the third trimester of pregnancy with fever, dull headache, neck soreness, diffuse body aches and purpuric skin lesions, but without joint effusions or vaginal discharge (39).

Meningitis may occur as an iatrogenic complication of spinal or combined spinal epidural analgesia, although this complication is rare. A recent review of publications in English from 1978 to 2007 identified 107 cases of meningitis as a sequelae of these procedures (40). Streptococcal species were identified in 43% of cases. Other causes included gram-negative infections in around 10% and staphylococci in 8%. The complication is rare, presumably because of the diligent use of aseptic techniques when administering epidural anaesthesia. Droplet contamination or needle contamination from incompletely sterilised skin is the most likely reason for contamination. Meningitis may be initially difficult to distinguish from the commoner complication of post-dural puncture that also presents with headache. Fever is usually present, sometimes accompanied by vomiting, confusion, and urinary retention. However, a recent study noted the presence of classic symptoms of meningitis (high fever, severe headache and nuchal rigidity) in only 14 out of 29 (48.3%) patients (41).

Listeriosis

Infection with the bacteria *Listeria monocytogenes* is more commonly reported in pregnant than non-pregnant women, particularly during the third trimester. The incidence of listeriosis in pregnancy is 12/100,000, compared with a rate of 0.7/100,000 in the general population (42). The condition is important obstetrically as it may result in fetal loss or disease in the newborn. Infection may result in miscarriage, preterm labour or intrauterine death in around 20% to 40% of cases and neonatal infection in around two-thirds of fetuses. The infection invariably occurs secondary to ingestion of high-risk food such as soft cheeses, unpasteurised milk, hot dogs and delicatessen meats. A recent study of listeriosis cases reported through the U.S. Listeria Initiative during 2004 to 2007 found around 17% were pregnancy associated (43). Maternal infection resulted in four neonatal deaths and 26 (20.3%) fetal losses. Invasive illnesses in newborns included meningitis (32.9%) and sepsis (36.5%).

The clinical presentation may resemble that of bacterial meningitis, but the condition more commonly presents in a more insidious way with malaise, a flu-like illness or gastrointestinal upset. In cases of listeria meningitis the CSF findings may mimic those of viral meningitis. A study from Norway found brainstem encephalitis in 19 of 172 patients with adult listeriosis (11%) but none of 40 pregnancy-related listeriosis cases (44). The diagnosis can only be made by culturing the organism from a sterile site such as blood, amniotic fluid or spinal fluid. Vaginal or stool cultures can be misleading

because some women are carriers without clinical disease (45). Gram stain is useful in only about one-third of cases, both because *Listeria* is an intracellular organism (46) and because the organism can resemble other species. Informing the microbiologist of suspicion of listerial infection can improve the specificity of Gram stains (47). Treatment is with high-dose ampicillin, 6 g a day or more (43).

Aseptic or Viral Meningitis

Aseptic meningitis is usually of viral origin but occasionally may be due to non-infective causes such as inflammatory conditions, for example, sarcoidosis, systemic lupus erythematosus, vasculitis or malignancy. It is most common in young children but can occur in adults. The incidence of aseptic meningitis in people aged 16 and over and has recently been reported as 7.6/100,000 (48). The condition is usually self-limiting, but may cause considerable morbidity, with moderate or high fever that may be resistant to antipyretics, and opiate analgesia that may be needed for several days to treat severe headache (49). Aseptic meningitis usually presents with headache, fever and neck stiffness. Mental confusion is less common than with bacterial meningitis, and a deterioration in mental status or the development of seizures may indicate progression to a meningoencephalitis (50).

Enteroviruses are by far the most common cause of viral meningitis and account for most cases at all ages (48,51,52). Enterovirus infection may be accompanied by mucocutaneous manifestations of enterovirus infection, including localised vesicles, herpangina and a generalised maculopapular rash.

In aseptic meningitis, the CSF usually shows normal opening pressure, a low WCC (<300) and normal glucose and protein (<100 mg/dL) concentrations. Some viruses, such as mumps, may cause the CSF glucose to be low. The gram stain will be negative and culture will be positive in around 50% of cases (53). Herpes viruses, arboviruses and GH virus can be identified on PCR assays and mumps and HIV with serology. As long as the latter is a later-generation assay including a p24 antigen as the antibody test alone may initially be negative in this manifestation of an HIV seroconversion illness.

HSV is the second most common cause of viral meningitis in adolescents and adults in the developed world (48) and meningeal symptoms are found in around one-third of women with a primary genital HSV-2 infection (54).

Acute HIV infection may cause aseptic meningitis; symptoms have been reported in up to 17% of cases of HIV infection at the time of seroconversion (55). Serology should be repeated 3 months after presentation in all cases of aseptic meningitis where initial serology is negative.

Chronic Meningitis

Tuberculosis, toxoplasmosis and cryptococcus infections are the commonest causes of chronic meningitis. There is no evidence that these infections are commoner in pregnancy, nor that pregnancy affects the course of disease caused by these organisms. CSF findings may include an elevated opening pressure, a moderately elevated WCC (50–400), a low glucose and an elevated protein (150 mg/dL to >1 g). (53,56). CSF culture and PCR studies are useful in the diagnosis of tuberculosis, and large-volume CSF collection (20–30 mL) may increase the likelihood of correctly diagnosing fugal or tuberculosis infection. Treatment should be prompt and guided by the microbiology department and will be partly dependent on the risk of adverse drug effects on the fetus. For example, streptomycin for TB treatment is contraindicated in pregnancy because of fetal ototoxicity and fluconazole should be avoided in the first trimester because of reported teratogenicity in animals.

Encephalitis in Pregnancy

Herpes simplex is the most common causative organism for viral encephalitis in the general population and the same is likely to apply to pregnant women, although the condition is rare and case reports are sporadic (57). Other relevant organisms are arbovirus, CMV and varicella zoster. Symptoms and signs include fever, headache, confusion, dysphasia, photophobia, hemiparesis and seizures. Brian MRI may show areas of hyperintensity and the EEG areas of slowing or epileptiform discharges. CSF PCR will establish the causative organism in most cases if arranged early. The treatment of choice for varicella or herpes infections is acyclovir which can be safely used in pregnancy.

Brian Abscess

Cerebral abscess is a life-threatening condition that has been rarely reported in pregnancy, with less than 15 case reports. Cases in pregnancy have been recently reported in association with ontological infection (58) and sinusitis (59).

Predisposing factors in general include infection, foreign bodies and immunosuppression. Presenting symptoms are often non-specific and include headache, seizures, confusion and focal neurologic deficits. MRI may indicate the site of the lesion and the diagnosis is confirmed by aspiration of purulent material. Treatment is with appropriate antibiotics, with surgical drainage reserved for large lesions.

CONCLUSION

Infectious disease in pregnancy in the United Kingdom is quite common and a leading cause of maternal and neonatal morbidity and mortality in the developing world. However, an increased immigrant population and air travel will increase the prevalence of infectious diseases not previously seen in the United Kingdom. Changes in immunity and physiology during pregnancy make pregnant women more susceptible to, or more severely affected by, infectious diseases. Most maternal infections present with non-specific symptoms. Antenatal screening and maintenance of high immunisation rates for common childhood diseases preconception are important public health preventive strategies. Early detection and intervention play a significant role in significantly reducing vertical transmission and preventing adverse fetal outcomes as seen in HIV and syphilis. Increased awareness of emerging infectious diseases with novel pathogens such as the 2009 Pandemic H1N1 influenza A virus and its disproportionate effects on pregnant women is important. Investigations and management of maternal infections can be complex requiring a multidisciplinary team approach. Ongoing research into the development of vaccines against toxoplasmosis and CMV remains a high priority. Further research into more effective in utero therapies for infected fetuses and long-term follow-up studies in affected infants are clearly needed.

CNS infections in pregnancy are uncommon but are associated with significant morbidity and mortality if diagnosed late or incorrectly treated. Diagnostic confusion with conditions that are more common in pregnancy that may cause neurological symptoms, for example, the headache of pre-eclampsia, may lead to delay in appropriate management. Obstetric staff should be aware of the presenting signs and symptoms of CSN infections in pregnancy and should have a low threshold for seeking a neurological opinion when there is diagnostic uncertainty.

REFERENCES

1. Arulkumaran S, Symonds IM, Fowlie A. Chapter 9: Infections in pregnancy. Oxford Handbook of Obstetrics and Gynaecology. 1st ed. Oxford: Oxford University Press, 2004.
2. Lewis G, ed 2007. The Confidential Enquiry Into Maternal and Child Health (CEMACH). Saving mother's lives: reviewing maternal deaths to make motherhood safer 2003-2005. The Seventh Report on Confidential Enquiries into Maternal Deaths in the United Kingdom. London: CEMACH, Dec 2007. Available at: http://www.publichealth.hscni.net/sites/default/files/Saving%20Mothers'%20Lives%202003-05%20.pdfLine.
3. Department of Health. Screening for Infectious Diseases in Pregnancy: Standards to support the UK Antenatal Screening Programme. August 2003. Available at: http://www.dh.gov.uk/prod_consum_dh/groups/dh_digitalassets/@dh/@en/documents/digitalasset/dh_4092049.pdf.
4. Khare MM. Infectious disease in pregnancy. Curr Obst Gynae 2005; 15(3):149–156.
5. Royal College of Obstetricians and Gynaecologists. Infection and pregnancy – study group statement. London: RCOG, June 2001. Available at: http://www.rcog.org.uk/womens-health/clinical-guidance/infection-and-pregnancy-study-group-statement.
6. M.M. Khare, M.D. Khare. Infections in pregnancy. In: Greer IA, Nelson-Piercy C and Walters B, eds. Maternal Medicine: Medical Problems in Pregnancy. Chapter 12. Churchill Livingstone: Elsevier, 2007:217–235.
7. Price LC. Infectious disease in pregnancy. Obst Gynae Rep Med 2008; 18(7):173–179.
8. Langford KS. Infectious disease and pregnancy. Curr Obst Gynae 2002; 12(3):125–130.
9. Tolfvenstam T, Broliden K. Parvovirus B19 infection. Sem Fet Neo Med 2009; 14(4):218–221.
10. De Jong E, De Haan T, Kroes A, et al. Parvovirus B19 infection in pregnancy. J Clin Virol 2006; 36(1):1–7.
11. Royal College of Obstetricians and Gynaecologists. Chickenpox in pregnancy. Green-top Guideline No. 13. London: RCOG, September 2007. Available at: http://www.rcog.org.uk/files/rcog-corp/uploaded-files/GT13ChickenpoxinPregnancy2007.pdf.
12. De Ruiter A, Mercey D, Anderson J, et al. British HIV Association and Children's HIV Association: guidelines for the management of HIV infection in pregnant women. HIV Med 2008; 9:452–502. Available at: http://www.bhiva.org/documents/Guidelines/Pregnancy/2008/PregnancyPub.pdf.
13. Royal College of Obstetricians and Gynaecologists. Management of HIV in pregnancy. Green-top Guideline No. 39, London: RCOG, June 2010. Available at: http://www.rcog.org.uk/files/rcog-corp/uploaded-files/GtG_no_39_HIV_in_pregnancy_June_2010_v2011.pdf.
14. HIV and infant feeding rapid advice: revised WHO principles and recommendations on infant feeding in the context of HIV – November 2009. ISBN: 9789241598873 WHO Website, NICE clinical guideline 62 – antenatal care 2008.
15. Taylor G, Anderson J, Clayden P, et al; BHIVA/CHIVA Writing Group. British HIV Association (BHIVA) and Children's HIV Association (CHIVA) position statement on infant feeding in the UK 2011. HIV Med 2011; 12(7):389–393; [Epub 21 March 2011].
16. British Association for Sexual Health and HIV (BASHH) 2007 National Guidelines for the Management of Genital Herpes. Available at: http://www.bashh.org/documents/115/115.pdf.
17. Royal College of Obstetricians and Gynaecologists. Management of genital herpes in pregnancy. Green-top Guideline No. 30. London: RCOG, September 2007. Available at: http://www.rcog.org.uk/files/rcog-corp/uploaded-files/GT30GenitalHerpes2007.pdf.

17a. Brown ZA, Benedetti J, Ashley R, et al. Neonatal herpes simplex virus infection in relation to asymptomatic maternal infection at the time of labor. NESM 1991; 324:1247–52.

17b. Prober CG, Sullender WM, Yasukawa LL, et al. Low risk of herpes simplex virus infections in neonates exposed to the virus at the time of vaginal delivery. NEJM. 1987; 316:240–4.

18. Azwa A, Barton SE. Aspects of Herpes simplex virus – a clinical review. J Fam Plann Reprod Health Care 2009; 35(4):237–242.

19. British Association of Sexual Health and HIV. National Guideline on the management of the Viral Hepatitides A, B & C, 2008. Available at: http://www.bashh.org/guidelines.

20. Department of Health and Royal College of Obstetricians and Gynaecologists. Pandemic H1N1 2009 influenza: clinical management guidelines for pregnancy. Revised 10 December 2009. Available at: http://www.dh.gov.uk/prod_consum_dh/groups/dh_digitalassets/@dh/@en/@ps/@sta/@perf/documents/digitalasset/dh_110048.pdf.

21. Health Protection Agency. Swine Influenza (Pandemic (H1N1) 2009 Influenza). Available at: http://www.hpa.org.uk/Topics/InfectiousDiseases/InfectionsAZ/SwineInfluenza/

22. British Association for Sexual Health and HIV. UK National Guidelines on the Management of Syphilis 2008. Available at: http://www.bashh.org/guidelines.

23. Royal College of Obstetricians and Gynaecologists. Prevention of early onset neonatal group B streptococcal disease: Green-top Guideline No. 36. London: RCOG, November 2003. Available at: http://www.rcog.org.uk/files/rcog-corp/uploaded-files/GT36GroupBStrep2003.pdf.

24. Centers for Disease Control and Prevention. 2002 Revised Guidelines for Prevention of Perinatal Group B Streptococcal Disease. August 16, 2002. Available at: http://www.cdc.gov/mmwr/preview/mmwrhtml/rr5111a1.htm.

25. Montoya JG, Remington JS. Management of *Toxoplasma gondii* infection during pregnancy. Clin Inf Dis 2008; 47:554–566.

26. Schantz-Dunn J, Nour NM. Malaria and pregnancy: a global health perspective. Rev Obstet Gynecol 2009; 2(3):186–192.

27. Royal College of Obstetricians and Gynaecologists. The diagnosis and treatment of malaria in pregnancy. Green-top Guideline No. 54B. London: RCOG, April 2010. Available at: http://www.rcog.org.uk/files/rcog-corp/GTG54bDiagnosisTreatmentMalaria0410.pdf.

28. Centers for Disease Control and Prevention. Guidelines for Treatment of Malaria in the United States. Updated May 18, 2009. Available at: http://www.cdc.gov/malaria/resources/pdf/treatmenttable73109.pdf.

29. Royal College of Obstetricians and Gynaecologists. The prevention of malaria in pregnancy. Green-top Guideline No. 54A. London: RCOG, April 2010. Available at: http://www.rcog.org.uk/files/rcog-corp/GTG54aPreventionMalariaPregnancy0410.pdf.

30. van de Beek D, de Gans J, Spanjaard L, et al. Clinical features and prognostic factors in adults with bacterial meningitis. N Engl J Med 2004; 351(18):1849–1859.

31. van de Beek D, de Gans J, Tunkel AR, et al. Community-acquired bacterial meningitis in adults. N Engl J Med 2006; 354 (1):44–53.

32. Spach DH, Jackson LA. Bacterial meningitis. Neurol Clin 1999; 17:711–735.

33. Landrum LM, Hawkins A, Goodman JR. Pneumococcal meningitis during pregnancy: a case report and review of literature. Infect Dis Obstet Gynecol 2009; 2009:63624.

34. Landrum LM, Hawkins A, Goodman JR, et al. Recurrent pneumococcal meningitis in pregnancy. Am J Obstet Gynecol 1962; 84 (12):1878–1880.

35. Hutchison CPT, Kenney A, Eykyn S. Maternal and neonatal death due to pneumococcal infection. Obstet Gynecol 1984; 63 (1):130–131.

36. Steiner ZP, Manor Y, Smorjik J, et al. Successful postmortem cesarean section in a case of fulminant pneumococcal meningitis. Israel J Med Sci 1978; 14(2):287–288.

37. Rennard M. Recurrent pneumococcal meningitis and pregnancy. Obstet Gynecol 1965; 25(6):815–818.

38. Tempest B. Pneumococcal meningitis in mother and neonate. Pediatrics 1974; 53(5):759–760.

39. Burgis JT, Nawaz H III. Disseminated gonococcal infection in pregnancy presenting as meningitis and dermatitis. Obstet Gynaecol 2006:798–801.

40. Sandkovsky U, Mihu MR, Adeyeye A, et al. Iatrogenic meningitis in an obstetric patient after combined spinal-epidural analgesia: case report and review of the literature. South Med J 2009; 102(3):287–290.

41. Moen V, Dahlgren N, Irestedt L. Severe neurological complications after central neuraxial blockades in Sweden 1990–1999. Anesthesiology 2004; 101:950–959.

42. Listeriosis. Atlanta: Centers for Disease Control and Prevention, 1999.

43. Jackson KA, Iwamoto M, Swerdlow D. Pregnancy-associated listeriosis. Epidemiol Infect 2010; 138(10):1503–1509; [Epub 17 February 2010].

44. Antal EA, Dietrichs E, Løberg EM, et al. Brain stem encephalitis in listeriosis. Scand J Infect Dis 2005; 37(3):190–194.

45. Southwick FS, Purich DL. Intracellular pathogenesis of listeriosis. N Engl J Med 1996; 334:770–776.

46. Silver HM. Listeriosis during pregnancy. Obstet Gynecol Surv 1998; 53:737–740.

47. Lamont RJ, Postlethwaite R. Carriage of *Listeria monocytogenes* and related species in pregnant and non-pregnant women in Aberdeen, Scotland. J Infect 1986; 13:187–193.

48. Kupila L, Vuorinen T, Vainionpää R, et al. Etiology of aseptic meningitis and encephalitis in an adult population. Neurology 2006; 66:75–80.

49. Rotbart HA, Brennan PJ, Fife KH, et al. Enterovirus meningitis in adults. Clin Infect Dis 1998; 27:896–898.

50. Sawyer MH, Rotbart H. Viral meningitis and aseptic meningitis syndrome. In: Scheld WM, Whitley RJ, Marra CM, eds. Infections of the Central Nervous System. 3rd ed. Philadelphia: Lippincott Williams & Wilkins, 2004:75–93.

51. Rantakallio P, Leskinen M, Von Wendt L. Incidence and prognosis of central nervous system infections in a birth cohort of 12,000 children. Scand J Infect Dis 1986; 18:287–294.

52. Davison KL, Ramsay ME. The epidemiology of acute meningitis in children in England and Wales. Arch Dis Child 2003; 88:662–664.

53. Coyle PK. Overview of acute and chronic meningitis. Neurol Clin 1999; 17:761–781.

54. Corey L, Adams HG, Brown ZA, et al. GH simplex virus infections: clinical manifestations, course, and complications. Ann Intern Med 1983; 98:958–972.

55. Boufassa F, Bachmeyer C, Carre N, et al. Influence of neurologic manifestations of primary human immunodeficiency virus infection on disease progression. J Infect Dis 1995; 171:1190–1195.

56. Davis LE, Garcia-Monco JC. Fungal infections of the central nervous system. Central nervous system tuberculosis. Neurol Clin 1999; 17(4):737–759.

57. Briton CB. CNS infections in pregnancy. In: Parthenon JM, ed. Neurologic Disorders in Pregnancy. London: Parthenon publishing, 2004.

58. Jacob CE, Kurien M, Varghese AM, et al. Treatment of otogenic brain abscess in pregnancy. Otol Neurotol 2009; 30(5):602–603.

59. Wax JR, Mancall A, Cartin A, et al. Sinogenic brain abscess complicating pregnancy. Am J Obstet Gynecol 2004; 191(5):1711–1712.

15

Idiopathic intracranial hypertension

Paul Riordan-Eva

INTRODUCTION

Since its first description as 'meningitis serosa' by Quincke in 1893, the syndrome of raised intracranial pressure without a specific identifiable cause has been known by a variety of names, including pseudotumour cerebri and benign intracranial hypertension, but idiopathic intracranial hypertension (IIH) is currently preferred, highlighting that it remains a diagnosis of exclusion and should not be regarded as benign with regard to visual outcome (1,2).

Pregnancy is not an independent risk factor, but IIH predominantly occurs in obese women of childbearing age, particularly those who are gaining weight (3). Pregnancy usually does not influence the severity of IIH but it limits treatment options (2,4,5). Similarly IIH does not usually adversely affect the outcome of pregnancy but it necessitates additional monitoring and may influence the timing and method of delivery, as well as the choice of anaesthesia (6). Optimal management of IIH in pregnancy requires close collaboration between obstetricians, neurologists, ophthalmologists, anaesthetists and sometimes neurosurgeons (7).

Other neuro-ophthalmic entities with particular relevance to pregnancy include skull base meningioma, pituitary macroadenoma and lymphocytic adenohypophysitis, all potentially causing rapid bilateral visual loss due to compression of the optic chiasm and/or optic nerves. These are discussed in other chapters of this book.

EPIDEMIOLOGY

IIH predominantly occurs in young obese adult females, being about eight times more common in females than males and rarely developing over age 45 years. The published annual age-adjusted incidence per 100,000 adult women aged up to 44 years ranges between 0.7 in Italy, 3.3 in the mid-western United States, 4.0 in Israel and 12.0 in Libya. It increases to 2.7 in Italy, 7.9 to 19.3 in the mid-western United States and 21.4 in Libya for overweight or obese adult women of the same age (8–12). IIH may be more aggressive, with worse visual outcome in black people (13).

DIAGNOSTIC CRITERIA

The diagnostic criteria for IIH continue to evolve but the essential criteria are that cerebrospinal fluid (CSF) pressure has been documented to be elevated with no identifiable cause, including normal CSF constituents, and any symptoms or signs can be explained by the raised CSF pressure (14). There are numerous causes of secondary raised intracranial pressure but those that must always be excluded are intracranial mass, hydrocephalus, cerebral venous sinus occlusion, severe anaemia and treatment with tetracycline or related compounds, or vitamin A or related compounds including retinoids (2,14).

IIH should not be diagnosed until all the essential diagnostic criteria have been fulfilled and other conditions excluded. Sometimes it is assumed that an obese young woman with headaches and swollen optic discs is sufficiently likely to have IIH that further investigation can be avoided, but obese young women are at risk of developing other conditions such as intracranial tumours. Cerebral venous sinus thrombosis has been reported to be present in 9% of patients with presumed IIH, as well as being associated with pregnancy (15). If the diagnostic criteria cannot be fulfilled for technical reasons, such as Chiari malformation precluding lumbar puncture, it is preferable to avoid making a diagnosis of IIH by using the seemingly equivalent but less dogmatic term 'intracranial hypertension of unknown cause', at least until a period of monitoring has shown that other diagnoses are unlikely.

The relationship between intracranial and systemic hypertension is complex. Accelerated hypertension, including that due to pre-eclampsia, may result in optic disc swelling due to direct vascular effects at the optic nerve head or raised intracranial pressure (papilloedema), and may exacerbate optic nerve damage from raised intracranial pressure from other causes such as IIH. Conversely, raised blood pressure may be secondary to raised intracranial pressure.

By definition, papilloedema is optic disc swelling due to raised intracranial pressure. Because optic disc swelling has many causes and examination of the optic discs rarely can distinguish between them, the term papilloedema should not be used until raised intracranial pressure has been identified, either by measurement of CSF pressure or by other investigations that indicate that CSF pressure is likely to be elevated, for instance head imaging showing an intracranial mass.

CLINICAL FEATURES
Symptoms

Most patients with IIH present with headache, which occurs in 90% of cases (16). Although in some cases the headaches have features to suggest raised intracranial pressure, such as being present on waking, being relieved by standing and being exacerbated by coughing, sneezing or straining, in many cases the features are non-specific and concern is generated by new onset or increase in severity or frequency, or the presence of abnormal neurological signs. In many patients with IIH, the headaches have features suggestive of migraine, tension headache or chronic daily headache (see chapter 13) and it is usually the identification of optic disc swelling that raises the possibility of raised intracranial pressure.

Momentary recurrent unilateral or bilateral loss of vision (transient visual obscurations), often precipitated by standing, bending or straining, occurs in up to 70% of patients but frequently is only identified on direct questioning. They are not a major prognostic factor with respect to visual loss. In the small proportion of patients without headache despite the raised intracranial pressure, persistent and often severe loss of vision may be the presenting feature. Intracranial noise, usually described as a whooshing sound synchronous with the pulse, is another symptom that occurs frequently but is often only revealed by direct questioning. Diplopia, usually due to unilateral or bilateral sixth nerve palsy as a false localising sign of raised intracranial pressure, occurs in approximately 40% of patients but is rarely the sole presenting feature. Although various focal neurological abnormalities other than sixth nerve palsy, such as unilateral or bilateral lower motor neurone seventh nerve palsy, have been described in IIH, presumably being due to the raised intracranial pressure, any such abnormality must raise concern about an alternative diagnosis.

A proportion of patients with IIH, reported to be up to 25% in one North American study, are asymptomatic at presentation, optic disc swelling being identified incidentally usually during routine examination by an optometrist (17).

Signs

Optic disc swelling is the crucial diagnostic sign in virtually all cases and its severity is an important prognostic factor. IIH without optic disc swelling (IIH without papilloedema – IIHWOP) has been reported but erroneous elevation of CSF pressure at lumbar puncture such as due to straining because of anxiety or discomfort needs to be excluded (14). Pallor of the optic discs (optic atrophy) indicates permanent optic nerve damage. Other fundal abnormalities due to raised intracranial pressure, often secondary to the optic disc swelling, such as retinal haemorrhages or exudates, may be present especially when intracranial pressure is very high or has risen rapidly (Fig. 15.1A–F).

Initial and continuing assessment of vision, which must include quantitative documentation of visual fields by computerised (e.g., Humphrey) or Goldmann perimetry (not just confrontation visual field testing), is a vital part of the management of IIH because it is the paramount determinant of how active treatment needs to be. Since visual acuity is relatively insensitive to optic nerve damage from raised intracranial pressure, impairment of visual acuity indicates severe optic nerve damage unless there are central retinal (macular) abnormalities or other reasons to explain it. Although enlargement of the blind spot, which largely relates to the severity of optic disc swelling, is commonly commented upon it is less important that other visual field changes, which usually consist of generalised or predominantly inferonasal visual field constriction. Results of visual field testing may vary widely due to various factors, including variation in the ability of the patient to perform the tests reliably. The possibility of non-organic visual loss needs to be borne in mind (18).

The usual ocular motility abnormality is unilateral or bilateral sixth nerve palsy but others may be present.

INVESTIGATIONS

Because of the possibility of life-threatening intracranial disease, including intracranial mass and, especially in pregnancy, cerebral venous sinus occlusion, urgent head imaging is usually required. Patients with severe optic disc swelling or severe or moderate impairment of vision require emergency investigation, often by admission to hospital so that treatment can be expedited.

No head imaging abnormalities are diagnostic of IIH but dilation of the optic nerve sheaths, posterior flattening of the globes and elevation of the optic discs are suggestive of raised intracranial pressure, and an empty sella suggests that it is

chronic (19,20). It has been suggested that transverse sinus stenosis (TSS) is the cause of IIH in some patients (21,22). However, there is evidence that intracranial hypertension can induce TSS, being reversed by lowering of intracranial pressure, and that in the majority of patients with IIH and tapered narrowing of the transverse sinus on CT venography (CTV) the associated bony grove is small or absent, indicating a pre-existing transverse sinus abnormality (23–25). Amongst patients with chronic headache without papilloedema, whether they present with chronic migraine or chronic tension-type headache, bilateral TSS on magnetic resonance venography (MRV) has been reported to occur in 7% to 9%, with approximately 70% of these patients being found to have raised intracranial pressure at lumbar puncture, leading to revision of the diagnosis to IIHWOP (26,27).

In non-pregnant women, the preferred technique for initial head imaging is usually contrast-enhanced computed tomography (CT) because of its ready availability and the ease of also performing CTV, which is as reliable as any other current imaging modalities for detecting cerebral venous sinus thrombosis. The distinction between thrombosis, congenital anomalies and arachnoid granulations of the cerebral venous sinuses can usually be made more simply and quickly by CTV than by non-contrast (e.g., phase contrast or time of flight) MRV, which in any case needs to be combined with MRI to determine whether any abnormality of the cerebral venous sinuses is due to thrombosis. How contrast-enhanced MRV compares with CTV has yet to be determined. In most cases of IIH, normal CT and CTV do not need to be supplemented by MRI and MRV, but contrast-enhanced MRI should be undertaken if there are atypical features.

In pregnancy CTV is contraindicated because of the necessary administration of contrast agent and the exposure to X rays, although the latter can be reduced by appropriate shielding. Thus, MRI and non-contrast MRV are preferable in pregnancy but even these should be avoided whenever possible in the first trimester (see chapter 2 'Imaging During Pregnancy'). Contrast-enhanced MRV probably should be avoided throughout pregnancy. In the absence of imaging contraindication, such as intracranial mass or Chiari malformation, lumbar puncture is indicated. It should be performed in the lateral decubitus position, with the legs extended and the patient as relaxed as possible when the CSF pressure is measured. Whether obesity directly elevates CSF pressure continues to be debated, with markedly conflicting results from the few published studies (28–30). It is generally thought that, under ideal conditions, lumbar CSF pressure needs to be greater than 25 cm to be elevated, with values between 20 and 25 cm being equivocal, and values below 20 cm being definitely normal, regardless of the patient's body mass index (BMI) (14). CSF pressure is known to fluctuate and occasionally repeat measurement or even CSF pressure monitoring is required.

Blood investigations rarely provide diagnostic clues, except for identifying anaemia, but are important to exclude underlying haematological abnormalities if cerebral venous thrombosis is identified. Prior to institution of acetazolamide therapy, serum potassium should be checked, particularly in patients already on diuretic therapy, and patients from susceptible ethnic groups should be tested for sickle cell disease.

TREATMENT

High BMI is clearly a risk factor for IIH and weight gain has an adverse effect on the development and course of IIH (31). In non-pregnant patients, there is evidence of benefit from weight

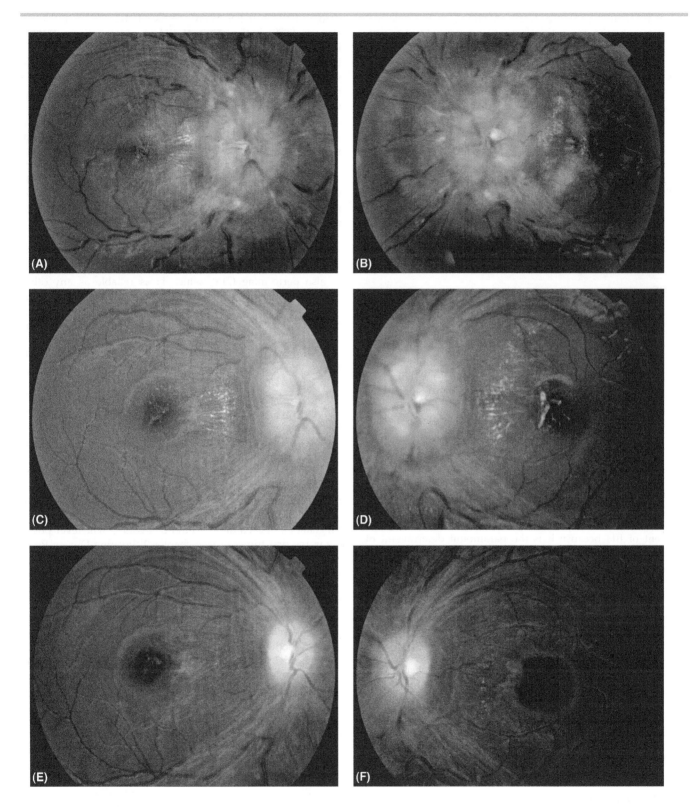

Figure 15.1 Fundal photographs showing regression of optic disc swelling and retinal exudates in a 16-year-old black woman who presented with IIH in her first pregnancy and was treated with oral acetazolamide following diagnostic lumbar puncture at which opening pressure was 56 cm. At presentation (17 weeks' gestation): (**A**) right eye, (**B**) left eye; 25 weeks' gestation: (**C**) right eye, (**D**) left eye; 36 weeks' gestation: (**E**) right eye, (**F**) left eye.

loss on severity of optic disc swelling in the short term and reduced need for treatment in the long term (32,33). In pregnancy weight loss is likely to be undesirable and usually the aim is to avoid excessive weight gain. However, weight loss is

desirable prior to pregnancy. Weighing at regular intervals during pregnancy and the involvement of dieticians preconceptually and during pregnancy may be helpful. Pregnancy limits the options for drug therapy because of potential adverse effects on the fetus. Based on clinical experience rather than published evidence, the standard first-line drug treatment for IIH outside pregnancy is acetazolamide, which reduces CSF production by inhibiting carbonic anhydrase. In high doses acetazolamide is teratogenic in rodents, producing a characteristic forelimb anomaly and exacerbating cerebral cortical dysgenesis, and in rabbits, causing axial skeletal malformations (34–36). However, there is evidence that acetazolamide in conventional doses is not harmful to the human fetus, such that it can be used with caution throughout pregnancy but should be avoided if possible in the first trimester (37). The usual dose is 500 mg – 1 g/day in two to four divided doses titrated against response and adverse effects. The occurrence of adverse effects, such as paraesthesiae, metallic taste with carbonated drinks, lethargy and depressed mood, varies between individuals but generally is dose dependent and may be less frequent with the slow-release formulation. A history of urinary tract calculi is a relative contraindication to acetazolamide because it predisposes to formation of calcium phosphate and calcium oxalate calculi. Alkalinising the urine may reduce the formation of uric acid and cystine stones. Acetazolamide predisposes to hypokalaemia and metabolic acidosis, which usually are not problematic unless there are other predisposing factors, such as diuretic therapy or diabetes mellitus, respectively, or there is greater potential for adverse consequences, such as in sickle cell anaemia in the case of metabolic acidosis.

Topiramate, usually 25 to 50 mg twice a day, is increasingly being used in the management of IIH outside pregnancy, having the threefold advantage of inhibiting carbonic anhydrase, being anorectic and being effective for chronic headache. It is a less potent carbonic anhydrase inhibitor than acetazolamide and thus probably has less effect on CSF production and intracranial pressure, but it seems to be as effective in the treatment of IIH, possibly due to greater weight loss (38,39). It has a similar range of side effects to acetazolamide. More often than acetazolamide, but still rarely, it causes acute bilateral glaucoma due to ciliary body swelling from an unpredictable hypersensitivity reaction that usually develops within a few days of starting treatment, and presents with ocular discomfort and redness, as well as reduced vision (40,41). With the higher doses used for migraine, topiramate has been reported to cause mild cognitive impairment (42).

Largely because of absence of evidence of safety, topiramate is relatively contraindicated in the first trimester of pregnancy because of the potential risk of fetal malformations. A review of the outcomes in 203 pregnancies from the U.K. Epilepsy and Pregnancy Register found a 9% risk of major congenital malformations associated with topiramate use (43). However, the rate was 4.3% (3 of 70 women) (CI, 1.7–13.3%) for monotherapy. Another study found no increase in prevalence of non-genetic structural defects in 41 children born to mothers who had taken topiramate during pregnancy, compared with 206 controls, but a significant increase in spontaneous abortions (11.3% vs. 2.8% in controls) (44). Presumably the majority of these women were taking topiramate for epilepsy control. Nearly half of the women were using polytherapy.

Furosemide, usually 40 to 80 mg daily, and bendroflumethiazide, usually 5 to 10 mg daily, are the standard medical treatments for non-pregnant IIH patients intolerant of acetazolamide and topiramate, but both are relatively contraindicated in pregnancy, conditions such as pulmonary oedema and congestive heart failure probably being the only valid indications for their use before delivery. Furosemide crosses the placenta and may be associated with a small increase in congenital abnormalities. It may reduce placental perfusion. High-dose parenteral steroids have a limited role in the acute management of patients presenting with rapidly worsening severe visual loss (fulminant IIH) (45,46). Otherwise systemic steroids are no longer used in the management of IIH.

Repeated (therapeutic) lumbar puncture to reduce CSF pressure has become less popular in the management of IIH, largely because in the majority of cases the effect on CSF pressure lasts less than 24 hours and improvement in headache lasts only a few days, with the additional risk that headache due to high CSF pressure will be replaced by headache due to low CSF pressure. However, some patients derive prolonged benefit, at least on headache severity, and repeated therapeutic lumbar puncture may be appropriate as a temporising measure when IIH has been exacerbated by pregnancy (5). It may also be useful in patients awaiting surgery. Rarely, temporary lumbar CSF drain is indicated (4).

The proportion of all IIH patients treated surgically is approximately 20% (47). The primary indications are progressive visual loss for which medical therapy is insufficient because of severity of visual loss, lack of efficacy or intolerable adverse effects. Surgery may also be undertaken for uncontrolled headache without progressive visual loss, but this is less likely to be appropriate in the antenatal period because of the risks to the fetus. However, there are several small case series of surgical management during the antenatal period for women with IIH that did not respond to other measures, without serious adverse effects on the pregnancy. The traditional surgical procedure is lumbo-peritoneal CSF shunt (LPS), which has been reported to be successful in a small number of pregnant patients, despite the potential risk, reported in patients undergoing the LPS for hydrocephalus, of obstruction of the peritoneal end of the catheter by the enlarging uterus in the third trimester (4,48–52). Adequate long-term control of CSF pressure is reported to be achieved after one procedure in approximately 40% of non-pregnant patients (47,53–55). Among the 60% requiring shunt revision about 10% of all patients account for over 50% of the revisions, some undergoing 10 or more revisions. Ventriculo-peritoneal CSF shunt (VPS) is reported to be safe and possibly more effective by reducing the risk of shunt obstruction, but it is technically more difficult because the cerebral ventricles are not dilated and there is the risk of cerebral complications (56,57). It is particularly indicated when LPS is contraindicated, such as in the presence of Chiari malformation that may be congenital or secondary to LPS. Results in pregnant patients have not been reported. Subtemporal or suboccipital decompression is occasionally performed in recalcitrant IIH cases but is unlikely to be appropriate in pregnancy. Premature elective delivery following maternal steroid therapy to mature the fetal lung may be appropriate in some cases.

In optic nerve sheath fenestration (ONSF), also known as optic nerve (sheath) decompression, an opening is created in the meninges of the orbital optic nerve just behind the globe. Although initially there may be drainage of CSF into the orbit, the probable long-term effect is occlusion of the subarachnoid space such that the raised CSF pressure is not transmitted to the optic nerve head, resulting in reduction in optic disc swelling and risk of further visual loss. There is no long-term reduction of CSF pressure. Although improvement in optic disc swelling in the fellow eye has been described, in general surgery on both eyes is likely to be necessary unless there is markedly asymmetric visual loss or a CSF shunt is also being performed. Most studies have reported that ONSF is safe and effective at stabilising vision in IIH (58–66). In one series, deterioration of vision occurred in 32% of eyes after technically successful surgery (67). In another series, 35% of patients required CSF shunting or subtemporal decompression for persistent headache or progressive visual loss (62). In general, the published literature suggests that the visual outcome is better after CSF shunting than after ONSF, but further surgery is more likely after CSF shunting (68). There has not been a randomised comparative study. There are no published reports on the outcome of ONSF in pregnancy, except for a single case report of severe visual loss due to IIH in the first trimester in pregnancy treated by external lumbar drain and bilateral ONSF, with improvement of vision in one eye but the other remaining completely blind (69).

The identification of TSS in some patients with IIH has led to stenting of the stenosed sinuses in refractory cases, with reports of promising results (70,71). However, there is evidence that the stenosis may be secondary to the raised intracranial pressure and further studies are required (23,24,72).

In the exceptional circumstance of pregnancy resulting in sufficiently severe IIH to pose a high risk to the mother of severe permanent visual loss, there may be justification for consideration of termination of the pregnancy.

FOLLOW-UP

How frequently a patient with IIH needs to undergo review during pregnancy and by whom it should be performed need to be determined on an individual basis. Patients presenting with severe disease initially require weekly, twice weekly or even daily review. More stable disease requires review every 1 to 3 months. Assessment within 4 weeks of expected or planned delivery is useful to provide information to the obstetrician, with whom contact needs to be maintained throughout the pregnancy, which can be difficult when the IIH is being managed in a major neurosciences unit and the pregnancy is being managed in a smaller local hospital. According to the skills of the relevant clinicians, whether patients with IIH are primarily under the care of a neurologist or an ophthalmologist varies between units.

DELIVERY
Mode of Delivery

Frequently there is concern on the part of the mother, the obstetrician, the anaesthetist, the neurologist and/or the ophthalmologist that increase in intracranial pressure due to pushing during the second stage of labour will result in permanent visual impairment. Although in practice this is not a significant risk, except possibly when the mother has severe acute papilloedema and already has marked visual loss, this concern commonly results in a decision to perform an elective caesarean section or to undertake an assisted second stage. However, there is no published evidence to support any alteration in the mode of delivery in IIH and indeed there are reported cases of vaginal deliveries with no untoward effects, even with persistent papilloedema, although whether these deliveries were assisted is unclear (4).

Analgesia and Anaesthesia

A diagnosis of IIH generates anxiety about the method of anaesthesia for delivery, including possible avoidance of general anaesthesia because it might further increase intracranial pressure (73). Extradural injection of bupivacaine has been shown to temporarily increase intracranial pressure and there is a theoretical risk that dilation of the lumbar thecal sac increases the risk of inadvertent spinal puncture, but epidurals have been reported to be successful even in the presence of an LPS (74–76). Spinal anaesthesia or an intrathecal catheter has also been advocated, both affording the opportunity to reduce intracranial pressure by draining CSF, but the duration of effect of intrathecal drugs may be markedly shortened if there is an LPS (77–79). It has been recommended that the position of an LPS should be identified by X ray prior to spinal or epidural anaesthesia to avoid damaging the shunt, and some have advocated that general anaesthesia should be used to avoid shunt damage (77). Overall, the relevant literature is limited to small case series or single case reports. The evidence base for neuroanaesthesia for pregnant patients is limited and there do not appear to be any published large studies to justify specific changes in anaesthetic practice for delivery in IIH (80). Needless to say, it is helpful to have a senior anaesthetist, who has been given sufficient advance notice, involved in the management of the patient.

NEONATAL PERIOD

There are single case reports, both occurring in preterm infants, of metabolic acidosis, hypocalcaemia and hypomagnesaemia, and of transient renal tubular acidosis, following acetazolamide therapy during pregnancy (81,82).

BREASTFEEDING

According to the British National Formulary, acetazolamide, furosemide and bendroflumethiazide are safe during breastfeeding, although the latter two may inhibit lactation. There is an empirical recommendation that topiramate is avoided because of its presence in breast milk, but a preliminary study of five neonates of mothers treated with topiramate for epilepsy showed very low blood levels during breastfeeding and no adverse effects (83).

BEFORE PREGNANCY

In women known to have IIH, it is prudent to maximise control of the disease prior to pregnancy. Weight should be optimised. Increasingly bariatric surgery is being considered for the morbidly obese with IIH, possibly providing better long-term results than CSF shunting, but recovery can be protracted (84–87). Polycystic ovary syndrome (PCOS) is reported to be five to eight times more prevalent amongst patients with IIH than in the general female population (88,89). Metformin, which is safe in pregnancy, combined with calorie-restricted, high-protein, low-carbohydrate diet appears to be beneficial in PCOS, including restoring normal menses, and may be beneficial for IIH before and during pregnancy (90–92). The potential risks of topiramate and acetazolamide during pregnancy need to be discussed and if possible a decision agreed as to whether treatment will be discontinued as soon as pregnancy is confirmed or even suspected, taking into account the individual's risk from exacerbation of the IIH, and how early ophthalmological review can be arranged if needed. Preferably planned discontinuation should have been achieved prior to conception.

SUMMARY

Since it predominantly occurs in women of childbearing age, it is important that obstetricians, neurologists, ophthalmologists, anaesthetists and possibly neurosurgeons are aware of how

IIH should be managed during pregnancy, particularly how treatment options, including around delivery, are affected by the need to avoid harm to the fetus as well as to the mother. In general, pregnancy does not influence the severity of IIH but this means that occasionally there will be women with fulminant disease during pregnancy, requiring aggressive medical and/or surgical therapy to minimise the severity of visual loss.

REFERENCES

1. Wall M, George D. Idiopathic intracranial hypertension: a prospective study of 50 patients. Brain 1991; 114:155–180.
2. Friedman DI. Papilledema. In: Miller NR, Newman NJ, eds. Walsh & Hoyt's Clinical Neuro-Ophthalmology. 6th ed. Philadelphia: Lippincott Williams & Wilkins, 2005:237–291.
3. Digre KB, Varner MW, Corbett JJ. Pseudotumor cerebri and pregnancy. Neurology 1984; 34:721–729.
4. Huna-Baron R, Kupersmith MJ. Idiopathic intracranial hypertension in pregnancy. J Neurol 2002; 249:1078–1081.
5. Tang RA, Dorotheo EU, Schiffman JS, et al. Medical and surgical management of idiopathic intracranial hypertension in pregnancy. Curr Neurol Neurosci Rep 2004; 4:398–409.
6. Peterson CM, Kelly JV. Pseudotumor cerebri in pregnancy. Case reports and review of literature. Obstet Gynecol Surv 1985; 40:323–329.
7. Evans RW. Management of pseudotumor cerebri during pregnancy. Headache 2000; 40:495–497.
8. Carta A, Bertuzzi F, Cologno D, et al. Idiopathic intracranial hypertension (pseudotumor cerebri): descriptive epidemiology, clinical features, and visual outcomes in Parma, Italy, 1990 to 1999. Eur J Ophthalmol 2004; 14:48–54.
9. Radhakrishnan K, Ahlskog JE, Cross SA, et al. Idiopathic intracranial hypertension (pseudotumor cerebri). Descriptive epidemiology in Rochester, Minn, 1976 to 1990. Arch Neurol 1993; 50:78–80.
10. Kesler A, Gadoth N. Epidemiology of idiopathic intracranial hypertension in Israel. J Neuroophthalmol 2001; 21:12–14.
11. Radhakrishnan K, Thacker AK, Bohlaga NH, et al. Epidemiology of idiopathic intracranial hypertension: a prospective and case-control study. J Neurol Sci 1993; 116:18–28.
12. Durcan FJ, Corbett JJ, Wall M. The incidence of pseudotumor cerebri. Population studies in Iowa and Louisiana. Arch Neurol 1988; 45:875–877.
13. Bruce BB, Preechawat P, Newman NJ, et al. Racial differences in idiopathic intracranial hypertension. Neurology 2008; 70:861–867.
14. Friedman DI, Jacobson DM. Diagnostic criteria for idiopathic intracranial hypertension. Neurology 2002; 59:1492–1495.
15. Lin A, Foroozan R, Danesh-Meyer HV, et al. Occurrence of cerebral venous sinus thrombosis in patients with presumed idiopathic intracranial hypertension. Ophthalmology 2006; 113:2281–2284.
16. Giuseffi V, Wall M, Siegel PZ, et al. Symptoms and disease associations in idiopathic intracranial hypertension (pseudotumor cerebri): a case-control study. Neurology 1991; 41:239–244.
17. Galvin JA, Van Stavern GP. Clinical characterization of idiopathic intracranial hypertension at the Detroit Medical Center. J Neurol Sci 2004; 223:157–160.
18. Ney JJ, Volpe NJ, Liu GT, et al. Functional visual loss in idiopathic intracranial hypertension. Ophthalmology 2009; 116:1808–1813.
19. Brodsky MC, Vaphiades M. Magnetic resonance imaging in pseudotumor cerebri. Ophthalmology 1998; 105:1686–1693.
20. Lim MJ, Pushparajah K, Jan W, et al. Magnetic resonance imaging changes in idiopathic intracranial hypertension in children. J Child Neurol 2010; 25:294–299.
21. Farb RI, Vanek I, Scott JN, et al. Idiopathic intracranial hypertension: the prevalence and morphology of sinovenous stenosis. Neurology 2003; 60:1418–1424.
22. Higgins JN, Gillard JH, Owler BK, et al. MR venography in idiopathic intracranial hypertension: unappreciated and misunderstood. J Neurol Neurosurg Psychiatry 2004; 75:621–625.
23. King JO, Mitchell PJ, Thomson KR, et al. Manometry combined with cervical puncture in idiopathic intracranial hypertension. Neurology 2002; 58:26–30.
24. McGonigal A, Bone I, Teasdale E. Resolution of transverse sinus stenosis in idiopathic intracranial hypertension after L-P shunt. Neurology 2004; 62:514–515.
25. Connor SE, Siddiqui MA, Stewart VR, et al. The relationship of transverse sinus stenosis to bony groove dimensions provides an insight into the aetiology of idiopathic intracranial hypertension. Neuroradiology 2008; 50:999–1004.
26. Bono F, Messina D, Gilberto C, et al. Bilateral transverse sinus stenosis predicts IIH without papilledema in patients with migraine. Neurology 2006; 67:419–423.
27. Bono F, Messina D, Gilberto C, et al. Bilateral transverse sinus stenosis and idiopathic intracranial hypertension without papilloedema in chronic tension-type headache. J Neurol 2008; 255:807–812.
28. Hannerz J, Greitz D, Ericson K. Is there a relationship between obesity and intracranial hypertension? Int J Obes Relat Metab Disord 1995; 19:240–244.
29. Corbett JJ, Mehta MP. Cerebrospinal fluid pressure in normal obese subjects and patients with pseudotumor cerebri. Neurology 1983; 33:1386–1388.
30. Bono F, Lupo MR, Serra P, et al. Obesity does not induce abnormal CSF pressure in subjects with normal cerebral MR venography. Neurology 2002; 59:1641–1643.
31. Daniels AB, Liu GT, Volpe NJ, et al. Profiles of obesity, weight gain, and quality of life in idiopathic intracranial hypertension (pseudotumor cerebri). Am J Ophthalmol 2007; 143:635–641.
32. Johnson LN, Krohel GB, Madsen RW, et al. The role of weight loss and acetazolamide in the treatment of idiopathic intracranial hypertension (pseudotumor cerebri). Ophthalmology 1998; 105:2313–2317.
33. Wong R, Madill SA, Pandey P, et al. Idiopathic intracranial hypertension: the association between weight loss and the requirement for systemic treatment. BMC Ophthalmol 2007; 7:15.
34. Hirsch KS, Wilson JG, Scott WJ, et al. Acetazolamide teratology and its association with carbonic anhydrase inhibition in the mouse. Teratog Carcinog Mutagen 1983; 3:133–144.
35. Sherman GF, Holmes LB. Cerebrocortical microdysgenesis is enhanced in c57BL/6J mice exposed in utero to acetazolamide. Teratology 1999; 60:137–142.
36. Nakatsuka T, Komatsu T, Fujii T. Axial skeletal malformations induced by acetazolamide in rabbits. Teratology 1992; 45:629–636.
37. Lee AG, Pless M, Falardeau J, et al. The use of acetazolamide in idiopathic intracranial hypertension during pregnancy. Am J Ophthalmol 2005; 139:855–859.
38. Dodgson SJ, Shank RP, Maryanoff BE. Topiramate as an inhibitor of carbonic anhydrase isoenzymes. Epilepsia 2004; 41: S35–S39.
39. Celebisoy N, Gökcay F, Sirin H, et al. Treatment of idiopathic intracranial hypertension: topiramate vs acetazolamide, an open-label study. Acta Neurol Scand 2007; 116:322–327.
40. Panday VA, Rhee DJ. Review of sulphonamide-induced acute myopia and acute bilateral angle-closure glaucoma. Compr Ophthalmol Update 2007; 8:271–276.
41. Leung DY, Leung H, Baig N, et al. Topiramate and asymptomatic ocular angle narrowing: a prospective pilot study. Eye 2009; 23:2079–2081.
42. Pandina GJ, Ness S, Polverejan E, et al. Cognitive effects of topiramate in migraine patients aged 12 through 17 years. Pediatr Neurol 2010; 42:187–195.
43. Hunt S, Russell A, Smithson WH, et al. Topiramate in pregnancy: preliminary experience from the UK Epilepsy and Pregnancy Register. Neurology 2008; 71:272–276.
44. Ornoy A, Zvi N, Arnon J, et al. The outcome of pregnancy following topiramate therapy: a study of 52 pregnancies. Reprod Toxicol 2008; 25:388–389.
45. Liu GT, Glaser GS, Schatz NJ. High-dose methylprednisolone and acetazolamide for visual loss in pseudotumor cerebri. Am J Ophthalmol 1994; 118:88–96.

46. Thambisetty M, Lavin PJ, Newman NJ, et al. Fulminant idiopathic intracranial hypertension. Neurology 2007; 68:229–232.

47. Burgett RA, Purvin VA, Kawasaki A. Lumboperitoneal shunting for pseudotumor cerebri. Neurology 1997; 49:734–739.

48. Kleinman G, Sutherling W, Martinez M, et al. Malfunction of ventriculoperitoneal shunts during pregnancy. Obstet Gynecol 1983; 61:753–754.

49. Hanakita J, Suzuki T, Yamamoto Y, et al. Ventriculoperitoneal shunt malfunction during pregnancy. Case report. J Neurosurg 1985; 63:459–460.

50. Samuels P, Driscoll DA, Landon MB, et al. Cerebrospinal fluid shunts in pregnancy. Report of two cases and review of the literature. Am J Perinatol 1988; 5:22–25.

51. Cusimano MD, Meffe FM, Gentili F, et al. Ventriculoperitoneal shunt malfunction during pregnancy. Neurosurgery 1990; 27:969–971.

52. Shapiro S, Yee R, Brown H. Surgical management of pseudotumour cerebri in pregnancy: case report. Neurosurgery 1995; 37:829–831.

53. Johnston I, Besser M, Morgan MK. Cerebrospinal fluid diversion in the treatment of benign intracranial hypertension. J Neurosurg 1988; 69:195–202.

54. Rosenberg ML, Corbett JJ, Smith C, et al. Cerebrospinal fluid diversion procedures in pseudotumor cerebri. Neurology 1993; 43:1071–1072.

55. Eggenberger ER, Miller NR, Vitale S. Lumboperitoneal shunt for the treatment of pseudotumor cerebri. Neurology 1996; 46:1524–1530.

56. McGirt MJ, Woodworth G, Thomas G, et al. Cerebrospinal fluid shunt placement for pseudotumor cerebri-associated intractable headache: predictors of treatment response and an analysis of long-term outcomes. J Neurosurg 2004; 101:627–632.

57. Bynke G, Zemack G, Bynke H, et al. Ventriculoperitoneal shunting for idiopathic intracranial hypertension. Neurology 2004; 63:1314–1316.

58. Corbett JJ, Nerad JA, Tse DT, et al. Results of optic nerve sheath fenestration for pseudotumor cerebri. The lateral orbitotomy approach. Arch Ophthalmol 1988; 106:1391–1397.

59. Sergott RC, Savino PJ, Bosley TM. Modified optic nerve sheath decompression provides long-term visual improvement for pseudotumor cerebri. Arch Ophthalmol 1988; 106:1384–1390.

60. Spoor TC, Ramocki, Madion MP, et al. Treatment of pseudotumor cerebri by primary and secondary optic nerve sheath decompression. Am J Ophthalmol 1991; 112:177–185.

61. Kelman SE, Heaps R, Wolf A, et al. Optic nerve decompression surgery improves visual function in patients with pseudotumor cerebri. Neurosurgery 1992; 30:391–395.

62. Acheson JF, Green WT, Sanders MD. Optic nerve sheath decompression for the treatment of visual failure in chronic raised intracranial pressure. J Neurol Neurosurg Psychiatry 1994; 57:1426–1429.

63. Goh KY, Schatz NJ, Glaser JS. Optic nerve sheath fenestration for pseudotumor cerebri. J Neuroophthalmol 1997; 17:86–91.

64. Herzau V, Baykal HE. Long-term outcome of optic nerve sheath fenestration in pseudotumor cerebri. Klin Monatsbl Augenheilkd 1998; 213:154–160.

65. Banta JT, Farris BK. Pseudotumor cerebri and optic nerve sheath decompression. Ophthalmology 2000; 107:1907–1912.

66. Chandrasekaran S, McCluskey P, Minassain D, et al. Visual outcomes for optic nerve sheath fenestration in pseudotumour cerebri and related conditions. Clin Experiment Ophthalmol 2006; 34:661–665.

67. Spoor TC, McHenry JG. Long-term effectiveness of optic nerve sheath decompression for pseudotumor cerebri. Arch Ophthalmol 1993; 111:632–635.

68. Binder DK, Horton JC, Lawton MT, et al. Idiopathic intracranial hypertension. Neurosurgery 2004; 54:538–552.

69. Zamecki KJ, Frohman LP, Turbin RE. Severe visual loss associated with idiopathic intracranial hypertension (IIH) in pregnancy. Clin Ophthalmol 2007; 1:99–103.

70. Higgins JNP, Cousins C, Owler BK, et al. Idiopathic intracranial hypertension: 12 cases treated by venous sinus stenting. J Neurol Neurosurg Psychiatry 2003; 74:1662–1666.

71. Donnet A, Metellus P, Levrier O, et al. Endovascular treatment of idiopathic intracranial hypertension: clinical and radiologic outcome of 10 consecutive patients. Neurology 2008; 70:641–647.

72. Friedman DI. Cerebral venous pressure, intra-abdominal pressure, and dural venous sinus stenting in idiopathic intracranial hypertension. J Neuroophthalmol 2006; 26:61–64.

73. Bagga R, Jain V, Gupta KR, et al. Choice of therapy and mode of delivery in idiopathic intracranial hypertension during pregnancy. Med Gen Med 2005; 7:42.

74. Palop R, Choed-Amphai E, Miller R. Epidural anesthesia for delivery complicated by benign intracranial hypertension. Anesthesiology 1979; 50:159–160.

75. Hilt H, Gramm HJ, Link J. Changes in intracranial pressure associated with extradural anaesthesia. Br J Anaesth 1986; 58:676–680.

76. Kim K, Orbegozo M. Epidural anesthesia for cesarean section in a parturient with pseudotumor cerebri and lumboperitoneal shunt. J Clin Anesth 2000; 12:213–215.

77. Abouleish E, Ali V, Tang RA. Benign intracranial hypertension and anesthesia for cesarean section. Anesthesiology 1985; 63:705–707.

78. Kaul B, Vallejo MC, Ramanathan S, et al. Accidental spinal analgesia in the presence of a lumboperitoneal shunt in an obese parturient receiving enoxaparin therapy. Anesth Analg 2002; 95:441–443.

79. Aly EE, Lawther BK. Anaesthetic management of uncontrolled intracranial hypertension during labour and delivery using an intrathecal catheter. Anaesthesia 2007; 62:178–181.

80. Wang LP, Paech MJ. Neuroanesthesia for the pregnant woman. Anesth Analg 2008; 107:193–200.

81. Merlob P, Litwin A, Mor N. Possible association between acetazolamide administration during pregnancy and metabolic disorders in the newborn. Eur J Obstet Gynecol Reprod Biol 1990; 35:85–88.

82. Ozawa H, Azuma E, Shindo K, et al. Transient renal tubular acidosis in a neonate following transplacental acetazolamide. Eur J Pediatr 2001; 160:321–322.

83. Ohman I, Vitols S, Luef G, et al. Topiramate kinetics during delivery, lactation, and in the neonate: preliminary observations. Epilepsia 2002; 43:1157–1160.

84. Amaral JF, Tsiaris W, Morgan T, et al. Reversal of benign intracranial hypertension by surgically induced weight loss. Arch Surg 1987; 122:946–949.

85. Sugerman HJ, Felton WL 3rd, Salvant JB Jr., et al. Effects of surgically induced weight loss on idiopathic intracranial hypertension in morbid obesity. Neurology 1995; 45:1655–1659.

86. Sugerman HJ, Felton WL 3rd, Sismanis A, et al. Gastric surgery for pseudotumor cerebri associated with severe obesity. Ann Surg 1999; 229:634–642.

87. Chandra V, Dutta S, Albanese CT, et al. Clinical resolution of severely symptomatic pseudotumor cerebri after gastric bypass in adolescents. Surg Obes Relat Dis 2007; 3:198–200.

88. Glueck CJ, Iyengar S, Goldenbarg N, et al. Idiopathic intracranial hypertension: associations with coagulation disorders and polycystic-ovary syndrome. J Lab Clin Med 2003; 142:35–45.

89. Glueck CJ, Aregawi D, Goldenberg N, et al. Idiopathic intracranial hypertension, polycystic-ovary syndrome, and thrombophilia. J Lab Clin Med 2005; 145:72–82.

90. Glueck CJ, Wang P, Fontaine R, et al. Metformin-induced resumption of normal menses in 39 of 43 (91%) previously amenorrheic women with the polycystic ovary syndrome. Metabolism 1999; 48:511–519.

91. Glueck CJ, Wang P, Fontaine R, et al. Metformin to restore normal menses in oligo-amenorrheic teenage girls with polycystic ovary syndrome (PCOS). J Adolesc Health 2001; 29:160–169.

92. Glueck CJ, Golnik KC, Aregawi D, et al. Changes in weight, papilledema, headache, visual field, and life status in response to diet and metformin in women with idiopathic intracranial hypertension with and without concurrent polycystic ovary syndrome or hyperinsulinemia. Transl Res 2006; 148:215–222.

16

Stroke in pregnancy

Victoria A. Mifsud

INTRODUCTION

Stroke is a relatively rare complication of pregnancy and the puerperium. However, it is potentially devastating due to the associated death and disability and it therefore represents a significant disease in this setting. Stroke is defined clinically by the World Health Organisation as rapidly developing clinical signs of focal (and sometimes global) disturbance of cerebral function, lasting more than 24 hours or leading to death with no apparent cause other than that of vascular origin (1). This encompasses a heterogeneity of underlying pathophysiologic mechanisms, but is largely subdivided into ischaemic and haemorrhagic. Ischaemic strokes are further subdivided into thrombotic or embolic, while haemorrhagic strokes are further subdivided into subarachnoid haemorrhage (SAH) or intracerebral haemorrhage (ICH). This classification, however, does not fully take into account entities, which, while not as common, still fall under the umbrella of stroke and which take on particular importance in pregnancy. These include cerebral venous sinus thrombosis (CVST), cerebrovascular events related to pre-eclampsia and eclampsia and reversible vasospastic angiopathy. This chapter addresses the epidemiology of stroke in pregnancy, causes of ischaemic and haemorrhagic stroke and management in specific situations, before discussing general treatment considerations.

EPIDEMIOLOGY

Stroke has long been noted in pregnancy. Hippocrates had written of apoplexy in association with childbirth and Meniere in 1828 referred to hemiplegia during pregnancy and childbirth which he ascribed to an excessive blood volume (2). Subsequently, there were several case reports of patients with a neurologic disorder in the puerperium where thrombosis of the cerebral venous sinuses was found at autopsy (2–5). Towards the end of the 19th century it was suggested that many neurologic symptoms of pregnancy were caused by cerebral venous sinus thrombosis (CVST). This assertion continued unchallenged for many years, but in many cases, reports of stroke in pregnancy were given a presumptive diagnosis of CVST without pathological confirmation, frequently before the advent of imaging techniques which could help confirm the diagnosis. It was in 1968 that this assumption was challenged when Cross and Jennet performed carotid angiography on a series of patients who presented to a neurosurgical unit in Glasgow with symptoms of a non-haemorrhagic stroke in pregnancy or the puerperium (6). They found that only 1 out of 31 patients (3.2%) had confirmed CVST on arteriography. They concluded that >70% of their patients had cerebral arterial disease with a confirmed major vessel occlusion in 55% of their patients. Furthermore, based on their series, they reported an incidence of non-haemorrhagic stroke in pregnancy and the puerperium of 1/20,000 deliveries.

Previously reported stroke incidences of 1/1666 (7) to 1/3000 (8) pregnancies which were based on largely unconfirmed diagnoses were clearly unreliable and most likely represented overestimations. Since then, however, despite the advent of modern imaging techniques, there are still wide variations in the reported incidence of stroke in pregnancy and the puerperium. This has been reported at 3.8 (9) to 34.2 (10) per100,000 deliveries (see Table 16.1) (6,9–22) as compared to a reported incidence of 10.7 per 100,000 women-years in non-pregnant women of childbearing age (15–44 years of age) (23). This wide variability is at least partly due to small sample sizes, potential selection bias in some series, differences in study design and marked variability of patient subgroups. As is evident from Table 16.1, in some cases CVST and arterial ischaemic events were grouped together (6,9,13,16), in others CVST was totally excluded (12,17), while in others CVST was taken as one group while arterial ischaemic and haemorrhagic strokes were grouped together (15,22).

Looking at the individual stroke subtypes in recent studies, overall ischaemic strokes were more frequent than haemorrhagic strokes, with a reported incidence of 3.8 (9) to 18 (16) per 100,000 deliveries for ischaemic strokes as compared to 2.9 (21) to 9 (13) per 100,000 deliveries for haemorrhagic strokes, except in Taiwan where the reported incidence of haemorrhagic strokes was significantly higher at 20.1 (18) and 31.4 (20) per 100,000 deliveries. In many cases there was not much of a difference between the ischaemic and haemorrhagic groups (11,12,24). In the non-pregnant population, however, ischaemic strokes account for about 83% of all strokes, while haemorrhagic strokes only account for 13%. This relatively increased proportion of haemorrhagic events in pregnancy and the puerperium suggests that this population is at an increased risk for haemorrhagic stroke. One study looking specifically at pregnancy-related haemorrhage found an incidence of 6.1/100,000 deliveries which is equivalent to 7.1 haemorrhages per 100,000 at-risk person-years and this was higher than the haemorrhage risk of 5/100,000 at-risk person-years observed in a control population of non-pregnant women aged 15 to 44 years (19). Despite the early assumption that CVST was the commonest form of ischaemic cerebrovascular event in pregnancy (2), in the studies where CVST and arterial ischaemic events were looked at separately, arterial events were more frequent than venous in developed countries. In fact, CVST has been estimated in the United States at about 11 to 12/100,000 deliveries (15,22). However, in other countries, the incidence of CVST in pregnancy and the puerperium may be higher. In Mexico City, 60% of all cases of CVST diagnosed over a 20-year period occurred in pregnancy or the puerperium (25) in an area where CVST is relatively frequent and makes up 8% of the cases on the hospital stroke register (26). In India, puerperal CVST was reported to account for 20% of strokes under the age of 40 and over a 10-year period, 138 out of 145 patients who presented with strokes in

Table 16.1 Incidence of Stroke in Pregnancy

	Cerebral venous thrombosis	Cerebral arterial infarction	Haemorrhage	Overall stroke incidence	Authors' reported/calculated relative risk during pregnancy and puerperium[a]
Cross et al. (6)	5/100,000 deliveries[b]		N/A	5/100,000 deliveries	
Wiebers and Whisnant (9)	0	3.8/100,000 deliveries[c]	0	3.8/100,000 deliveries	Similar
Simolke et al. (11)	2.2/100,000 deliveries	7.8/100,000 deliveries	6.7/100,000 deliveries	16.7/100,000 deliveries	
Sharshar et al. (12)	N/A	4.3/100,000 deliveries	4.6/100,000 deliveries	8.9/100,000 deliveries[d]	Similar for infarction Increased risk for haemorrhage
Kittner et al. (13)	11/100,000 deliveries		9/100,000 deliveries	20/100,000 deliveries	Inf:OR 0.7 in preg; 8.7 PP Hge:OR 2.5 in preg; 28.3 PP Inf + Hge: OR 2.4
Witlin et al. (14)	11.3/100,000 deliveries	6.3/100,000 deliveries	7.6/100,000 deliveries	25.2/100,000 deliveries	
Lanska and Kryscio (15)	11.4/100,000 deliveries	17.7/100,000 deliveries		29.1/100,000 deliveries	
Lanska and Kryscio (22)	11.6/100,000 deliveries	13.1/100,000 deliveries		24.6/100,000 deliveries	
Jaigobin and Silver (16)	18/100,000 deliveries		8/100,000 deliveries	26/100,000 deliveries[e]	
Ros et al. (17)	N/A	4.0/100,000 deliveries	6.2/100,000 deliveries (2.4 SAH, 3.8 ICH)	8.2/100,000 deliveries[f]	
Jeng et al. (18)	10/100,000 deliveries	16/100,000 deliveries	20.1/100,000 deliveries (2 SAH, 18.1 ICH)	46.2/100,000 deliveries[e]	
James et al. (10)				34.2/100,000 deliveries[g]	Threefold risk compared to previous reported stroke risk in young women
Bateman et al. (19)	N/A	N/A	6.1/100,000 deliveries		
Liang et al. (20)	4.5/100,000 deliveries	12/100,000 deliveries	31.4/100,000 deliveries	47.9/100,000 deliveries	
Bashiri et al. (21)	1.2/100,000 deliveries	5.2/100,000 deliveries	2.9/100,000 deliveries	9.2/100,000 deliveries	

Abbreviations: Hge = Haemorrhage; Inf = Infarct; PP = Post-partum; SAH = Subarachnoid Haemorrhage
[a]Compared to non-pregnant women of same age group.
[b]Only 1/31 patients had demonstrable CVT; >70% arterial occlusion.
[c]Only 1 observed case of pregnancy-related stroke in 25-year period.
[d]Excluding all cases of CVT.
[e]Adjusted for local referrals only and excluding all tertiary referrals.
[f]Excluding all cases of CVT.
[g]Cannot give accurate rates for each subgroup as 46% were only classified at time of discharge as 'pregnancy-related cerebrovascular events'.

the puerperium were diagnosed with CVST (27). Recent studies have demonstrated hyperhomocysteinaemia and low folate levels in both a Mexican and an Indian population and this may be related to the increased risk of CVST in these groups (26,28). In a study of Taiwanese women, the incidence of all strokes in pregnancy and the puerperium was estimated at 46.6/100,000 deliveries and CVST accounted for 22.4% of these (18), that is, 10.4/100,000 deliveries.

The incidence and type of stroke were also related to the stage of pregnancy (Table 16.2) (6,10–13,15–19,22,25). Cross and Jennet noted that as many ischaemic strokes occurred in the puerperium as in the second and third trimester together and only one stroke was noted in the first trimester (6). Most studies revealed a marked preponderance for CVST to occur in the post-partum period, while arterial infarctions occurred at any time during pregnancy with an increased risk in the third trimester and in the post-partum period (11,12,16). Two studies looked at the risk of ischaemic stroke occurring around the time of delivery separately from the remainder of pregnancy and the post-partum period (10,17) and they both demonstrated an increased risk in the peripartum period which increases further in the rest of the puerperium. A similar pattern was observed for CVST (10). Haemorrhagic strokes were also most common in the post-partum period (10,13,17,19), with some increased risk in the peripartum period and the third trimester (10–12,17). In a population-based study in the Washington/Maryland area in the United States, the relative risk for stroke during pregnancy was 0.7 for ischaemic and 2.5 for haemorrhagic strokes. However, this rose to 5.4 for ischaemic and 18.2 for haemorrhagic strokes in the 6 weeks post-delivery (including abortions) (13).

Pregnancy-related stroke, unfortunately, is still associated with significant mortality. Four to eight percent of all maternal deaths are thought to be the result of stroke (29–31) while studies reported over a 30-year period and across continents demonstrate mortality rates of 0% to 38% for women who sustain a stroke in pregnancy or the puerperium (6,10–12,14–16,22,32). Mortality depends largely on stroke subtype and while the mortality is quite low for ischaemic strokes, it is significantly higher for ICH (12,16). Amongst women who sustain pregnancy-related strokes, 42% to 63% remain with residual neurologic deficits (11,12,32) while 22% of stroke survivors were discharged to a facility other than home, as compared to 3% of all post-partum women. Apart from the maternal mortality and morbidity associated with maternal stroke, this was also associated with premature delivery and increased fetal mortality (12). Furthermore, if the stroke is secondary to maternal thrombophilia, this may also be associated with an increased risk of fetal loss, pre-eclampsia and placental abruption. Compared to strokes unrelated to pregnancy, patients with pregnancy-related stroke tend to be 10 years younger. However, the risk of pregnancy-related stroke increased with age – especially over the age of 35 (10,17) – with a risk of stroke of 58.1/100,000 deliveries in the 35- to 39-year-olds and 90.5/100,000 deliveries in the 40-year-olds. However, there was a small additional risk in the very young, such that the risk in women under 20 years of age was greater than that in the 20- to 34-year age group (10). In patients with CVST, an increased risk was noted in the very young – 15- to 24-year-olds – compared to the 25- to 34-year-olds, with the younger ones being 3.7 times more likely to sustain a CVST than their older counterparts (15).

The risk of stroke is also related to race and ethnicity. In an analysis of the U.S. Nationwide Inpatient Sample for the years 2000 and 2001 (10), African-American women had the highest risk of stroke at 52.5/100,000 deliveries, followed by white women at 31.7/100,000 deliveries and then by Hispanic women at 26.1/100,000. When controlled for age and race, white women aged over 35 years were 2.2 times as likely to have stroke as those under the age of 35 years, but African-American women aged 35 years or over were 4.5 times as likely to have a stroke as white women less than 35 years old.

Multiple births were also associated with a dramatically increased risk of stroke with one study reporting a 12 times increased risk of stroke (33). In one small study, a history of a previous stroke was associated with a 1.8% absolute risk of recurrence during pregnancy and the puerperium and the relative risk of recurrence was higher in the post-partum period (RR 9.7) than during pregnancy (RR 2.2) (34). However, in another small study, women who sustained a stroke unrelated to pregnancy and a small group of women who sustained a stroke in pregnancy or the puerperium were followed during subsequent pregnancies and none of them suffered a recurrent thrombotic event during pregnancy or after delivery (35). It was therefore shown that women with a previous ischaemic arterial or venous stroke have a low risk of recurrence during subsequent pregnancies, with the post-partum period affording a slightly increased risk. The only prognostic factor significantly associated with recurrence (even in non-pregnant women) was the finding of a definite cause for the initial stroke (34). In fact, in women with a history of stroke and thrombophilia, the recurrence may be as high as 20% (36). The risk of recurrence of CVST during pregnancy in women who had previously sustained CVST also appears to be low, as in a small study 22 pregnancies were observed in 14 women who had previously sustained CVST and there was no evidence of CVST or extracerebral venous thrombosis in any of them (37). Several medical problems have been associated with an increased risk of stroke, including diabetes (10,33), hypertension (15,22,38), pre-eclampsia (12,13,16,18,20,33,39) and metabolic disorders including fluid, electrolyte and acid-base abnormalities (10,22). In an analysis of the U.S. Nationwide Inpatient Sample (10) between 2000 and 2001, several conditions were shown to be strongly associated with a risk of pregnancy-related stroke. These include thrombophilia [odds ratio (OR) 16.0], systemic lupus erythematosus (SLE) (OR 15.2), sickle cell disease (OR 9.1), heart disease (OR 3.2) and migraine headaches (OR 16.9). Substance abuse, smoking and anaemia were all associated with increased risk. Some complications of pregnancy, including post-partum haemorrhage (OR 1.8), pre-eclampsia and gestational hypertension (OR 4.4), transfusion (OR 10.3) and pregnancy-related infection (OR 25) were all significantly associated with pregnancy-related stroke (10). Other causes included extracranial vertebral artery dissection, post-partum cerebral angiopathy and disseminated intravascular coagulation (DIC) associated with amniotic fluid embolism (12). Several studies have shown caesarean section to be strongly associated with stroke (22,33,38). However, it is unclear whether the caesarean section itself is a causative risk factor for stroke because of the increased thrombotic and cardiovascular risk of surgery, or whether caesarean section is performed more frequently in association with stroke because these patients requiring caesarean section tend to have risk factors which put them at risk of stroke, for example, pre-eclampsia.

PREGNANCY AS A HYPERCOAGULABLE STATE

Normal pregnancy is associated with a significant increase in procoagulant activity due to a rise in concentration of most clotting factors, especially factor VII, factor VIII, factor X,

Table 16.2 Timing of Stroke in Pregnancy

	Cerebral venous thrombosis n (%)	Cerebral arterial infarction n (%)	Haemorrhage n (%)
Cross et al. (6)	T1: 1 (3.2%) T2: T3: } 15 (48.4%) PP[a]: 15 (48.4%) – ½ in 1st wk PP; ½ PP day 11–16		N/A
Simolke et al. (11)	T1: 0 T2: 0 T3: 0 PP: 2 (100%) – in 2 weeks PP	T1: 1 (14.3%) T2: 2 (28.57%) T3: 2 (28.57%) PP: 2 (28.57%) – in 1st wk PP	T1: 0 T2: 0 T3: 5 (83.3%) PP: 1 (16.7%)
Cantu and Barinagarrementeria (25)	T1: 1 (1.6%) T2: 2 (3.2%) T3: 2 (3.2%) PP: 57 (92.0%) – 21 in 1st wk PP 36 in wks 2 and 3 PP	N/A	N/A
Sharshar et al. (12)	N/A	T1: 1 (6.7%) T2: 2 (13.3%) T3: 5 (33.3%) PP: 7 (46.7%)	T1: 0 T2: 2 (12.5%) T3: 10 (62.5%) PP: 4 (25%) – incl 1 in labour
Kittner et al. (13)	T1: 0 T2: 1 (5.9%) T3: 5 (29.4%) PP: 11 (64.7%) – incl 1 case of CVT PP		T1: 0 T2: 3 (21.4%) T3: 2 (14.3%) PP: 9 (64.3%) – incl 1 post-abort at 16/40
Lanska and Kryscio (15)	T1: T2: } 7 (22.6%) T3: PP: 9 (29%) Unspecified: 16 (48.4%)	T1: T2: } 17 (31.5%) T3: PP: 21 (38.9%) Unspecified: 16 (29.6%)	
Lanska and Kryscio (22)	T1: T2: } 0 T3: PP: 87 (51.2%) Unspecified: 83 (48.8%)	T1: T2: } 2 (1.1%) T3: PP: 65 (35.5%) Unspecified: 116 (63.4%)	
Jaigobin and Silver (16)	T1: 0 T2: 0 T3: 1 (12.5%) PP: 7 (87.5%)	T1: 3 (21.4%) T2: 1 (7.1%) T3: 4 (28.6%) PP: 6 (42.9%)	T1: 1 (7.7%) (0 ICH 1 SAH) T2: 6 (46.2%) (3 ICH 3 SAH) T3: 2 (15.4%) (1 ICH 1 SAH) PP: 4 (30.7%) (2 ICH 2 SAH)
Ros et al. (17)	N/A	T1+T2: N/A T3: 5 (19.2%) Peri-P[b]: 6 (23.1%) PP: 15 (57.7%)	T1+T2: N/A T3: 4 (13.3%) Peri-P[b]: 12 (40%) PP: 14 (46.7%)
James et al. (10)	T1: T2: } 20 (40%) T3: At delivery: 10 (20%) PP: 20 (40%)	T1: T2: } 184 (29%) T3: At delivery: 234 (31%) PP: 348 (45%)	T1: T2: } 91 (13%) T3: At delivery: 194 (27%) PP: 422 (60%)
Jeng et al. (18)	T1: 2 (18%) T2: 1 (9%) T3: 0 PP: 8 (73%)	T1: 2 (13%) T2: 4 (25%) T3: 4 (25%) PP: 6 (38%)	T1: ICH 2 (11%) SAH 0 T2: ICH 5 (26%) SAH 0 T3: ICH 6 (32%) SAH 1 (33%) PP: ICH 6 (32%) SAH 2 (67%)
Bateman et al. (19)	N/A	N/A	T1: T2: } 122 (41.6%) T3: PP: 171 (58.4%)

T1, 1st trimester; T2, 2nd trimester; T3, 3rd trimester.
[a]PP: Puerperium. [b]Peri-P: Peripartum period from 2 days before to 1 day after delivery.

factor XII and von Willebrand factor (40). This rise occurs mainly in late gestation and is accompanied by a marked increase in fibrinogen up to twice non-pregnant levels (41). Pregnancy, however, is also associated with a reduction in activity of physiologic anticoagulants. Protein S falls progressively throughout gestation (42) but it is uncertain whether this contributes to the hypercoagulable state (41). Antithrombin and protein C levels appear to be unaffected by pregnancy (42), but an acquired protein C resistance occurs in pregnancy and at term. Forty-five percent of pregnant women have an acquired activated protein C (APC) sensitivity ratio below the fifth percentile of the normal range for non-pregnant women of similar age (43). It is thought that APC resistance plays a key role in pregnancy-related vascular complications (41).

In addition, plasma fibrinolytic activity is reduced during pregnancy and remains low during labour and delivery but returns to normal shortly after delivery. Tissue plasminogen activator (tPA) activity decreases during pregnancy and this is due to a gradual increase in production of plasminogen activator inhibitor-1 as well as due to increasing levels of plasminogen activator inhibitor-2 – originally discovered in the placenta (41,44). Fibrinolytic activity is further inhibited by the presence of thrombin-activatable fibrinolysis inhibitor (TAFI), which increases in the third trimester (45). The increase in procoagulant activity, together with the reduction in fibrinolysis, results in the hypercoagulable state of pregnancy. Coagulation and fibrinolysis tend to return to normal by about 3 or 4 weeks after delivery (46).

ISCHAEMIC STROKE

Pregnancy-related stroke is essentially a stroke occurring in women of childbearing age, that is, up to about 45 years of age. The incidence of stroke in non-pregnant women of this age group has been reported as 10.7/100,000 women-years (23). Thus, although pregnancy confers an increased risk of stroke as compared to the non-pregnant counterparts, one must not assume that the pregnancy is the cause of stroke. When a pregnant women presents with a stroke, general causes of stroke in the young adult should be considered, together with a few pregnancy-specific causes.

Causes of Arterial Ischaemic Stroke in the Young Adult

The causes of ischaemic stroke in young adults of both genders have been reported in various series and registries across various continents. Thus, although they vary widely, the relative frequencies of the various causes of stroke in young adults have been determined to some extent as seen in Table 16.3 (47–53).

In pregnancy, however, most series looking at stroke have either been too small, have not had the benefit of the results of a full aetiological work-up or have simply consisted of retrospective chart review. Thus the relative frequencies of the various stroke aetiologies in pregnancy are not really known. In most conditions it is uncertain whether pregnancy is coincidental or whether the physiologic and haematologic changes of pregnancy play a role in the occurrence of the stroke.

Apart from the general causes of ischaemic strokes, there are a few conditions which are specific to pregnancy, such as amniotic fluid embolism, choriocarcinoma and eclampsia. In addition, there are a few conditions which are not specific to pregnancy but which have been linked to the pregnant state (apart from also being associated with some other conditions). These include peripartum cardiomyopathy and reversible vasospastic angiopathy.

Table 16.3 Reported Causes/Frequencies of Ischaemic stroke in the Young Adult

Cardioembolic: 15.4–29.3%
Large artery atherosclerosis:1.9–21.6%
Small vessel disease: 0–20.5%
Undetermined aetiology: 9.8–33%
Extracranial carotid and vertebral dissection: 3.3–24%
Migraine: 0.8–14.6%
Antiphospholipid antibody syndrome: 1.5–3.8%
Other haematologic disorders: 2.3–5.6%
Drug abuse: 0.5–4%
Inflammatory vasculopathies
 Intracranial vasculitis
 SLE
 Takayasu's
 Behcet's
Non-inflammatory non-atherosclerotic vasculopathies
 Moyamoya
 Fibromuscular dysplasia
 Post-radiation vasculopathy
Mitochondrial cytopathies
Infection related
 HIV
 Syphilis
Trauma
Peri-procedural

Causes of Ischaemic Stroke in Pregnancy

Non-Pregnancy-Specific Causes of Stroke

Cardioembolic. Potential cardiac sources of embolism have been divided into those which afford high risk and those which afford medium-risk of stroke. One such example of this type of classification is used in the TOAST criteria (54). Some specific cardiac conditions and their relation to the risk of stroke are discussed individually in a little more detail.

i) Rheumatic heart disease Mitral stenosis is the commonest form of valvular rheumatic heart disease seen in pregnancy (55,56). Mitral stenosis is thought to be associated with increased stroke risk even in the absence of atrial fibrillation (AF), although good estimates of absolute stroke risk independent of AF are not available (57). However, it is frequently associated with AF, which affords the major risk of cardioembolic stroke seen with mitral stenosis and which has been estimated, in the non-pregnant population, to increase the stroke risk to at least 5%/year (57). The tachycardia and hypervolaemia seen as a result of the physiologic changes of pregnancy tend to exacerbate the impact of the mitral valve obstruction, raising the left atrial pressure. Thus, AF may develop in pregnancy even in patients with mild to moderate stenosis who, before pregnancy, are asymptomatic from their mitral stenosis and are in sinus rhythm (55). This increases their risk of cardioembolic stroke and may require anticoagulation (see section 'Treatment of Ischaemic Stroke').

ii) Patent foramen ovale A patent foramen ovale (PFO) is the persistence of an embryonic opening in the interatrial septum which arises from the lack of normal fusion of the atrial septum primum and secondum, which normally occurs in infancy by 1 year of age. It may or may not be associated with an atrial septal aneurysm (ASA) which is defined as a >10 mm excursion of a mobile interatrial septum. PFO is a relatively common finding and known to be present in about 25% of the general population (58). However, it has been found at a higher frequency of about 40% of young patients with cryptogenic stroke (59–62), suggesting that it may be a true risk factor for stroke, especially in the young. This is further supported by the fact that patients with cryptogenic stroke and a PFO consistently have a lower prevalence of conventional risk factors than patients with cryptogenic stroke but no PFO (62). The PFO may provide a potential conduit for paroxysmal embolisation. Thrombi which form in the venous circulation may pass to the left side of the heart and from there to the general arterial circulation, especially if there is reversal of shunt from right to left. There have even been a few case reports demonstrating thrombi trapped in a PFO on echocardiography (63–65). However, the exact link between PFO and stroke remains somewhat controversial. Reported estimates of the annual stroke recurrence in patients with PFO and cryptogenic stroke vary considerably from 1.5% to about 12% depending on the study population (60,66–70). Long-term follow-up of such patients has not convincingly shown an increased risk of stroke recurrence in patients with a PFO and a cryptogenic stroke on medical treatment (60,71,72).

In some studies, the presence of an ASA or of large right-to-left intracardiac shunting in combination with a PFO has been shown to significantly increase the risk of recurrent stroke (66–68,73–77), but this has not always been borne out (60,78,79). Thus, taking all of this information into consideration, the importance of a PFO with or without an ASA for a first stroke or recurrent cryptogenic stroke remains in question (80).

There has only been one randomised study comparing the use of warfarin versus aspirin in patients with PFO and this did not show any significant difference in the rates of recurrent stroke between the two groups. However, this was a substudy of a larger trial and not designed to detect superiority of one treatment in patients with PFO (60). Closure of the interatrial septal defect is another treatment option and transcatheter closure appears to have rare short-term complications which tend to be minor (81–91). However, no randomised trials have been reported comparing different medical therapies or comparing medical treatment versus surgical or transcatheter closure. Non-randomised studies in which closure was compared with medical treatment alone indicate trends towards better outcomes with closure (80). The expert panel of the American Heart Association (AHA) concluded in the 2011 guidelines for secondary stroke prevention that there are insufficient data to establish whether anticoagulation is equivalent or superior to aspirin for secondary stroke prevention in patients with PFO and the use of antiplatelet therapy is reasonable.

The 2006 recommendations added that warfarin is reasonable for high-risk patients who have other indications for oral anticoagulation such as those with an underlying hypercoagulable state or evidence of venous thrombosis (92). In pregnancy, the hypercoagulable state, together with the pressure of the enlarged uterus on the iliac vessels may predispose to the formation of clots in the venous system. Furthermore, Valsalva manoeuvre at the time of delivery may also result in shunt reversal and may therefore predispose to paradoxical embolism in the presence of a PFO and there have been a number of reports of PFO-related stroke in pregnancy or the puerperium (93–96). In view of this, although antiplatelet agents are probably reasonable, an argument may be made to consider anticoagulation for secondary stroke prevention in the case of a cryptogenic ischaemic event in pregnancy in the presence of a PFO. The usual principles guiding the use of anticoagulants in pregnancy would apply if this treatment option is chosen (see section 'Treatment of Ischaemic Stroke').

iii) Congenital heart disease Stroke is not very common in patients with congenital heart disease (97). In fact, in two studies looking at the risk of adverse maternal outcomes,

including stroke, in pregnant patients with a history of congenital heart disease, there was only one stroke in a series of 405 pregnancies in 318 women (98) and no strokes in another series of 90 pregnancies in 53 women (99). The major mechanism of stroke in these patients is thought to be paradoxical embolism through an anatomically abnormal communication between the venous and arterial circulation (97). Although this occurs infrequently, it may be encountered if systemic vasodilatation and/or elevation of pulmonary resistance promote transient right-to-left shuntings (55). The European guidelines for the treatment of adult congenital heart disease refer to a potential increased risk of stroke in pregnancy in patients with atrial septal defect (ASD), atrioventricular septal defect and patients with Ebstein's anomaly because of the presence of intracardiac shunting (100). Thromboembolic events may also occur in the context of atrial tachycardias or atrial stasis associated with transvenous pacing or even as a result of infective endocarditis in some types of repaired and unrepaired congenital heart disease (24). Anticoagulation may be required to prevent cardioembolic stroke and the usual principles guiding the use of anticoagulation in pregnancy should be followed (see section 'Treatment of Ischaemic Stroke' below).

iv) Prosthetic heart valves As a result of the hypercoagulable state, pregnancy in a woman with a mechanical heart valve carries an increased risk of valve thrombosis of 3% to 14% (55) with a consequent increased risk of cardioembolic stroke. Thus permanent anticoagulation is required to reduce this risk.

The optimal management of thromboprophylaxis in the case of mechanical heart valves is somewhat controversial as there is conflicting evidence as to whether unfractionated heparin (UFH) and low–molecular weight heparin (LMWH) are as effective as warfarin for stroke prevention in such cases (101). The evidence-based guidelines of the American College of Chest Physicians (ACCP) (101) and the guidelines of the AHA (80) differ slightly in their recommendations and suggest a number of possible management strategies:

1. UFH or LMWH may be used for full anticoagulation throughout pregnancy. If UFH is used, it is important that the dosing is adjusted according to activated partial thromboplastin time (APTT). If LMWH is used, weight-adjusted dosing should be used, administered twice a day and adjusted according to anti-factor Xa levels. The heparin is usually stopped temporarily shortly before delivery and anticoagulation with heparin or with warfarin is resumed after delivery. When choosing between UFH and LMWH, the ACCP guidelines (101) tend to recommend LMWH over UFH since this is associated with a lower risk of osteoporosis and with a lower risk of heparin-induced thrombocytopenia (HIT).

2. In patients considered to be at high risk of embolisation, for example, in the case of older mechanical valves, or in patients with a history of thromboembolism, it may be preferable to use UFH or LMWH in early pregnancy until the 13th week of gestation and then to continue on warfarin for most of the pregnancy, even though exposure to vitamin K antagonists in the second and third trimesters has been associated with a very small risk of fetal abnormalities (see section 'Treatment of Ischaemic Stroke'). Furthermore, use of warfarin in pregnancy can result in a fetal coagulopathy. Thus, to avoid delivering an anticoagulated infant, with the associated risks to the child, warfarin is usually stopped about 3 weeks prior to delivery at which point the patient is switched back to UFH or LMWH. This is stopped temporarily around the

time of delivery and anticoagulation resumed post-partum. An alternative strategy is to continue on warfarin throughout pregnancy, planning for a caesarean section at 38 weeks and interrupting anticoagulation only very briefly for about 2 or 3 days before delivery. Although this has been associated with good fetal and maternal outcomes, experience with this strategy is quite limited. When warfarin is used in the case of prosthetic heart valves, the target International Normalised Ratio (INR) should be 3.0 with a range of 2.5 to 3.5.

3. In some high-risk cases, it may even be considered justified to use warfarin throughout pregnancy, despite the risks of teratogenicity and fetal loss associated with warfarin in the first trimester of pregnancy. The target INR should be 3.0 with a range of 2.5 to 3.5. In these cases, warfarin is switched to UFH or LMWH about 3 weeks prior to delivery or for a few days prior to a planned caesarean section at 38 weeks as in (2) above to avoid a fetal coagulopathy.

4. In some particularly high-risk cases, low-dose aspirin 75 to 100 mg daily is sometimes recommended in addition to warfarin to further reduce the risk of thrombosis, although this will increase the risk of bleeding.

It is important that such difficult decisions which may impact significantly on the outcome of the pregnancy are very carefully discussed with the patient and that she is made fully aware of the risks associated with the various management options. If planning to use UFH or LMWH in the early stages of pregnancy, the recommendation of the guidelines of the ACCP (101) is to perform frequent pregnancy tests and to switch the mother to heparin as soon as pregnancy is detected. If this strategy is used, the mother must be made fully aware of the importance of early detection and of the need to replace warfarin by the 6th week of gestation. Alternatively, one may switch to heparin prior to conception.

The stroke rate associated with bioprosthetic valves is significantly lower and antiplatelet therapy is usually sufficient to prevent thromboembolism unless other risk factors such as AF and previous embolism are present (57).

v) Atrial Fibrillation Although AF is very rare in women of childbearing age with no structural heart disease or endocrine abnormalities (102), lone AF precipitated by pregnancy has been reported in women with absolutely no other risk factors (102,103). Anticoagulation may be required in the context of AF, according to the associated risk factor profile.

vi) Peripartum cardiomyopathy Peripartum cardiomyopathy (PPCM) is an idiopathic form of dilated cardiomyopathy that usually develops during the last month of pregnancy or the first 5 months post-partum (104) in women without pre-existing cardiac dysfunction. Although not strictly meeting current criteria, cases of pregnancy-associated cardiomyopathy with similar features have been described presenting as early as at the 17th week of gestation (105). The aetiologic mechanisms are not well defined but recent data suggest a role for unbalanced oxidative stress-mediated proteolytic cleavage of prolactin in the peri/post-partum period into a cardiotoxic angiostatic and proapoptotic 16 kDa protein, with subsequent impaired cardiac microvascularisation (106). Several other aetiologies have been considered including inflammation possibly mediated via pro-inflammatory cytokines, viral infection of the heart and an autoimmune response against maternal myocardium possibly due to introduction of fetal cells into the maternal circulation (107). However, none of these mechanisms are very well supported by clinical evidence as there has been marked variability

in the results of endomyocardial biopsies and in the finding of autoantibodies against myocardium (108).

Women with PPCM present with symptoms of heart failure secondary to left ventricular systolic dysfunction. In 78% of patients, symptoms develop in the first 4 months after delivery, 9% present in the last month of pregnancy and only 13% present either prior to 1 month before delivery or more than 4 months post-partum (107). The left ventricle may not be dilated, but the ejection fraction is nearly always reduced to <45%. It is not uncommon for patients to develop left ventricular thrombi (109) especially with an ejection fraction of <35%, with consequent risk of cardioembolic stroke (110,111).

The chances of recovery of cardiac function after pregnancy correlate well with the degree of left ventricular dilatation and systolic function seen on early echo (112).

Arteriopathies. i) Atherosclerosis Premature atherosclerosis is seen in about 2% to 20% of strokes in this age group and occurs particularly in patients with the traditional risk factors of hypertension, diabetes, hypercholesterolaemia, smoking and a family history of atherosclerotic disease, especially when multiple risk factors are present in combination (113), though other more novel risk factors including hyperhomocysteinaemia and elevated lipoprotein (a) levels have been shown to contribute to atherosclerosis in the young (114). Inflammation and possibly infection may also be atherogenic and in fact women with chronic inflammatory disorders such as rheumatoid arthritis, SLE and systemic sclerosis have been shown to have accelerated atherosclerosis when compared with healthy age-matched controls (115).

ii) Non-atheromatous arteriopathies Non-atheromatous arteriopathies also form an important proportion of strokes in this age group.

Cervical arterial dissection. Cervical arterial dissection is probably the most common non-atheromatous vasculopathy and is thought to account for 10% to 25% of strokes in the under 45 age group (47,116). It has been reported in pregnancy and in the post-partum period (12,13,117–123). Dissections are usually classified as traumatic or spontaneous. However, it is likely that some degree of mechanical stress or trauma is also involved in the cases thought to be spontaneous and that the provoking insult can be trivial and is often either forgotten by the patient or not thought to be significant, such as a bout of violent coughing or awkward head movements. In about 1% to 5% of patients with spontaneous cervical artery dissection there may be underlying vessel wall/connective tissue abnormalities such as in Ehlers Danlos type IV, Marfan syndrome and osteogenesis imperfecta, which predispose the vessel wall to dissection. About 5% of patients will have a family member with a history of arterial dissection (116). The association with fibromuscular dysplasia (FMD) is stronger and dissection is seen in about 15% of FMD patients.

Although the first symptom in some patients with dissection may be sudden onset of a stroke, in most cases, the patient will first develop some headache or neck pain, possibly with some referred pain to the eye and possibly associated with mild ptosis and meiosis of an ipsilateral Horner syndrome, and will subsequently develop signs of cerebral or retinal ischaemia after a lag of hours to days. There are frequently multiple embolic transient ischaemic attacks (TIAs) with complete resolution before persistent stroke symptoms occur. In a small case series of six patients with post-partum dissection, all patients presented with unilateral or bilateral headache and/or neck pain 5 to 18 days after delivery. Two patients had no further symptoms, one only had an associated Horner syndrome and the remaining three sustained symptoms of cerebral ischaemia – TIA in two and stroke in the third (122). Although dissection in pregnancy and the post-partum period appears to be rare, this illustrates the variable presentation and the need for a high index of suspicion if the diagnosis of dissection is to be made.

There is not enough evidence in the literature to unequivocally guide treatment of this condition as there have not been any randomised controlled trials comparing the use of antiplatelets with anticoagulants in these cases. Two metaanalyses of case series reported no significant difference in death or disability between either treatment modality (124,125). However it was felt that these series were small, included both retrospective and prospective series and were subject to report bias (126). A further small prospective nonrandomised and non-blinded comparison of treatment of cervical dissection with antiplatelets or anticoagulants reported a similar incidence of stroke recurrence independent of which treatment modality was used (127), suggesting that there may not be much difference in efficacy between the two. In fact the 2011 guidelines of the AHA for the prevention of stroke and TIA conclude that antithrombotic therapy for at least 3 to 6 months is reasonable for patients with cervical arterial dissection who have symptoms of stroke or TIA, but they go on to state that the relative efficacy of antiplatelet agents compared with anticoagulants is unknown (80). This treatment choice must be tailored for the individual and in cases where anticoagulation would pose an increased risk of haemorrhage, such as in strokes with large areas of infarction, the choice may be swayed in favour of antiplatelet agents rather than anticoagulation (128). There are no specific recommendations in the case of pregnancy. However, the above information should be taken into consideration together with any potential risks to the fetus, based on the timing in pregnancy, when selecting antiplatelets versus anticoagulation in pregnancy (see section 'Treatment of Ischaemic Stroke' below).

Stenting is usually reserved for those who continue to have new symptoms despite maximal medical therapy (80). In those patients with cervical arterial dissection who do not develop signs of a stroke or TIA, but develop local symptoms, that is, headache, neck or eye pain, Horner syndrome, lower cranial palsies, etc., antiplatelets are usually considered adequate for stroke prevention, unless symptoms continued to progress despite treatment.

Recurrence of cervical artery dissection is rare and has been reported to recur in 0.9% to 4% of cases (129,130). There are two cases reported of pregnancy after a previous cervical arterial dissection. In one case the initial dissection had not occurred in the context of pregnancy and had occurred 2 years prior to the reported pregnancy. By this time the patient was on low-dose aspirin for secondary stroke prevention and had remained on this throughout pregnancy. She underwent an uneventful normal pregnancy and normal vaginal delivery with epidural analgaesia and though she did not require any assistance, the plan was to intervene to minimise expulsive effort, if required (131). The second patient presented with symptoms of a dissection 9 days after delivering her third child by normal spontaneous vaginal delivery. Bilateral carotid artery dissections were diagnosed and she was initially treated with anticoagulation for 6 to 7 months and then switched to antiplatelets. She subsequently underwent another uncomplicated pregnancy. She remained on low-dose aspirin until the 32nd week of gestation and underwent an elective caesarean section at 39 weeks (120).

Fibromuscular Dysplasia. FMD is a relatively uncommon non-atherosclerotic, non-inflammatory vascular disease that results in arterial narrowing and aneurysms of small and medium-sized vessels (132). It most commonly affects the renal vasculature followed by the extracranial carotid and the extracranial vertebral arteries (132) but it has been described in almost every arterial bed (133). It occurs most frequently in women between 20 and 60 years of age (134). Although cerebrovascular FMD tends to present a little later with a mean age of 50, it has been reported at any age with a range of 0 to 90 (135).

FMD is an angiopathy which is characterised by fibrosis, frequently associated with smooth muscle hyperplasia (136) and which is classified into three main categories according to the layer of the arterial wall affected – intimal, medial or adventitial (137). Arterial narrowing and aneurysm formation occur and may be complicated by arterial dissection. The commonest forms result in segmental narrowing with poststenotic dilatation causing the characteristic beading or 'string of beads' on vascular imaging. Less commonly, FMD may result in a concentric long smooth narrowing of the involved section of the blood vessels (132).

The most common location for extracranial FMD is the internal carotid artery (ICA) – most frequently at the level of C1/C2 and in the most recent report of the International Fibromuscular Disease Registry, the extracranial carotid was involved in 55.3% of patients while the vertebral circulation was affected in 16.6% (138). Involvement of the carotid arteries is usually bilateral and sometimes seen together with involvement of the vertebrals (139) although any single artery may be involved in isolation. Intracranial involvement is rare with only sporadic cases reported (140).

Cerebrovascular FMD may be asymptomatic (132) and is detected as an incidental finding or during evaluation of a carotid bruit. It may present with non-specific symptoms such as headache, neck pain, dizziness or a swooshing sound in the ears (135), or in a proportion of cases it may present with focal symptoms of stroke or TIA, SAH, Horner syndrome or cranial nerve palsies. The underlying mechanism includes one or more of hypoperfusion distal to severe stenosis, thromboembolism secondary to the FMD or to associated dissection or aneurysm rupture (141). Thus, FMD may be a cause of stroke in pregnancy. However, pregnancy does not appear to increase the risk of developing FMD (141). There is one report of pregnancy in a patient previously diagnosed with FMD (142). The patient was put on antiplatelet agents in the third trimester but still presented with focal neurologic symptoms suggestive of a mild stroke in the 39th week of pregnancy. She was delivered by caesarean section. Few generalisations may be made from a single case report.

Diagnosis of FMD as a cause of stroke is made on vascular imaging which most commonly reveals the characteristic string of beads or long area of narrowing, sometimes in association with dissection or with intracranial aneurysms. If the patient has experienced stroke or TIA as a result of arterial stenosis, then balloon angioplasty should be considered if feasible. If a dissection occurs during the procedure, then stenting is usually required (141).

If the focal symptoms were the result of a spontaneous dissection complicating FMD, then the patient is usually treated medically as is usual for dissections, but if the patient continues to be symptomatic despite medical treatment, stenting is usually required (141).

A ruptured aneurysm requires emergency treatment with coil embolisation or clipping, according to size, shape, location, etc. However, an asymptomatic aneurysm is usually monitored and considered for treatment as per the usual criteria for aneurysms based on size, location, prior history of rupture, etc. Asymptomatic FMD which is discovered during the course of routine investigation is usually associated with a good prognosis and does not require intervention. However, the patients are usually started on low-dose aspirin for primary stroke prevention (141) and monitored for disease progression. When cervicocranial FMD is diagnosed, it is important to exclude coexistant renovascular FMD which may itself result in refractory hypertension.

Reversible cerebral vasoconstriction syndrome. Reversible cerebral vasoconstriction syndrome (RCVS) is a clinical syndrome which was initially eponymously referred to as the Call–Fleming syndrome and which is seen in various clinical settings, ranging from migraine to the use of vasoactive substances to late pregnancy and the puerperium (143). Post-partum angiopathy, which, as its name implies, occurs in the post-partum period is a classical cerebral vasoconstriction syndrome and the trend is now to refer to it under the umbrella term of RCVS. In two-third of cases it presents in the first post-partum week and in 50% to 70% of cases it is associated with the use of vasoconstrictor medication, such as ergot alkaloids for post-partum haemorrhage or bromocriptine to inhibit lactation (144).

This syndrome is characterised by severe, usually thunderclap, headaches, with or without seizures and with or without focal neurologic deficits. Arterial vasospasm is seen on vascular imaging and reversibility, usually over a 4- to 12-week period, is an essential feature for final confirmation of the diagnosis (145). The appearance of segmental vasoconstriction (beading) of the large- and medium-sized intracranial arteries has resulted in quite a lot of confusion and has resulted in the condition being sometimes called a 'benign vasculitis'. The reversibility of the lesions, however, demonstrates this not to be the case. It is thought that in the case of post-partum angiopathy the hormonal changes of pregnancy may result in a vasoactive state which induces vasospasm.

The classical presentation of post-partum angiopathy is of a patient, who develops a thunderclap headache, up to 4 weeks post-delivery. There are frequently no associated neurologic symptoms at presentation. If she presents at this early stage, she is frequently worked up for SAH but unless she has developed a small focal cortical SAH imaging and lumbar puncture are negative. The vasospasm causes the headaches and if the patient presents with multiple, recurrent thunderclap headaches, it is almost pathognomonic of RCVS (144). The headache tends to start posteriorly and may be excruciating, resulting in severe distress.

As the disease progresses the patient may develop seizures. Focal cortical SAHs and ICHs may occur and tend to occur early in the course of the disease – usually within the first week (146). Subsequently, spasm of the blood vessels may result in focal neurologic deficits which may be transient, suggestive of a TIA, or which may be due to infarction with the clinical presentation of stroke.

The degree of vasospasm is highly variable at the peak of the disease and the clinical manifestations may range from simple recurrent thunderclap headaches with no associated focal neurologic symptoms to thunderclap headaches associated with progressive focal neurologic deficits due to progressive infarction with seizures. The infarction is frequently seen in the internal watershed territories as a result of the spasm.

CT or MRI may reveal signs of infarction and vascular imaging – magnetic resonance angiography (MRA), CT angiogram (CTA) or angiography – may reveal the characteristic beading of the vasospastic angiopathy. Sometimes, it may take several days for the beading to appear on vascular imaging and in the context of the classical history, one must maintain a high index of suspicion and if necessary repeat dedicated vascular imaging within a few days to help confirm the diagnosis. The vasospasm tends to be self-limiting over an approximately 8- to 12-week period.

The exact underlying pathology is not clearly understood, but the syndrome may sometimes overlap with posterior reversible encephalopathy syndrome (PRES) and classical imaging findings of PRES may be seen in association with this condition. When PRES occurs, it tends to develop early in the course of the disease.

Treatment usually consists of supportive therapy and although there is no clear evidence for their use, calcium antagonists are usually used in the non-pregnant population until the spasm subsides. Some will use nimodipine in the acute phase, while others tend to use the more long-acting verapamil for 8 to 12 weeks and until the vasospasm is seen to have resolved on repeat imaging. It appears that the vasospasm resolves spontaneously with or without treatment. In the rare cases when RCVS occurs in a patient in the advanced stages of pregnancy, rather than in the post-partum period, the need for these medications before the child is delivered should be carefully considered. They are both classified as category C drugs, and should only be used if the benefits outweigh the risks.

Since other life-threatening conditions such as aneurysmal SAH, CVST and pituitary apoplexy may all present with thunderclap headaches, it is important to exclude these other conditions, especially when the clinical picture is not yet clear. Thus, most of these patients undergo initial CT brain looking for an SAH and if this is normal they frequently undergo a lumbar puncture to rule out this serious diagnosis. If this is negative they will then frequently require an MRI of the brain with MRA and possibly with magnetic resonance venography (MRV) to rule out a venous sinus thrombosis.

Vasculitis is frequently cited as a differential of the radiologic appearance and enters the differential diagnosis. However, the clinical course of vasculitis tends to be different with a longer history of smouldering headache rather than a presentation with recurrent thunderclap headaches prior to onset of focal neurologic deficits. The older literature used to consider the RCVS to be a 'benign vasculitis' and there are therefore several reports of treatment with steroids. More recent literature, however, does not consider this to be an inflammatory condition and there does not seem to be a role for the use of steroids in this condition (145).

Moyamoya disease. Moyamoya disease is an occlusive arteriopathy of the distal internal carotid arteries (ICAs) or of the proximal middle cerebral or anterior cerebral arteries. This results in progressive stenosis and even occlusion of these arteries in the Circle of Willis and is associated with nearby formation of a fine network of abnormal collateral vessels which characteristically look like a puff of smoke on angiography – hence the name moyamoya which is a Japanese word meaning 'puff of smoke'. Moyamoya disease refers to the idiopathic form of the condition which is thought to have a genetic predisposition. It was first described and is seen most commonly in East Asia – especially in Japan – but since the disease was first described, several idiopathic cases have also been recognised throughout the rest of the world though at a much lower frequency. There is a female predominance, initially reported at 1.8:1 and more recently at 2.18:1 (147).

A similar occlusive vasculopathy associated with the characteristic puff of smoke appearance of collaterals may be seen in association with other underlying conditions and in these cases the condition is referred to as moyamoya syndrome. Some underlying conditions to consider are neurofibromatosis, radiation-induced vasculopathy, autoimmune disorders, brain tumours and particularly Sickle cell disease, which is so important due to its prevalence.

Adults with moyamoya may present with signs of ischaemia and may therefore present with clinical features of TIAs or infarction but, unlike in children, about half will present with ICH, which may be intracerebral, subarachnoid or intraventricular (148).

In view of the female predominance, moyamoya is naturally encountered regularly in pregnant women. There appears to be no evidence that pregnancy increases the risk of stroke in moyamoya (149,150); however, cases of stroke in pregnant patients with moyamoya have been reported. When these cases were analysed, it was concluded that when stroke occurred in pregnancy in patients who were known to suffer from moyamoya, they had a better prognosis than those who presented with pregnancy-related stroke as the first presentation of moyamoya (149). They also had a relatively low incidence of pregnancy-related stroke (150). Almost all of the maternal deaths in pregnancy-related stroke linked to moyamoya were due to ICH rather than infarction.

There are no guidelines as to the best mode of delivery for patients with moyamoya. A recent survey of the practice across various centres in Japan revealed that although the majority of patients with previously diagnosed moyamoya are delivered by caesarean section, about 24% of patients underwent vaginal delivery and no attacks were witnessed in either case, suggesting that there was no reason to avoid vaginal delivery in patients with previously diagnosed moyamoya (150). Extracranial-intracranial (EC-IC) bypass surgery is sometimes performed to attempt to allow the moyamoya vessels to regress and hopefully to reduce the risk of haemorrhage (151). There is, as yet, no clear evidence that surgery does in fact reduce the risk of bleeding, but surgery is frequently performed as the only possible interventional treatment which may afford some benefit. In this survey, whether the patient had previously undergone EC-IC bypass or not did not influence the mode of delivery. Furthermore, it is not clear whether previous surgery contributed to the better outcomes in patients previously diagnosed with moyamoya before becoming pregnant.

When patients present with a stroke in pregnancy as the first presentation of moyamoya, the outcome appears to be much worse, and the mode of delivery would probably have to be dictated by the patient's condition. Patients with known moyamoya should be counselled regarding the potential risks of pregnancy.

Haematological conditions. i) Sickle cell disease Sickle cell disease (SCD) increases the risk of stroke. Ischaemic stroke accounts for 54% of all strokes in SCD. It follows a bimodal distribution with the greatest incidence between 2 and 19 years of age and another peak after the age of 30. Between 20 and 29 years of age, most strokes tend to be haemorrhagic rather than ischaemic (134). By the age of 45, patients with SCD have a 24% chance of sustaining a clinical stroke, but the risk is lower for patients with Haemoglobin SC (HbSC) disease and lowest for those with HbS-β thalassaemia (134).

The abnormal haemoglobin (Hb) tends to polymerise, especially under situations of low oxygen tension and under other conditions of stress, altering the architecture and flexibility of the erythrocyte and causing sickling. This process also results in increased erythrocyte surface expression of adhesion molecule receptors (152). The lack of deformability of the sickled red blood cells (RBCs) together with the increased stickiness leads to obstructive adhesion of the sickle cells to

each other and to the vascular endothelium (153). This results in vaso-occlusion which leads to ischaemia with infarction, reperfusion injury and endothelial cell damage with an associated inflammatory reaction (154). In addition, the damaged erythrocytes undergo haemolysis and there is evidence to suggest that this results in changes which contribute to development of a progressive vasculopathy (155).

Ischaemic strokes in SCD are predominantly large-artery strokes and are associated with large-artery stenosis or occlusion affecting mainly the distal ICA, the proximal middle cerebral artery (MCA) or anterior cerebral artery (ACA) and the Circle of Willis (156,157) and infarction is frequently seen in a border zone distribution (158,159). Histological studies have demonstrated intimal thickening, fibroblast and smooth muscle cell proliferation and thrombus formation in the affected arteries (157,158). Small-vessel infarcts are also seen and sludging and intravascular sickling in the smaller blood vessels may play a part (159). These are particularly seen as silent infarcts on MRI (160). A proportion of patients with SCD will develop an intracranial occlusive vasculopathy with basal fine collaterals making SCD an important cause of moyamoya syndrome. An extracranial vasculopathy has also been described, causing stenosis or occlusion of the extracranial ICA (161).

SCD may also be a cause of venous sinus thrombosis as a result of the increased viscosity and tendency to adhesion (162,163).

In the Cooperative Study of Sickle Cell Disease, risk factors for stroke included having had a prior TIA, low steady-state Hb, frequent episodes of acute chest syndrome, an episode of acute chest syndrome in the previous 2 weeks and an elevated systolic blood pressure (134).

There is no clear evidence that pregnancy increases the risk of a stroke in a patient with SCD. In one study, comparing pregnant women with SCD with pregnant women without from the U.S. Nationwide Inpatient Sample from the Healthcare Cost and Utilization Project of the Agency for Healthcare Research and Quality for the years 2000 to 2003, there was a tendency towards a possible increased risk of stroke in the patients with SCD, but the OR did not reach statistical significance (164). However, in the Nationwide Inpatient Sample 2000 to 2001, having SCD was significantly associated with an increased risk of stroke in pregnancy with an OR of 9.1, on univariate analysis (10). In the 2000 to 2003 sample, there was a 4.9-fold risk of developing CVST with a p-value <0.001 (164). In addition, SCD was shown to increase the risk of eclampsia (OR 3.2), which itself increases the risk of stroke in pregnancy (164).

Transfusion is the cornerstone of treatment for an acute stroke in patients with SCD, and patients admitted with an acute stroke should undergo immediate emergency exchange transfusion to reduce the concentration of HbS to below 30% (165,166). Based on practice in children, this would usually be followed up with a continued transfusion regimen to maintain the HbS concentration at less than 30% (166). However, this practice in the paediatric population is based on a retrospective multicentre review of children withstroke and there have been no randomised controlled trials. The role of chronic transfusion for the prevention of recurrent stroke after a first ischaemic stroke in adulthood has not been defined (80,165). If it is deemed that chronic transfusion therapy is required for secondary stroke prevention, it is not clear at this point, for how long this would need to be maintained, or the intensity of the transfusion. The SWiTCH study of hydroxyurea for stroke prevention in children was stopped prematurely in 2010 when interim analysis revealed a high number of strokes in the hydroxyurea group (155). The analysis also concluded that it was unlikely that hydroxyurea with regular phlebotomy would be more beneficial than the combination of chronic transfusion therapy with deferasirox, an oral iron chelator to control iron overload. In the long term, any chronic transfusion therapy would need to be associated with iron chelation measures. One chelator desferrioxamine has been given a category C risk for use in pregnancy and should be withheld during pregnancy due to the risk of teratogenicity (167). Deferasirox has been given a category B risk in pregnancy due to toxicity in animal studies. If a pregnant patient is on chronic transfusion therapy for secondary prevention of a stroke, she is not routinely given iron supplementation in pregnancy, unless blood testing reveals low iron stores. Although it has been common practice in some countries to use prophylactic transfusions throughout pregnancy in an effort to prevent fetal and maternal complications, studies have failed to demonstrate significant benefit (168,169). The use of antiplatelet agents or anticoagulants for secondary prevention of stroke in SCD has not been specifically evaluated but their use within the usual guidelines for secondary stroke prevention is considered reasonable provided there are no contraindications (165).

Between the age of 20 and 29 years the risk of haemorrhage is higher than the risk of ischaemic stroke (134). Low steady-state Hb and an elevated leukocyte count were seen to increase the risk of haemorrhagic stroke (134). Patients may develop intraparenchymal, intraventricular or SAH. This increased risk of haemorrhage is partly accounted for by the development of moyamoya syndrome in some cases of SCD, with the associated risk of rupture of the fragile collaterals as well as by the increased incidence of aneurysms and arteriovenous malformations (AVMs) in patients with SCD.

ii) Antiphospholipid antibody syndrome The antiphospholipid antibody syndrome (APS) is an autoimmune disorder characterised by arterial or venous thrombosis and/or obstetric morbidity in the context of persistent circulating antiphospholipid antibodies (APLs). The antibodies are directed against protein antigens that bind negatively charged phospholipids and prothrombin, but the mechanism by which they contribute to the risk of venous and arterial thrombosis is not yet fully understood (170). The APS is most often primary if there is no underlying rheumatologic condition, but it is considered to be secondary if there is an associated underlying rheumatologic condition, especially SLE. It has been found that the different antibodies in different concentrations and in different circumstances have different significance with regard to thrombotic risk and this risk is modified by the presence of other vascular risk factors (171) - especially smoking and use of the oral contraceptive pill (OCP) (172) - and probably by the presence or absence of SLE (173).

The Sydney revised criteria for diagnosis of the APS (174) call for the presence of at least one of the specified clinical criteria and one of the laboratory criteria for a firm diagnosis of APS to be made. The clinical criteria are as follows: (*i*) at least one episode of arterial, venous or small-vessel thrombosis in any organ and (*ii*) pregnancy morbidity including one of unexplained fetal loss after 10 weeks of gestation; one or more premature births before 34 weeks of gestation because of eclampsia, pre-eclampsia or placental insufficiency; or three or more episodes of unexplained fetal loss before the 10th week of gestation. The laboratoty criteria include (*i*) lupus anticoagulant (LA) present on two occasions at least 12 weeks apart, (*ii*) medium or high titres of anticardiolipin antibodies (aCL) IgG or IgM, at least 12 weeks apart and (*iii*) anti-β_2-glycoprotein-1 (β_2GP1) IgG or IgM antibodies at a titre above the 99th percentile on two occasions at least 12 weeks apart.

The antibodies have not been shown to be significant unless they are persistent on repeated determinations. Thus, according to the criteria for the diagnosis of the APS (174), the APLs must be retested at the end of 12 weeks and found to be still persistent to fulfil the laboratory criteria for the diagnosis of the APS. Also, some antibodies have been found to afford a higher risk of thrombosis than others, such that it is not just the presence of the antibodies but their concentration and overall profile which are also important. Thus the combination of antibodies increases the risk of thrombosis, especially the presence of all three antibodies LA + aCL + anti-β_2-GP1 together, which is associated with the highest risk of recurrent thrombosis and virtually always persistent on repeated assay (175). Persistent isolated LA has also been most strongly associated with increased stroke risk (176), whereas anti-β_2-GP1 alone has been associated with the lowest (177). Therefore, the detection of LA on two samples 12 weeks apart is enough to fulfil the laboratory criteria for the diagnosis of APS, while aCL must be present at moderate to high levels (>40 GPL or MPL) and anti-β_2-GP1 must be in the 99th percentile to be considered significant. Persistent isolated aCL at medium to high titres are also included as a high-risk profile, whereas low-level titres are not (173).

These have important implications when selecting appropriate individualised treatment for each patient. Transient APLs, especially at low titres are not thought to be significant and such patients should be treated as antibody negative.

APS is well known to obstetricians because of the important association with recurrent early fetal loss (<10 weeks) as well as the association with unexplained late fetal loss, intrauterine growth retardation (IUGR) and pre-eclampsia. It is an acquired thrombophilia and clearly associated with venous thrombosis – including CVST (178,179). Despite debate and conflicting results in different studies, a recent consensus report concluded that APLs are also established risk factors for ischaemic stroke in adults with and without SLE (180), although their role in recurrent stroke is less clear, except in association with SLE – mainly due to inclusion into large studies of patients who were antibody positive on a single estimation of aPLs but did not necessarily have the APS (180).

APS is therefore considered an important cause of stroke in women of childbearing age and therefore in pregnancy and the puerperium. It may cause arterial stroke, which would present in the usual way with abrupt onset of focal neurologic deficits, but which may be associated with a history of obstetric problems. Livedo reticularis and thrombocytopenia are sometimes a feature of APS and if present in the context of stroke may give a clue regarding the underlying aetiology. In the presence of LA, the APTT may be prolonged and may also provide a clue to the underlying aetiology. This prolongation of APTT is an in vitro effect and is not associated with prolonged clotting, but rather with thrombophilia.

A recent international task force report has very clearly outlined appropriate primary and secondary prevention strategies for thrombosis in APL positive patients with and without APS and with and without SLE. Risk factor modification applies to all patients with APS (173). However, debate persists about the appropriate secondary prevention after stroke and other arterial events. This group's overall recommendation refers to the non-pregnant population. They recommend that patients with definite APS and arterial thrombosis should be treated with warfarin, with a target INR of >3.0 or with a combination of warfarin (INR 2–3) and low-dose aspirin, although not all members of the panel agreed and it was felt that these recommendations were made on relatively low-quality evidence (173). However, the most recent guidelines for the secondary prevention of stroke from the AHA recommend oral anticoagulation with a target INR of 2 to 3 for patients with APS who sustain a stroke or TIA (80). There are no specific guidelines for treatment of stroke or TIA in the context of the APS in pregnancy. However, the guidelines of the AHA for the secondary prevention of stroke recommend that pregnant women with a stroke or TIA and a hypercoagulable state should remain on anticoagulation throughout pregnancy (80).

If a patient is already on warfarin pre-pregnancy, the recommendation of the ACCP is to perform frequent pregnancy tests and to switch to therapeutic doses of unfractionated or LMWH as soon as pregnancy is detected, in view of the risk of teratogenicity with warfarin (101). If this strategy is adopted then the patient must understand the importance of switching to heparin by the 6th week of gestation. Alternatively, the patient may be started on full anticoagulation treatment doses of UFH or LMWH before conception (see section 'Treatment of Ischaemic Stroke'). There is no guidance as to whether patients who were on a combination of warfarin and aspirin pre-pregnancy should be switched to a combination of therapeutic heparin and low-dose aspirin during pregnancy.

Patients with the APS and a history of venous thrombosis, including CVT, are usually on lifelong anticoagulation with warfarin with a target INR of 2 to 3 (173). Thus, as is usual practice, if a patient is on anticoagulation with warfarin pre-pregnancy for secondary prevention of venous thrombosis, she should be switched to therapeutic doses of LMWH or UFH as soon as pregnancy is detected or prior to conception (see section 'Treatment of Ischaemic Stroke'). The importance of discontinuation of warfarin by the 6th week of gestation must be stressed with the patient.

Similarly, if a patient with APS and no history of thrombosis develops the first episode of venous thrombosis, including CVST, in pregnancy then she should be treated with therapeutic doses of LMWH or UFH during pregnancy and continued post-partum on indefinite anticoagulation with warfarin ± low-dose aspirin.

If a patient is known to have APS and has a history of recurrent fetal loss, but has no history of thrombosis, treatment with a combination of low-dose aspirin and prophylactic doses of LMWH or prophylactic to intermediate doses of subcutaneous UFH throughout pregnancy to help prevent fetal loss is recommended (101).

For patients who test positive for APLs but do not have a high-risk antibody profile, do not meet lab criteria for APS and have no history of arterial or venous thrombosis, it is recommended that they do not require thromboprophylaxis during pregnancy but should receive prophylactic heparin in the puerperium (173).

iii) Inherited thrombophilias The commonest inherited thrombophilias are protein C, protein S or antithrombin deficiency, activated protein C resistance as a result of factor V Leiden mutation, prothrombin G20210A mutation and the methylene tetrahydrofolate reductase (MTHFR) mutation. Their association with arterial ischaemic stroke is controversial and while they have been weakly linked to arterial ischaemic stroke in various case reports, case series and meta-analyses (181–191), especially in those under 50 years of age with no other cerebrovascular risk factors, other data have suggested otherwise (192–199). In this context, the usefulness of looking for an inherited thrombophilia in patients with arterial stroke

has been called into question (200). However, until the link is clarified further, it is reasonable to continue to seek thrombophilic conditions in young patients with an acute arterial stroke, especially when there are no traditional cerebrovascular risk factors and provided the results are interpreted within the whole clinical context.

The inherited thrombophilias, however, have been clearly shown to be associated with CVST (201–204). A significant association has been described for factor V Leiden mutation and G20210A prothrombin mutation (202–204) with estimated ORs of 3.4 and 9.3, respectively (201). There has been some controversy about the association with the MTHFR mutation, but recent work has suggested that adult CVST may be associated with this genetic defect (203) as well as with hyperhomocysteinaemia (26,28,202,205) which may be inherited as well as acquired. A strong association has also been found with protein C and protein S deficiency, with estimated ORs of 11.1 and 12.5, respectively (201,204), as well as with antithrombin deficiency (204). It has been suggested that the importance of each inherited thrombophilic defect in contributing to thrombosis may be different according to the site of thrombosis, with a different pattern for CVST as compared to lower limb deep vein thrombosis or to thrombosis at other unusual sites (204,206). It is now believed that venous thrombosis is a multifactorial problem and that in the context of an underlying inherited thrombophilia, pregnancy and the puerperium, which are themselves hypercoagulable states, may interact to precipitate the development of CVST (207,208). Hereditary thrombophilias have also been linked to a risk of fetal loss, a subject beyond the scope of this chapter.

Evidence-based guidelines of the ACCP outline recommendations for the management of venous thrombosis and thrombophilia in pregnancy (101). There are no specific guidelines for the prevention of CVST, in the context of thrombophilia, but it is reasonable to generalise from the guidelines for general prevention of venous thromboembolism in pregnancy. When anticoagulation with heparin is required in pregnancy, the ACCP guidelines recommend using LMWH over UFH, whenever possible, since efficacy is similar but LMWH carries a lower risk of osteoporosis and of HIT.

1. Patients with a history of thrombophilia and a history of venous thrombosis who are on long-term anticoagulation with warfarin should be switched to full-dose anticoagulation with heparin – preferably LMWH during pregnancy. LMWH is given in weight-adjusted full-treatment doses, administered in two doses per day, and adjusted according to anti-factor Xa activity. It is recommended that those on long-term vitamin K antagonists who are attempting pregnancy should remain on the vitamin K antagonists while performing frequent pregnancy tests, switching to LMWH (or sometimes UFH) when pregnancy is achieved (101). It is essential that these patients fully understand the importance of early detection and the need to discontinue warfarin by the 6th week of gestation. In some cases, switching to the chosen heparin prior to conception may be an alternative strategy.

2. For pregnant women with a laboratory confirmed thrombophilia, who have a past history of a single previous episode of venous thrombosis but who are not receiving long-term anticoagulation, the recommendation is to use prophylactic dose or intermediate dose LMWH (or prophylactic or intermediate dose UFH) followed by post-partum anticoagulation with oral or subcutaneous agents for 4 to 6 weeks after delivery (101).

An alternative strategy for those with a 'low-risk' thrombophilia is to withhold pharmacologic prophylaxis, but to offer clinical surveillance for thrombosis throughout pregnancy with close clinical monitoring and immediate investigation of any symptoms suspicious of venous thrombosis or pulmonary embolism. The patients should still be treated post-partum with oral or subcutaneous anticoagulation for 4 to 6 weeks after delivery (101).

This strategy of surveillance, however, should not be adopted for those patients with 'higher risk' thrombophilias including antithrombin deficiency, compound heterozygosity for prothrombin G20210A variant and factor V Leiden or homozygosity for these conditions. Such patients should always be treated antepartum with prophylactic or intermediate dose LMWH or UFH followed by post-partum anticoagulation as above (101).

Also, if the previous thrombotic event was CVST then prophylaxis with LMWH in subsequent pregnancies is recommended (201) rather than surveillance.

3. For those pregnant patients with antithrombin deficiency but no history of venous thrombosis, the recommendation is to use antepartum prophylactic anticoagulation preferably with LMWH but possibly with UFH, followed by post-partum prophylaxis (101).
4. For pregnant patients with all other types of thrombophilia but no history of venous thrombosis one may choose antepartum clinical surveillance or treatment with prophylactic LMWH or UFH – always followed by post-partum anticoagulation – based on an individual risk assessment (101).

Pregnancy-Specific Causes of Stroke

Pre-eclampsia/Eclampsia. Pre-eclampsia is one of the hypertensive disorders of pregnancy (see chapter 10). There has been some debate over the precise definition across various countries but in 2000 the National High Blood Pressure Education Working Group in the United States defined pre-eclampsia as the development of sustained hypertension ($\geq$140/90 mmHg) together with the development of proteinuria of $\geq$0.3 g/24 hr after 20 weeks of gestation in a patient with no prior history of hypertension (209). Patients who were previously hypertensive and who develop proteinuria are considered to have pre-eclampsia superimposed on chronic hypertension (209). Pre-eclampsia is further classified into mild or severe. Patients with more severe blood pressure (in the region of $\geq$160 (210) or $\geq$170 (211)/110 mmHg) or with heavy proteinuria [$\geq$1 g to $\geq$5 g/24 hr in different guidelines (210–212)], or who develop symptoms of organ involvement, such as right upper quadrant or epigastric pain, oliguria of <500 mL/24 hr, pulmonary oedema, thrombocytopaenia, persistent headache, altered mental status, blurred vision or blindness or who develop signs of fetal compromise including severe fetal growth restriction are considered to have severe pre-eclampsia (210). Eclampsia is defined as the development of new-onset seizures in patients with pre-eclampsia (210), in whom there is no other obvious explanation for the seizures. Severe pre-eclampsia or eclampsia may be complicated by the HELLP syndrome (haemolysis, elevation of liver enzymes and low platelets) or by DIC. Pre-eclampsia usually occurs after gestational week 20 [though it may occur earlier in cases of trophoblastic disease (213,214)] and it most frequently occurs close to term, and may occur post-partum. It has been observed, however, that pre-eclampsia which develops before 34 or 35 weeks of gestation is not only associated

with worse fetal outcome due to fetal immaturity but also associated with increased maternal mortality, with the highest risk at 20 to 28 weeks of gestation (215). In fact it has been proposed that early and late pre-eclampsia may represent two separate disease entities (216,217). Thus, although not initially included in the 2002 Practice Bulletin of the American College of Obstetricians & Gynaecologists (210) and not included in the British (211) or Australian (218) guidelines, a position statement from the American Society of Hypertension in 2008 included the timing of onset of pre-eclampsia as a marker of severity, classifying pre-eclampsia that develops at <35 weeks as severe. However, a patient with seemingly mild disease may still progress to eclampsia or severe pre-eclampsia rapidly and unpredicatably, and therefore still requires careful management. Also, although most cases of eclampsia in the post-partum period occur within the first 48 hours of delivery and cases of late post-partum eclampsia are classically described as occurring up to 4 weeks post-partum, one case has been reported as late as 8 weeks post-partum (219).

Pre-eclampsia/Eclampsia is a complex multisystem disorder due to a complex interaction of various factors but it is thought to be primarily a disorder of placental implantation together with an abnormal exaggerated maternal systemic inflammatory immune response (220) to placentation and later to the shedding of syncytial fragments into the maternal circulation (221). This results in placental hypoxic-reoxygenation injury and oxidative stress, which leads to release of placental factors including antioxidants, cytokines, apoptotic factors and anti-angiogenic factors. These interact with maternal factors to cause a maternal systemic inflammatory response and endothelial cell injury (221). In fact, women with pre-existing factors which predispose to endothelial dysfunction, such as pre-existing hypertension, renal disease, obesity and dyslipidaemia are at a higher risk of developing this abnormal maternal response (222). This systemic inflammatory response leads to endothelial cell dysfunction associated with altered vascular reactivity, widespread vasoconstriction, increased systemic vascular resistance, enhanced platelet aggregation, activation of the coagulation system and disruption of the normal systemic volume and blood pressure controls (209). This may result in a maternal multisystem disorder with the clinical features of pre-eclampsia and eclampsia, or in fetal effects with growth retardation, reduced amniotic fluid, hypoxia secondary to placental insufficiency and even perinatal death (223).

The pathophysiology behind the neurologic manifestations of pre-eclampsia and eclampsia are not completely understood and the mechanism by which stroke occurs in this setting is not clear. However, based on the available data, various hypotheses have been proposed. It is possible that in some instances a sudden rise in blood pressure may result in vasoconstriction of the cerebral microvasculature as a compensatory autoregulatory response, which could result in ischaemia (224). However, it has been suggested that ischaemic stroke may be due to a complex interaction between endotheliopathy and coagulopathy (225) and the presence of a genetic tendency to thrombophilia may further contribute to an ischaemic event. Furthermore, the endothelial dysfunction described above frequently results in diminished autoregulatory capacity and enhanced permeability of the blood-brain barrier (226). Impairment of dynamic cerebral autoregulation has, in fact, been demonstrated in a small series of patients with eclampsia (227) and it is thought that the upper limit of autoregulation in such patients may be

Table 16.4   Frequency of Ischaemic and Haemorrhagic Strokes in Eclampsia

Study	Total no. of strokes reported (excluding CVT)	No. of ischaemic strokes reported (excluding CVT)	No. (%) of ischaemic strokes with pre/eclampsia (excluding CVT)	No. of haemorrhagic strokes (excluding SAH when possible)	No. (%) of haemorrhagic strokes with pre/eclampsia (excluding SAH when possible)
Wiebers and Whisnant (9)	1	1	0	0	0
Simolke et al. (11)	15	9	0	6	2 (33.3%)
Sharshar et al. (12)	31	15	7 (47%)	16	7 (44%)
Awada et al. (257)	12	9	1 (11%)	3	0
Kittner et al. (13)	31	17	4 (23.5%)	14	2 (14.3%)
Witlin and Friedman (14)	11	5	2 (40%)	6	0
Lanska and Kryscio (15)	54		5 (9.3%)		
Lanska and Kryscio (22)	183		57 (31%)		
Jaigobin and Silver (16)	19	13	3 (23%)	6	1 (17%)
Skidmore and Williams (39)	32	21	3 (14%)	11	4 (36.4%)
Jeng et al. (18)	35	16	1 (6.3%)	19	7 (37%)
Liang et al. (20)	29	8	2 (25%)	21	5 (24%)
Bashiri et al. (21)	14	9	5 (55.6%)	5	3 (60%)

reduced. It has also been shown that patients with severe pre-eclampsia have a high cerebral perfusion pressure (228,229), which could result in barotrauma and damage to the cerebral blood vessels (230). In these circumstances, when systemic blood pressure exceeds the upper level of autoregulation, forced vasodilatation may occur, which may result in leaking of tight junctions, interstitial extravasation of protein and fluid, leading to formation of vasogenic oedema and micro-haemorrhages (230), as one would see in pre-eclampsia/eclampsia-related PRES. However, it may also lead to rupture and haemorrhage (230) causing a haemorrhagic stroke. Eclampsia-induced coagulation disorders may also play a role in genesis of haemorrhage (12). Vasospasm of the cerebral proximal large arteries on cerebral angiography has been reported in some cases of eclampsia (231,232). This may represent an autoregulatory response to the severe hypertension. However, cases of coexistent pre-eclampsia/eclampsia-related PRES and post-partum cerebral angiopathy (or RCVS) have been reported (233) suggesting that there may be some overlap between the two conditions. Certainly any severe significant associated vasospasm in the case of coexisting RCVS or post-partum angiopathy could result in associated ischaemic stroke or even focal haemorrhage.

Pre-eclampsia occurs in about 3% to 8% of all pregnancies (217,234,235) but the rate is significantly higher in cases of multiple pregnancies (236) and especially in patients with a history of pre-eclampsia in a previous pregnancy (237). Other risk factors include primiparity (238,239), race, with black women being at higher risk (240), high pre-pregnancy body mass index, a family history of eclampsia and underlying medical conditions, such as diabetes, renal disease, presence of APLs (239), insulin resistance (223), pre-existing hypertension (234,241–243) and thrombophilias (244). Other less established risk factors include maternal age, paternal factors and history of previous abortions (245,246). An association has been noted between migraines and pre-eclampsia, but a cause-and-effect relationship has not been established (247). Eclampsia is less frequent, and has been reported as affecting 2–10/10,000 deliveries in Europe and the United States (248–254), but is reported at a much higher frequency in developing countries (255,256). Pre-eclampsia and eclamp-

sia remain a significant cause of maternal and fetal morbidity and mortality.

Pre-eclampsia and eclampsia constitute the commonest risk factor for stroke in pregnancy and the puerperium. In various population-based studies and case series, it has been reported as accounting for 6% to 55% of pregnancy-related ischaemic strokes and 14% to 60% of pregnancy-related haemorrhagic strokes (Table 16.4) (9,11–16,18,20,21,22,39,257). In an analysis of the U.S. Nationwide Inpatient Sample between 2000 and 2001, eclampsia and pre-eclampsia were associated with a fourfold increased risk in stroke (ischaemic and haemorrhagic combined) with an OR of 4.4 (10). In the case of ischaemic strokes, however, these numbers must be interpreted with caution as some cases reported as ischaemic stroke may actually have been cases of PRES, which is frequently seen in pre-eclampsia and eclampsia.

ICH is clearly an important cause of morbidity and mortality in pre-eclampsia and eclampsia. In a large study looking at the Pregnancy Mortality Surveillance System in the United States between 1979 and 1992, 20% of all pregnancy-related deaths were due to pre-eclampsia/eclampsia with cerebrovascular events accounting for 38.7% of these (215). The majority of these deaths were due to ICH (34.7%), while cerebral oedema accounted for 3% and only 1% were due to cerebral embolism. Also in a series of 28 patients with stroke secondary to pre-eclampsia/eclampsia, 89% sustained a haemorrhage, mortality was as high as 53% and all surviving patients but three were left with significant morbidity (230). ICH or stroke is also the commonest cause of death in patients with the HELLP syndrome, accounting for 26.4% of deaths in one series (258).

The commonest neurologic presentation of pre-eclampsia/eclampsia is PRES, which was initially described as the reversible posterior leukoencephalopathy syndrome (RPLS) (259). The classical clinical features are of headache and nausea with visual loss or visual disturbances, ranging from visual agnosia to cortical blindness or even hemianopia, associated with agitation or alteration in level of consciousness, which may proceed to stupor and coma, and seizures. The onset may be subacute, with seizures developing later, but the patient may also present with a seizure at onset. Other focal neurologic deficits may also develop, including dysphasia, hemiparesis and ataxia. If treated rapidly, the encephalopathy is usually reversible and the patients usually recover completely within a matter of hours to days. However, in a subset of cases, neurologic signs may persist, suggesting associated underlying infarction or haemorrhage. Mortality in this syndrome is usually due to the mortality associated with any underlying haemorrhage, if severe. However, in a very small proportion of patients, the vasogenic oedema is so severe as to result in a significant rise in intracranial pressure (ICP) with the risk of fatal transtentorial herniation (260).

The classical brain imaging changes are of bilateral symmetrical subcortical changes, compatible with vasogenic oedema, seen predominantly in the posterior regions – that is, in the occipital and parietal lobes – but which may also involve the frontal and temporal lobes in about 50% of cases (261,262). Although the oedema largely affects the white matter, grey matter, including basal ganglia and thalamus, and cortical lesions are also seen in 25% to 94% of cases (261–263) and brainstem and cerebellar involvement is also frequent. The changes do not follow a vascular distribution and tend to straddle watershed territories. These imaging characteristics are predominantly compatible with vasogenic oedema and therefore associated with free diffusion on apparent diffusion coefficient (ADC) maps and diffusion weighted imaging (DWI) MRI. One characteristic feature of PRES is that the neuro-imaging features resolve, probably over several days to weeks, although in one series of patients with PRES from multiple causes, the earliest neuroimaging resolution was seen in 5 days (261). However, in a proportion of patients, some areas of cytotoxic oedema, which show up as areas of restricted diffusion on DWI MRI, and which imply areas of irreversible ischaemic injury, are sometimes seen. In a proportion of cases, resolution is not complete and some residual lesions are seen on follow-up MRI consistent with areas of infarction, focal gliosis or laminar necrosis (262,264).

The treatment of pre-eclampsia/eclampsia is covered in chapter 10 and entails control of seizures, control of blood pressure and delivery. In cases of mild pre-eclampsia, delivery may be delayed in cases of severe prematurity, provided the mother remains stable and there are no signs of fetal distress. However, in cases of severe pre-eclampsia/eclampsia, immediate delivery is essential. Magnesium sulphate has been shown to be superior to anticonvulsants and to diazepam in the control of eclamptic seizures and is also useful in the treatment of pre-eclampsia.

It is important to remember that seizures in pregnancy are not always due to eclampsia and other diagnoses must be considered. CVST is a very important differential diagnosis since it commonly also presents with headache and seizures and though hypertension and proteinuria are not a feature of this condition, both of these are relatively common in pregnancy and may coexist. Furthermore, ICH is not uncommon in pre-eclampsia/eclampsia. Thus, if the clinical picture is classical for eclampsia, with hypertension and proteinuria, perhaps preceded by pre-eclampsia, then in the hyperacute phase, it is reasonable to treat as eclampsia with magnesium sulphate and antihypertensives. However, if the patient does not respond rapidly to standard treatment for eclampsia, or if the clinical picture is not classical for eclampsia without associated hypertension or proteinuria, urgent CT scan of the brain with CT venogram should be sought to rule out an underlying haemorrhage, CVST or other diagnosis. This is important since treatment of the seizures would be different in the case of a different neurologic diagnosis and would

require the use of standard anticonvulsants, such as intravenous phenytoin. In addition, it is essential not to miss the diagnosis of CVST, as this would require immediate treatment with anticoagulation to prevent further propagation of thrombosis and to help prevent further venous infarction, thus aiming to prevent further disability and even mortality. In one study of 24 pregnant women who presented with various neurologic disorders, 10 patients presented with seizures and were suspected to have eclampsia, but only two of these patients actually turned out to have eclampsia on further investigation. Thus the assumption that seizures in pregnancy and the puerperium represented eclampsia resulted in delay in diagnosis in 8 out of these 10 patients (14).

Amniotic fluid embolism. Amniotic fluid embolism is a rare condition which has been reported as occurring in about 1/8000 to 1/80,000 pregnancies (265) but in a recent U.K. Amniotic Fluid Embolism Register held between 2005 and 2009, it was found to occur in 1/50,000 pregnancies (266). Mortality has gradually dropped over time and it now accounts for about 13% of direct maternal deaths in the United Kingdom as well as in the United States, France, Canada and Australia, but in other parts of the world, mortality is still higher and in Singapore, amniotic fluid embolism accounts for about 30% of maternal deaths (266).

Amniotic fluid embolism occurs when amniotic fluid enters the maternal circulation via the uterine veins. It results in a multisystem disorder involving mainly the cardiovascular, pulmonary and haematological systems. It is thought that an immunologic process resulting in activation of complement and of the clotting cascade results in pulmonary collapse, severe pulmonary vasoconstriction and thrombosis deaths (266). A form of anaphylactic reaction to the fetal cells that enter the maternal circulation has also been proposed (265).

The commonest presentation of amniotic fluid embolism is the sudden onset of dyspnoea with respiratory distress, hypotension, circulatory collapse, cardiac arrest, seizures and DIC, with profound fetal distress (265,267). Some premonitory symptoms may occur in about 47% of patients but these are rather non-specific and include numbness, tingling, paraesthesia in the finger tips, light-headedness, chest pain, breathlessness and feeling cold (265). In about 32% of cases, fetal distress may occur before any evident changes in the mother (268).

Amniotic fluid embolism is one of the pregnancy-specific causes of stroke (12) and in one series only 15% of mothers who sustained amniotic fluid embolism, or 39% of the survivors, survived neurologically intact (265), while in another series only 2 out of 31 survivors (6.5%) had long-term neurologic deficits (268). However, as described above, the presentation is not usually that of a straightforward stroke. Neurologic deficits have been described in survivors as a result of cerebral hypoperfusion with resultant ischaemia, secondary to the severe hypotension and even cardiac arrest. Another mechanism is paradoxical embolisation of amniotic fluid to the brain in patients with a PFO or ASD. In one recent case report, a mother who was clinically diagnosed with amniotic fluid embolism was noted to have a hemiparesis, dysphasia and a homonymous hemianopia on extubation, with bilateral anterior and posterior circulation infarcts confirmed on MRI. She was documented to have an ASD and it was thought most likely that she had sustained a paradoxical embolism, accounting for all the features of the case (269). In reports of another case, a large mass was visualised on echo passing from the right atrium to the left and straddling a PFO in a patient with a syndrome consistent with a severe amniotic fluid embolism. This patient was treated with cardiopulmonary bypass until the pulmonary resistance improved and the visualised clot was surgically removed. On histological examination of this clot, there were clearly fetal squamous cells that were positive for cytokeratin, suggesting that it had formed as the result of amniotic embolism. Although this patient did not actually sustain a stroke, this case proves that paradoxical embolism of amniotic material via a PFO or ASD may occur (270–272).

Choriocarcinoma. Choriocarcinoma may develop after any type of pregnancy (273) and occurs in about 1 in 50,000 deliveries (274). Choriocarcinoma may metastasise to the brain and may present with focal signs and symptoms of a space-occupying lesion, which may be confused for a stroke (275). However, it has a predilection to invade blood vessels and may cause (*i*) infarction by local arterial occlusion (276) or by embolic arterial occlusion (277), (*ii*) intraparenchymal haemorrhage by invasion through a blood vessel wall (275,278–281) or (*iii*) SAH by formation of a metastatic arterial aneurysm (282–284). Formation of a carotid-cavernous fistula by invasion of metastases has also been described (282). The stroke may sometimes be the first presentation of an otherwise unsuspected choriocarcinoma. In these case reports, diagnosis was sometimes made on histological examination of the vessel wall on evacuation of the haematoma. Treatment of the stroke is primarily the treatment of the cerebral metastases with chemotherapy, together with supportive care and rehabilitation. The majority of patients respond well to chemotherapy even in the presence of cerebral or pulmonary meatstases.

CEREBRAL VENOUS SINUS THROMBOSIS

CVST is a relatively uncommon cause of stroke, accounting for about 0.5% to 1% of all strokes (201) and about 2% of strokes in pregnancy and the puerperium (10). Pregnancy and the puerperium with the associated hypercoagulable state constitute an important risk factor for CVST and the association between pregnancy and CVST has been consistently reported (10,11,15,16,21,22,25). As mentioned earlier, the reported incidence in the United States is approximately 11–12/100,000 deliveries (15,23) but it may be significantly higher in other parts of the world with estimates calculated at 10 times higher in some developing countries (25,285). In the International Study on Cerebral Venous and Dural Sinus Thrombosis (ISCVT), a large international observational cohort study, pregnancy and the puerperium were associated with CVST in 12.3% of all cases of CVST in the study and with 17% of the cases of CVST in women (286), while in a study from Mexico about half of the cases of CVST occurred in association with pregnancy and the puerperium (25). It has been noted that women with gender-specific risk factors, including pregnancy and the puerperium, who develop CVST tend to be younger than their non-pregnant counterparts without such risk factors (286).

The greatest risk for CVST is in the puerperium and to a lesser extent in the third trimester of pregnancy – especially peripartum (10,13,16,22,25,287). The hypercoagulable state of pregnancy persists for about 6 weeks into the puerperium and it is thought that this is what underlies the increased risk of CVST. It is thought that this is probably made worse after delivery as a result of volume depletion and trauma as well as by instrumentation, caesarean section and infection (201). In one study, the risk of developing peripartum or post-partum

CVST was associated with increasing maternal age, larger hospital size and with delivery by caesarean section, as well as with comorbidities such as hypertension, infections – other than influenza and pneumonia – and with excess vomiting (22).

Inherited thrombophilias, as mentioned above, have been associated with an increased risk of venous thromboembolism, including CVST, and it is thought that the combination of pregnancy and an inherited thrombophilia, such as antithrombin deficiency, protein C or protein S deficiency, activated protein C resistance secondary to factor V Leiden mutation or G20210 prothrombin mutation (288–292), act synergistically to increase the risk of venous thromboembolic events in pregnancy and the puerperium (207) and may predispose to thrombosis in 'unusual sites' such as CVST (293). It also seems that in some cases, having an inherited thrombophilic defect predisposes to a venous thrombosis early in pregnancy and sometimes even in the first trimester (293,294), which is relatively unusual as VTE most commonly occurs in the third trimester or in the post-partum period.

A similar interaction with other acquired prothrombotic risk factors is also likely to occur and CVST in the puerperium has been reported with hyperhomocysteinaemia, which may be hereditary or acquired (28), as well as in association with aCLs (295). The risk seems to be even greater when multiple thrombophilic defects and prothrombotic risk factors are found in combination (296,297). The presence of a hyperviscosity or hypercoagulable state will further increase the risk of CVST, thus coexistant conditions such as SCD, malignancy, paroxysmal nocturnal haemoglobinuria and polycythaemia may all precipitate CVST in pregnancy or the puerperium, as is the case with conventional risk factors such as sepsis, dehydration or severe anaemia (298).

CVST may present with focal features and therefore may sometimes have a stroke-like presentation. When focal features occur, it is usually as a result of focal cerebral damage secondary to venous infarction and/or haemorrhage. The exact features will therefore depend on the location of the affected area. It is not unusual for multifocal or progressive focal neurologic deficits to occur. Hemiparesis and dysphasia are common symptoms, but other cortical features may be seen and if the deep venous system is involved, there may be associated thalamic infarction and swelling with agitation and amnesia.

Focal features secondary to venous infarction are usually accompanied by features due to raised ICP which results from occlusion of venous drainage. Thus headache tends to occur in 90% of cases of CVST (299) and tends to be diffuse. However, it may also have migrainous features and rarely may even be thunderclap in onset (300), necessitating differentiation from a SAH. The headache is frequently associated with papilloedema and may be associated with a sixth nerve palsy as a false localising sign of raised ICP. Sometimes the patient presents only with features of raised ICP without ever developing focal features of venous infarction. In these cases, the headache may become chronic and is usually associated with papilloedema. However, isolated headache without papilloedema may sometimes occur and in these cases the diagnosis of CVST may require a higher index of suspicion and is not infrequently delayed. In the case of CVST in pregnancy and the puerperium, however, patients tend to progress quite rapidly from onset of headache to more worrying features – and tend to present with headache of a few days' duration with focal neurologic deficits, ± alteration of level of consciousness ± seizures.

Dural sinus thrombosis tends to be associated with significant venous obstruction and may therefore be associated with significant cerebral oedema. In addition, focal venous infarction may itself be associated with post-infarct swelling and there may also be associated space occupation if there is significant haemorrhage. Thus, CVST may be associated with significant elevation in ICP which may sometimes prove fatal.

It is important to note that one of the more dangerous presentations of CVST is of a patient presenting with seizures and alteration of level of consciousness in late pregnancy or in the post-partum period. This is very similar to a possible presentation of eclampsia. It is thus important to have a high index of suspicion and to be aware that not every seizure in pregnancy and the puerperium is due to eclampsia. If usual associated features of eclampsia, such as proteinuria and oedema are absent, or if the patient being treated for eclampsia does not make a very rapid recovery with magnesium sulphate or develops focal neurologic features, the possibility of CVST must be considered and investigated appropriately with immediate scanning (see chapter 2).

Venous sinus thrombosis may be confirmed on imaging. If there is focal venous infarction or haemorrhage, the fact that the infarcts tend not to respect arterial territories and tend to be superficial and lobar raises the suspicion of venous infarction. Thrombus in the dural sinuses may sometimes be visualised on cross-sectional imaging but frequently dedicated venous imaging is required to confirm the venous sinus thrombosis. MRV is preferred over CTV in pregnancy since it can visualise the cerebral venous system without requiring contrast and without radiation exposure, thus minimising danger to the fetus. Isolated cortical vein thrombosis is more difficult to identify with certainty and needs MRI for diagnosis.

Treatment of acute venous sinus thrombosis requires full-dose anticoagulation. If the acute venous thrombosis occurs in pregnancy, then the treatment of choice is weight-adjusted full-treatment doses of LMWH, administered in two doses per day and adjusted according to anti-factor Xa activity, or, in certain circumstances, UFH, with the dose adjusted according to APTT (101,201). This should continue throughout pregnancy and the puerperium, although one may switch to oral anticoagulation with warfarin in the post-partum phase. If the acute venous thrombosis occurs during the puerperium, treatment is usually started with LMWH followed by oral anticoagulation with warfarin aiming for an INR of 2 to 3. Treatment should be continued for the duration for the pregnancy and for at least 6 weeks post-partum. The total duration of treatment should be no less than 6 months (101,201). Since the major underlying problem is venous occlusion, it is important to treat with anticoagulation even in the presence of initial haemorrhagic infarction, since this is the result of the raised venous pressure and may not settle unless propagation of the venous occlusion can be halted. Benefit and relative safety of treatment with anticoagulation have been demonstrated (301,302). However, patients who do present with significant haemorrhage at time of diagnosis tend to have poor outcomes, with and without anticoagulation.

In some cases, progression of venous thrombosis continues despite treatment with full-dose anticoagulation. In these cases, if there is clinical deterioration despite treatment, one may consider neuroradiologic intervention and treatment with intra-sinus administration of thrombolytics or direct mechanical thrombectomy. This is reserved for life-threatening cases, not responding to usual measures and must be performed at a specialised centre with the necessary expertise.

The patient needs very close neurologic monitoring and should be nursed in a specialised neurology or stroke unit. If seizures occur anticonvulsants are required to prevent further seizures. The choice of anticonvulsant may be guided by the mother's condition and the stage of pregnancy. There is a risk of developing hydrocephalus which may require urgent neurosurgical intervention. It is also important to be aware that CVST may be associated with significant raised ICP so monitoring of visual acuity is essential. If there is any deterioration of vision, then measures should be instituted to manage the intracranial hypertension.

It is essential to test for inherited or acquired thrombophilias. Initial testing should be carried out at the time of diagnosis, before starting anticoagulation. However, protein C and S levels are not reliable in the acute phase or in pregnancy and the puerperium, so these are usually tested about 4 weeks after the initial course of anticoagulation is completed. It is important to test for the known hereditary and acquired thrombophilias described above, and not to simply ascribe the venous thrombosis to the pregnant or puerperal state (299), since as mentioned above, various risk factors for venous thrombosis often coexist and interact to precipitate the acute event. If an associated thrombophilic state is diagnosed, then one may require lifelong anticoagulation, depending on the risk profile of the thrombophilia (see section 'Thrombophilias' above), but if no other cause for the thrombosis is found and it is thought to be purely related to the pregnant/puerperal state, possibly precipitated by a transient risk factor, such as sepsis, then the patient would not require indefinite anticoagulation but would need prophylaxis with LMWH during subsequent pregnancies (201).

Some small studies have followed the risk of recurrence of CVST in subsequent pregnancies, after experiencing a CVST and this risk appears to be low (34,37,303). It is therefore felt that one episode of CVST should not be a contraindication to further pregnancies. However, appropriate prophylactic regimens with LMWH during pregnancy and the puerperium should be followed (201).

Although CVST may be so severe as to be fatal, in most cases, if the patient survives the acute phase, the outcome tends to very good. It has been consistently reported that patients who develop CVST in the context of pregnancy or the puerperium tend to do better than their counterparts without this risk factor, and make a better recovery (25,286,304).

PITUITARY APOPLEXY

Pituitary apoplexy is the clinical syndrome of acute haemorrhage, infarction or haemorrhagic infarction, usually into an existing pituitary adenoma or, rarely, into a physiologically enlarging pituitary, as in pregnancy (see chapter 18). A case of apoplexy into lymphocytic hypophysitis has also been reported (305). The symptoms of apoplexy may result from the sudden expansion of the pituitary, as a result of the acute haemorrhage or ischaemia, with local mass effect on surrounding structures, or from acute resultant pituitary dysfunction with pituitary insufficiency. Thus, the patient may present with symptoms ranging from a combination of acute onset of headache with nausea and vomiting, visual field deficits, including blindness, and ophthalmoplegia, which result from mass effect on the parasellar regions and the cavernous sinus, to decreased level of consciousness, coma and circulatory collapse secondary to the acute pituitary insufficiency, leading to severe adrenal insufficiency and shock. This may be life-threatening. The headache may be so abrupt in onset as to suggest an SAH and patients are frequently initially misdiagnosed and worked up for a possible SAH (306) if the correct diagnosis is not immediately considered. There are a few rare reports of pituitary apoplexy causing carotid ischaemia by compression or spasm of the intracavernous portion of the carotid artery. This results in ischaemic stroke in the distribution of the carotid artery with associated focal neurologic deficits, including hemiparesis (307). Vasospam may sometimes occur as a result of seepage of necrotic material or blood into the subarachnoid space (308).

Apoplexy may occur into known pituitary tumours, but in about 80% of cases it is the first presentation of a previously undiagnosed pituitary lesion (309). It is thought that pregnancy predisposes to pituitary apoplexy because of the physiological expansion of the pituitary as a result of the hormonal changes in pregnancy.

MRI is the investigation of choice but sometimes the urgency of the situation may require immediate CT scanning at initial presentation to help exclude other causes for the clinical picture. It is important to bear in mind that routine axial CT scan may sometimes exclude the sella and may not detect a pituitary lesion unless the area of interest is specified (310). It is therefore important to have a high index of suspicion.

Pituitary apoplexy is a medical emergency and resuscitation and haemodynamic stabilisation of the patient are the first priority. Even patients who appear clinically well require close monitoring to ensure that they remain haemodynamically stable. High-dose steroids are required as replacement therapy for the glucocorticoid deficiency, but also to help prevent swelling and further compression of the parasellar structures. Treatment is usually started with hydrocortisone 50 mg intravenously 6 hourly (311), though this is commonly switched to dexamethasone once the patient is more stable. Any concerns regarding the use of steroids in pregnancy must be balanced against the mother's condition and clinical need. If pituitary apoplexy occurs in pregnancy, however, it tends to occur late in pregnancy when the use of steroids is not considered to pose a risk to the fetus. Other hormonal deficiencies require investigation and replacement as appropriate. Assessment of the patient's vision, including acuity and visual fields is essential and requires close monitoring to ensure that any deterioration of vision is immediately noted.

Management of the pituitary lesion itself most often depends on the patient's general condition, level of consciousness and the presence of visual impairment. In cases where the patient presents with mild symptoms and has no significant visual loss, no progressive deterioration in vision and no deterioration in level of consciousness, or in cases where the patient responds very rapidly to steroids, some will advocate conservative management (312,313). However, patients with persistent or deteriorating neurologic symptoms, hypothalamic dysfunction or patients showing rapid deterioration require urgent surgical decompression of the pituitary lesion (306,311). If trans-sphenoidal surgery is deemed necessary, then it is usually recommended within the first week of the acute event to maximise chances of improvement. Trans-sphenoidal surgery is not contraindicated in pregnancy and has been carried out successfully during gestation (138,314–317).

The classical eponymous syndrome Sheehan syndrome refers to ischaemic necrosis of the pituitary due to severe post-partum haemorrhage. Although few patients with this syndrome develop symptoms acutely with a presentation of pituitary apoplexy, most patients with Sheehan syndrome have mild disease and some degree of hypopituitarism may not be diagnosed for several years (318).

INTRACRANIAL HAEMORRHAGE

ICH may be divided into intraparenchymal haemorrhage and SAH. As mentioned above, ICH has been reported in 3 to 9/100,000 pregnancies (10–14,16,17,21) except in Taiwan where the haemorrhage rate is in the region of 20 (18) to 31 (20)/100,000 deliveries (Table 16.1). One large American study, which utilised the Nationwide Inpatient Sample between 1993 and 2001, demonstrated an increased rate of ICH in pregnancy compared to non-pregnant women in the same age group since the rate of pregnancy-related haemorrhage was 6.1/100,000 deliveries, which was equivalent to 7.1 haemorrhages per 100,000 at-risk person-years while the rate in non-pregnant women was 5/100,000 person-years (19). Haemorrhage may occur at any time in pregnancy, but in most series it was most likely to occur in the post-partum period or possibly late in pregnancy (10–13,17–19). In the Nationwide Inpatient Sample between 1993 and 2001, the rate of ICH in the antenatal period was similar to that in non-pregnant patients of the same age but increased significantly in the post-partum period (19). However, the timing of bleeding in pregnancy does seem to depend to some extent on the underlying aetiology, and in one study of pregnancy-related haemorrhages caused exclusively by aneurysms and arteriovenous malformations (AVMs), 92% of bleeds occurred antenatally and only 8% in the post-partum period (319). There appears to be a tendency for aneurysms to bleed more with advancing gestational age (319,320), but with regard to AVMs, while some report an increasing tendency to bleed with increasing gestational age (319), others report the major risk of haemorrhage from AVMs in the second trimester, as well as occurring around delivery and early in the post-partum period (16,320).

ICH accounts for 25% to 51% of pregnancy-related strokes (10,12,13,16). Mortality of pregnancy-related ICHs has been reported at about 20% to 25% (12,16,19) and in the analysis of the Nationwide Inpatient Sample, deaths as a result of pregnancy-related ICH accounted for 7.1% of all pregnancy-related mortality for the study period. In fact, SAH has been cited as the third leading non-obstetric cause of death in pregnant women (321). Morbidity is also worse for ICHs with about 30% to 63% of patients who sustain a pregnancy-related ICH being discharged to another medical facility – usually a nursing home or rehabilitation facility – rather than being discharged home (19,39). Risk factors for pregnancy-related ICH noted in various studies include age above 35 years, African-American race, pre-existing or pregnancy-induced hypertension, coagulopathy, thrombocytopaenia, cigarette smoking, use of illicit drugs, especially cocaine, and excessive alcohol use (12,13,19).

The commonest causes of ICH in pregnancy are pre-eclampsia/eclampsia and cerebral vascular malformations, especially AVMs and aneurysms, but also including cavernomas (see chapter 17). Other reported causes include cocaine-induced vasculopathy, DIC or other coagulopathy, vasculitis, moyamoya syndrome or disease, choriocarcinoma or other tumour, sarcoid vasculopathy and infective endocarditis. The cause remains undetermined in a proportion of cases. The RCVS may sometimes result in a focal intraparenchymal haemorrhage. Pre-eclampsia/eclampsia has been reported to account for 15% to 44% of cases of pregnancy-related ICH and AVMs have been reported to account for 7%

to 38% of haemorrhages (12,13,16,18,19,39) in various cases series looking at all pregnancy-related stroke. However, in case series focusing on pregnancy-related ICH caused only by aneurysms and AVMs, aneurysms accounted for 64% to 77% of haemorrhages, while AVMs accounted for 23% to 36% (319,320).

Some of these cases series included SAH, while others excluded this condition. The commonest causes of SAH are rupture of a berry aneurysm or bleeding of an AVM, though other potential causes include trauma and eclampsia (322). RCVS may result in SAH but this is usually a localised small volume and focal cortical SAH of little clinical significance. Although one of the leading causes of SAH, AVMs are much more likely to cause intraparenchymal than SAH. There has been some controversy about the risk of bleeding from AVMs in pregnancy. Early reports had suggested that AVMs in pregnancy are associated with a fourfold increased risk of bleeding (320). However, more recent studies suggest that the risk of haemorrhage from an AVM in pregnancy is no different to that in the general population (323).

The clinical signs and symptoms of an ICH will depend on the type of haemorrhage and on the severity. SAH typically presents with thunderclap headache, with or without decreased level of consciousness and with or without focal symptoms and signs. Sometimes there may be a seizure at onset. The patient usually exhibits nuchal rigidity. Even if the patient appears to be showing relatively rapid signs of improvement, if the history is suggestive of a possible SAH, this must be excluded by emergency scanning, followed, if negative, by a lumbar puncture. If SAH is confirmed, MRA or other form of angiography is required to ascertain the underlying cause of the haemorrhage, seeking an underlying aneurysm or AVM (see section 'Investigation'). The patient will usually need to be nursed in a neurosurgical high dependency or critical care unit and is closely monitored for any neurologic deterioration. If the patient is on any antiplatelet agents, these are stopped immediately.

In the non-pregnant population, nimodipine is usually used prophylactically in cases of SAH to prevent the onset of vasospasm. This has been classified as a class C (see Editorial Note on the FDA classification of drugs and pregnancy) drug since teratogenic effects have been noted in animals, but the effects on humans is unclear although no harmful effects have been noted yet. However, nimodipine has been trialled in humans for pre-eclampsia, although magnesium was found to be superior (324), and it has also been used in pregnancy in patients with bipolar disorder (325) with no adverse fetal effects recorded. It is therefore considered that nimodipine may be used to prevent vasospasm if the benefit is felt to outweigh the risk. This decision may be partly affected by the stage in pregnancy and the characteristics of the haemorrhage. If vasospasm does set in, then it must be aggressively treated with triple-H therapy (hypervolaemic, hypertensive, haemodilutional therapy), together with nimodipine. Neurointerventional treatment such as angioplasty of a focal area of spasm may be a possible alternative. Depending on the stage of pregnancy and on the patient's general condition prophylactic anticonvulsants in a patient who has not experienced a seizure may be deferred, unless the mother is deemed to be at high risk. Treatment of the underlying aneurysm or AVM is covered elsewhere in the book and is an important consideration (see chapter 6c).

An intraparenchymal haemorrhage of relatively small volume will present with abrupt onset of focal neurologic deficit suggestive of a stroke, usually in association with a significant headache. The patient may show signs of progressive deterioration over a few hours, if the size of the haemorrhage expands. However, a haemorrhage of large volume at onset may present with headache, impaired level of consciousness, focal neurologic deficits and seizures. In this setting, the priority is to ensure that the patient is haemodynamically stable and to proceed to brain scanning at the earliest opportunity. This is usually an emergency situation, so CT scanning with abdominal shielding if the patient is in the antenatal period is usually more readily available and easier to perform than MRI. The patient will usually need supportive care and may need to be nursed in a neurosurgical high dependency unit or a stroke unit. Where possible, the primary treatment should be aimed at the underlying cause of the haemorrhage, for example, treatment of the underlying pre-eclampsia/eclampsia or the underlying coagulopathy. Neurosurgical decisions should be based on usual neurosurgical principles (319). Thus intervention for clot evacuation in case of neurologic deterioration, where the haemorrhage is causing significant mass effect, or ventricular drainage in case of development of hydrocephalus may be required, but these decisions must be tailor-made to the patient and her condition. If an underlying lesion is identified, then treatment must be considered (see chapter 6c). It is recommended that any decision regarding the need for early delivery of the baby and the mode of delivery should be made primarily on obstetric considerations (319,326).

There have been reports of women undergoing subsequent uneventful pregnancies after an episode of pregnancy-related ICH. In one study of 52 patients with pregnancy-related ICH, 9 patients subsequently became pregnant again and none of them experienced recurrent haemorrhage. It was concluded that the decision regarding future pregnancies should not be influenced by the neurologic condition but should be individualised on obstetric grounds (326).

INVESTIGATION

An overview is presented here with specific investigations already discussed in relevant sections.

If a lady who is pregnant or in the puerperium develops sudden onset of a neurologic deficit suggestive of a stroke, she will need immediate medical attention and should be treated as an emergency. A full and detailed history of the acute event, together with past medical and obstetric history, history of risk factors, family history, medication and drug history is essential. Neurologic, general and obstetric examination looking for clues as to the diagnosis and a possible underlying cause is important. It is important to perform fundoscopy, which may reveal pailloedema in cases of pre-eclampsia/eclampsia, venous sinus thrombosis, or other causes of raised ICP, or which may reveal irregular blood vessels or retinal microvascular ischaemic changes, suggestive of a vasculitic process. One must consider potential non-stroke differential diagnoses such as migraine, seizure with Todd's paralysis, hypoglycaemia with focal neurologic deficits and tumour. At the same time, the various characteristics of the stroke syndromes in pregnancy or the puerperium, as described above, should be borne in mind to help reach a likely diagnosis and probable differential as to the underlying aetiology.

Brain scanning is essential to help distinguish between ischaemic stroke and haemorrhage. Over all one tends to prefer MRI rather than CT scanning in pregnancy to avoid radiation exposure. However, in an emergency situation, if MRI is not readily available, then CT scan with abdominal shielding is performed. In the case of the post-partum patient, where there is no contraindication to CT scanning, this is the usual initial investigation of choice to help exclude an acute haemorrhage. In the early hours of an ischaemic stroke there may only be subtle changes on the CT scan to suggest an underlying ischaemic process and repeat imaging is usually required to confirm the diagnosis.

As discussed above, in the case of young women, who sustain a stroke in pregnancy and the puerperium, there is a wide range of potential underlying causes for an ischaemic stroke. MRI with DWI is extremely sensitive to even minute areas of ischaemia and may expose patterns of ischaemia that are not readily obvious on clinical examination and which may not be visible even on delayed CT scan. This may guide diagnosis and further investigation. Thus, for example, in a patient with clinical signs and symptoms of a localised infarct, MRI with DWI may unexpectedly reveal a shower of multiple asymptomatic areas of infarction in both hemispheres, suggesting a cardioembolic source or some other diffuse process, rather than the localised infarct suggested by the clinical examination; alternatively, it may reveal a very superficial pattern of haemorrhagic infarction, suggesting venous rather than arterial infarction, etc.

In this age group, arteriopathies are also important causes of ischaemic stroke, and visualisation of the intracranial blood vessels is desirable. Thus MRI with intracranial MRA provides a non-invasive examination of the blood vessels without radiation exposure and without the need for contrast dye, both of which may be detrimental to the fetus. If the clinical picture is suggestive of a venous sinus thrombosis then MRV is essential. In the post-partum period, CTA or CT venogram (CTV) may be preferred for clearer imaging of the vasculature.

Intraparenchymal haemorrhage is readily visible on the initial plain CT scan. MRI may be required to look for an underlying lesion such as a tumour or a cavernoma or an AVM. Sometimes as underlying lesion may be obscured by the haematoma on an early MRI and this may need to be delayed to at least 6 weeks post-haemorrhage to allow time for the volume of blood to decrease in size.

SAH may be visible on the initial CT scan, but if the clinical picture is highly suggestive of an SAH with thunderclap headache at onset but a negative CT scan, lumbar puncture looking for xanthochromia and blood degradation products is the gold standard and must be performed to completely exclude an SAH in these circumstances. It is true that post-partum cerebral angiopathy (or the RCVS) also presents with thunderclap headache, often with a negative CT scan, but it is a criterion for diagnosis of this syndrome that SAH as a cause for the symptoms and the vasospasm is excluded. Thus, even when suspecting RCVS, lumbar puncture should definitely be performed in cases of CT negative thunderclap headache. Xanthochromia is caused by breakdown products of Hb, reflecting a bleed into the subarachnoid space at some time prior to the time of the lumbar puncture. This process usually takes a few hours, so it is usual to wait 12 hours from the onset of symptoms before performing the procedure, to allow time for blood degradation products to start to form, thus avoiding any confusion with blood introduced traumatically at the time of the lumbar puncture (327). The cerebrospinal fluid (CSF) may be inspected visually for xanthochromia but must be sent for bilirubin analysis by spectrophotometry (327). If SAH is confirmed then the source of bleeding must be carefully sought. If the patient is post-partum, then CTA is the usual first-line investigation, but if this is negative it is usually followed by digital subtraction angiography (DSA). If the patient is pregnant at time of presentation, then initial screening with MRA may be reasonable, since this will usually detect aneurysms at least 3 mm in size and larger. However, if the responsible aneurysm or malformation is not found on MRA, angiography would be essential, as re-bleeding of an unsecured aneurysm could be catastrophic with fatal consequences or severe resulting disability.

Ultrasound carotid doppler examination is commonly used to visualise the extracranial carotid arteries in the neck and to exclude cervical carotid artery stenosis or occlusion. It may sometimes suggest the presence of a cervical artery dissection and may indicate the presence of a more distal stenosis. The vertebral flow is commonly also visualised along part of its course in the neck. However, if an underlying arteriopathy, including cervical artery dissection, is suspected, more detailed examination of the extracranial blood vessels is required. In the post-partum patient, CTA may be the first investigation of choice for clear delineation of the extracranial vasculature starting from their origins. However, if the patient is still pregnant and visualisation is required, it may be reasonable to start with MRA as the initial investigation to avoid radiation exposure. However, it may be necessary to proceed to CTA or formal DSA, if clinical doubt remains and further imaging is required for a definite diagnosis as the risks of missing a dissection could be devastating.

Initial blood investigations should include routine tests such as full blood count, including platelet count and haematocrit, Erythrocyte Sedimentation Rate (ESR), renal and liver function tests, fasting blood glucose, fasting lipid profile and clotting screen. Urine dipstick for proteinuria is essential to assess whether the patient may be pre-eclamptic or eclamptic depending on the clinical picture.

Tests for aCLs, LA and, in selected cases, anti-β_2GP1 antibodies are essential. If any of these are positive, then they must be repeated after 3 months to ensure that they are persistently positive and truly significant (see section 'Antiphospholipid Antibody Syndrome'). Other tests for inherited thrombophilias are usually also performed in this age group and include protein C, protein S and antithrombin levels, activated protein C resistance and DNA for factor V Leiden mutation, GP20210A prothrombin mutation and MTHFR mutation. Elevated homocysteine is an important potential risk factor and serum levels may be estimated. There is some debate as to whether the coagulation factors should be measured in arterial strokes since they are so much more clearly associated with venous thrombosis rather than with arterial. However, there probably appears to be a weak link with arterial stroke, especially in those under the age of 50, so it is still usual to test for these factors in young patients with arterial ischaemic strokes, especially in the absence of traditional risk factors (see section 'Inherited Thrombophilias'). However, they are extremely important in the case of venous thrombosis. Testing is usually performed at presentation, even though the results of some of the coagulation factors may be transiently reduced in the acute phase of a stroke and even though pregnancy itself results in alteration of some coagulation factors. If there is an abnormality of the levels of coagulation factors, they must be repeated about 3 months post-partum. Of course, pregnancy or the acute phase of a stroke will not alter the presence or absence of a genetic prothrombotic mutation.

Cardiac imaging is usually required, especially if a cardioembolic source is suspected. Transthoracic echocardiogram gives best views of the ventricles, but if used in combination with bubble contrast administered intravenously, it may be used to assess the integrity of the interatrial septum for the presence of a PFO. Transoesophageal echocardiogram gives better views of the atria and of the interatrial septum. It is therefore sometimes used first line in the evaluation of a PFO, or may be used after transthoracic echo to confirm the presence and morphology of a PFO detected with bubble contrast. It is also the preferred investigation if views of the left atrial appendage are required to rule out atrial clot or in cases of suspected bacterial endocarditis.

Further investigation will be guided by the individual's history and clinical examination. Thus, for example, in a patient with a history suggestive of a rheumatological condition, testing for other antibodies such as antinuclear antibodies, extractable nuclear antigens, antineutrophilic cytoplasmic antibodies, anti-double-stranded DNA antibodies and complement levels may be required; in a patient with probable FMD a renal angiogram may be required.

TREATMENT OF ISCHAEMIC STROKE

Pregnancy has been considered a relative contraindication to thrombolysis and has largely been an exclusion criterion for participation in trials for thrombolysis of acute ischaemic stroke. Thus, there is no evidence from randomised controlled trials regarding the use of thrombolysis in pregnancy-related stroke. In the non-pregnant population, the National Institute of Neurological Disorders and Stroke (NINDS) trial had shown that treatment with intravenous recombinant tissue plasminogen activator (tPA) within 3 hours of onset of stroke symptoms was associated with a significant increase in better recovery at the end of 3 months in treated patients (39% vs. 26%) (328). However, this was associated with a significant increased risk of haemorrhage of 6.4% in the treated group versus 0.6% in the placebo group. Despite this, there was no increased mortality in the treated group at the end of 3 months. A modest improvement was also seen when treated between 3 and 4.5 hours of symptom onset (329). There are a few case reports of thrombolysis of ischaemic stroke in pregnancy (330–334), and many more reported cases of the use of thrombolytics for other non-stroke diagnoses, including myocardial infarction, pulmonary embolism, thrombosed artificial heart valves and superior vena cava syndrome in pregnancy with relatively good maternal outcomes (335). The major maternal concerns regarding the use of thrombolytics in pregnancy include the risk of ICH, the risk of extracranial haemorrhage and the possibility of placental or uterine haemorrhage or haematoma. The major fetal concerns relate to the risk of effects on the placenta with possible premature labour, placental abruption or fetal loss, together with the risk of teratogenicity (334). Women with pregnancy-related stroke who were treated with intravenous or intra-arterial tPA in pregnancy, mainly responded well to the treatment and enjoyed good recovery (330–334). One patient died of a malignant MCA infarct secondary to dissection complicating angiography when an interventional approach to treatment was used. Three patients experienced asymptomatic ICHs, but there were no symptomatic ICHs resulting in any clinical deterioration (330,334).

TPA is classified as a category C drug, which implies that its effects on the human fetus are not known. However, it does not cross the placenta and there has been no evidence of teratogenicity in animal studies (336). One paper reported a case series of 22 cases of thrombolysis in pregnancy (10 for strokes and 12 for non-stroke diagnoses) with a literature review of the use of thrombolysis in pregnancy (334). Out of these 22 cases, healthy babies were delivered in 11 cases (50%) at term or preterm. Of the remainder, one baby died 14 days after delivery, there were two spontaneous abortions in the first trimester and four terminations of pregnancy. There was not enough information about the fetal outcome in the remainder of these pregnancies. The number of reported cases is too small to reach any firm conclusions regarding the safety of tPA in pregnancy and the potential effects on the fetus remain largely unknown. However, it appears that thrombolysis of acute ischaemic stroke in pregnancy may be relatively safe, although the risks and benefits to both mother and fetus must be carefully considered in taking such a decision. Intra-arterial thrombolysis delivers a smaller dose of drug to the mother and may therefore be associated with reduced risk to the mother and fetus. However, it is not suitable in all cases of stroke and is used primarily in cases of distal ICA or proximal MCA occlusion or in basilar thrombosis. It is not as readily available as intravenous thrombolysis since it requires specialised interventional expertise. Furthermore, it requires the use of angiography and although abdominal shielding is used it will entail some degree of radiation exposure to the fetus, as well as exposure to contrast. However, it may offer an alternative to intravenous thrombolysis in selected cases. Mechanical clot disrupters/clot retrieval systems are used in a similar setting as intra-arterial thrombolysis and require the same expertise and are associated with the same exposure to radiation and contrast. They may be preferred in pregnancy since they may be employed without the use of thrombolytic agents, but there are no data regarding their specific use in pregnancy. In light of the limited evidence, the 2008 guidelines of the ACCP concluded that the safety of thrombolysis in pregnancy was still unclear and it was recommended that thrombolysis in pregnancy should only be used in cases of life-threatening thromboembolism (101).

When a pregnant woman develops symptoms suggestive of an acute stroke, she should be treated as an emergency and should be reviewed immediately in an emergency department. It is clearly the first priority to ensure that she is cardiovascularly and haemodynamically stable and a rapid blood glucose estimation should be performed. She should be evaluated in a monitored setting with continuous cardiac monitoring, frequent blood pressure monitoring and frequent neurologic observations. A proper history is essential to help establish the diagnosis and to ascertain the exact time of onset of the stroke, or at least when the patient was last known to be well. When a precise time of onset is not available, the time when she was last seen well is taken to represent the time of onset of the stroke.

Especially if the patient is being considered for thrombolysis, or if the patient is deteriorating in any way, initial investigation must take place extremely rapidly. In the case of thrombolysis, treatment may only be given within 4.5 hours of onset of symptoms and within that time, the earlier treatment is begun, the better the outcomes and probably the safer the treatment. Thus, there really is no time to lose. The door-to-needle time refers to the time between reaching hospital (door) and starting thrombolytic therapy (needle) and spans the initial evaluation, initial investigations, consideration of results, reaching a diagnosis, taking the decision to start thrombolysis and proceeding to actually give the initial bolus. In the United Kingdom the gold standard for the door-to-needle time is 30 minutes, while in the United States, this is usually 60 minutes. However, one must never sacrifice safety for speed. If the patient receives thrombolysis then she is precluded from receiving antiplatelets or anticoagulants for 24 hours after the administration of thrombolysis and these agents should only be started if haemorrhage is excluded on the follow-up scan performed 24 hours post-thrombolysis.

If the patient is not considered to be a suitable candidate for thrombolysis, then secondary prevention becomes an immediate consideration. Antiplatelets are the cornerstone of secondary stroke prevention, except in clinical situations where anticoagulation is deemed necessary, for example, in cardioembolic strokes, in some thrombophilic states and in some cases of arterial dissection. Specific situations that require anticoagulation are addressed in the individual sections above.

In general, patients who would normally be treated with antiplatelets if they sustained a stroke in the non-pregnant state are also considered suitable for antiplatelet agents if they sustain a pregnancy-related stroke. Antiplatelets are also generally indicated in pregnancy if a patient had sustained a non-cardioembolic, non-pregnancy-related stroke prior to pregnancy.

Aspirin is the most commonly used antiplatelet agent in pregnancy-related stroke. It is considered safe in the second and third trimester; but, there is some controversy around its use in the first trimester of pregnancy. Animal studies have suggested an increased risk of fetal malformations and there have been multiple reports of congenital malformations in association with aspirin use in pregnancy. In fact, it has been classified as a category D drug, which means that there is some evidence of risk in humans, but that in some circumstances its benefits may outweigh the risks. However, a meta-analysis of the reports of malformations with first-trimester aspirin use did not show an increased overall risk of teratogenicity except perhaps for an increased risk of gastroschisis (337). One population-based case-controlled study of the use of aspirin in early pregnancy also showed no association with birth defects (338). Furthermore, early aspirin use is advocated in early pregnancy in the case of patients with APS with fetal loss (339,340) and in women at high risk of eclampsia (341), suggesting its relative safety.

In this setting, with limited data and no randomised case-controlled trials, the 2011 guidelines of the AHA for the prevention of stroke or TIA recommend using UFH or LMWH in the first trimester followed thereafter by low-dose aspirin throughout pregnancy in patients who would normally be considered suitable for antiplatelet agents outside of pregnancy (80). However, the eighth edition of the evidence-based clinical practice guidelines of the ACCP suggests that although the safety of aspirin in the first trimester remains uncertain, there is no clear evidence of harm to the fetus and that even if aspirin does cause any fetal anomalies by exposure in the first trimester, their incidence is extremely rare. This group therefore recommends that if there is a clear indication for aspirin with no satisfactory alternative agent, then patients should be offered aspirin even in the first trimester (101).

There is even less information on the use of clopidogrel in pregnancy. In practice, a poll of stroke neurologists in the United States showed that 51% of these practitioners would choose aspirin as their treatment of choice throughout pregnancy for secondary stroke prevention in patients who had previously sustained a non-cardioembolic stroke unrelated to pregnancy (342). A small percentage of practitioners, however, chose clopidogrel despite the lack of information about its effects in pregnancy.

For patients who require full-dose anticoagulation in pregnancy, the picture is a little more clear. Vitamin K antagonists, such as warfarin, do cross the placenta and their use throughout pregnancy has been associated with congenital anomalies and development of an embryopathy (343). This appears to result mainly from exposure to warfarin in the first trimester. Interestingly, however, this risk seems to be eliminated if warfarin is replaced at or before the 6th week of gestation (344) and is relatively high if the fetus is exposed to warfarin or other vitamin K antagonists between the 6th and 12th week of gestation. Exposure to warfarin during any trimester has been associated with structural central nervous system (CNS) abnormalities but these appear to be very rare (345). There also appears to be a small risk of mild neurodevelopmental problems, but their clinical significance is quite uncertain (346). Exposure to Vitamin K antagonists is also associated with fetal loss and fetal haemorrhagic complications. A fetal coagulopathy with excessive anticoagulation of the fetus, and therefore risk of bleeding, may occur if the mother is on warfarin at the time of delivery.

LMWH and UFH do not cross the placenta and there is no evidence that they may cause teratogenicity or fetal bleeding. They are therefore considered safe for the fetus (101).

In most cases, if the patient is already on warfarin at the time that she falls pregnant, the warfarin should be switched to UFH or LMWH before the 6th week of gestation and for the remainder of the pregnancy, until very close to delivery. In fact, the recommended strategy is that if a woman on warfarin is attempting to conceive, frequent pregnancy tests should be performed and the warfarin switched to UFH or LMWH as soon as pregnancy is detected (101). In this setting, it is essential that the patient is counselled regarding the risks of teratogenicity and fetal loss with warfarin and understands the importance of discontinuing warfarin before the 6th week of gestation. An alternative strategy would be to start treatment with heparin prior to conception.

LMWH is associated with a lower risk of osteoporosis and of HIT. Thus, if possible, use of LMWH is preferred to UFH in pregnancy (101). If aiming for full anticoagulation with heparin, weight-adjusted LMWH should be administered in two doses per day and the dose should be adjusted according to anti-factor Xa levels. If UFH is used, then the dose should be adjusted to maintain a therapeutic APTT.

If a patient is on heparin in pregnancy, it must be stopped very close to delivery and anticoagulation resumed post-partum.

If the patient is being maintained on long-term warfarin throughout pregnancy, for medical reasons, then this must be discontinued close to delivery to avoid delivering an anticoagulated child with the associated risks. In most cases warfarin is stopped about 3 weeks before delivery (101), or in the middle of the third trimester (80) and it is substituted with LMWH or UFH. This is then stopped very close to delivery and anticoagulation resumed after delivery.

CONCLUSION

Stroke in pregnancy and the puerperium is relatively rare but important because of the associated morbidity and mortality. Potential causes in this group of patients are diverse, but certain specific potential diagnoses should be considered. Patients who present with symptoms and signs of a stroke will need urgent evaluation and treatment. Such patients should be cared for jointly by a stroke specialist and obstetrician.

REFERENCES

1. Hatano S. Experience from a multicentre stroke register: a preliminary report. Bull World Health Organ 1976; 54(5):541–553 [Epub 1 Jan 1976].
2. Carroll JD, Leak D, Lee HA. Cerebral thrombophlebitis in pregnancy and the puerperium. Q J Med 1966; 35(139):347–368 [Epub 1 Jul 1966].

3. Symonds C. Cerebral thrombophlebitis. Br Med J 1940; 2: 348–352.

4. Martin J, Sheehan H. Primary thrombosis of cerebral veins (following childbirth). Br Med J 1941; 1:349–353.

5. Martin J. Thrombosis in the superior longitudinal sinus following childbirth. Br Med J 1941; 2:537–540.

6. Cross JN, Castro PO, Jennett WB. Cerebral strokes associated with pregnancy and the puerperium. Br Med J 1968; 3(5612):214–218 [Epub 27 Jul 1968].

7. Goldman JA, Eckerling B, Gans B. Intracranial venous sinus thrombosis in pregnancy and puerperium. Report of fifteen cases. J Obstet Gynaecol Br Commonw 1964; 71:791–796 [Epub 1 Oct 1964].

8. Huggenberg H, Kesselring F. Postpartum cerebral complications. Gynaecologia. International monthly review of obstetrics and gynecology. Revue internationale mensuelle d'obstetrique et de gynecologie Monatsschrift fur Geburtshilfe und Gynakologie 1958; 146(312–317):312.

9. Wiebers DO, Whisnant JP. The incidence of stroke among pregnant women in Rochester, Minn, 1955 through 1979. JAMA 1985; 254(21):3055–3057 [Epub 6 Dec 1985].

10. James AH, Bushnell CD, Jamison MG, et al. Incidence and risk factors for stroke in pregnancy and the puerperium. Obstet Gynecol 2005; 106(3):509–516 [Epub 2 Sept 2005].

11. Simolke GA, Cox SM, Cunningham FG. Cerebrovascular accidents complicating pregnancy and the puerperium. Obstet Gynecol 1991; 78(1):37–42 [Epub 1 Jul 1991].

12. Sharshar T, Lamy C, Mas JL. Incidence and causes of strokes associated with pregnancy and puerperium. A study in public hospitals of Ile de France. Stroke in Pregnancy Study Group. Stroke 1995; 26(6):930–936 [Epub 1 Jun 1995].

13. Kittner SJ, Stern BJ, Feeser BR, et al. Pregnancy and the risk of stroke. N Engl J Med 1996; 335(11):768–774 [Epub 12 Jul 1996].

14. Witlin AG, Friedman SA, Egerman RS, et al. Cerebrovascular disorders complicating pregnancy – beyond eclampsia. Am J Obstet Gynecol 1997; 176(6):1139–1145; discussion 45–48 [Epub 1 Jun 1997].

15. Lanska DJ, Kryscio RJ. Stroke and intracranial venous thrombosis during pregnancy and puerperium. Neurology 1998; 51 (6):1622–1628 [Epub 17 Dec 1998].

16. Jaigobin C, Silver FL. Stroke and pregnancy. Stroke 2000; 31 (12):2948–2951 [Epub 11 Jan 2000].

17. Ros HS, Lichtenstein P, Bellocco R, et al. Increased risks of circulatory diseases in late pregnancy and puerperium. Epidemiology 2001; 12(4):456–460 [Epub 21 Jun 2001].

18. Jeng JS, Tang SC, Yip PK. Incidence and etiologies of stroke during pregnancy and puerperium as evidenced in Taiwanese women. Cerebrovasc Dis 2004; 18(4):290–295 [Epub 28 Aug 2004].

19. Bateman BT, Schumacher HC, Bushnell CD, et al. Intracerebral hemorrhage in pregnancy: frequency, risk factors, and outcome. Neurology 2006; 67(3):424–429 [Epub 9 Aug 2006].

20. Liang CC, Chang SD, Lai SL, et al. Stroke complicating pregnancy and the puerperium. Eur J Neurol 2006; 13(11):1256–1260 [Epub 14 Oct 2006].

21. Bashiri A, Lazer T, Burstein E, et al. Maternal and neonatal outcome following cerebrovascular accidents during pregnancy. J Matern Fetal Neonatal Med 2007; 20(3):241–247 [Epub 18 Apr 2007].

22. Lanska DJ, Kryscio RJ. Risk factors for peripartum and postpartum stroke and intracranial venous thrombosis. Stroke 2000; 31 (6):1274–1282 [Epub 3 Jun 2000].

23. Petitti DB, Sidney S, Quesenberry CP Jr., et al. Incidence of stroke and myocardial infarction in women of reproductive age. Stroke 1997; 28(2):280–283 [Epub 1 Feb 1997].

24. Warnes CA, Williams RG, Bashore TM, et al. ACC/AHA 2008 guidelines for the management of adults with congenital heart disease: a report of the American College of Cardiology/American Heart Association Task Force on Practice Guidelines (Writing Committee to Develop Guidelines on the Management of Adults With Congenital Heart Disease). Developed in collaboration with the American Society of Echocardiography, Heart Rhythm Society, International Society for Adult Congenital

Heart Disease, Society for Cardiovascular Angiography and Interventions, and Society of Thoracic Surgeons. J Am Coll Cardiol 2008; 52(23):e1–e121 [Epub 29 Nov 2008].

25. Cantu C, Barinagarrementeria F. Cerebral venous thrombosis associated with pregnancy and puerperium. Review of 67 cases. Stroke 1993; 24(12):1880–1884 [Epub 1 Dec 1993].

26. Cantu C, Alonso E, Jara A, et al. Hyperhomocysteinemia, low folate and vitamin B12 concentrations, and methylene tetrahydrofolate reductase mutation in cerebral venous thrombosis. Stroke 2004; 35(8):1790–1794 [Epub 12 Jun 2004].

27. Srinivasan K. Ischemic cerebrovascular disease in the young. Two common causes in India. Stroke 1984; 15(4):733–735 [Epub 1 Jul 1984].

28. Nagaraja D, Noone ML, Bharatkumar VP, et al. Homocysteine, folate and vitamin B(12) in puerperal cerebral venous thrombosis. J Neurol Sci 2008; 272(1–2):43–47 [Epub 12 Jul 2008].

29. Chang J, Elam-Evans LD, Berg CJ, et al. Pregnancy-related mortality surveillance – United States, 1991-1999. MMWR Surveill Summ 2003; 52(2):1–8 [Epub 27 Jun 2003].

30. Kaunitz AM, Hughes JM, Grimes DA, et al. Causes of maternal mortality in the United States. Obstet Gynecol 1985; 65(5):605–612 [Epub 1 May 1985].

31. Rochat RW, Koonin LM, Atrash HK, et al. Maternal mortality in the United States: report from the Maternal Mortality Collaborative. Obstet Gynecol 1988; 72(1):91–97 [Epub 1 Jul 1988].

32. Wang KC, Chen CP, Yang YC, et al. Stroke complicating pregnancy and the puerperium. Zhonghua Yi Xue Za Zhi (Taipei) 1999; 62(1):13–19 [Epub 4 Mar 1999].

33. Ros HS, Lichtenstein P, Bellocco R, et al. Pulmonary embolism and stroke in relation to pregnancy: how can high-risk women be identified? Am J Obstet Gynecol 2002; 186(2):198–203.

34. Lamy C, Hamon JB, Coste J, et al. Ischemic stroke in young women: risk of recurrence during subsequent pregnancies. French Study Group on Stroke in Pregnancy. Neurology 2000; 55(2):269–274 [Epub 26 Jul 2000].

35. Coppage KH, Hinton AC, Moldenhauer J, et al. Maternal and perinatal outcome in women with a history of stroke. Am J Obstet Gynecol 2004; 190(5):1331–1334 [Epub 29 May 2004].

36. Soriano D, Carp H, Seidman DS, et al. Management and outcome of pregnancy in women with thrombophylic disorders and past cerebrovascular events. Acta Obstet Gynecol Scand 2002; 81 (3):204–207 [Epub 23 Apr 2002].

37. Mehraein S, Ortwein H, Busch M, et al. Risk of recurrence of cerebral venous and sinus thrombosis during subsequent pregnancy and puerperium. J Neurol Neurosurg Psychiatry 2003; 74 (6):814–816 [Epub 20 May 2003].

38. Lanska DJ, Kryscio RJ. Peripartum stroke and intracranial venous thrombosis in the National Hospital Discharge Survey. Obstet Gynecol 1997; 89(3):413–418 [Epub 1 Mar 1997].

39. Skidmore FM, Williams LS, Fradkin KD, et al. Presentation, etiology, and outcome of stroke in pregnancy and puerperium. J Stroke Cerebrovasc Dis 2001; 10(1):1–10 [Epub 2 Oct 2007].

40. Bremme KA. Haemostatic changes in pregnancy. Best Pract Res Clin Haematol 2003; 16(2):153–168 [Epub 24 May 2003].

41. Brenner B. Haemostatic changes in pregnancy. Thromb Res 2004; 114(5–6):409–414 [Epub 28 Oct 2004].

42. Gilabert J, Fernandez JA, Espana F, et al. Physiological coagulation inhibitors (protein S, protein C and antithrombin III) in severe preeclamptic states and in users of oral contraceptives. Thromb Res 1988; 49(3):319–329 [Epub 1 Feb 1988].

43. Mathonnet F, de Mazancourt P, Bastenaire B, et al. Activated protein C sensitivity ratio in pregnant women at delivery. Br J Haematol 1996; 92(1):244–246 [Epub 1 Jan 1996].

44. Kruithof EK, Tran-Thang C, Gudinchet A, et al. Fibrinolysis in pregnancy: a study of plasminogen activator inhibitors. Blood 1987; 69(2):460–466 [Epub 1 Feb 1987].

45. Thornton P, Douglas J. Coagulation in pregnancy. Best Pract Res Clin Obstet Gynaecol 2010; 24(3):339–352 [Epub 26 Jan 2010].

46. Dahlman T, Hellgren M, Blomback M. Changes in blood coagulation and fibrinolysis in the normal puerperium. Gynecol Obstet Investig 1985; 20(1):37–44 [Epub 1 Jan 1985].

47. Bogousslavsky J, Regli F. Ischemic stroke in adults younger than 30 years of age. Cause and prognosis. Arch Neurol 1987; 44 (5):479–482 [Epub 1 May 1987].

48. Adams HP Jr., Kappelle LJ, Biller J, et al. Ischemic stroke in young adults. Experience in 329 patients enrolled in the Iowa Registry of stroke in young adults. Arch Neurol 1995; 52(5):491–495 [Epub 1 May 1995].

49. Kristensen B, Malm J, Carlberg B, et al. Epidemiology and etiology of ischemic stroke in young adults aged 18 to 44 years in northern Sweden. Stroke 1997; 28(9):1702–1709 [Epub 26 Sept 1997].

50. Lee TH, Hsu WC, Chen CJ, et al. Etiologic study of young ischemic stroke in Taiwan. Stroke 2002; 33(8):1950–1955 [Epub 3 Aug 2002].

51. Nedeltchev K, der Maur TA, Georgiadis D, et al. Ischaemic stroke in young adults: predictors of outcome and recurrence. J Neurol Neurosurg Psychiatry 2005; 76(2):191–195 [Epub 18 Jan 2005].

52. Varona JF, Guerra JM, Bermejo F, et al. Causes of ischemic stroke in young adults, and evolution of the etiological diagnosis over the long term. Eur Neurol 2007; 57(4):212–218 [Epub 3 Feb 2007].

53. Putaala J, Metso AJ, Metso TM, et al. Analysis of 1008 consecutive patients aged 15 to 49 with first-ever ischemic stroke: the Helsinki young stroke registry. Stroke 2009; 40(4):1195–1203 [Epub 28 Feb 2009].

54. Adams HP Jr., Bendixen BH, Kappelle LJ, et al. Classification of subtype of acute ischemic stroke. Definitions for use in a multicenter clinical trial. TOAST. Trial of Org 10172 in Acute Stroke Treatment. Stroke 1993; 24(1):35–41 [Epub 1 Jan 1993].

55. Siu SC, Colman JM. Heart disease and pregnancy. Heart 2001; 85 (6):710–715 [Epub 23 May 2001].

56. Brady K, Duff P. Rheumatic heart disease in pregnancy. Clin Obstet Gynecol 1989; 32(1):21–40 [Epub 1 Mar 1989].

57. Palacio S, Hart RG. Neurologic manifestations of cardiogenic embolism: an update. Neurol Clin 2002; 20(1):179–193, vii [Epub 5 Jan 2002].

58. Homma S, Sacco RL. Patent foramen ovale and stroke. Circulation 2005; 112(7):1063–1072 [Epub 17 Aug 2005].

59. Lamy C, Giannesini C, Zuber M, et al. Clinical and imaging findings in cryptogenic stroke patients with and without patent foramen ovale: the PFO-ASA Study. Atrial Septal Aneurysm. Stroke 2002; 33(3):706–711 [Epub 2 Mar 2002].

60. Homma S, Sacco RL, Di Tullio MR, et al. Effect of medical treatment in stroke patients with patent foramen ovale: patent foramen ovale in Cryptogenic Stroke Study. Circulation 2002; 105(22):2625–2631 [Epub 5 Jun 2002].

61. Handke M, Harloff A, Olschewski M, et al. Patent foramen ovale and cryptogenic stroke in older patients. N Engl J Med 2007; 357 (22):2262–2268 [Epub 30 Nov 2007].

62. Kent DM, Thaler DE. Is patent foramen ovale a modifiable risk factor for stroke recurrence? Stroke 2010; 41(10 suppl):S26–S30 [Epub 12 Oct 2010].

63. Nellessen U, Daniel WG, Matheis G, et al. Impending paradoxical embolism from atrial thrombus: correct diagnosis by transesophageal echocardiography and prevention by surgery. J Am Coll Cardiol 1985; 5(4):1002–1004 [Epub 1 Apr 1985].

64. Schreiter SW, Phillips JH. Thromboembolus traversing a patent foramen ovale: resolution with anticoagulation. J Am Soc Echocardiogr 1994; 7(6):659–662 [Epub 1 Nov 1994].

65. Hust MH, Staiger M, Braun B. Migration of paradoxic embolus through a patent foramen ovale diagnosed by echocardiography: successful thrombolysis. Am Heart J 1995; 129(3):620–622 [Epub 1 Mar 1995].

66. Mas JL, Arquizan C, Lamy C, et al. Recurrent cerebrovascular events associated with patent foramen ovale, atrial septal aneurysm, or both. N Engl J Med 2001; 345(24):1740–1746 [Epub 14 Dec 2001].

67. Mas JL, Zuber M. Recurrent cerebrovascular events in patients with patent foramen ovale, atrial septal aneurysm, or both and cryptogenic stroke or transient ischemic attack. French Study Group on Patent Foramen Ovale and Atrial Septal Aneurysm. Am Heart J 1995; 130(5):1083–1088 [Epub 1 Nov 1995].

68. De Castro S, Cartoni D, Fiorelli M, et al. Morphological and functional characteristics of patent foramen ovale and their embolic implications. Stroke 2000; 31(10):2407–2413 [Epub 7 Oct 2000].

69. Bogousslavsky J, Garazi S, Jeanrenaud X, et al. Stroke recurrence in patients with patent foramen ovale: the Lausanne Study. Lausanne Stroke with Paradoxal Embolism Study Group. Neurology 1996; 46(5):1301–1305 [Epub 1 May 1996].

70. Cujec B, Mainra R, Johnson DH. Prevention of recurrent cerebral ischemic events in patients with patent foramen ovale and cryptogenic strokes or transient ischemic attacks. Can J Cardiol 1999; 15(1):57–64 [Epub 20 Feb 1999].

71. Almekhlafi MA, Wilton SB, Rabi DM, et al. Recurrent cerebral ischemia in medically treated patent foramen ovale: a meta-analysis. Neurology 2009; 73(2):89–97 [Epub 15 May 2009].

72. Meissner I, Khandheria BK, Heit JA, et al. Patent foramen ovale: innocent or guilty? Evidence from a prospective population-based study. J Am Coll Cardiol 2006; 47(2):440–445 [Epub 18 Jan 2006].

73. Cabanes L, Mas JL, Cohen A, et al. Atrial septal aneurysm and patent foramen ovale as risk factors for cryptogenic stroke in patients less than 55 years of age. A study using transesophageal echocardiography. Stroke 1993; 24(12):1865–1873 [Epub 1 Dec 1993].

74. Homma S, Di Tullio MR, Sacco RL, et al. Characteristics of patent foramen ovale associated with cryptogenic stroke. A biplane transesophageal echocardiographic study. Stroke 1994; 25(3):582–586 [Epub 1 Mar 1994].

75. Steiner MM, Di Tullio MR, Rundek T, et al. Patent foramen ovale size and embolic brain imaging findings among patients with ischemic stroke. Stroke 1998; 29(5):944–948 [Epub 22 May 1998].

76. Hausmann D, Mugge A, Becht I, et al. Diagnosis of patent foramen ovale by transesophageal echocardiography and association with cerebral and peripheral embolic events. Am J Cardiol 1992; 70(6):668–672 [Epub 1 Sept 1992].

77. Van Camp G, Schulze D, Cosyns B, et al. Relation between patent foramen ovale and unexplained stroke. Am J Cardiol 1993; 71(7):596–598 [Epub 1 Mar 1993].

78. Di Tullio MR, Sacco RL, Sciacca RR, et al. Patent foramen ovale and the risk of ischemic stroke in a multiethnic population. J Am Coll Cardiol 2007; 49(7):797–802 [Epub 20 Feb 2007].

79. Serena J, Marti-Fabregas J, Santamarina E, et al. Recurrent stroke and massive right-to-left shunt: results from the prospective Spanish multicenter (CODICIA) study. Stroke 2008; 39(12):3131–3136 [Epub 27 Sept 2008].

80. Furie KL, Kasner SE, Adams RJ, et al. Guidelines for the prevention of stroke in patients with stroke or transient ischemic attack: a guideline for healthcare professionals from the american heart association/american stroke association. Stroke 2011; 42(1):227–276 [Epub 23 Oct 2010].

81. Balbi M, Casalino L, Gnecco G, et al. Percutaneous closure of patent foramen ovale in patients with presumed paradoxical embolism: periprocedural results and midterm risk of recurrent neurologic events. Am Heart J 2008; 156(2):356–360 [Epub 29 Jul 2008].

82. Casaubon L, McLaughlin P, Webb G, et al. Recurrent stroke/TIA in cryptogenic stroke patients with patent foramen ovale. Can J Neurol Sci 2007; 34(1):74–80 [Epub 14 Mar 2007].

83. Harrer JU, Wessels T, Franke A, et al. Stroke recurrence and its prevention in patients with patent foramen ovale. Can J Neurol Sci 2006; 33(1):39–47 [Epub 6 Apr 2006].

84. Kiblawi FM, Sommer RJ, Levchuck SG. Transcatheter closure of patent foramen ovale in older adults. Catheter Cardiovasc Interv 2006; 68(1):136–142; discussion 43–44 [Epub 7 Jun 2006].

85. Kutty S, Brown K, Asnes JD, et al. Causes of recurrent focal neurologic events after transcatheter closure of patent foramen ovale with the CardioSEAL septal occluder. Am J Cardiol 2008; 101(10):1487–1492 [Epub 13 May 2008].

86. Post MC, Van Deyk K, Budts W. Percutaneous closure of a patent foramen ovale: single-centre experience using different

types of devices and mid-term outcome. Acta Cardiologica 2005; 60(5):515–519 [Epub 3 Nov 2005].

87. Slavin L, Tobis JM, Rangarajan K, et al. Five-year experience with percutaneous closure of patent foramen ovale. Am J Cardiol 2007; 99(9):1316–1320 [Epub 5 May 2007].

88. von Bardeleben RS, Richter C, Otto J, et al. Long term follow up after percutaneous closure of PFO in 357 patients with paradoxical embolism: difference in occlusion systems and influence of atrial septum aneurysm. Int J Cardiol 2009; 134(1):33–41 [Epub 22 Aug 2008].

89. Wahl A, Krumsdorf U, Meier B, et al. Transcatheter treatment of atrial septal aneurysm associated with patent foramen ovale for prevention of recurrent paradoxical embolism in high-risk patients. J Am Coll Cardiol 2005; 45(3):377–380 [Epub 1 Feb 2005].

90. Wahl A, Kunz M, Moschovitis A, et al. Long-term results after fluoroscopy-guided closure of patent foramen ovale for secondary prevention of paradoxical embolism. Heart 2008; 94(3):336–341 [Epub 20 Jul 2007].

91. Windecker S, Wahl A, Nedeltchev K, et al. Comparison of medical treatment with percutaneous closure of patent foramen ovale in patients with cryptogenic stroke. J Am Coll Cardiol 2004; 44(4):750–758 [Epub 18 Aug 2004].

92. Sacco RL, Adams R, Albers G, et al. Guidelines for prevention of stroke in patients with ischemic stroke or transient ischemic attack: a statement for healthcare professionals from the American Heart Association/American Stroke Association Council on Stroke: co-sponsored by the Council on Cardiovascular Radiology and Intervention: the American Academy of Neurology affirms the value of this guideline. Stroke 2006; 37(2):577–617 [Epub 25 Jan 2006].

93. Kozelj M, Novak-Antolic Z, Grad A, et al. Patent foramen ovale as a potential cause of paradoxical embolism in the postpartum period. Eur J Obstet Gynecol Reprod Biol 1999; 84(1):55–57 [Epub 21 Jul 1999].

94. Vij M, Mowbray D. Pregnancy outcome in patients with patent foramen ovale and cerebral embolism. Eur J Obstet Gynecol Reprod Biol 2008; 140(1):147–148 [Epub 28 Dec 2007].

95. Giberti L, Bino G, Tanganelli P. Pregnancy, patent foramen ovale and stroke: a case of pseudoperipheral facial palsy. Neurol Sci 2005; 26(1):43–45 [Epub 7 May 2005].

96. Schrale RG, Ormerod J, Ormerod OJ. Percutaneous device closure of the patent foramen ovale during pregnancy. Catheter Cardiovasc Interv 2007; 69(4):579–583 [Epub 14 Feb 2007].

97. Hirsch R, Streifler J. Congenital heart disease and stroke. Semin Cerebrovasc Dis Stroke 2005; 5(1):13–20.

98. Balint OH, Siu SC, Mason J, et al. Cardiac outcomes after pregnancy in women with congenital heart disease. Heart 2010; 96(20):1656–1661 [Epub 13 Oct 2010].

99. Khairy P, Ouyang DW, Fernandes SM, et al. Pregnancy outcomes in women with congenital heart disease. Circulation 2006; 113(4):517–524 [Epub 2 Feb 2006].

100. Baumgartner H, Bonhoeffer P, De Groot NM, et al. ESC Guidelines for the management of grown-up congenital heart disease (new version 2010). Eur Heart J 2010; 31(23):2915–2957 [Epub 31 Aug 2010].

101. Bates SM, Greer IA, Pabinger I, et al. Venous thromboembolism, thrombophilia, antithrombotic therapy, and pregnancy: American College of Chest Physicians Evidence-Based Clinical Practice Guidelines. 8th ed. Chest 2008; 133(6 suppl):844S–886S [Epub 24 Jul 2008].

102. Gowda RM, Punukollu G, Khan IA, et al. Lone atrial fibrillation during pregnancy. Int J Cardiol 2003; 88(1):123–124 [Epub 28 Mar 2003].

103. Cacciotti L, Camastra GS, Ansalone G. Atrial fibrillation in a pregnant woman with a normal heart. Intern Emerg Med 2010; 5 (1):87–88 [Epub 17 Sept 2009].

104. Elliott P, Andersson B, Arbustini E, et al. Classification of the cardiomyopathies: a position statement from the European Society Of Cardiology Working Group on Myocardial and Pericardial Diseases. Eur Heart J 2008; 29(2):270–276 [Epub 6 Oct 2007].

105. Elkayam U, Akhter MW, Singh H, et al. Pregnancy-associated cardiomyopathy: clinical characteristics and a comparison between early and late presentation. Circulation 2005; 111 (16):2050–2055 [Epub 27 Apr 2005].

106. Hilfiker-Kleiner D, Kaminski K, Podewski E, et al. A cathepsin D-cleaved 16 kDa form of prolactin mediates postpartum cardiomyopathy. Cell 2007; 128(3):589–600 [Epub 10 Feb 2007].

107. Sliwa K, Hilfiker-Kleiner D, Petrie MC, et al. Current state of knowledge on aetiology, diagnosis, management, and therapy of peripartum cardiomyopathy: a position statement from the Heart Failure Association of the European Society of Cardiology Working Group on peripartum cardiomyopathy. Eur J Heart Fail 2010; 12(8):767–778 [Epub 3 Aug 2010].

108. Pyatt JR, Dubey G. Peripartum cardiomyopathy: current understanding, comprehensive management review and new developments. Postgrad Med J 2011; 87(1023):34–39 [Epub 12 Oct 2010].

109. Sliwa K, Skudicky D, Bergemann A, et al. Peripartum cardiomyopathy: analysis of clinical outcome, left ventricular function, plasma levels of cytokines and Fas/APO-1. J Am Coll Cardiol 2000; 35(3):701–705 [Epub 15 Mar 2000].

110. Ford RF, Barton JR, O'Brien JM, et al. Demographics, management, and outcome of peripartum cardiomyopathy in a community hospital. Am J Obstet Gynecol 2000; 182(5):1036–1038 [Epub 20 May 2000].

111. Fett JD, Christie LG, Carraway RD, et al. Five-year prospective study of the incidence and prognosis of peripartum cardiomyopathy at a single institution. Mayo Clin Proc 2005; 80(12):1602–1606 [Epub 14 Dec 2005].

112. Witlin AG, Mabie WC, Sibai BM. Peripartum cardiomyopathy: a longitudinal echocardiographic study. Am J Obstet Gynecol 1997; 177(5):1129–1132 [Epub 16 Dec 1997].

113. Leijdekkers VJ, Vahl AC, Leenders JJ, et al. Risk factors for premature atherosclerosis. Eur J Vasc Endovasc Surg 1999; 17 (5):394–397 [Epub 18 May 1999].

114. Knoflach M, Kiechl S, Penz D, et al. Cardiovascular risk factors and atherosclerosis in young women: atherosclerosis risk factors in female youngsters (ARFY study). Stroke 2009; 40(4):1063–1069 [Epub 13 Feb 2009].

115. Tyrrell PN, Beyene J, Feldman BM, et al. Rheumatic disease and carotid intima-media thickness: a systematic review and meta-analysis. Arterioscler Thromb Vasc Biol 2010; 30(5):1014–1026 [Epub 13 Feb 2010].

116. Schievink WI. Spontaneous dissection of the carotid and vertebral arteries. N Engl J Med 2001; 344(12):898–906 [Epub 22 Mar 2001].

117. Bruninx G, Roland H, Matte JC, et al. Carotid dissection during childbirth. J Mal Vasc 1996; 21(2):92–94 [Epub 1 Jan 1996].

118. Lepojarvi M, Tarkka M, Leinonen A, et al. Spontaneous dissection of the internal carotid artery. Acta Chir Scand 1988; 154 (10):559–566 [Epub 1 Oct 1988].

119. Wiebers DO, Mokri B. Internal carotid artery dissection after childbirth. Stroke 1985; 16(6):956–959 [Epub 1 Nov 1985].

120. Abisaab J, Nevadunsky N, Flomenbaum N. Emergency department presentation of bilateral carotid artery dissections in a postpartum patient. Ann Emerg Med 2004; 44(5):484–489 [Epub 3 Nov 2004].

121. Gasecki AP, Kwiecinski H, Lyrer PA, et al. Dissections after childbirth. J Neurol 1999; 246(8):712–715 [Epub 25 Aug 1999].

122. Arnold M, Camus-Jacqmin M, Stapf C, et al. Postpartum cervicocephalic artery dissection. Stroke 2008; 39(8):2377–2379 [Epub 7 Jun 2008].

123. Tuluc M, Brown D, Goldman B. Lethal vertebral artery dissection in pregnancy: a case report and review of the literature. Arch Pathol Lab Med 2006; 130(4):533–535 [Epub 6 Apr 2006].

124. Lyrer P, Engelter S. Antithrombotic drugs for carotid artery dissection. Cochrane Database Syst Rev 2003; (3):CD000255 [Epub 15 Aug 2003].

125. Menon R, Kerry S, Norris JW, et al. Treatment of cervical artery dissection: a systematic review and meta-analysis. J Neurol Neurosurg Psychiatry 2008; 79(10):1122–1127 [Epub 28 Feb 2008].

126. Kasner SE, Dreier JP. A fresh twist on carotid artery dissections. Neurology 2009; 72(21):1800–1801 [Epub 27 Mar 2009].

127. Georgiadis D, Arnold M, von Buedingen HC, et al. Aspirin vs anticoagulation in carotid artery dissection: a study of 298 patients. Neurology 2009; 72(21):1810–1815 [Epub 27 Mar 2009].

128. Engelter ST, Brandt T, Debette S, et al. Antiplatelets versus anticoagulation in cervical artery dissection. Stroke 2007; 38 (9):2605–2611 [Epub 28 Jul 2007].

129. Touze E, Gauvrit JY, Moulin T, et al. Risk of stroke and recurrent dissection after a cervical artery dissection: a multicenter study. Neurology 2003; 61(10):1347–1351 [Epub 26 Nov 2003].

130. Bassetti C, Carruzzo A, Sturzenegger M, et al. Recurrence of cervical artery dissection. A prospective study of 81 patients. Stroke 1996; 27(10):1804–1807 [Epub 1 Oct 1996].

131. O'Rourke N, Wollman L, Camann W. Bilateral spontaneous vertebral artery dissection: management during labor and vaginal delivery. Int J Obstet Anesthesia 2004; 13(1):44–46 [Epub 24 Aug 2004].

132. Olin JW, Pierce M. Contemporary management of fibromuscular dysplasia. Curr Opin Cardiol 2008; 23(6):527–536 [Epub 3 Oct 2008].

133. Slovut DP, Olin JW. Fibromuscular dysplasia. N Engl J Med 2004; 350(18):1862–1871 [Epub 30 Apr 2004].

134. Ohene-Frempong K, Weiner SJ, Sleeper LA, et al. Cerebrovascular accidents in sickle cell disease: rates and risk factors. Blood 1998; 91(1):288–294 [Epub 7 Feb 1998].

135. Mettinger KL. Fibromuscular dysplasia and the brain. II. Current concept of the disease. Stroke 1982; 13(1):53–58 [Epub 1 Jan 1982].

136. Alimi Y, Mercier C, Pellissier JF, et al. Fibromuscular disease of the renal artery: a new histopathologic classification. Ann Vasc Surg 1992; 6(3):220–224. [Epub 1 May 1992].

137. Harrison EG Jr, McCormack LJ. Pathologic classification of renal arterial disease in renovascular hypertension. Mayo Clin Proc Mayo Clin 1971; 46(3):161–167. [Epub 1 Mar 1971].

138. Ohtsubo T, Asakura T, Kadota K, et al. [A report of a trans-sphenoidal operation during pregnancy for a pituitary adenoma]. No Shinkei Geka 1991; 19(9):867–870 [Epub 1 Sept 1991].

139. Corrin LS, Sandok BA, Houser OW. Cerebral ischemic events in patients with carotid artery fibromuscular dysplasia. Arch Neurol 1981; 38(10):616–618 [Epub 1 Oct 1981].

140. Osborn AG, Anderson RE. Angiographic spectrum of cervical and intracranial fibromuscular dysplasia. Stroke 1977; 8(5):617–626 [Epub 1 Sept 1977].

141. Olin JW, Sealove BA. Diagnosis, management, and future developments of fibromuscular dysplasia. J Vasc Surg 2011; 53(3):826–36 e1 [Epub 18 Jan 2011].

142. Ezra Y, Kidron D, Beyth Y. Fibromuscular dysplasia of the carotid arteries complicating pregnancy. Obstet Gynecol 1989; 73(5 pt 2):840–843 [Epub 1 May 1989].

143. Singhal AB, Bernstein RA. Postpartum angiopathy and other cerebral vasoconstriction syndromes. Neurocrit Care 2005; 3 (1):91–97 [Epub 15 Sept 2005].

144. Ducros A, Bousser MG. Reversible cerebral vasoconstriction syndrome. Pract Neurol 2009; 9(5):256–267 [Epub 19 Sept 2009].

145. Singhal AB, Hajj-Ali RA, Topcuoglu MA, et al. Reversible cerebral vasoconstriction syndromes: analysis of 139 cases. Arch Neurol 2011; 68(8):1005–1012 [Epub 13 Apr 2011].

146. Ducros A, Boukobza M, Porcher R, et al. The clinical and radiological spectrum of reversible cerebral vasoconstriction syndrome. A prospective series of 67 patients. Brain 2007; 130 (pt 12):3091–3101 [Epub 21 Nov 2007].

147. Baba T, Houkin K, Kuroda S. Novel epidemiological features of moyamoya disease. J Neurol Neurosurg Psychiatry 2008; 79 (8):900–904 [Epub 14 Dec 2007].

148. Fukui M, Kono S, Sueishi K, et al. Moyamoya disease. Neuropathology 2000; 20(suppl):S61–S64 [Epub 19 Oct 2000].

149. Komiyama M, Yasui T, Kitano S, et al. Moyamoya disease and pregnancy: case report and review of the literature. Neurosurgery 1998; 43(2):360–368; discussion 8–9 [Epub 8 Aug 1998].

150. Takahashi JC, Miyamoto S. Moyamoya disease: recent progress and outlook. Neurol Med Chir 2010; 50(9):824–832 [Epub 5 Oct 2010].

151. Houkin K, Kamiyama H, Abe H, et al. Surgical therapy for adult moyamoya disease. Can surgical revascularization prevent the recurrence of intracerebral hemorrhage? Stroke 1996; 27(8):1342–1346 [Epub 1 Aug 1996].

152. Verduzco LA, Nathan DG. Sickle cell disease and stroke. Blood 2009; 114:5117–5125.

153. Gavins F, Yilmaz G, Granger DN. The evolving paradigm for blood cell-endothelial cell interactions in the cerebral microcirculation. Microcirculation 2007; 14:667–681.

154. Platt OS. Sickle cell anemia as an inflammatory disease. J Clin Invest 2000; 106:337–338.

155. Rees DC, Williams TN, Gladwin MT. Sickle-cell disease. Lancet 2010; 376:2018–2031.

156. Stockman JA, Nigro MA, Mishkin MM, et al. Occlusion of large cerebral vessels in sickle cell anaemia. N Engl J Med 1972; 287:846–849.

157. Merkel KH, Ginsberg PL, Parker JC, et al. Cerebrovascular disease in sickle cell anaemia: a clinical, pathological and radiological correlation. Stroke 1978; 9:45–52.

158. Rothman SM, Fulling KH, Nelson JS. Sickle cell anaemia and central nervous system infarction: a neuropathological study. Ann Neurol 1986; 20:684–690.

159. Pavlakis SG, Bello J, Prohvnik I, et al. Brain infarction in sickle cell anaemia: magnetic resonance imaging correlates. Ann Neurol 1988; 23:125–130.

160. Moser FG, Miller ST, Bello JA, et al. The spectrum of brain MR abnormalities in sickle-cell disease: a report from the Cooperative Study of Sickle Cell Disease. Am J Neuroradiol 1996; 17:965–972.

161. Deane CR, Goss D, Bartram J, et al. Extracranial internal carotid arterial disease in children with sickle cell anaemia. Haematologica 2010; 95:1287–1292.

162. Sebire G, Tabarki B, Saunders DE, et al. Cerebral venous sinus thrombosis in children: risk factors, presentation, diagnosis and outcome. Brain 2005; 128:477–489.

163. Oguz M, Aksungur EH, Soyupak SK, et al. Vein of Galen and sinus thrombosis with bilateral thalamic infarcts in sickle cell anemia: CT follow-up and angiographic demonstration. Neuroradiology 1994; 36:155–156.

164. Villers MS, Jamison MG, DeCastro LM, et al. Morbidity associated with sickle cell disease in pregnancy. Am J Obstet Gynecol 2008; 199:125.e1–125.e5.

165. Lottenberg R, Hassell KL. An evidence-based approach to the treatment of adults with sickle cell disease. Hematology 2005; 1:58–65.

166. Stuart MJ, Nagel RL. Sickle-cell disease. Lancet 2004; 364:1343–1360.

167. Hassell K. Pregnancy and sickle cell disease. Haematol/Oncol Clin North Am 2005; 19:903–916.

168. Koshy M, Burd L, Wallace D, et al. Prophylactic re-cell transfusions in pregnant patients with sickle cell disease. N Engl J Med 1988; 319:1447–1452.

169. Ngo C, Kayem G, Habibi A, et al. Pregnancy in sickle cell disease: maternal and fetal outcomes in a population receiving prophylactic partial exchange transfusions. Eur J Obstet Gynaecol Reprod Biol 2010; 152:138–142.

170. Giannakopoulos B, Passam F, Rahgozar S, et al. Current concepts on the pathogenesis of the antiphospholipid syndrome. Blood 2007; 109:422–430.

171. Roubey RAS. Risky business: the interpretation, use, and abuse of antiphospholipid antibody tests in clinical practice. Lupus. 2010; 19:440–445.

172. Urbanus RT, Siegerink B, Roest M, et al. Antiphospholipid antibodies and risk of myocardial infarction and ischaemic stroke in young women in the RATIO study: a case-control study. Lancet Neurol 2009; 8:998–1005.

173. Ruiz-Irastorza G, Cuadrado MJ, Brey R, et al. Evidence-based recommendations for the prevention and long-term management of thrombosis in antiphospholipid antibody-positive patients: report of a task force at the 13th International Congress on antiphospholipid antibodies. Lupus 2011; 20:206–218.

174. Miyakis S, Lockshin MD, Atsumi T, et al. International consensus statement on an update of the classification criteria for definite antiphospholipid syndrome (APS). J Thromb Haemost 2006; 4:295–306.

175. Pengo V, Ruffatti A, Legnani C, et al. Clinical course of high-risk patients diagnosed with antiphospholipid syndrome. J Thromb Haemostasis 2010; 8:237–242.

176. Galli M, Luciani D, Bertolini G, et al. Lupus anticoagulants are stronger risk factors for thrombosis than anticardiolipin antibodies in the antiphospholipid syndrome: a systematic review of the literature. Blood 2003; 101:1827–1832.

177. Galli M, Luciani D, Bertolini G, et al. Anti-β_2-glycoprotein I, antiprothrombin antibodies, and the risk of thrombosis in the antiphospholipid syndrome. Blood 2003; 102:2717–2723.

178. Provenzale JM, Ortel TL. Anatomic distribution of venous thrombosis in patients with antiphospholipid antibody: imaging findings. Am J Roentgenol 1995; 165:365–368.

179. Nagai S, Horie Y, Akai T, et al. Superior sagittal sinus thrombosis associated with primary antiphospholipid syndrome – case report. Neurol Med Chir (Tokyo) 1998; 38:34–39.

180. Brey RL, Muscal E, Chapman J. Antiphospholipid antibodies and the brain: a consensus report. Lupus 2011; 20:153–157.

181. Davous P, Horellou MH, Conard J, et al. Cerebral infarction and familial protein S deficiency. Stroke 1990; 21:1760–1761.

182. Simioni P, de Ronde P, Prandoni P, et al. Ischaemic stroke in young patients with activated protein C resistance. A report of three cases belonging to three different kindreds. Stroke 1995; 26:885–890.

183. De Stefano V, Chiusolo P, Paciaroni K, et al. Prothrombin G20210A mutant genotype is a risk factor for cerebrovascular ischemic disease in young patients. Blood 1998; 91:3562–3565.

184. Margaglione M, D'Andrea G, Giuliani N, et al. Inherited prothrombotic conditions and premature ischemic stroke: sex difference in the association with factor V Leiden. Arterioscler Thromb Vasc Biol 1999; 19:1751–1756.

185. Kim RJ, Becker RC. Association between factor V Leiden, prothrombin G20210A, and methylenetetrahydrofolate reductase C677T mutations and events of the arterial circulatory system: a meta-analysis of published studies. Am Heart J 2003; 146:948–957.

186. Pezzini A, Del Zotto E, Magoni M, et al. Inherited thrombophilic disorders in young adults with ischemic stroke and patent foramen ovale. Stroke 2003; 34:28–33.

187. Casas JP, Hingorani AD, Bautista LE, et al. Meta-analysis of genetic studies in ischemic stroke. Arch Neurol 2004; 61:1652–1661.

188. Aznar J, Mira Y, Corella D, et al. V Leiden and prothrombin G20210A mutations in young adults with cryptogenic ischemic stroke. Thromb Haemost 2004; 91:1031–1034.

189. Mahmoodi BK, Brouwer J-LP, Veeger NJGM, et al. Hereditary deficiency of Protein C or Protein S confers increased risk of arterial thromboembolic events at a young age. Results from a large family cohort study. Circulation 2008; 118:1659–1667.

190. Hooda A, Khandelwal PD, Saxena P. Protein S deficiency: recurrent ischemic stroke in young. Ann Ind Acad Neurol 2009; 12:183–184.

191. Leung TW, Yip S-F, Lam C-W, et al. Genetic predisposition of white matter infarction with protein S deficiency and R335C mutation. Neurology 2010; 75:2185–2189.

192. Ridker PM, Hennekens CH, Lindpaintner K, et al. Mutation in gene coding for coagulation factor V and the risk of myocardial infarction, stroke, and venous thrombosis in apparently healthy men. N Engl J Med 1995; 332:912–917.

193. Longstreth WT, Rosendaal FR, Siscovick DS, et al. Risk of stroke in young women and two prothrombotic mutations: factor V Leiden and prothrombin gene mutation (G20210A). Stroke 1998; 29:577–580.

194. Ridker PM, Hennekens CH, Miletich JP. G20210A mutation in prothrombin gene and risk of myocardial infarction, stroke, and venous thrombosis in a large cohort of US men. Circulation 1999; 99:999–1004.

195. Voetsch B, Damasceno BP, Massaro A, et al. Inherited thrombophilia as a risk factor for the development of ischemic stroke in young adults. Thromb Haemost 2000; 83:229–233.

196. Lopaciuk S, Bykowska K, Kwiecinski H, et al. Factor V Leiden, prothrombin gene G20210A variant, and methylenetetrahydrofolate reductase C677T genotype in young adults with ischemic stroke. Clin Appl Thromb Haemost 2001; 7:346–350.

197. Hankey GJ, Eikelboom JW, van Bockxmeer FM, et al. Inherited thrombophilia in ischemic stroke and its pathogenic subtypes. Stroke 2001; 32:1793–1799.

198. Madonna P, de Stefano V, Coppola A, et al. Hyperhomocysteinaemia and other inherited prothrombotic conditions in young adults with a history of ischemic stroke. Stroke 2002; 33:51–56.

199. Juul K, Tybjærg-Hansen A, Steffensen R, et al. Factor V Leiden: The Copenhagen City Heart Study and 2 meta-analyses. Blood 2002; 100:3–10.

200. Morris JG, Singh S, Fisher M. Testing for inherited thrombophilias in arterial stroke. Can it cause more harm than good? Stroke 2010; 41:2985–2990.

201. Saposnik G, Barinagarrementería F, Brown RD, et al. Diagnosis and management of cerebral venous thrombosis: a statement for healthcare professionals from the American Heart Association/American Stroke Association. Stroke 2011; 42:1158–1192.

202. Dentali F, Crowther M, Ageno W. Thrombophilic abnormalities, oral contraceptives, and risk of cerebral vein thrombosis: a meta-analysis. Blood 2006; 107:2766–2773.

203. Marjot T, Yadav S, Hasan N, et al. Genes associated with adult cerebral venous thrombosis. Stroke 2011; 42:913–918.

204. Bombeli T, Basic A, Fehr J. Prevalence of hereditary thrombophilia in patients with thrombosis in different venous systems. Am J Haematol 2002; 70:126–132.

205. Martinelli I, Battaglioli T, Pedotti P, et al. Hyperhomocysteinaemia in cerebral vein thrombosis. Blood 2003; 102:1363–1366.

206. Wysokinska EM, Wysokinski WE, Brown RD, et al. Thrombophilia differences in cerebral venous sinus and lower extremity deep venous thrombosis. Neurology 2008; 70:627–633.

207. Rosendaal FR. Venous thrombosis: a multicausal disease. Lancet 1999; 353:1167–1173.

208. Stam J. Thrombosis of the cerebral veins and sinuses. N Engl J Med 2005; 352:1791–1798.

209. National High Blood Pressure Education Program Working Group on High Blood Pressure in Pregnancy. Report of the National High Blood Pressure Education Program Working Group on High Blood Pressure in Pregnancy. Am J Obstet Gynecol 2000; 183:S1–S22.

210. ACOG Committee on Practice Bulletins – Obstetrics. ACOG Practice Bulletin No. 33: diagnosis and management of preeclampsia and eclampsia. Obstet Gynecol 2002; 99:159–167.

211. Tuffnell DJ, Shennan AH, Waugh JJS, et al. on behalf of the Guidelines and Audit Committee of the Royal College of Obstetricians and Gynaecologists. Guideline No 10(A): management of severe pre-eclampsia/eclampsia. London: Royal College of Obstetricians and Gynaecologists 2006; Reviewed 2010.

212. Lindheimer MD, Taler SJ, Cunningham FG. Hypertension in pregnancy. ASH position article. J Am Soc Hypertens 2008; 2:484–494.

213. Brittain PC, Bayliss P. Partial hydatidiform molar pregnancy presenting with severe preeclampsia prior to twenty weeks gestation: a case report and review of the literature. Mil Med 1995; 160:42–44.

214. Ramsey PS, Van Winter JT, Gaffey TA, et al. Eclampsia complicating hydatidiform molar pregnancy with a coexisting, viable fetus. A case report. J Reprod Med 1998; 43:456–458.

215. Mackay AP, Berg CJ, Atrash HK. Pregnancy-related mortality from preeclampsia and eclampsia. Obstet Gynecol 2001; 97:533–538.

216. von Dadelszen P, Magee LA, Roberts JM. Subclassification of Preeclampsia. Hypertens Pregnancy 2003; 22:143–148.

217. Vatten LJ, Skjaerven R. Is pre-eclampsia more than one disease? BJOG 2004; 111:298–302.

218. Lowe SA, Brown MA, Dekker GA, et al. Guidelines for the management of hypertensive disorders of pregnancy 2008. Aust N Z J Obstet Gynecol 2009; 49:242–246.

219. Minnerup J, Kleffner I, Wersching H, et al. Late onset postpartum eclampsia: it is really never too late —a case of eclampsia 8 weeks after delivery. Stroke Res Treat 2010; 2010 pii: 798616 [Epub 1 Sept 2009].

220. Brown CM, Garovic VD. Mechanisms and management of hypertension in pregnant women. Curr Hypertens Rep 2011 Jun 8 [Epub ahead of print].

221. James JL, Whitley GS, Cartwright JE. Pre-eclampsia: fitting together the placental, immune and cardiovascular pieces. J Pathol 2010; 221:363–378.

222. Cudihy D, Lee RV. The pathophysiology of pre-eclampsia: current clinical concepts. J Obstet Gynaecol 2009; 29:576–582.

223. Sibai B, Dekker G, Kupferminc M. Pre-eclampsia. Lancet 2005; 365:785–799.

224. Shah AK, Rajamani K, Whitty JE. Eclampsia: a neurological perspective. J Neurol Sci 2008; 271:158–167.

225. Bushnell CD, Hurn P, Colton C, et al. Advancing the study of stroke in women. Summary and recommendations for future research from and NINDS-Sponsored Multidisciplinary Working Group. Stroke 2006; 37:2387–2399.

226. Cipolla MJ. Cerebrovascular function in pregnancy and eclampsia. Hypertension 2007; 50:14–24.

227. Oehm E, Reinhard M, Keck C, et al. Impaired dynamic cerebral autoregulation in eclampsia. Ultrasound Obstet Gynecol 2003; 22:395–398.

228. Riskin-Mashiah S, Belfort MA, Saade GR, et al. Cerebrovascular reactivity in normal pregnancy and eclampsia. Obstet Gynecol 2001; 98:827–832.

229. Williams KP, Wilson S. Variation in cerebral perfusion pressure with different hypertensive states in pregnancy. Am J Obstet Gynecol 1998; 179:1200–1203.

230. Martin JN, Thigpen BD, Moore RC, et al. Stroke and severe preeclampsia and eclampsia: a paradigm shift focusing on systolic blood pressure. Obstet Gynecol 2005; 105:246–254.

231. Trommer BL, Homer D, Mikhael MA. Cerebral vasospasm and eclampsia. Stroke 1988; 19:326–329.

232. Lewis LK, Hinshaw DB, Will AD, et al. CT and angiographic correlation of severe neurological disease in toxaemia of pregnancy. Neuroradiology 1988; 30:59–64.

233. Singhal AB. Postpartum angiopathy with reversible posterior leukoencephalopathy. Arch Neurol 2004; 61:411–416.

234. Ros HS, Cnattingius S, Lipworth L. Comparison of risk factors for preeclampsia and gestational hypertension in a population-based cohort study. Am J Epidemiol 1998; 147:1062–1070.

235. Hauth JC, Ewell MG, Esterlitz JR, et al. for the Calcium for Preeclampsia Prevention Study Group. Pregnancy outcomes in healthy nulliparas who developed hypertension. Obstet Gynecol 2000; 95:24–28.

236. Sibai B, Hauth J, Caritis S, et al. for the National Institute of Child Health and Human Development Network of Maternal-Fetal Medicine Units. Hypertensive disorders in twin versus singleton gestations. Am J Obstet Gynecol 2000; 182:938–942.

237. Hnat MD, Sibia B, Caritis S, et al. for the National Institute of Child Health and Human Development Network of Maternal-Fetal Medicine Units. Perinatal outcome in women with recurrent preeclampsia compared with women who develop preeclampsia as nulliparas. Am J Obstet Gynecol 2002; 186:422–426.

238. Hartikainen A-L, Aliharmi RH, Rantakallio PT. A cohort study of epidemiological associations and outcomes of pregnancies with hypertensive disorders. Hypertens Pregnancy 1998; 17:31–41.

239. Duckitt K, Harrington D. Risk factors for pre-eclampsia at antenatal booking: systematic review of controlled studies. BMJ 2005; 330:565–567.

240. Sibai BM, Ewell M, Levine RJ, et al. for the Calcium for Preeclampsia Prevention (CPEP) Study Group. Am J Obstet Gynecol 1997; 177:1003–1010.

241. Sibai BM, Anderson GD. Pregnancy outcome of intensive therapy in severe hypertension in first trimester. Obstet Gynecol 1986; 67:517–522.

242. McCowan LME, Buist RG, North RA, et al. Perinatal morbidity in chronic hypertension. BJOG 1996; 103:123–129.

243. Sibai BM, Lindheimer M, Hauth J, et al. for the National Institute of Child Health and Human Development network of maternal-fetal medicine units. N Engl J Med 1998; 339:667–671.

244. van Pampus MG, Dekker GA, Wolf H, et al. High prevalence of hemostatic abnormalities in women with a history of severe preeclampsia. Am J Obstet Gynecol 1999; 180:1146–1150.

245. Trogstad L, Magnus P, Stoltenberg C. Pre-eclampsia: risk factors and causal models. Best Pract Res Clin Obstet Gynaecol 2011; 25:329–342.

246. Hutcheon JA, Lisonkova S, Joseph KS. Epidemiology of pre-eclampsia and the other hypertensive disorders of pregnancy. Best Pract Res Clin Obstet Gynecol 2011; 25:391–403.

247. Bushnell CD, Jamison M, James AH. Migraines during pregnancy linked to stroke and vascular diseases: US population based case-control study. BMJ 2009; 338:b664.

248. Ekholm E, Salmi MM, Erkkola R. Eclampsia in Finland in 1990-1994. Acta Obstet Gynecol Scand 1999; 78:877–882.

249. Knight M. on behalf of UKOSS. Eclampsia in the United Kingdom 2005. BJOG 2007; 114:1072–1078.

250. Kullberg G, Lindeberg S, Hanson U. Eclampsia in Sweden. Hypertens Pregnancy 2002; 21:13–21.

251. Andersgaard AB, Herbst A, Johansen M, et al. Eclampsia in Scandinavia: incidence, substandard care, and potentially preventable cases. Acta Obstet Gynecol 2006; 85:929–936.

252. Zwart JJ, Richters A, Öry F, et al. Eclampsia in the Netherlands. Obstet Gynecol 2008; 112:820–827.

253. Wallis AB, Saftlas AF, Hsia J, et al. Secular trends in the rates of preeclampsia, eclampsia, and gestational hypertension, United States, 1987-2004. Am J Hypertens 2008; 21:521–526.

254. Zhang J, Meikle S, Trumble A. Severe maternal morbidity associated with hypertensive disorders in pregnancy in the United States. Hypertens Pregnancy 2003; 22:203–212.

255. Moodley J, Naicker RS, Mankowitz E. Eclampsia – a method of management. A preliminary report. S Afr Med J 1983; 63:530–535.

256. Duley L. The global impact of pre-eclampsia and eclampsia. Semin Perinatol 2009; 33:130–137.

257. Awada A, al Rajeh S, Duarte R, et al. Stroke & Pregnancy. Int J Gynecol Obstet 1995; 48:157–161.

258. Isler CM, Rinehart BK, Terrone DA, et al. Maternal mortality associated with HELLP (hemolysis, elevated liver enzymes, and low platelets) syndrome. Am J Obstet Gynecol 1999; 181:924–928.

259. Hinchey J, Chaves C, Appignani B, et al. A reversible posterior leukoencephalopathy syndrome. N Engl J Med 1996; 334:494–500.

260. Cunningham FG, Twickler D. Cerebral edema complicating eclampsia. Am J Obstet Gynecol 2000; 182:94–100.

261. Lee VH, Wijdicks EFM, Manno EM, et al. Clinical spectrum of reversible posterior leukoencephalopathy syndrome. Arch Neurol 2008; 65:205–210.

262. Liman TG, Bohner G, Heuschmann PU, et al. The clinical and radiological spectrum of posterior reversible encephalopathy syndrome: the retrospective Berlin PRES study. J Neurol 2011 Jun 30 [Epub ahead of print].

263. Casey SO, Sampaio RC, Michel E, et al. Posterior reversible encephalopathy syndrome: utility of fluid-attenuated inversion recovery MR imaging in the detection of cortical and subcortical lesions. Am J Neuroradiol 2000; 21:1199–1206.

264. Koch S, Rabinstein A, Falcone S, et al. Diffusion-weighted imaging shows cytotoxic and vasogenic edema in eclampsia. Am J Neuroradiol 2001; 22:1068–1070.

265. Clark SL, Hankins GDV, Dudley DA, et al. Amniotic fluid embolism: analysis of the national registry. Am J Obstet Gynecol 1995; 172:1158–1169.

266. Tuffnell DJ, Togobo M. Amniotic fluid embolism. Obstet Gynaecol Reprod Med 2011; 21:217–220.

267. Gist RS, Stafford IP, Leibowitz AB, et al. Amniotic fluid embolism. Anesth Analg 2009; 108:1599–1602.

268. Tuffnell DJ. United Kingdom amniotic fluid embolism register. BJOG 2005; 112:1625–1629.

269. Kumar V, Khatwani M, Aneja S, et al. Paradoxical amniotic fluid embolism presenting before caesarean section in a woman

with an atrial septal defect. International J Obstet Anesth 2010; 19:94–98.

270. Kumar S, Wong G, Maysky M, et al. Amniotic fluid embolism complicated by paradoxical embolism and disseminated intravascular coagulation. Am J Crit Care 2010; 19:379–382.

271. Vellayappan U, Attias MD, Shulman MS. Paradoxical embolization by amniotic fluid seen on transesophageal echocardiography. Anesth Analg 2009; 108:1110–1112.

272. Lee PHU, Shulman MS, Vellayappan U, et al. Surgical treatment of an amniotic fluid embolism with cardiopulmonary collapse. Ann Thorac Surg 2010; 90:1694–1696.

273. Ngan S, Seckl MJ. Gestational trophoblastic neoplasia management: an update. Curr Opin Oncol 2007; 19:486–491.

274. Seckl MJ, Sebire N, Berkowitz RS. Gestational trophoblastic disease. Lancet 2010; 376:717–729.

275. Gurwitt LJ, Long JM, Clark RE. Cerebral metastatic choriocarcinoma. A postpartum cause of 'stroke'. Obstet Gynecol 1975; 45:583–588.

276. Saad N, Tang YM, Sclavos E, et al. Metastatic choriocarcinoma: a rare cause of stroke in the young adult. Australas Radiol 2006; 50:481–483.

277. Aguilar MJ, Rabinovitch R. Metastatic chorionepithelioma simulating multiple strokes. Neurology 1964; 14:933–937.

278. Vaughan HG, Howard RG. Intracranial haemorrhage due to metastatic chorionepithelioma. Neurology 1962; 12:771–777.

279. Suresh TN, Santosh V, Shastry Kolluri VR, et al. Intracranial haemorrhage resulting from unsuspected choriocarcinoma metastasis. Neurol India 2001; 49:231–236.

280. van den Doel EMH, van Merriënboer FJJM, Tulleken CAF. Cerebral haemorrhage from unsuspected choriocarcinoma. Clin Neurol Neurosurg 1985; 87:287–290.

281. Huang C-Y, Chen C-A, Hsieh C-Y, et al. Intracerebral haemorrhage as initial presentation of gestational choriocarcinoma: a case report and literature review. Int J Gynecol Cancer 2007; 17:1166–1171.

282. Weir B, MacDonald N, Mielke B. Intracranial vascular complications of choriocarcinoma. Neurosurgery 1978; 2:138–142.

283. Pullar M, Blumbergs PC, Phillips GE, et al. Neoplastic cerebral aneurysm from metastatic gestational choriocarcinoma. Case report. J Neurosurg 1985; 63:644–647.

284. Hove B, Andersen BB, Christiansen TM. Intracranial oncotic aneurysms from choriocarcinoma. Case report and review of the literature. Neuroradiology 1990; 32:526–528.

285. Prakash C, Bansal BC. Cerebral venous thrombosis. J Indian Acad Clin Med 2000; 5:55–61.

286. Coutinho JM, Ferro JM, Canhão P, et al. Cerebral venous and sinus thrombosis in women. Stroke 2009; 40:2356–2361.

287. Jeng J-S, Tang S-C, Yip P-K. Stroke in women of reproductive age: comparison between stroke related and unrelated to pregnancy. J Neurol Sci 2004; 221:25–29.

288. Vicente V, Rodriguez C, Soto I, et al. Risk of thrombosis during pregnancy and post-partum in hereditary thrombophilia. Am J Haematol 1994; 46:151–167.

289. Galan HL, McDowell AB, Johnson PR, et al. Puerperal cerebral venous thrombosis associated with decreased free protein S: a case report. J Reprod Med 1995; 40:859–862.

290. Zuber M, Toulon P, Marnet L, et al. Factor V Leiden mutation in cerebral venous thrombosis. Stroke 1996; 27:1721–1723.

291. Martinelli I, Sacchi E, Landi G, et al. High risk of cerebral-vein thrombosis in carriers of a prothrombin-gene mutation and in users of oral contraceptives. N Engl J Med 1998; 338:1793–1797.

292. Cakmak S, Derex L, Berruyer M, et al. Cerebral vein thrombosis. Clinical outcome and systematic screening of prothrombotic factors. Neurology 2003; 60:1175–1178.

293. McAuley WJ, Hunt BJ, Ahmad HN, et al. First trimester superior sagittal sinus venous thrombosis and antithrombin deficiency. J Obstet Gynecol 2005; 25:808–810.

294. Hirsch DR, Mikkola KM, Marks PW, et al. Pulmonary embolism and deep vein thrombosis during pregnancy or oral contraceptive use: prevalence of Factor V Leiden. Am Heart J 1996; 131:1145–1148.

295. Carhuapoma JR, Mitsias P, Levine SR. Cerebral venous thrombosis and anticardiolipin antibodies. Stroke 1997; 28:2363–2369.

296. Folkeringa N, Brouwer JLP, Korteweg FJ, et al. High risk of pregnancy-related venous thromboembolism in women with multiple thrombophilic defects. Br J Haematol 2007; 138:110–116.

297. Brey RL, Coull BM. Cerebral venous thrombosis. Role of activated protein C resistance and Factor V gene mutation. Stroke 1996; 27:1719–1720.

298. Helms AK, Kittner SJ. Pregnancy and stroke. CNS Spectr 2005; 10:580–587.

299. Ferro JM, Canhão P, Stam J, et al. for the ISCVT Investigators. Prognosis of cerebral vein and dural sinus thrombosis. Results of the International Study on Cerebral Vein and Dural Sinus Thrombosis (ISCVT). Stroke 2004; 35:664–670.

300. Cumurciuc R, Crassard I, Sarov M, et al. Headache as the only neurological sign of cerebral venous thrombosis: a series of 17 cases. J Neurol Neurosurg Psychiatry 2005; 76:1084–1087.

301. Einhäupl KM, Villringer A, Meister W, et al. Heparin treatment in sinus venous thrombosis. Lancet 1991; 338:597–600.

302. de Bruijn SF, Stam J. Randomised, placebo-controlled trial of anticoagulation treatment with low-molecular-weight heparin for cerebral sinus thrombosis. Stroke 1999; 30:484–488.

303. Preter M, Tzourio C, Ameri A, et al. Long-term prognosis in cerebral venous thrombosis. Follow-up of 77 patients. Stroke 1996; 27:243–245.

304. Stolz E, Rahimi A, Gerriets T, et al. Cerebral venous thrombosis: an all or nothing disease? Prognostic factors and long term outcome. Clin Neurol Neurosurg 2005; 107:99–107.

305. Lee MS, Pless M. Apoplectic lymphocytic hypophysitis. Case report. J Neurosurg 2003; 98:183–185.

306. Semple P, Webb M, de Villiers J, et al. Pituitary apoplexy. Neurosurgery 2005; 56:65–73.

307. Das NK, Behari DS, Banerji D. Pituitary apoplexy associated with acute cerebral infarct. J Clin Neurosci 2008; 15:1418–1420.

308. Mohindra S, Kovai P, Chhabra R. Fatal bilateral ACA territory infarcts after pituitary apoplexy: a case report and literature review. Skull Base 2010; 20:285–288.

309. de Heide LJM, van Tol KM, Doorenbos B. Pituitary apoplexy presenting during pregnancy. Netherlands J Med 2004; 62:393–396.

310. Murad-Kejbou S, Eggenberger E. Pituitary apoplexy: evaluation, management, and prognosis. Curr Opin Ophthalmol 2009; 20:456–461.

311. Nawa R, Abdel Mannan D, Selman W, et al. Pituitary tumour apoplexy: a review. J Intensive Care Med 2008; 23:75–90.

312. Maccagnan P, Macedo CL, Kayath MJ, et al. Conservative management of pituitary apoplexy: a prospective study. J Clin Endocrinol Metab 1995; 80:2190–2197.

313. Ayuk J, McGregor J, Mitchell RD, et al. Acute management of pituitary apoplexy – surgery or conservative management? Clin Endocrinol 2004; 61:747–752.

314. Ross RJM, Chew SL, Perry L, et al. Diagnosis and selective cure of Cushing's disease during pregnancy by transsphenoidal surgery. Eur J Endocrinol 1995; 132:722–726.

315. Verdugo C, Alegría J, Grant C, et al. Cushing's disease treatment with transsphenoidal surgery during pregnancy. Rev Med Chil 2004; 132:75–80.

316. Casson IF, Davis JC, Jeffreys RV, et al. Successful management of Cushing's disease during pregnancy by transsphenoidal adenectomy. Clin Endocrinol (Oxf) 1987; 27:423–428.

317. Lunardi P, Rizzo A, Missori P, et al. Pituitary apoplexy in an acromegalic woman operated on during pregnancy by transphenoidal approach. Int J Gynaecol Obstet 1991; 34:71–74.

318. Keleştimur F. Sheehan's syndrome. Pituitary 2003; 6:181–188.

319. Dias MS, Sekhar LN. Intracranial haemorrhage from aneurysms and arteriovenous malformations during pregnancy and the puerperium. Neurosurgery 1990; 27:855–866.

320. Robinson JL, Hall CS, Sedzimir CB. Arteriovenous malformations, aneurysms, and pregnancy. J Neurosurg 1974; 41:63–70.

321. Barno A, Freeman DW. Maternal deaths due to spontaneous subarachnoid hemorrhage. Am J Obstet Gynecol 1976; 125:384–392.

322. Shah AK. Non-aneurysmal primary subarachnoid haemorrhage in pregnancy-induced hypertension and eclampsia. Neurology 2003; 61:117–120.

323. Horton JC, Chambers WA, Lyons SL, et al. Pregnancy and the risk of haemorrhage from cerebral arteriovenous malformations. Neurosurgery 1990; 27:867–872.

324. Belfort MA, Saade GR, Moise KJ, et al. Nimodipine in the management of preeclampsia: maternal and fetal effects. Am J Obstet Gynecol 1994; 171:417–424.

325. Yingling DR, Utter G, Vengalil S, et al. Calcium channel blocker, nimodipine, for the treatment of bipolar disorder during pregnancy. Am J Obstet Gynecol 2002; 187:1711–1712.

326. Amias AG. Cerebral vascular disease in pregnancy. I. Haemorrhage. J Obstet Gynaecol Br Commonwealth 1970; 77:100–120.

327. Cruickshank A, Auld P, Beetham R, et al. Revised national guidelines for analysis of cerebrospinal fluid for bilirubin in suspected subarachnoid haemorrhage. Ann Clin Biochem 2008; 45:238–244.

328. The NINDS rt-PA Stroke Study Group. Tissue plasminogen activator for acute ischemic stroke. The National Institute of Neurological Disorders and Stroke rt-PA Stroke Study Group. N Engl J Med 1995; 333(24):1581–1587.

329. Hacke W, Kaste M, Bluhmki E, et al. Thrombolysis with alteplase 3 to 4.5 hours after acute ischemic stroke. N Engl J Med 2008; 359(13):1317–1329.

330. Elford K, Leader A, Wee R, et al. Stroke in ovarian hyperstimulation syndrome in early pregnancy treated with intra-arterial rt-PA. Neurology 2002; 59:1270–1272.

331. Dapprich M, Boessenecker W. Fibrinolysis with alteplase in a pregnant woman with stroke. Cerebrovasc Dis 2002; 13:290.

332. Johnson DM, Kramer DC, Cohen E, et al. Thrombolytic therapy for acute stroke in late pregnancy with intra-arterial recombinant tissue plasminogen activator. Stroke 2005; 36:e53–e55.

333. Wiese KM, Talkad A, Mathews M, et al. Intravenous recombinant plasminogen activator in a pregnant woman with cardioembolic stroke. Stroke 2006; 37:2168–2169.

334. Murugappan A, Coplin WM, Al-Sadat AN, et al. Thrombolytic therapy of acute ischemic stroke during pregnancy. Neurology 2006; 66:768–770.

335. Turrentine MA, Braems G, Ramirez M. Use of thrombolytics for the treatment of thromboembolic disease during pregnancy. Obstet Gynecol Surv 1995; 50:534–541.

336. DeKeyser J, Gdovinova Z, Uyttenboogaart M, et al. Intravenous alteplase for stroke. Beyond the guidelines and in particular clinical situations. Stroke 2007; 38:2612–2618.

337. Kozer E, Nikfar S, Costei A, et al. Aspirin consumption during the first trimester of pregnancy and congenital anomalies: a meta-analysis. Am J Obstet Gynecol 2002; 187:1623–1630.

338. Norgard B, Puho E, Czeizel AE, et al. Aspirin use during early pregnancy and the risk of congenital abnormalities: a population-based case-control study. Am J Obstet Gynecol 2005; 192:922–923.

339. Rai R, Cohen H, Dave M, et al. Randomised controlled trial of aspirin and aspirin plus heparin in pregnant women with recurrent miscarriage associated with phospholipid antibodies (or antiphospholipid antibodies). BMJ 1997; 314:253.

340. Mak A, Cheung MW-L, Cheak AA, et al. Combination of heparin and aspirin is superior to aspirin alone in enhancing live births in patients with recurrent pregnancy loss and positive anti-phospholipid antibodies: a meta-analysis of randomized controlled trials and meta-regression. Rheumatology 2010; 49:281–288.

341. Bujold E, Roberge S, Lacasse Y, et al. Prevention of preeclampsia and intrauterine growth restriction with aspirin started in early pregnancy: a meta-analysis. Obstet Gynecol 2010; 116:402–414.

342. Helms AK, Drogan O, Kittner SJ. First trimester stroke prophylaxis in pregnant women with a history of stroke. Stroke 2009; 40:1158–1161.

343. Chan KY, Gilbert-Barness E, Tiller G. Warfarin embryopathy. Pediatr Pathol Mol Med 2003; 22:277–283.

344. Chan WS, Anand S, Ginsberg JS. Anticoagulation of pregnant women with mechanical heart valves: a systematic review of the literature. Arch Int Med 2000; 160(2):191–196 [Epub 27 Jan 2000].

345. Schaefer C, Hannemann D, Meister R, et al. Vitamin K antagonists and pregnancy outcome. A multi-centre prospective study. Thromb Haemostasis 2006; 95:917–1051.

346. van Driel D, Wesseling J, Sauer PJ, et al. In utero exposure to coumarins and cognition at 8 to 14 years old. Pediatrics 2001; 107:123–129.

17

Vascular malformations of the brain in pregnancy

David P. Breen, Catharina J. M. Klijn, and Rustam Al-Shahi Salman

INTRODUCTION

Intracranial haemorrhage, including both spontaneous (non-traumatic) intracerebral haemorrhage (ICH) and subarachnoid haemorrhage (SAH), is a well recognised complication of pregnancy and the puerperium. Incidence rates vary from 6 to 31 per 100,000 deliveries (Table 17.1) (1–8). This compares to an incidence of intracranial haemorrhage in women of reproductive age who are not pregnant of approximately 5 per 100,000 women-years (9). The Confidential Enquiry into Maternal Deaths in the United Kingdom found intracranial haemorrhage to be the third leading cause of indirect maternal deaths (in other words, deaths caused by pre-existing or new health conditions aggravated by pregnancy), after cardiac and psychiatric causes (10).

Vascular malformations of the brain are a leading cause of intracranial haemorrhage during pregnancy and the early post-partum period. Intracranial haemorrhage can also be caused by eclampsia, coagulopathy, arterial dissection, intracranial venous thrombosis, pituitary apoplexy and rarer causes such as bleeding into metastases from a choriocarcinoma. Intracranial vascular malformations are an even more common problem prior to conception, when neurologists, neurosurgeons and obstetricians worry about the risk of haemorrhage during pregnancy if the malformation is left untreated. Given the widening availability and liberal use of brain imaging in high-income countries, detection of some incidental intracranial vascular malformations is rising (11,12), making the dilemma of their management an increasingly common problem.

This chapter reviews published evidence relating to the incidence and risk of SAH and ICH from intracranial aneurysms, arteriovenous malformations (AVMs), cavernous malformations and developmental venous anomalies (DVAs). We also consider the evidence for strategies for treating intracranial vascular malformations and managing labour which are commonly followed in clinical practice to try to minimise the risks to mother and child. The investigation and management of ICH in pregnancy and the puerperium is covered in chapter 6c.

INTRACRANIAL ANEURYSMS
Classification

Intracranial aneurysms are localised defects of an arterial wall. Pouch-like saccular aneurysms – previously called 'berry' aneurysms – are the predominant morphological type, most of which arise at or near bifurcations of major arteries on the Circle of Willis. More than three-quarters of saccular aneurysms involve the anterior cerebral circulation, and roughly one-fifth are accompanied by at least one other intracranial aneurysm. Fusiform aneurysms (non-saccular dilatations, which involve the entire vessel wall for a short distance), dissecting aneurysms (caused by a tear in the intima of the arterial wall, resulting in a mural haematoma) and mycotic aneurysms (caused by septic emboli, often due to infective endocarditis) are much rarer than saccular aneurysms. Most unruptured intracranial aneurysms are asymptomatic, although they can produce cranial neuropathies by external compression (e.g., oculomotor nerve palsy – usually with dilatation of the pupil – due to a posterior communicating artery aneurysm and optic neuropathy due to an ophthalmic artery aneurysm).

Incidence of Rupture of Intracranial Aneurysms and Its Outcome in Women Who Are Not Pregnant

The prevalence of unruptured intracranial aneurysms in people without a pertinent family history is 2.3% [95% confidence interval (CI) 1.7–3.1] (13). In a meta-analysis of 19 studies (including 4705 patients and 6556 unruptured aneurysms), the overall risk of rupture of untreated aneurysms in studies with a mean follow-up of less than 5 years was 1.2% (95% CI, 1.0–1.5) for every patient-year at risk; in studies with a mean follow-up between 5 and 10 years this risk was 0.6% (95% CI, 0.5–0.7); and in studies with a mean follow-up of more than 10 years it was 1.3% (95% CI, 0.9–1.8) (14). The annual incidence of SAH in the general population ranges from 4.2 to 22.7 per 100,000 (depending on the geographical region), and the incidence in women is 1.24 times (95% CI, 1.09–1.42) higher than in men (15).

The risk of haemorrhage from unruptured intracranial aneurysms has been quite well characterised over the short term, but there is still some uncertainty about long-term risk. The principal factors that seem to raise the risk of intracranial aneurysm rupture are increasing patient age, female gender, Japanese or Finnish descent, increasing aneurysm size, symptomatic aneurysms (which cause symptoms by compression of adjacent neural tissue, rather than SAH) and aneurysm location on the posterior circulation (14,16).

The outcome after aneurysmal SAH is poor. In a recent meta-analysis, up to half of people with aneurysmal SAH in the general population died within the first month, although case-fatality rates have decreased over the past three decades. The range of follow-up varied amongst the studies (1–12 months after SAH), but overall 19% of patients were left dependant (17).

Incidence of Aneurysm Rupture and Its Outcome During Pregnancy or the Puerperium

Reliable data on the incidence of aneurysmal rupture during pregnancy are limited due to the rarity of intracranial haemorrhage during pregnancy, the failure of many studies to distinguish SAH from ICH (and other types of intracranial haemorrhage) and the variable extent of investigation for the underlying cause of intracranial haemorrhage in these studies.

Table 17.1   Main Studies of Intracranial Haemorrhage in Pregnancy

| Study | Country | Number of events per 100,000 deliveries | | | Investigations performed to identify cause |
		Intracranial haemorrhage	ICH	SAH	
Jaigobin et al., 2000 (1)	Canada	26	12	14	Neuroimaging, angiography and craniotomy
James et al., 2005 (5)	United States	–	7.7	–	Not specified
Jeng et al., 2004 (2)	Taiwan	20.1	18.1	2.0	Neuroimaging and angiography
Liang et al., 2006 (3)	Taiwan	31.4	–	–	Neuroimaging
Kittner et al., 1996 (6)	United States	–	9	–	Neuroimaging and autopsy data (if available)
Ros et al., 2001 (4)	Sweden	6.2	3.8	2.4	Neuroimaging and angiography
Sharshar et al., 1995 (7)	France	–	4.6	–	Neuroimaging
Wiebers et al., 1995 (8)	United States	–	0	–	Neuroimaging

There are conflicting views on whether pregnancy increases the risk of aneurysmal SAH at all. There is a theoretical risk that haemodynamic changes in pregnancy contribute to aneurysm instability. Alterations in the arterial wall during pregnancy (18), metabolic and endocrine factors (19), and the increase of circulating blood volume (up to 50% by the third trimester) are all hypothetical reasons why extra stress might be placed on already weakened vessel walls.

Estimates of the incidence of aneurysmal SAH during pregnancy and the puerperium vary. A retrospective, hospital-based study in Canada reported seven cases of SAH during pregnancy or the first 6 weeks post-partum among 50,711 deliveries, representing an incidence of ~14 per 100,000 pregnancies (1). Three of these SAHs were caused by ruptured aneurysms (all affecting the posterior communicating artery). This incidence may be an overestimate because of selection bias, since approximately two-thirds of patients with intracranial haemorrhage in this cohort were referred from outside the hospital's catchment area because of its specialist obstetric and neurological services.

A Swedish group retrospectively studied more than 650,000 women (with more than one million pregnancies) over an 8-year period (4). They found eight cases of SAH, although the causes were not described. Compared to women in early pregnancy and women who were not pregnant, the relative risk of SAH from 2 days before to 1 day after delivery was 47 (95% CI, 19–98), but the absolute risk was small and this excess risk declined over the subsequent 6-week post-partum period. A large Dutch study in a single University Hospital found no such increase in the risk of aneurysmal SAH in women during pregnancy, delivery or the puerperium in comparison to women who were not pregnant (20).

One study reported a 27–40% case fatality following SAH in pregnancy (21). In a review of 118 previously reported cases of aneurysmal haemorrhage during pregnancy or the puerperium, fetal death occurred in 17% of the cases in which fetal outcome was reported (22).

Treatment of Aneurysms

Ruptured aneurysms are treated to prevent re-bleeding, provided there is a chance of a good outcome and it is technically possible to occlude the aneurysm. The International Subarachnoid Aneurysm Trial demonstrated that for patients whose aneurysm was amenable to either treatment with endovascular coiling or neurosurgical clipping, coiling produced better short-term (23) and long-term outcomes (24). There is no evidence to suggest that management should differ between pregnant and non-pregnant women. Both endovascular coiling and surgical clipping have been described in pregnant women with aneurysmal SAH (22,25).

Recommendations for Pregnancy and Mode of Delivery

Ideally, women with unruptured aneurysms should be counselled before conception in order to discuss treatment options, taking into account their views and the size and characteristics of their aneurysm. In the general population, screening for intracranial aneurysms may be appropriate for people with two first-degree relatives affected by aneurysms, or with polycystic kidney disease (although no randomised controlled trial data exist to support screening in either situation) (13). Screening prior to conception in other situations cannot be recommended. If an intracranial aneurysm has been occluded, it need not be a consideration during pregnancy and should not influence the mode of delivery.

Recommendations on the preferred mode of delivery for women with an unruptured intracranial aneurysm cannot be made, given the absence of high-quality evidence. Reasoned opinion has led some to recommend vaginal delivery unless the aneurysm has been diagnosed at term, or there has been neurosurgical intervention in the week prior to delivery (26). Others advise against a prolonged labour because of the risk of rupture due to the Valsalva effect of bearing-down, thus advocating elective caesarean section or vaginal delivery with epidural anaesthesia and instrumental delivery (if necessary) (27). It seems wise to avoid home births or a prolonged labour, although the evidence base for this advice is not strong. Elective caesarean section is not mandatory. Decisions should be made by a clinician with expertise in the management of unruptured aneurysms on an individual patient basis, and should take into account the known risk factors for aneurysm rupture (14,16).

ARTERIOVENOUS MALFORMATIONS
Classification

A pial AVM consists of a tangled cluster of blood vessels (called a 'nidus') in which blood shunts directly from arteries to veins in the absence of a normal capillary bed. Pial AVMs are supplied by the internal carotid or vertebrobasilar circulation. If an AVM is large, it may also recruit dural blood supply from the external carotid circulation and is then classified as a mixed AVM. AVMs that consist of a direct shunt from the external carotid circulation within the dura are called dural AV fistulas (DAVFs), and they are believed to be secondary to trauma, surgery, thrombosis of an adjacent venous sinus or veno-occlusive disease and will not be further discussed. Pial or mixed AVMs tend to be detected in the fourth or fifth decade of life, and manifest with ICH, seizure or non-haemorrhagic focal neurological deficits, in descending order of frequency (28,29). Aneurysms can occur in association with AVMs.

Incidence of AVM Rupture and Its Outcome in Women Who Are Not Pregnant

Contemporary population-based studies show that the annual incidence of first-ever haemorrhage from an AVM is ~0.5 per 100,000 adults (including pregnant women) (28,29). Studies at tertiary referral centres found the risk of haemorrhage from a known, unruptured AVM to be between 1% and 8% per year, and re-bleed rates between 5% and 34% per year; the risk of re-bleed is greater for AVMs with exclusive deep venous drainage or deep brain location (30,31). The 30-day case-fatality after AVM haemorrhage was 18% (95% CI, 4–43%) in a population-based study of cases between 1965 and 1992 (32), but was lower (11%; 95% CI, 6–19%) in a contemporary population-based study (33).

Incidence of Rupture and Its Outcome During Pregnancy or the Puerperium

Various studies have attempted to establish whether particular trimesters of pregnancy or mode of delivery influence the incidence of AVM rupture. Unfortunately, none of these studies is prospective or population based, and bias most probably plays a role. In particular, the occurrence of haemorrhage may discourage some women from becoming pregnant again, or may even be fatal, so preventing future pregnancies.

One study reported five ruptured AVMs during pregnancy among 50,711 deliveries, representing an incidence of ~10 per 100,000 deliveries (1). Two retrospective studies failed to find a higher risk of AVM haemorrhage during pregnancy (34,35). Another retrospective study of 191 women of childbearing age compared crude rates of first or recurrent haemorrhage during pregnancy with rates at other times (without a statistical analysis): compared to the bleeding rate of 4.5% per year when these women were not pregnant, there appeared to be a higher rate of haemorrhage during the second trimester (17% per year) but not at other stages of gestation (36). However, these studies used women's lifetimes prior to pregnancy as their own controls and various selection biases were at play (such as referral for stereotactic radiotherapy and survival following previous AVM haemorrhage), which makes the results difficult to interpret. For now, it seems that the risk of AVM haemorrhage during pregnancy is not substantially increased, but further research on representative samples of women with AVMs and well-chosen control groups is crucial to reliably quantify the risk.

In one study of nine women with intracranial haemorrhage due to a ruptured AVM, three women died, one had a spontaneous abortion just before her haemorrhage and one infant died (37). Another study found that maternal mortality was 28% and fetal mortality was 14% after an AVM-related intracranial haemorrhage (22).

Treatment

Treatments used to obliterate AVMs include surgical excision, endovascular embolisation, stereotactic radiotherapy or a combination of these methods. Ruptured AVMs tend to be treated. The vascular anatomy of AVMs and the anatomical location of their nidus influence both the risk of re-bleeding and decisions about whether and how to treat the AVM. The treatment of unruptured AVMs in an effort to prevent a first haemorrhage is more controversial. Treatment of unruptured AVMs appears to be an independent determinant of poor outcome in the short term (38), and a randomised controlled trial is underway to address the effects of treatment in this setting in men and women who are not pregnant (www.arubastudy.org).

In the same way as for unruptured intracranial aneurysms, decisions about treatment of AVMs should ideally be made prior to conception. Small studies have described good outcomes for both mother and baby following the treatment of AVMs during pregnancy (22,39), providing some reassurance for patients with AVMs that are thought to have a high risk of (re-)haemorrhage during pregnancy.

Recommendations for Pregnancy and Mode of Delivery

Women should discuss AVM treatment with a neurovascular specialist before conception, taking into account their views and the predicted risk of haemorrhage from their AVM. If an AVM has been obliterated, it need not be a consideration during pregnancy and need not influence the mode of delivery.

There are currently no grounds on which to recommend that women with AVMs should be sterilised in view of their risk of haemorrhage, as described in one older study (40). With this in mind, the older literature makes uncomfortable reading: in a report of 126 women who sought advice concerning the risks of AVM haemorrhage during pregnancy, avoidance of pregnancy was recommended to 101 of them (36 of whom were subsequently sterilised, and 20 of whom had a termination of pregnancy) (32). Even now, some clinicians continue to strongly advise against pregnancy for a woman with an unruptured AVM to become pregnant, despite the lack of evidence to support this.

We are unable to make recommendations on the preferred mode of delivery for women with an unruptured AVM, given the absence of high-quality evidence. Reasoned opinion has led some to recommend elective caesarean section and avoidance of a prolonged second stage of labour for women with an unruptured AVM (27). As with unruptured intracranial aneurysms, it seems wise to avoid home births or a prolonged labour, although the evidence base for this advice is not strong. Elective caesarean section is not mandatory. Decisions regarding mode of delivery in these women should be based on obstetric considerations.

CAVERNOUS MALFORMATIONS
Classification

Cavernous malformations are composed of capillary sinusoids, lined with endothelium devoid of tight junctions, embedded in a connective tissue matrix, without intervening brain parenchyma. The overall prevalence of asymptomatic cavernous malformations is ~0.15% from MR imaging studies of people without neurological symptoms (11). Multiple malformations are common, especially in the familial form of the disorder, which is inherited in an autosomal dominant manner (with incomplete penetrance due to the frequently asymptomatic nature of cavernous malformations). Three causative genes have been identified (41). Genetic counselling should be sought in patients in whom the family history is suggestive of familial occurrence. Cavernous malformations are mostly asymptomatic, but can present with intracranial haemorrhage (which is usually intracerebral, low volume and mild in its clinical severity (42)), non-haemorrhagic neurological deficits or epilepsy. Cavernomas can also occur in the spinal cord, but there is no evidence to indicate whether these cavernomas should influence mode of delivery or obstetric anaesthesia.

Incidence of Rupture and Its Outcome in Women Who Are Not Pregnant

Knowledge about the prognosis of cavernous malformations is limited by existing reports being hospital based and usually

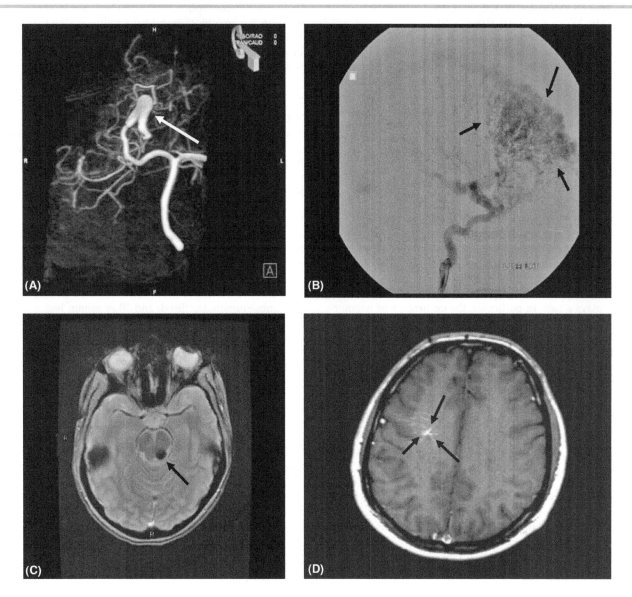

Figure 17.1 (**A**) Intracranial aneurysm (*arrow*) on the posterior cerebral artery, diagnosed on digital subtraction angiography in a 30-year-old woman in the puerperium. (**B**) AVM (*arrows*) in the left frontal lobe, diagnosed on digital subtraction angiography prior to a 30-year-old woman undergoing in-vitro fertilisation. (**C**) Cavernous malformation (*arrow*) in the left posterior pons, diagnosed on gradient echo imaging in a 28-year-old woman, who subsequently underwent an uneventful pregnancy, delivery and puerperium. (**D**) DVA (*arrows*) in the right frontal lobe, diagnosed on contrast-enhanced magnetic resonance imaging in a 25-year-old asymptomatic woman.

retrospective with average follow-up durations of 5 years at most. One ongoing population-based study has not yet reported (28). On the basis of the existing literature, the risk of first-ever bleeding is 0.4% to 0.6% per year (43,44), and the risk of re-bleeding ranges from 3.8% to 33.9% per year depending on the study. Brainstem cavernous malformations appear to carry a higher risk of re-bleeding (45,46).

Incidence of Rupture and Its Outcome During Pregnancy or the Puerperium

Suggestions that pregnancy may provoke bleeding from a cavernous malformation are mainly based on case reports (47,48). In one hospital-based series of 145 patients with cavernous malformations, three women presented with intracranial haemorrhage during pregnancy (47). In another series of 66 patients, 6 women presented with intracranial haemor-

rhage, 2 of which occurred in the first trimester of pregnancy (49). None of these small studies found pregnancy to be an independent predictor of haemorrhage in multivariable analyses. There have been no reported deaths in pregnancy from intracranial haemorrhage related to a cavernous malformation, and there seems to be no evidence to advise against pregnancy in women with cavernous malformation because of the risk of haemorrhage.

Treatment

Most cavernous malformations are not treated. Those with aggressive modes of presentation or a poor predicted prognosis are treated depending on their surgical accessibility: cavernous malformations in supratentorial lobar and some brainstem locations are excised surgically (50). Stereotactic radiotherapy is used in some parts of the world to treat surgically inaccessible cavernous malformations (51), but many are sceptical about its beneficial effects.

Since experience of managing cavernous malformations (with or without intracranial haemorrhage) in pregnancy is limited, we cannot recommend their treatment prior to pregnancy, and decisions should be tailored to each woman.

Recommendations for Pregnancy and Mode of Delivery

In the same way as for intracranial aneurysms and AVMs, women should discuss cavernous malformation treatment before conception, taking into account their views and the predicted risk of haemorrhage. If a cavernous malformation has been surgically resected, it need not be a consideration during pregnancy and need not influence the mode of delivery.

In the face of less than a handful of case reports suggesting cavernous malformation haemorrhage might be caused by pregnancy or vaginal delivery, we do not support the view of some authors that pregnancy may be contraindicated or caesarean section may be indicated for women with cavernous malformations that are large, have recently bled, or are in brainstem or deep locations (41). It would be inappropriate to recommend caesarean section as the preferred mode of delivery for women with a cavernous malformation. Decisions regarding the mode of delivery in these women should be based on obstetric considerations.

DEVELOPMENTAL VENOUS ANOMALIES
Classification

A DVA is a variation in the normal venous drainage of an area of brain, which is thought to be congenital, and may be associated with cavernous malformations. They are characteristically found along the lateral ventricles (draining into a subependymal or cortical vein), but can occur anywhere in the brain or spinal cord. Almost all DVAs are found incidentally. On contrast-enhanced MRI, the serpentine appearance of the peripheral draining veins resembles a caput medusae (Fig. 17.1).

Incidence of Rupture, Outcome and Treatment

Symptomatic intracranial haemorrhage from DVAs is non-existent in most follow-up studies (52), but in those that have described associated bleeds, the annual rate of haemorrhage has been between 0.15% and 0.34% (52–54). In case reports of intracranial haemorrhage due to rupture of DVAs (55–57), it is unclear whether the haemorrhage in these cases was in fact caused by an undetected cavernous malformation. There have been no reports of significant maternal or fetal morbidity due to intracranial haemorrhage related to a DVA. Surgical excision of DVAs is generally regarded as hazardous, because they drain normal brain, and their excision can result in venous infarction.

Recommended Mode of Delivery

We can find no evidence to recommend caesarean section instead of vaginal delivery in women with a DVA, with or without a history of intracranial haemorrhage.

CONCLUSIONS

The shortage of evidence about whether pregnancy and certain modes of delivery influence haemorrhage from intracranial vascular malformations is a challenge for expectant mothers, obstetricians, neurosurgeons, neurologists and researchers. In general, it seems that any influence of pregnancy or the puerperium on the risk of ICH from vascular malformations is not large when compared to the effect of known risk factors (Table 17.2). Pregnancy, or the wish to become pregnant, is generally not a reason to screen for vascular malformations, unless there are other indications for screening. The advice to screen for intracranial vascular malformations in these women should be similar to that given in the general population.

Table 17.2 Summary of Data on Intracranial Vascular Malformations in the General Population and in Pregnancy

Type of malformation	Asymptomatic prevalence, %	Risk factors for haemorrhage	Increased risk of rupture			Suggestions for pregnancy and delivery
			Pregnancy	Delivery	Puerperium	
Aneurysm	~2	Patient: increasing age, female gender, Japanese or Finnish descent Aneurysm: increasing size, symptomatic, posterior circulation location	±	±	0	None, if previously treated. Discuss treatment prior to conception. Avoid home births. Avoid prolonged labour. Caesarean section is not mandatory; mode of delivery can be based on obstetric considerations.
AVM	~0.05	Deep venous drainage, deep location, nidal and feeder aneurysms	±	±	±	None, if previously treated. Discuss treatment prior to conception. Avoid home births. Avoid prolonged labour. Caesarean section is not mandatory; mode of delivery can be based on obstetric considerations.
Cavernous	~0.16	Brainstem location	–	0	0	None, if previously treated. Discuss treatment prior to conception. Mode of delivery determined by obstetric, not neurological considerations.
DVA	~0.04	?	0	0	0	None

±, contradictory evidence from well-designed studies; –, evidence from case reports; 0, no evidence.

Ideally, treatment options for intracranial vascular malformations should be discussed prior to conception. Intervention may be warranted in women with aneurysms and AVMs to prevent haemorrhage, and this should be undertaken prior to conception if possible. Pregnant women with an intracranial vascular malformation should ideally be managed by a multidisciplinary team (including a neurologist or neurosurgeon with expertise in vascular malformations).

ACKNOWLEDGEMENTS

RASS is funded by a Medical Research Council clinician scientist fellowship.

REFERENCES

1. Jaigobin C, Silver FL. Stroke and pregnancy. Stroke 2000; 31:2948–2951.
2. Jeng JS, Tang SC, Yip PK. Incidence and etiologies of stroke during pregnancy and puerperium as evidenced in Taiwanese women. Cerebrovasc Dis 2004; 18:290–295.
3. Liang CC, Chang SD, Lai SL, et al. Stroke complicating pregnancy and the puerperium. Eur J Neurol 2006; 13:1256–1260.
4. Salonen Ros H, Lichtenstein P, Bellocco R, et al. Increased risks of circulatory diseases in late pregnancy and puerperium. Epidemiology 2001; 12:456–460.
5. James A, Bushnell CD, Jamison M, et al. Incidence and risk factors for stroke in pregnancy and the puerperium. Obstet Gynecol 2005; 106:509–516.
6. Kittner SJ, Stern BJ, Feeser BR, et al. Pregnancy and the risk of stroke. N Eng J Med 1996; 335:768–774.
7. Sharshar T, Lamy C, Mas J. Incidence and causes of strokes associated with pregnancy and puerperium: a study in public hospitals of Ile de France. Stroke 1995; 26:930–936.
8. Wiebers DO, Whisnant JP. The incidence of stroke among pregnant women in Rochester Minn, 1955 through 1979. JAMA 1985; 254:3055–3057.
9. Pettiti DB, Sidney S, Quesenberry CP, et al. Incidence of stroke and myocardial infarction in women of reproductive age. Stroke 1997; 28:280–283.
10. Confidential Enquiry into Maternal and Child Health (CEMACH). Saving Mother's Lives 2003-2005: reviewing maternal deaths to make motherhood safer. London: CEMACH, 2007.
11. Al-Shahi Salman R, Whiteley W, Warlow C. Screening using whole body MRI scanning: who wants an incidentaloma? J Med Screen 2007; 14:2–4.
12. Gabriel RA, Kim H, Sidney S, et al. Ten-year detection rate of brain arteriovenous malformations in a large, multiethnic, defined population. Stroke 2010; 41:21–26.
13. Rinkel GJE. Intracranial aneurysm screening: indications and advice for practice. Lancet Neurol 2005; 4:122–128.
14. Wermer MJ, van der Schaaf IC, Algra A, et al. Risk of rupture of unruptured intracranial aneurysms in relation to patient and aneurysm characteristics: an updated meta-analysis. Stroke 2007; 38:1404–1410.
15. de Rooij NK, Linn FH, van der Plas JA, et al. Incidence of subarachnoid haemorrhage: a systematic review with emphasis on region, age, gender and time trends. J Neurol Neurosurg Psychiatry 2007; 78:1365–1372.
16. International Study of Unruptured Intracranial Aneurysms Investigators. Unruptured intracranial aneurysms: natural history, clinical outcome, and risks of surgical and endovascular treatment. Lancet 2003; 362:103–110.
17. Nieuwkamp DJ, Setz LE, Algra A, et al. Changes in case fatality of aneurysmal subarachnoid haemorrhage over time, according to age, sex, and region: a meta-analysis. Lancet Neurol 2009; 8:635–642.
18. Manalo-Estrella P, Barker AE. Histopathological findings in human aortic media associated with pregnancy. Arch Pathol 1967; 83:336–341.
19. Weir BK, Drake CG. Rapid growth of residual aneurismal neck during pregnancy: case report. J Neurosurg 1991; 75:780–782.
20. Tiel Groenestege AT, Rinkel GJE, van der Bom JG, et al. The risk of aneurysmal subarachnoid haemorrhage during pregnancy, delivery, and the puerperium in the Utrecht population: case-crossover study and standardized incidence ratio estimation. Stroke 2009; 40:1148–1151.
21. Mas JL, Lamy C. Stroke in pregnancy and the puerperium. J Neurol 1998; 245:1431–1459.
22. Dias MS, Sekhar LN. Intracranial haemorrhage from aneurysms and arteriovenous malformations during pregnancy and the puerperium. Neurosurgery 1990; 27:855–865.
23. Molyneux AJ, Kerr RS, Yu LM, et al. International subarachnoid aneurysm trial (ISAT) of neurosurgical clipping versus endovascular coiling in 2143 patients with unruptured intracranial aneurysms: a randomised comparison of effects on survival, dependency, seizures, re-bleeding, subgroups, and aneurysm occlusion. Lancet 2005; 366:809–817.
24. Molyneux AJ, Kerr RSC, Birks J, et al. Risk of recurrent subarachnoid haemorrhage, death, or dependance and standardised mortality ratios after clipping or coiling of an intracranial aneurysm in the International Subarachnoid Aneurysm Trial (ISAT): long-term follow-up. Lancet Neurol 2009; 8:427–433.
25. Kizilkilic O, Albayram S, Adeletli I, et al. Endovascular treatment of ruptured intracranial aneurysms during pregnancy: report of three cases. Arch Gynecol Obstet 2003; 268:325–328.
26. Treadwell SD, Thanvi B, Robinson TG. Stroke in pregnancy and the puerperium. Postgrad Med J 2008; 84:238–245.
27. Davie CA, O'Brien P. Stroke and pregnancy. J Neuro Neurosurg Psychiatry 2008; 79:240–245.
28. Al-Shahi R, Bhattacharya JJ, Currie DG, et al. Prospective, population-based detection of intracranial vascular malformations in adults: the Scottish Intracranial Vascular Malformation Study (SIVMS). Stroke 2003; 34:1163–1169.
29. Stapf C, Mast H, Sciacca RR, et al. The New York Islands AVM Study: design, study progress, and initial results. Stroke 2003; 34: e29–e33.
30. Al-Shahi R, Warlow C. A systematic review of the frequency and prognosis of arteriovenous malformations of the brain in adults. Brain 2001; 124:1900–1926.
31. Stapf C, Mast H, Sciacca RR, et al. Predictors of hemorrhage in patients with untreated brain arteriovenous malformations. Neurology 2006; 66:1350–1355.
32. Brown RD Jr., Wiebers DO, Torner JC, et al. Incidence and prevalence of intracranial vascular malformations in Olmsted County, Minnesota, 1965 to 1992. Neurology 1996; 46:949–952.
33. van Beijnum J, Lovelock CE, Cordonnier C, et al. Outcome after spontaneous and arteriovenous malformation-related intracerebral haemorrhage: population-based studies. Brain 2009; 132:537–543.
34. Horton JC, Chambers WA, Lyons SL, et al. Pregnancy and the risk of hemorrhage from cerebral arteriovenous malformations. Neurosurgery 1990; 27:867–872.
35. Fujita K, Tsunoda H, Shigemutsu S, et al. Clinical study on the intracranial arteriovenous malformations associated with pregnancy. Nippon Sank Fujinka Gakkai Zasshi 1995; 47:1359–1364.
36. Forster DM, Kunkler IH, Hartland P. Risk of cerebral bleeding from arteriovenous malformations in pregnancy: the Sheffield experience. Stereotact Funct Neurosurg 1993; 61(suppl 1):20–22.
37. Sadasivan B, Malik GM, Lee C, et al. Vascular malformations and pregnancy. Surg Neurol 1990; 33:305–313.
38. Mohr JP, Stapf C, Sciacca RR, et al. Natural history versus treatment outcome in patients with unruptured brain arteriovenous malformation (AVM). Stroke 2004; 35:328.
39. Trivedi RA, Kirkpatrick PJ. Arteriovenous malformations of the cerebral circulation that rupture in pregnancy. J Obstet Gynaecol 2003; 23:484–489.
40. Robinson JL, Hall C, Sedzimir CB. Arteriovenous malformations, aneurysms, and pregnancy. J Neurosurg 1974; 41:63–70.
41. Labauge P, Denier C, Bergametti F, et al. Genetics of cavernous angiomas. Lancet Neurol 2007; 6:237–244.
42. Cordonnier C, Al-Shahi Salman R, Bhattacharya JJ, et al. Differences between intracranial vascular malformation types in the characteristics of their presenting haemorrhages: prospective,

population-based study. J Neurol Neurosurg Psychiatry 2008; 79:47–51.

43. Kondziolka D, Lunsford LD, Kestle JR. The natural history of cerebral cavernous malformations. J Neurosurg 1995; 83:820–824.

44. Aiba T, Tanaka R, Koike T, et al. Natural history of intracranial cavernous malformations. J Neurosurg 1995; 83:56–59.

45. Kim DS, Park YG, Choi JU, et al. An analysis of the natural history of cavernous malformations. Surg Neurol 1997; 48:9–17.

46. Hasegawa T, McInerney J, Kondziolka D, et al. Long-term results after stereotactic radiosurgery for patients with cavernous malformations. Neurosurgery 2002; 50:1190–1197.

47. Pozatti E, Acciarri N, Togretti F, et al. Growth, subsequent bleeding, and de novo appearance of cerebral cavernous angiomas. Neurosurgery 1996; 38:662–670.

48. Flemming KD, Goodman BP, Meyer FB. Successful brainstem cavernous malformation resection after repeated haemorrhages during pregnancy. Surg Neurol 2003; 60:545–547.

49. Robinson JR, Swad IA, Little JR. Natural history of the cavernous angiomas. J Neurosurg 1991; 75:709–714.

50. Bertalanffy H, Benes L, Miyazawa T, et al. Cerebral cavernomas in the adult: review of the literature and analysis of 72 surgically treated patients. Neurosurg Rev 2002; 25:1–53.

51. Kondziolka D, Flickinger JC, Lunsford LD. Radiosurgery for cavernous malformations. Prog Neurol Surg 2007; 20:220–230.

52. Hon JML, Bhattacharya JJ, Counsell CE, et al. The presentation and clinical course of intracranial developmental venous anomalies in adults: a systematic review and prospective, population-based study. Stroke 2009; 40:1980–1985.

53. McLaughlin MR, Kondziolka D, Flickinger JC, et al. The prospective natural history of cerebral venous malformations. Neurosurgery 1998; 43:195–200.

54. Naff NJ, Wermer J, Hoenig-Rigamonti K, et al. A longitudinal study of patients with venous malformations; documentation of a negligible hemorrhagic risk and benign natural history. Neurology 1998; 50:1709–1714.

55. Toledano M, Portilla Cuenca JC, Porras Estrades LF, et al. Pseudo-emesis gravidarum caused by complicated cerebral venous angiomas. Neurologica 2006; 21:92–95.

56. Rubin SM, Jackson GM, Cohen AW. Management of the pregnant patient with a cerebral venous angioma: a report of two cases. Obstet Gynecol 1991; 78:929–931.

57. Yamamoto M, Inagawa T, Kamiya K, et al. Intracerebral haemorrhage due to venous thrombosis in venous angioma—case report. Neurol Med Chir (Tokyo) 1989; 29:1044–1046.

18

Pituitary disease in pregnancy

Dorota Dworakowska and Simon J. B. Aylwin

INTRODUCTION

As is the case with many organ systems, in pregnancy the pituitary gland undergoes profound changes in its anatomy and physiology. The normal endocrine milieu is altered and both corpus luteum and the placenta become additional sources of hormone secretion. As a consequence of physiological hormonal changes, the evaluation and assessment of pituitary functions in pregnant women differs from the non-pregnant state. Pregnancy can be regarded as a state of mild physiological acromegaly and the circulating cortisol and adrenocorticotropic hormone (ACTH) levels reach values in the range seen in Cushing's disease. The alteration in physiology has consequences both for the evaluation of endocrine status and also for the management of concurrent endocrine disturbance.

Management of pituitary disorders during pregnancy is specific and remains focused on balance between benefits and risks for both mother and fetus. In this chapter, we focus on the normal anatomical and physiological changes during pregnancy and review the literature related to the management of known and suspected pituitary disease, pituitary adenomas, lymphocytic hypophysitis, Sheehan's syndrome and hypopituitarism.

NORMAL ANATOMICAL AND PHYSIOLOGICAL CHANGES IN THE PITUITARY GLAND DURING PREGNANCY

Anatomy and Pituitary MRI During Pregnancy

Radiological and post-mortem studies demonstrate an increase in the cranio-caudal height of the pituitary gland throughout pregnancy (overall increase of 130% in comparison to non-pregnant). The upper limit for the height of the normal pituitary gland increases to12 mm in the immediate post-partum period (1,2). Pituitary MRI shows enlargement of the anterior pituitary gland, with the stalk remaining centrally positioned whilst the posterior pituitary gland is not visualised in the third trimester (3). A gradual, slight increase in size is observed in each pregnancy. In non-lactating woman, it takes up to 1 year for pituitary to shrink to near pre-pregnancy size (3–5).

MRI of the pituitary is the recommended modality of imaging if required; however, it is relatively contraindicated in the first trimester due to a theoretical risk to the fetus. The potential benefit and the unknown risks of MRI at any gestation should be weighed on an individual basis. Use of contrast agent gadopentetate dimeglumine (gadolinium) is contraindicated in pregnancy (6). The usual approach for pregnant patients is to consider postponing MRI till after birth. If not possible, MRI without a contrast agent should be the choice (7). Because of the increase in size of the normal pituitary, it may be more challenging to distinguish normal from a homogeneously enlarged pituitary mass, particularly without contrast. Where MRI is required for non-endocrine evaluation

in pregnancy, incidental pituitary abnormalities can be over-diagnosed and need follow-up imaging months after parturition.

Prolactin

Increased oestrogen level induces lactotroph hyperplasia and hypertrophy, resulting in 10-fold increased prolactin (PRL) secretion during pregnancy (8). Progesterone also stimulates PRL secretion (9). As in non-pregnant women, maternal pituitary PRL secretion is stimulated by thyrotropin-releasing hormone (TRH), arginine, meals and sleep (10). Additional lactotrophs are recruited through transdifferentiation from somatotroph cells (11,12). Serum levels of PRL start to fall gradually a week post-partum as the lactotroph hyperplasia regresses. PRL levels rise briskly in response to suckling during lactation and remain elevated in breastfeeding individuals, gradually falling over a period of several months (13).

TSH

Serum levels of human chorionic gonadotropin (hCG) produced by placenta peak at 9 to 13 weeks of gestation. hCG shares a common alpha-subunit with thyroid-stimulating hormone (TSH) and therefore shows structural similarity, leading to direct stimulation of the thyroid TSH receptor and a consequent decrease in maternal TSH (14). TSH levels start to rise after hCG levels fall at the end of the first trimester (14). Increased oestrogen levels lead to a significant increase in thyroxine (T4)-binding globulin (TBG) levels that reach a plateau after 12 to 14 weeks of gestation, and total thyroid hormone levels are concomitantly increased (15). The increased requirement for thyroxine (T4) production or replacement during pregnancy is related to increased TBG, the placental degradation of T4, increased maternal clearance of T4 and perhaps due to transfer of T4 from mother to fetus (15,16).

ACTH

Pregnancy affects the hypothalamic-pituitary-adrenal axis leading to increased urinary free cortisol (UFC), total and free plasma cortisol, ACTH and corticosteroid-binding globulin (CBG) levels (7). However, the corticotroph number in pituitary remains unaltered.

The causes of increased ACTH may include placental synthesis and release of biologically active corticotropin-releasing hormone (CRH) and ACTH, pituitary desensitisation to cortisol feedback, or enhanced pituitary responses to corticotropin-releasing factors (6). Plasma levels of ACTH rise steadily in the first trimester of pregnancy and again at the end of the third trimester. Levels fall rapidly after delivery and return to pre-pregnancy levels within 24 hours post- delivery (17).

The increase in free cortisol levels in pregnancy may be explained by the following: resistance to cortisol action, anti-glucocorticoid effects of elevated progesterone, altered set point for pituitary ACTH, and autonomic secretion of ACTH from the placenta (7). Increased levels of placental oestrogen result in an increase in CBG production in the liver. Diurnal variation in cortisol secretion is maintained throughout pregnancy, but it may be partially blunted (6,18–20).

This physiological state of hypercortisolism in pregnancy has no impact on the fetus due to the action of the 11-beta-hydroxysteroid dehydrogenase-2 enzyme (11-βHSD-2) in the placenta which converts cortisol into inactive metabolites (6,20,21). Cortisol and ACTH rise during the stress of labour and fall in the post-partum period to non-pregnant levels (18). The insensitivity of plasma cortisol to feedback inhibition persists beyond normal pregnancy in a significant proportion of healthy women for 2 to 3 weeks, and is absent by the 5th post-natal week (22).

GH-IGF1

Pregnancy can be regarded a state of mild physiological acromegaly. Maternal pituitary growth hormone (GH) secretion falls after the first trimester of pregnancy. As pregnancy progresses, total GH levels remain stable throughout pregnancy due to secretion of a GH variant (GH-V) by the placenta. GH-V stimulates insulin-like growth factor 1 (IGF1) thereby decreasing the pituitary GH secretion (23). GH-V is detectable by the 5th week of pregnancy, and levels increase exponentially and peak at 35 to 37 weeks (24). GH-V is secreted continuously with a non-pulsatile manner, and is regulated neither by GH-releasing factor nor by ghrelin (25,26), is not suppressible by high glucose levels and routine radioimmunoassay (RIA) and immunoradiometric assay (IRMA) methods may be variable in detecting GH-V (27).

LH/FSH

Pituitary gonadotropin synthesis and release are inhibited during pregnancy with decreased follicle-stimulating hormone/luteinizing hormone (FSH/LH) responses to gonadotropin-releasing hormone (GnRH) stimulation (28). Maternal serum LH and FSH start to decrease by 6 to 7 weeks of pregnancy and remain undetectable in the second trimester, as a result of suppression of elevated sex steroids (17-β-estradiol and progesterone) and regulatory peptides (10).

Vasopressin

The set point for serum osmolality is lower in pregnant women by about 10 mOsm/kg (275–280 mOsm/Kg compared to 285–295 mOsm/Kg in non-pregnant women), with serum sodium decreased by about 4 to 5 mmol/mL. This decrease lasts until the 10th week of gestation and does not change later on (29–31). Levels of vasopressin in the plasma do not change, although there is a higher rate of synthesis and secretion of vasopressin by the posterior pituitary to compensate increased clearance by the placental enzyme vasopressinase (30,31). The osmostat is restored to pre-pregnancy levels by 2 to 3 weeks post-partum (30,32).

PITUITARY ADENOMAS

All patients with pituitary tumours have an increased risk of developing visual fields abnormalities due to chiasmal compression since the normal pituitary gland enlarges during pregnancy. In addition there is an increased risk of infarction or haemorrhage because of enhanced vascularity during pregnancy. The main challenge during pregnancy is to determine which patients may be safely followed up until delivery and those who need intervention during gestation. Medical management of pathological hormone excess may also need to be modified during pregnancy.

Prolactinoma

Case Description

A 25-year-old woman initially presented with inability to conceive, secondary amenorrhea, galactorrhea and persistent headache, and subsequently was diagnosed with macroadenoma (1.7 cm) with elevated serum PRL level. She was given bromocriptine, which normalised her menstruation and the PRL level, followed by conception during treatment. Pregnancy remained uneventful until 27 weeks when she developed severe headache and total loss of vision in the left eye and partial loss of vision in the right eye. MRI showed enlargement of macroadenoma up to 2.5 cm with compression on optic chiasm and she underwent trans-sphenoidal adenectomy. After surgery, her vision improved and she delivered vaginally at 39 weeks (33).

Prolactinomas (PRL-omas) are the most frequent of all pituitary tumours and account for 50% of functioning pituitary tumours. PRL excess leads to suppression of gonadotrophin secretion and direct inhibition of gonadal steroidogenesis causing anovulatory cycles and subfertility (34). Because of the interference of PRL-omas with fertility, these tumours are almost always recognised before pregnancy and need careful follow-up during pregnancy. Risk to the mother from a PRL-oma is determined by the size of the tumour, whereas risk to the fetus is related to the risks of treatment of the adenoma during pregnancy. The main goal of treatment during pregnancy is to avoid the clinical consequences of optic chiasm compression. PRL increases in normal pregnancy and therefore cannot be used as a tumour marker. Therefore, monitoring is primarily clinical unless chiasmal compression is suspected, in which case MRI of pituitary is justified.

The initial size of the PRL-oma is a reliable indicator of the degree of risk during pregnancy. Pregnancy leads to clinically significant increase in the size of PRL-omas in 1% to 2% of microadenomas (<10 mm at diagnosis), 15% to 35% of macroadenomas (>10 mm at diagnosis) and in 4% to 7% of macroadenomas cases previously treated with surgery and/or radiotherapy (7,35–39).

In patients with microadenomas, close clinical observation accompanied by visual field testing in each trimester is recommended (7,40). Dopamine agonists can be stopped safely as the risk of clinically relevant tumour expansion is low (7). There is no need for routine imaging of the micro-PRL-oma during pregnancy unless clinically indicated in unusual patients.

During pregnancy, the treatment of macroadenomas is more controversial and should be individualised. The first approach allows continuation of medical therapy with dopamine agonists to reduce the risk of tumour growth. This option may be preferred when the duration of dopamine agonist therapy before conception was short or when the original tumour had substantial extrasellar expansion (7). Other authors suggest that because in the first trimester of pregnancy the growth of the pituitary macroadenoma is likely to be less than in other trimesters (and this is a period of the most important fetal organogenesis), medical therapy should be temporarily withdrawn (34). In patients where the PRL-oma size has been successfully controlled prior to pregnancy, many can be managed for the duration of pregnancy without dopamine agonist treatment.

In each approach for macro-PRL-oma, clinical monitoring, including visual field assessment, is needed. For small volume treated residual from treated macroadenoma assessment every 3 months is indicated. For the relatively few patients with known previous macroadenoma where regression and control has not been previously confirmed, or known unresponsive tumour or no treatment, visual fields should be assessed every 6 weeks (7,40). MRI pituitary should be performed if there are symptoms of tumour enlargement or deterioration in visual fields. Tumours that previously responded to dopamine agonists will remain responsive if treatment needs to be subsequently re-introduced. Surgical resection of PRL-omas in pregnancy is recommended only if there is a poor response with tumour growth despite dopamine agonist therapy, or intolerance to dopamine agonist therapy (37,38).

Surgical de-bulking of the tumour and/or radiotherapy may be considered before conception in patients with substantial suprasellar extension at diagnosis and those where clinical increase in size occurred in a previous pregnancy. However, both surgery and radiotherapy can lead to gonadotropin deficiency (34,36,38).

MRI pituitary should be repeated 2 to 3 months postpartum, or 2 months after cessation of lactation, to re-assess baseline tumour size. There are reports in the literature that PRL levels may decrease or even normalise post-partum with PRL-oma resolution although the exact mechanism leading to this remains unclear (37,41,42).

There is no evidence that the suckling reflex in the postpartum period increases tumour growth in PRL-omas and breastfeeding is not contraindicated (38). Dopamine agonists may impair lactation; however, it seems wise for patients who have to maintain dopamine agonists to prevent tumour growth, to continue their treatment (37).

Effect of Dopamine Agonist Therapy on Pregnancy and the Fetus
Bromocriptine has a well-established role for PRL-oma treatment before and during pregnancy. It is known to cross the placenta (38). A substantial number of pregnancies have occurred during treatment with bromocriptine in early pregnancy and the risk of fetal malformation has not been shown to be different from the normal population. There are data from about 100 women who were treated with bromocriptine throughout pregnancy with only two minor adverse events reported (43,44). Nine years of follow-up of children born to mothers who were taking bromocriptine during the early part of pregnancy has not shown any adverse effects (43,45,46).

Cabergoline may be an effective and safe alternative to bromocriptine during pregnancy, and is better tolerated (47). Cabergoline has also been shown to cross the placenta in animals, but there are no current data in humans. Use of cabergoline in early pregnancy has been studied in 350 pregnancies and there have been no significant adverse effects reported. Follow-up of children born to mothers who were treated with Cabergoline in the initial part of pregnancy has also not shown any adverse effects (37,48,49).

Pergolide has also been shown to cross the placenta in animal studies. Although no causal relationship between pergolide and congenital abnormalities has been established, currently there is very little safety information available about use of pergolide in pregnancy (34,38). Quinagolide is a non-ergot derived dopamine agonist used in the treatment of PRL-omas. Ectopic pregnancy, miscarriages and fetal malformations were reported during quinagolide usage (50). On the other hand, in the group of patient with PRL-oma resistant to bromocriptine, quinagolide efficacy was not related with any congenital abnormalities (51). Since data regarding pergolide and quinagolide are limited, they should be considered a last line of medical treatment during pregnancy (7,34). Other non-ergot dopamine agonists are not licensed for treatment of PRL-oma.

Conclusion

- In microadenomas, due to the low risk of tumour growth, clinical follow-up without treatment is considered appropriate.
- In macroadenomas, pregnancy should be planned after the control of tumour growth. Close follow-up or dopamine agonist treatment throughout pregnancy may be preferred depending on the tumour and patient preference, or dopamine agonists can be recommened after the first trimester. Pre-gestational treatment duration and tumour size should be taken into consideration while making a decision about treatment.
- There is no need for routine imaging of the PRL-oma during pregnancy, and PRL measurement is of little help.
- Breastfeeding is not associated with further tumour growth. In patients who required dopamine agonists to treat or prevent tumour growth lactation may be impaired.

Corticotroph Adenoma

Case Description

A 20-year-old patient developed early symptoms of recurrent Cushing's disease during follow-up. Her original presentation was at 14 years of age with typical paediatric cortisol excess, increased weight with cessation of vertical growth. She had typical biochemical features of pituitary dependent Cushing's disease and underwent pituitary resection with ACTH-positive adenoma identified and complete cortisol deficiency post-operatively consistent with cure. During follow-up her normal cortisol axis recovered and she stopped glucocorticoid supplementation. She was on an oral contraceptive. When features of possible early recurrence arose, contraception was interrupted to allow evaluation of possible cortisol excess. She had an elevated 24-hour urinary cortisol excretion and an unsuppressed cortisol after 1-mg overnight dexamethasone tests. However, on her next visit she reported a confirmed pregnancy, casting doubt as to the validity of the test results. After careful consideration, she proceeded with the pregnancy without therapy and was monitored cautiously. Hypertension developed requiring the use of labetolol but there was no clinical progression and she underwent normal full-term vaginal delivery. Subsequent evaluation showed consistently elevated 24-hour urinary cortisol values, loss of diurnal variation, confirming recurrent Cushing's disease and further ACTH staining tumour was resected during a further surgical procedure.

Pregnancy is rare in patients with Cushing's syndrome (CS) because hypercortisolemia and hyperandrogenaemia lead to impaired fertility, although cases have been described (52,53). The aetiologies of CS in pregnancy are similar to those found in non-pregnant women, but benign adrenal tumours are the most frequent cause in contrast to in non-pregnant patients [50% gestational CS were caused by adrenal disease, whereas 40% were caused by pituitary adenoma or Cushing's disease (CD)] (7,38). Cyclical CD due to an ACTH-producing pituitary adenoma with fluctuating ACTH levels was also reported in pregnancy (54). The diagnosis may be difficult to establish with confidence because of overlapping clinical and biochemical features of mild cortisol excess in pregnancy (6).

Effect of Cushing's Syndrome on Pregnancy and Maternal and Fetal Well-Being

CS in pregnancy is associated with maternal morbidity and mortality due to gestational diabetes, hypertension, preeclampsia, congestive heart failure, pulmonary oedema and premature labour (6,38,55–59). Poor wound healing, multiple fractures and psychiatric problems in pregnant women with CS have also been reported (55,60–62). Fetal loss and complications are increased due to the same mechanisms, and there is an increase in spontaneous abortions, stillbirths, early neonatal deaths and intrauterine growth retardation (6,56,63,64). Premature birth occurs in almost half of the cases (55). There are, however, reported cases of Cushing's disease and syndrome in the literature with uneventful pregnancies and normal fetal outcome (52) or resolution of hypercortisolemia after delivery (61,65).

Diagnosis of Cushing's Syndrome in Pregnancy

The features of CS diagnosed during gestation have similarities to normal pregnancy such as weight gain, hypertension, glucose intolerance and striae. Hirsutism and acne may indicate excessive androgen production. The presence of hypokalemia, muscle weakness, pathological fractures and large purple abdominal striae are important feature of CS (60,66).

Diagnostic tests for CS are less reliable during pregnancy. A dexamethasone suppression test can give rise to false-positive results due to blunted response to dexamethasone (67–69). Urine 24-hour free cortisol (UFC) has been suggested as the best choice for screening of CS during pregnancy (68). UFC levels are unchanged during the first trimester, but levels may be increased up to three-fold in the second and third trimesters in normal pregnancy (19). UFC greater than three times the upper limit should be considered abnormal in the last two trimesters (68).

Demonstrating a normal diurnal variation in cortisol secretion (including salivary cortisol levels) may be a helpful method to differentiate between hypercortisolism of pregnancy and CS (70,71). Inferior petrosal sinus sampling should not be a routine investigation method because of radiation exposure and increased thrombotic events, although it has been used in a small number of pregnant patients with suspected CD. The direct jugular approach is preferred to minimise radiation to the fetus (56,62,72,73). There are case reports in the literature of IPSS use in pregnancy, with no adverse effects seen (7,56,73).

Plasma ACTH levels can be used for the differential diagnosis of ACTH- and non-ACTH-dependent CS; however, one should be aware of the predominance of adrenal aetiology in CS in pregnancy and the physiological increase of ACTH during gestation (74). ACTH levels may not be suppressed in pregnant patients with adrenal CS, unlike in non-pregnant ones. This may be attributed to the production of ACTH by the placenta or stimulation of ACTH by placental CRH. Detectable ACTH levels may not exclude adrenal aetiology. A high-dose dexamethasone suppression test for distinction of CD and ectopic ACTH may be helpful (7). The HPA axis becomes resistant in the third trimester of pregnancy, and higher doses of CRH are needed to evoke sufficient ACTH and cortisol response (56,62,75,76).

MRI pituitary is rarely helpful in the diagnosis of CD, since CD is usually caused by a microadenoma, and the growth of the pituitary gland during normal pregnancy can mask the visualisation of the microadenomas. In cases where surgery is planned, MRI may be needed (74).

Treatment

Treatment for CS in pregnancy remains controversial; there are several cases showing a significant reduction in the number of live births in women with no treatment compared to women who had treatment for CS (56,64,70).

Trans-sphenoidal surgery in pregnant patients with CD has been reported to be successful in several cases, with resection of the tumour and subsequent achievement of remission of CD (56,62,72,77,78). The risks associated with surgical resection in the second trimester are thought to outweigh the risks to the mother and fetus if not treated. Medical adrenolytic therapy may be used in severe CD patients, when surgery cannot be performed or the condition is diagnosed in the third trimester. Metyrapone has been used during pregnancy (11 cases reported) but may cause adrenal insufficiency in the neonate (58,65,79–82) and can increase the incidence of preeclampsia and hypertension in mothers (65,79). Ketoconazole has been used in pregnancy (3 cases reported) to control hypercortisolism and has shown no adverse effects despite its potential anti-androgenic effects on the fetus (56,66,83,84). Intrauterine growth restriction, fetal hypoadrenalism and co-arctation of the aorta with metyrapone, and transient neonatal hypoglycaemia with ketoconazole have been reported in individual cases (56,65,66). Neither treatment is without hazard. Unlike ketoconazole, however, metyrapone does not have an inhibitory effects on androgen synthesis (85).

Patients treated for CD during pregnancy, by either surgery or medical therapy, should be monitored and treated for possible adrenal insufficiency when necessary.

Conclusion

- If CD is diagnosed during the first trimester, medical therapy should be considered in the context of severe hypercortisolemia until the removal of the tumour in the second trimester.
- Surgery is the treatment of choice for pregnant women with CD during the second trimester if intervention is required.
- For cases with delayed diagnosis late in the third trimester, medical treatment may be preferred, and the surgery may be postponed to the post-partum period.
- Patients treated for CD during pregnancy, by either surgery or medical therapy, should be monitored and treated for possible adrenal insufficiency when necessary.

Acromegaly

Case Presentation

A 29-year-old woman with a long-lasting history of oligo-amenorrhea, fell pregnant shortly after being diagnosed with acromegaly. MRI demonstrated a macroadenoma of the pituitary with suprasellar extension and compression of the optic chiasm leading to incomplete bitemporal hemianopia. Trans-sphenoidal surgery was performed during the second trimester, impaired visual fields became normal and subsequent biochemical tests suggested remission. She delivered a healthy full-term infant via caesarean section after an uncomplicated pregnancy. The infant's development was unremarkable. Post-partum assessment showed persistent acromegaly activity and the patient was judged to therapy (86).

Effect of Acromegaly on Pregnancy

Acromegaly can cause oligo-amenorrhea and may interfere with fertility. The anovulatory cycles are caused by suppression of gonadotrophs or because of hyperprolactinae-mia (70,86). There is an increased risk of gestational diabetes mellitus in pregnant women with acromegaly. GH antagonises insulin action leading to carbohydrate intolerance through increased resistance to insulin. Hypertension and cardiomyopathy (induced by the pre-existing acromegaly) may be exacerbated in pregnancy (70). Pregnancy may improve acromegaly. In some pregnancies with uncontrolled acromegaly, the disease has been reported to improve (87).

Effect of Pregnancy on Acromegaly

In pregnant women with acromegaly, tumour enlargement has been reported in cases with pre-existing invasive macroadenomas (25,35,88,89). A majority of patients with enlargement reported headaches and one patient reported visual field changes (11). It is unclear if tumour enlargement occurs due to lactotroph hyperplasia in the normal pituitary or enlargement of the tumour itself. There are a number of series reporting women with acromegaly at various stages of treatment completing pregnancies without evidence of tumour growth (11,37,90).

Biochemical confirmation of acromegaly is difficult during pregnancy due to higher levels of IGF1 in pregnant women and secretion of GH-V by the placenta. Placental GH-V does not show suppression to oral glucose loading and cannot be measured separately (26,70). To diagnose acromegaly in pregnancy, specific RIAs for GH-V are required to differentiate pituitary and placental secretion of GH (11). IGF1 levels are unhelpful in the diagnosis and follow-up of acromegaly during pregnancy (25).

Pituitary GH is secreted in a pulsatile manner, compared to the non-pulsatile secretory profile of the placental variant (23). Seventy percent of pregnant women with acromegaly show a paradoxical GH response to TRH (25,91) while TRH has no effect on placental GH-V (25). These two differences have been used to establish acromegaly in pregnancy (70). The use of an oral glucose tolerance test for suppression of GH during pregnancy is not well established, although it has been used in some reports (11,92,93). The increased and less pulsatile GH levels might be a clue for the diagnosis of acromegaly during pregnancy (25).

Treatment of Acromegaly in Pregnancy

Dopamine agonists can control the disease in 10% of acromegaly cases (94). The drug is more effective on tumours with GH and PRL co-secretion. Bromocriptine has been used in previously treated or untreated acromegalic patients during pregnancy (95–97). Bromocriptine used throughout pregnancy for treatment of acromegaly has not been shown to lead to adverse fetal or maternal outcome (98,99).

The somatostatin analogue, octreotide, has been used throughout pregnancy for different indications: nesidioblastosis (hyperinsulinemic hypoglycaemia), TSH-secreting pituitary adenoma or acromegaly, and seems to be safe (100–103). There are some reports in the literature about treatment with octreotide or octreotide-LAR during the entire pregnancy in acromegaly with no adverse obstetric or fetal outcomes reported (11,93,102,104–111). Maternal-fetal transfer of octreotide has been detected in patients with acromegaly, and TSH-secreting adenoma without any effect on TSH, thyroid hormone or IGF1 in the newborn (102,107).

The current practice is to advice contraception in patients treated with octreotide or to stop octreotide if pregnancy is desired. Restarting octreotide in pregnancy should be considered only if there is a significant tumour growth during pregnancy for which surgical resection is not possible (70).

Pegvisomant has been used in two pregnant patients with acromegaly until confirmation of pregnancy without untoward effects. Maternal IGF1 was controlled well, and transplacental passage of the drug was absent or minimal. The effect on the fetal GH axis is unlikely, and there is no evidence of substantial secretion into breast milk (112,113).

Conclusion

- In known acromegaly, definitive treatment with surgery should be undertaken prior to conception.
- Interruption of medical therapy during pregnancy is unlikely to affect the long-term outcome of acromegaly if the long-term course of the disease is considered.
- Breastfeeding is not contraindicated for acromegalic women with uneventful pregnancies.

NON-FUNCTIONING PITUITARY ADENOMAS

The majority of clinically non-functioning pituitary adenomas (NFPAs) arise from gonadotrophs and are rare in women of reproductive age. If an NFPA is suspected, then other conditions such as low-grade acromegaly should be ruled out. Adenomas greater than 1.2 cm in size are thought to have a higher risk of growth causing visual compromise during pregnancy (35).

If a patient with a known pituitary tumour becomes pregnant, then surgery may be considered during the second trimester in the presence of deteriorating visual fields. Dopamine agonists or conservative management may be preferred in the third trimester. Tumour de-bulking is indicated in patients with NFPA who wish to become pregnant (37).

Thyrotrophinomas

There are only three case reports in the literature about thyrotrophinomas (TSH-omas) in pregnancy (100,114,115). Two of these cases involved treatment with octreotide during pregnancy to reduce tumour size (114,115). There were no adverse incidents reported with the use of octreotide. If there is evidence of tumour growth in pregnancy, surgical resection in the second trimester should be considered (100,114). As with other pituitary tumours, patients with TSH-omas also need close follow-up for mass-related symptoms of tumour.

It is important to control the hyperthyroidism in this condition with anti-thyroid drugs to reduce the risk of spontaneous abortions, premature births and congenital malformations associated with uncontrolled hyperthyroidism in pregnancy (114).

LYMPHOCYTIC HYPOPHYSITIS

Lymphocytic hypophysitis (LyH) is an autoimmune disorder characterised by lymphocytic infiltration and destruction of the pituitary gland leading to various degrees of pituitary dysfunction. Women presenting during pregnancy or the post-partum period usually manifest with symptoms of hypopituitarism, diabetes insipidus and/or symptoms of mass lesion such as headache and visual field defects (7,116). LyH does not have adverse effects on the fetus or gestational outcome (117), and in many instances the mass lesion will resolve spontaneously post-partum although recovery of disturbed pituitary function is uncommon.

The hormone deficiencies include deficiency of hormones produced by the anterior, posterior or both lobes. ACTH deficiency is followed by TSH and both are likely to require treatment. PRL deficiency may cause a failure to lactate (70,117). Hyperprolactinaemia affects around 30% of LyH cases and is likely to represent stalk compression (118,119).

Diagnosis of LyH is based on the clinical setting, biochemical features and imaging findings. Pathological diagnosis may be deferred unless there are other indications for surgical intervention. Radiological features include diffuse thickening of the pituitary stalk, enhanced contrast enhancement of the gland and loss of the neurohypophyseal 'bright spot' (120). One case series of patients with LyH followed up with imaging studies revealed the development of empty sella during follow-up (117,121–124).

Treatment of LyH includes replacement of deficient pituitary hormones including treatment of diabetes insipidus. In cases with visual fields and/or neurological impairment surgery may be considered, although glucocorticoids are routinely used to reduce mass effect. Surgery is recommended if patients are unable to tolerate the high doses of steroids, or show a poor response (117). There is no consensus for the dose and length of treatment with corticosteroids, but high doses are usually used. Since most patients improve after parturition, steroid therapy or surgical intervention would be seldom required. Spontaneous recovery has been reported in some cases (125,126).

SHEEHAN'S SYNDROME

Sheehan's syndrome (SS) is described as post-partum hypopituitarism due to pituitary necrosis caused by severe hypotension or shock secondary to massive bleeding during or after delivery. Any significant blood loss leading to hypotension can lead to vasospasm, occlusion or thrombosis of blood vessels supplying the pituitary gland, causing ischaemic necrosis and varying degrees of hypopituitarism (127). SS was found to be the sixth leading cause of GH deficiency among 1034 GH-deficient patients (7,128). However, since it is rarely a pathological diagnosis, the distinction between SS and LyH can be difficult.

The diagnostic criteria of SS include the following: typical obstetric history of severe post-partum vaginal bleeding, severe hypotension or shock for which blood transfusion and/or fluid replacement was necessary, failure of post-partum lactation and/or to resume regular menses after delivery, anterior pituitary failure (partial or panhypopituitarism) and an empty sella on CT scan or MRI that does not show pituitary enlargement (7,129). Persistent hypotension, hypoglycaemia, failure to lactate, unexplained extreme fatigue, nausea or loss of libido in the context of a significant obstetric haemorrhage may raise the suspicion of ischaemic necrosis of the pituitary gland (70,129). Even though failure of post-partum lactation is a classical symptom of SS, hyperprolactinaemia was also reported (130,131). Amenorrhea from the immediate post-partum period can be seen, but this may be accompanied with normal gonadotrophin levels and pregnancies have also been reported following SS (132).

SS detected in the acute phase is rare (133–135), but most of the SS cases are diagnosed during the early post-partum period in western countries. There is no correlation between severity of hypopituitarism and degree of empty sella. Hypopituitarism requires biochemical diagnosis since the radiological features of pituitary infarction are variable and cannot be used for diagnosis (7,70,136). Panhypopituitarism occurs in 55% to 86% of cases with SS, with GH deficiency in all patients with SS (136–139). Diabetes insipidus (DI) is very rare in patients with SS, but partial DI has been reported occasionally (140–144). Many asymptomatic women have been noted to have impaired urine concentrating abilities when tested (143,144).

Treatment of SS includes replacement of deficient hormone(s), with initially high doses of glucocorticoids for the first few days as would be used in any major medical emergency, which may be lifesaving. Maintenance therapy includes glucocorticoids and thyroxine, with the dose adjustment related with clinical symptoms. Most patients will be treated with oestrogen and GH replacement in due course.

MANAGEMENT OF HYPOPITUITARISM IN PREGNANCY

In patients with gonadotrophin deficiency treated by gonadotrophin replacement and conception through normal intercourse, there is a pregnancy rate of 47% and overall birth rate of 42% (145). The rate of spontaneous abortion, midtrimester intrauterine death, poor placental function and maternal morbidity has been reported to be increased (146), although with modern endocrine and obstetric care, the risks are likely to be less than in previous reports. Pregnancies in women with hypopituitarism are regarded as 'high risk' and monitored closely.

A poorer outcome was observed in cases with childhood onset of hypopituitarism (versus women who developed hypopituitarism after the age of 13) and in women with multiple hormonal deficiencies (versus simple hypogonadotrophic hypogonadism) (147). Most of the women are unable to breastfeed post-partum (145,146).

Cortisol Deficiency

Newly occurring features of adrenal insufficiency are nonspecific (emesis, fatigue and mild hyponatremia) and may not be recognised since they can also be seen in a normal pregnancy. Adrenal insufficiency is associated with increased morbidity and mortality during pregnancy if undiagnosed or left untreated (148). New onset of cortisol deficiency in pregnancy is uncommon and is usually the result of autoimmune hypophysitis or pituitary infarction with necrosis. They can have an insidious onset during pregnancy or in the post-partum period and can present with hypotension, hypoglycaemia and vomiting (117,129). However, in most cases the patient will have recognised pre-pregnancy hypopituitarism (6).

The biochemical diagnosis of cortisol deficiency in pregnancy also presents challenges. An early morning cortisol level of >525 nmol/L (19 µg/dL) excludes cortisol deficiency in the first and second trimester (6). This value cannot be used reliably in the third trimester as there is normally a threefold rise in cortisol levels in the third trimester. ACTH levels have diagnostic value but only if they are very high or very low in pregnancy (149,150). A standard ACTH stimulation test is preferred as a diagnostic test during pregnancy, although cut-off values are not determined to diagnose adrenal insufficiency in pregnant women (7). It can be used to rule out cortisol deficiency in the third trimester if the stimulated 30 minutes value is at least 828 nmol/L (30 µg/dL) (149–154), but this test does not detect early hypopituitarism. An insulin tolerance test is contraindicated during pregnancy (75), but can be used in the post-partum period to confirm onset of hypocortisolism during pregnancy (6).

Women with known adrenal insufficiency that is appropriately treated can expect to have uneventful pregnancies (6). Hydrocortisone is the preferred steroid in pregnancy due to its short half-life and its susceptibility to degradation by the 11-βHSD-2 in the placenta, reducing fetal transfer of hydrocortisone (6).

Patients receiving glucocorticoid replacement may need to increase their hydrocortisone dose by 50% during the last trimester of pregnancy, although this is not required routinely. At the start of established labour, the hydrocortisone dose should be increased to doses used peri-operatively (100 mg IM/IV 6 hourly) until 24- to 48-hour post-partum (155,156). Glucocorticoids may pass to breast milk, but the amounts are insufficient to affect neonatal adrenal functions (6). Hydrocortisone can be continued safely during breastfeeding (157,158). Patients with adequate treatment for corticotroph deficiency can expect to have an uneventful pregnancy with no adverse effects on the fetus (6,159).

Standard advice to patients with steroid insufficiency should be reinforced in pregnancy: to increase the dose in the event of inter-current illnesses, to self-administer intra-muscular hydrocortisone in the event of gastrointestinal symptoms or vomiting and to present to hospitals early in the course of any illness. During periods of severe acute illness an initial bolus dose of 100 to 200 mg of IV hydrocortisone should be followed by 100 mg boluses very 6 to 8 hourly until the acute illness is resolved (160).

Thyroid

The replacement with L-T4, with free T4 in the upper half of the normal range for the age, is recommended during pregnancy in patients with hypothyroidism (161). In pituitary disease, however, the level of TSH does not contribute. Women with known *primary* hypothyroidism before pregnancy are typically advised to increase the L-T4 dose by 25 to 50 µg as soon as pregnancy is confirmed (16,70). Similar advice is appropriate for individuals with secondary pituitary hypothyroidism. We would recommend testing fT4 each 6 to 8 weeks. The aim is to maintain fT4 in the upper level of the reference range. Approximately one-third of the maternal thyroid hormone crosses to the fetus, and it plays an important role in fetal neurodevelopment in the first half of pregnancy prior to fetal pituitary-thyroid axis development (161,162). The dose of thyroxine replacement needs to be re-evaluated after delivery, and is usually adjusted downwards if it has been increased during pregnancy.

Growth Hormone

In GH-deficient patients, for planned pregnancies, GH should be used at least until confirmation of pregnancy, which helps preparation of the uterus for conception and results in better fertilisation results (7).

Gestational GH therapy in the first two trimesters of pregnancy was reported to be safe for the mother and the fetus without important adverse events and obstetric complications (163).

After the early stage of pregnancy, current practice is to continue therapy until 14 to 18 weeks, although there are no randomised data to address this issue. By the 24th week of gestation, the placental variant is secreted in adequate amounts to generate a normal to high IGF1 level (26).

Diabetes Insipidus

Symptoms of DI can also develop during pregnancy and in the early post-partum period due to destruction of the posterior pituitary by autoimmune hypophysitis, pituitary infarction or rarely due to an enlarging pituitary adenoma (164). Placental vasopressinase is associated with increased vasopressin (AVP) degradation, which may unmask borderline DI or worsen DI during pregnancy (165). The majority of DI cases (58%) deteriorate, 20% improve and 15% remain the same during pregnancy. In individuals with severe symptoms and where desmopressin (DDAVP) treatment is considered, a water deprivation test may be required to make a firm diagnosis.

Desmopressin seems safe during pregnancy and breastfeeding, without any adverse incidents (7,164,166,167). Monitoring and dose titration should be done bearing in mind that normal plasma osmolality and sodium level during pregnancy is lower than in non-pregnant women due to volume expansion and resetting of the osmostat in pregnancy (164,166).

During pregnancy, patients should be allowed to drink to thirst. Fluid balance must be closely monitored in women with DI during labour as they are in danger of getting fluid overloaded and hyponatremic due to excessive parenteral fluid administration (168).

There are case reports of severe vasopressin-resistant DI in association with: acute fatty liver, pre-eclampsia and disorders in coagulation, which resolves within the first few weeks of post-partum (169,170).

DI diagnosed during pregnancy and in the post-partum period should be re-evaluated. It is recommended that DDAVP be discontinued in the immediate post-partum period and symptoms re-evaluated as well as baseline osmolality before continuing with DDAVP (7).

Conclusions

- Patients with hypopituitarism, treated with thyroxine and hydrocortisone, should be monitored by an endocrinologist and may need to increase their replacement doses during gestation.
- There is no clear consensus regarding growth hormone replacement, and some recommend discontinuation whereas other clinicians continue to mid-pregnancy.
- Asymptomatic DI may become symptomatic during pregnancy, and DDAVP dose may need to be increased.

REFERENCES

1. Gonzalez JG, Elizondo G, Galdivar D, et al. Pituitary gland growth during normal pregnancy: an in vivo study using magnetic resonance imaging. Am J Med 1988; 85(2):217–220.
2. Dinc H, Esen F, Demirci A. Pituitary dimensions and volume measurements in pregnancy and post partum. MR assessment. Acta Radiol 1998; 39(1):64–69.
3. Elster AD, Sanders TG, Vines FS, et al. Size and shape of the pituitary gland during pregnancy and post partum: measurement with MR imaging. Radiology 1991; 181(2):531–535.
4. Scheithauer BW, Sano T, Kovacs KT, et al. The pituitary gland in pregnancy: a clinicopathologic and immunohistochemical study of 69 cases. Mayo Clin Proc 1990; 65(4):461–474.
5. Thorner MO. Changes in the anatomy and function of the maternal anterior pituitary gland during pregnancy. Mayo Clin Proc 1990; 65(4):597–599.
6. Lindsay JR, Nieman LK. The hypothalamic-pituitary-adrenal axis in pregnancy: challenges in disease detection and treatment. Endocr Rev 2005; 26(6):775–799.

7. Karaca Z, Tanriverdi F, Unluhizarci K, et al. Pregnancy and pituitary disorders. Eur J Endocrinol 2010; 162(3):453–475.

8. Rigg LA, Lein A, Yen SS. Pattern of increase in circulating prolactin levels during human gestation. Am J Obstet Gynecol 1977; 129(4):454–456.

9. Bohnet HG, Naber NG, del Pozo E, et al. Effects of synthetic gestagens on serum prolactin and growth hormone secretion in amenorrheic patients. Arch Gynecol 1978; 226(3):233–240.

10. Foyouzi N, Frisbaek Y, Norwitz ER. Pituitary gland and pregnancy. Obstet Gynecol Clin North Am 2004; 31(4):873–892, xi.

11. Herman-Bonert V, Seliverstov M, Melmed S. Pregnancy in acromegaly: successful therapeutic outcome. J Clin Endocrinol Metab 1998; 83(3):727–731.

12. Stefaneanu L, Whittom R, Smyth H, et al. Pituitary lactotrophs and somatotrophs in pregnancy: a correlative in situ hybridization and immunocytochemical study. Virchows Arch B Cell Pathol Incl Mol Pathol 1992; 62(5):291–296.

13. Tyson JE, Hwang P, Guyda H, et al. Studies of prolactin secretion in human pregnancy. Am J Obstet Gynecol 1972; 113(1):14–20.

14. Glinoer D. The regulation of thyroid function in pregnancy: pathways of endocrine adaptation from physiology to pathology. Endocr Rev 1997; 18(3):404–433.

15. Burrow GN, Fisher DA, Larsen PR. Maternal and foetal thyroid function. N Engl J Med 1994; 331(16):1072–1078.

16. Mandel SJ, Larsen PR, Seely EW, et al. Increased need for thyroxine during pregnancy in women with primary hypothyroidism. N Engl J Med 1990; 323(2):91–96.

17. Okamoto E, Takai T, Makino T, et al. Immunoreactive corticotropin-releasing hormone, adrenocorticotropin and cortisol in human plasma during pregnancy and delivery and postpartum. Horm Metab Res 1989; 21(10):566–572.

18. Cousins L, Rigg L, Hollingsworth D, et al. Qualitative and quantitative assessment of the circadian rhythm of cortisol in pregnancy. Am J Obstet Gynecol 1983; 145(4):411–416.

19. Carr BR, Parker CR Jr., Madden JE, et al. Maternal plasma adrenocorticotropin and cortisol relationships throughout human pregnancy. Am J Obstet Gynecol 1981; 139(4):416–422.

20. Seckl JR, Cleasby M, Nyirenda MJ. Glucocorticoids, 11beta-hydroxysteroid dehydrogenase, and foetal programming. Kidney Int 2000; 57(4):1412–1417.

21. Holmes MC, Abrahamsen CT, French KL, et al. The mother or the foetus? 11beta-hydroxysteroid dehydrogenase type 2 null mice provide evidence for direct foetal programming of behavior by endogenous glucocorticoids. J Neurosci 2006; 26(14):3840–3844.

22. Owens PC, Smith R, Brinsmead MW, et al. Postnatal disappearance of the pregnancy-associated reduced sensitivity of plasma cortisol to feedback inhibition. Life Sci 1987; 41(14):1745–1750.

23. Eriksson L, Frankenne F, Eden S, et al. Growth hormone 24-h serum profiles during pregnancy – lack of pulsatility for the secretion of the placental variant. Br J Obstet Gynaecol 1989; 96 (8):949–953.

24. Chellakooty M, Vangsgaard K, Larsen T, et al. A longitudinal study of intrauterine growth and the placental growth hormone (GH)-insulin-like growth factor I axis in maternal circulation: association between placental GH and foetal growth. J Clin Endocrinol Metab 2004; 89(1):384–391.

25. Beckers A, Stevenaert A, Foidart JM, et al. Placental and pituitary growth hormone secretion during pregnancy in acromegalic women. J Clin Endocrinol Metab 1990; 71(3):725–731.

26. Frankenne F, Closset J, Gomez F, et al. The physiology of growth hormones (GHs) in pregnant women and partial characterization of the placental GH variant. J Clin Endocrinol Metab 1988; 66(6):1171–1180.

27. Igout A, Frankenne F, L'Hermite-Balériaux M, et al. Somatogenic and lactogenic activity of the recombinant 22 kDa isoform of human placental growth hormone. Growth Regul 1995; 5(1):60–65.

28. Reyes FI, Winter JS, Faiman C. Pituitary gonadotropin function during human pregnancy: serum FSH and LH levels before and after LHRH administration. J Clin Endocrinol Metab 1976; 42 (3):590–592.

29. Braunstein GD, Asch RH. Predictive value analysis of measurements of human chorionic gonadotropin, pregnancy specific beta 1-glycoprotein, placental lactogen, and cystine aminopeptidase for the diagnosis of ectopic pregnancy. Fertil Steril 1983; 39 (1):62–67.

30. Davison JM, Sheills EA, Barron WM, et al. Changes in the metabolic clearance of vasopressin and in plasma vasopressinase throughout human pregnancy. J Clin Invest 1989; 83 (4):1313–1318.

31. Davison JM, Vallotton MB, Lindheimer MD. Plasma osmolality and urinary concentration and dilution during and after pregnancy: evidence that lateral recumbency inhibits maximal urinary concentrating ability. Br J Obstet Gynaecol 1981; 88(5):472–479.

32. Lindheimer MD, Davison JM. Osmoregulation, the secretion of arginine vasopressin and its metabolism during pregnancy. Eur J Endocrinol 1995; 132(2):133–143.

33. Abid S, Sadiq I, Anwar S, et al. Pregnancy with macroprolactinoma. J Coll Physicians Surg Pak 2008; 18(12):787–788.

34. Casanueva FF, Molitch ME, Schlechte JA, et al. Guidelines of the Pituitary Society for the diagnosis and management of prolactinomas. Clin Endocrinol (Oxf) 2006; 65(2):265–273.

35. Kupersmith MJ, Rosenberg C, Kleinberg D. Visual loss in pregnant women with pituitary adenomas. Ann Intern Med 1994; 121(7):473–477.

36. Turner H, John W. Oxford Handbook of Endocrinology and Diabetes. 2nd ed. Oxford University Press, 2009.

37. Bronstein MD, Salgado LR, de Castro Musolino NR. Medical management of pituitary adenomas: the special case of management of the pregnant woman. Pituitary 2002; 5(2):99–107.

38. Molitch ME. Medical management of prolactin-secreting pituitary adenomas. Pituitary 2002; 5(2):55–65.

39. Rossi AM, Vilska S, Heinonen PK. Outcome of pregnancies in women with treated or untreated hyperprolactinemia. Eur J Obstet Gynecol Reprod Biol 1995; 63(2):143–146.

40. Melmed S, Casanueva FF, Hoffman AR, et al. Diagnosis and treatment of hyperprolactinemia: an Endocrine Society clinical practice guideline. J Clin Endocrinol Metab 2011; 96(2):273–288.

41. Crosignani PG, Mattei AM, Severini V, et al. Long-term effects of time, medical treatment and pregnancy in 176 hyperprolactinemic women. Eur J Obstet Gynecol Reprod Biol 1992; 44(3):175–180.

42. Rasmussen C, Bergh T, Nillius SJ, et al. Return of menstruation and normalization of prolactin in hyperprolactinemic women with bromocriptine-induced pregnancy. Fertil Steril 1985; 44 (1):31–34.

43. Raymond JP, Goldstein E, Konopka P, et al. Follow-up of children born of bromocriptine-treated mothers. Horm Res 1985; 22 (3):239–246.

44. Konopka P, Raymond JP, Merceron RE, et al. Continuous administration of bromocriptine in the prevention of neurological complications in pregnant women with prolactinomas. Am J Obstet Gynecol 1983; 146(8):935–938.

45. Krupp P, Monka C. Bromocriptine in pregnancy: safety aspects. Klin Wochenschr 1987; 65(17):823–827.

46. Turkalj I, Braun P, Krupp P. Surveillance of bromocriptine in pregnancy. JAMA 1982; 247(11):1589–1591.

47. Laloi-Michelin M, Ciraru-Vigneron N, Meas T. Cabergoline treatment of pregnant women with macroprolactinomas. Int J Gynaecol Obstet 2007; 99(1):61–62.

48. Robert E, Musatti L, Piscitelli G, et al. Pregnancy outcome after treatment with the ergot derivative, cabergoline. Reprod Toxicol 1996; 10(4):333–337.

49. Ricci E, Parazzini F, Motta T, et al. Pregnancy outcome after cabergoline treatment in early weeks of gestation. Reprod Toxicol 2002; 16(6):791–793.

50. Webster J. A comparative review of the tolerability profiles of dopamine agonists in the treatment of hyperprolactinaemia and inhibition of lactation. Drug Saf 1996; 14(4):228–238.

51. Morange I, Barlier A, Pellegrini I, et al. Prolactinomas resistant to bromocriptine: long-term efficacy of quinagolide and outcome of pregnancy. Eur J Endocrinol 1996; 135(4):413–420.

52. Yawar A, Zuberi LM, Haque N. Cushing's disease and pregnancy: case report and literature review. Endocr Pract 2007; 13 (3):296–299.

53. Lado-Abeal J, Rodriguez-Arnao J, Newell-Price JD, et al. Menstrual abnormalities in women with Cushing's disease are correlated with hypercortisolemia rather than raised circulating androgen levels. J Clin Endocrinol Metab 1998; 83(9):3083–3088.

54. Miyoshi T, Otsuka F, Suzuki J, et al. Periodic secretion of adrenocorticotropin in a patient with Cushing's disease manifested during pregnancy. Endocr J 2005; 52(3):287–292.

55. Guilhaume B, Sanson ML, Billaud L, et al. Cushing's syndrome and pregnancy: aetiologies and prognosis in twenty-two patients. Eur J Med 1992; 1(2):83–89.

56. Lindsay JR, Jonklaas J, Oldfield EH, et al. Cushing's syndrome during pregnancy: personal experience and review of the literature. J Clin Endocrinol Metab 2005; 90(5):3077–3083.

57. Murakami S, Saitoh M, Kubo T, et al. A case of mid-trimester intrauterine foetal death with Cushing's syndrome. J Obstet Gynaecol Res 1998; 24(2):153–156.

58. Blanco C, Maqueda E, Rubio JA, et al. Cushing's syndrome during pregnancy secondary to adrenal adenoma: metyrapone treatment and laparoscopic adrenalectomy. J Endocrinol Invest 2006; 29(2):164–167.

59. Lo CY, Lo CM, Lam KY. Cushing's syndrome secondary to adrenal adenoma during pregnancy. Surg Endosc 2002; 16 (1):219–220.

60. Tajika T, Shinozaki T, Watanabe H, et al. Case report of a Cushing's syndrome patient with multiple pathologic fractures during pregnancy. J Orthop Sci 2002; 7(4):498–500.

61. Aron DC, Schnall AM, Sheeler LR. Spontaneous resolution of Cushing's syndrome after pregnancy. Am J Obstet Gynecol 1990; 162(2):472–474.

62. Mellor A, Harvey RD, Pobereskin LH, et al. Cushing's disease treated by trans-sphenoidal selective adenomectomy in mid-pregnancy. Br J Anaesth 1998; 80(6):850–852.

63. Chico A, Manzanares JM, Halperin I, et al. Cushing's disease and pregnancy: report of six cases. Eur J Obstet Gynecol Reprod Biol 1996; 64(1):143–146.

64. Bevan JS, Gough MH, Gillmer MD, et al. Cushing's syndrome in pregnancy: the timing of definitive treatment. Clin Endocrinol (Oxf) 1987; 27(2):225–233.

65. Close CF, Mann MC, Watts JF, et al. ACTH-independent Cushing's syndrome in pregnancy with spontaneous resolution after delivery: control of the hypercortisolism with metyrapone. Clin Endocrinol (Oxf) 1993; 39(3):375–379.

66. Prebtani AP, Donat D, Ezzat S. Worrisome striae in pregnancy. Lancet 2000; 355(9216):1692.

67. Odagiri E, Ishiwatari N, Abe Y, et al. Hypercortisolism and the resistance to dexamethasone suppression during gestation. Endocrinol Jpn 1988; 35(5):685–690.

68. Nieman LK, Biller BMK, Findling JW, et al. The diagnosis of Cushing's syndrome: an Endocrine Society Clinical Practice Guideline. J Clin Endocrinol Metab 2008; 93(5):1526–1540.

69. McLean M, Smith R. Corticotropin-releasing hormone in human pregnancy and parturition. Trends Endocrinol Metab 1999; 10 (5):174–178.

70. Molitch ME. Pituitary disorders during pregnancy. Endocrinol Metab Clin North Am 2006; 35(1):99–116, vi.

71. Allolio B, Hoffmann J, Linton EA, et al. Diurnal salivary cortisol patterns during pregnancy and after delivery: relationship to plasma corticotrophin-releasing-hormone. Clin Endocrinol (Oxf) 1990; 33(2):279–289.

72. Coyne TJ, Atkinson RL, Prins JB. Adrenocorticotropic hormone-secreting pituitary tumor associated with pregnancy: case report. Neurosurgery 1992; 31(5):953–955; discussion 955.

73. Pinette MG, Pan YQ, Oppenheim D, et al. Bilateral inferior petrosal sinus corticotropin sampling with corticotropin-releasing hormone stimulation in a pregnant patient with Cushing's syndrome. Am J Obstet Gynecol 1994; 171(2):563–564.

74. Polli N, Pecori Giraldi F, Cavagnini F. Cushing's disease and pregnancy. Pituitary 2004; 7(4):237–241.

75. Schulte HM, Weisner D, Allolio B. The corticotrophin releasing hormone test in late pregnancy: lack of adrenocorticotrophin and cortisol response. Clin Endocrinol (Oxf) 1990; 33 (1):99–106.

76. Suda T, Iwashita M, Ushiyama T, et al. Responses to corticotropin-releasing hormone and its bound and free forms in pregnant and nonpregnant women. J Clin Endocrinol Metab 1989; 69(1):38–42.

77. Casson IF, Davis JC, Jeffreys RV, et al. Successful management of Cushing's disease during pregnancy by transsphenoidal adenectomy. Clin Endocrinol (Oxf) 1987; 27(4):423–428.

78. Ross RJ, Chew SL, Perry L, et al. Diagnosis and selective cure of Cushing's disease during pregnancy by transsphenoidal surgery. Eur J Endocrinol 1995; 132(6):722–726.

79. Cabezon C, Bruno OD, Cohen M, et al. Twin pregnancy in a patient with Cushing's disease. Fertil Steril 1999; 72(2):371–372.

80. Connell JM, Cordiner J, Davics DL, et al. Pregnancy complicated by Cushing's syndrome: potential hazard of metyrapone therapy. Case report. Br J Obstet Gynaecol 1985; 92(11):1192–1195.

81. Gormley MJ, Hadden DR, Kennedy TL, et al. Cushing's syndrome in pregnancy–treatment with metyrapone. Clin Endocrinol (Oxf) 1982; 16(3):283–293.

82. Hana V, Dokoupilova M, Marek J, et al. Recurrent ACTH-independent Cushing's syndrome in multiple pregnancies and its treatment with metyrapone. Clin Endocrinol (Oxf) 2001; 54 (2):277–281.

83. Berwaerts J, Verhelst J, Mahler C, et al. Cushing's syndrome in pregnancy treated by ketoconazole: case report and review of the literature. Gynecol Endocrinol 1999; 13(3):175–182.

84. Amado JA, Pesquera C, Gonzalez EM, et al. Successful treatment with ketoconazole of Cushing's syndrome in pregnancy. Postgrad Med J 1990; 66(773):221–223.

85. Biller BM, Grossman AB, Stewart PM, et al. Treatment of adrenocorticotropin-dependent Cushing's syndrome: a consensus statement. J Clin Endocrinol Metab 2008; 93(7):2454–2462.

86. Sahli R, Christ E. [Pregnancy in active acromegaly]. Dtsch Med Wochenschr 2008; 133(45):2328–2331.

87. Lau SL, McGrath S, Evain-Brion D, et al. Clinical and biochemical improvement in acromegaly during pregnancy. J Endocrinol Invest 2008; 31(3):255–261.

88. Goluboff LG, Ezrin C. Effect of pregnancy on the somatotroph and the prolactin cell of the human adenohypophysis. J Clin Endocrinol Metab 1969; 29(12):1533–1538.

89. Okada Y, Morimoto I, Ejima K, et al. A case of active acromegalic woman with a marked increase in serum insulin-like growth factor-1 levels after delivery. Endocr J 1997; 44(1):117–120.

90. Colao A, Merola B, Ferone D. Acromegaly. J Clin Endocrinol Metab 1997; 82(9):2777–2781.

91. Chang-DeMoranville BM, Jackson IM. Diagnosis and endocrine testing in acromegaly. Endocrinol Metab Clin North Am 1992; 21(3):649–668.

92. Hisano M, Sakata M, Watanabe N, et al. An acromegalic woman first diagnosed in pregnancy. Arch Gynecol Obstet 2006; 274 (3):171–173.

93. Mozas J, Ocón E, López de la Torre M, et al. Successful pregnancy in a woman with acromegaly treated with somatostatin analog (octreotide) prior to surgical resection. Int J Gynaecol Obstet 1999; 65(1):71–73.

94. Newman CB. Medical therapy for acromegaly. Endocrinol Metab Clin North Am 1999; 28(1):171–190.

95. Jaspers C, Haase R, Pfingsten H, et al. Long-term treatment of acromegalic patients with repeatable parenteral depot-bromocriptine. Clin Investig 1993; 71(7):547–551.

96. Miyakawa I, Taniyama K, Koike H, et al. Successful pregnancy in an acromegalic patient during 2-Br-alpha-ergocryptine (CB-154) therapy. Acta Endocrinol (Copenh) 1982; 101(3):333–338.

97. Yap AS, Clouston WM, Mortimer RH, et al. Acromegaly first diagnosed in pregnancy: the role of bromocriptine therapy. Am J Obstet Gynecol 1990; 163(2):477–478.

98. Bigazzi M, Ronga R, Lancranjan I, et al. A pregnancy in an acromegalic woman during bromocriptine treatment: effects

on growth hormone and prolactin in the maternal, foetal, and amniotic compartments. J Clin Endocrinol Metab 1979; 48 (1):9–12.

99. Espersen T, Ditzel J. Pregnancy and delivery under bromocriptine therapy. Lancet 1977; 2(8045):985–986.

100. Blackhurst G, Strachan MW, Collie D, et al. The treatment of a thyrotropin-secreting pituitary macroadenoma with octreotide in twin pregnancy. Clin Endocrinol (Oxf) 2002; 57 (3):401–404.

101. Boulanger C, Vezzosi D, Bennet A, et al. Normal pregnancy in a woman with nesidioblastosis treated with somatostatin analog octreotide. J Endocrinol Invest 2004; 27(5):465–470.

102. Fassnacht M, Capeller B, Arlt W, et al. Octreotide LAR treatment throughout pregnancy in an acromegalic woman. Clin Endocrinol (Oxf) 2001; 55(3):411–415.

103. Neal JM. Successful pregnancy in a woman with acromegaly treated with octreotide. Endocr Pract 2000; 6(2):148–150.

104. Atmaca A, Dagdelen S, Erbas T. Follow-up of pregnancy in acromegalic women: different presentations and outcomes. Exp Clin Endocrinol Diabetes 2006; 114(3):135–139.

105. Biermasz NR, Romijn JA, Pereira AM, et al. Current pharmacotherapy for acromegaly: a review. Expert Opin Pharmacother 2005; 6(14):2393–2405.

106. Caron P, Broussaud S, Bertherat J, et al. Acromegaly and pregnancy: a retrospective multicenter study of 59 pregnancies in 46 women. J Clin Endocrinol Metab 2010; 95(10):4680–4687.

107. Caron P, Gerbeau C, Pradayrol L. Maternal-foetal transfer of octreotide. N Engl J Med 1995; 333(9):601–602.

108. Hierl T, Ziegler R, Kasperk C. Pregnancy in persistent acromegaly. Clin Endocrinol (Oxf) 2000; 53(2):262–263.

109. Mikhail N. Octreotide treatment of acromegaly during pregnancy. Mayo Clin Proc 2002; 77(3):297–298.

110. Shimatsu A, Usui T, Tagami T, et al. Suppressed levels of growth hormone and insulin-like growth factor-1 during successful pregnancy in persistent acromegaly. Endocr J 2010; 57 (6):551–553.

111. Takeuchi K, Funakoshi T, Oomori S, et al. Successful pregnancy in an acromegalic women treated with octreotide. Obstet Gynecol 1999; 93(5 pt 2):848.

112. Brian SR, Bidlingmaier M, Wajnrajch MP, et al. Treatment of acromegaly with pegvisomant during pregnancy: maternal and foetal effects. J Clin Endocrinol Metab 2007; 92(9):3374–3377.

113. Qureshi A, Kalu E, Ramanathan G, et al. IVF/ICSI in a woman with active acromegaly: successful outcome following treatment with pegvisomant. J Assist Reprod Genet 2006; 23(11–12): 439–442.

114. Chaiamnuay S, Moster M, Katz MR, et al. Successful management of a pregnant woman with a TSH secreting pituitary adenoma with surgical and medical therapy. Pituitary 2003; 6 (2):109–113.

115. Caron P, Gerbeau C, Pradayrol L, et al. Successful pregnancy in an infertile woman with a thyrotropin-secreting macroadenoma treated with somatostatin analog (octreotide). J Clin Endocrinol Metab 1996; 81(3):1164–1168.

116. Asa SL, Bilbao JM, Kovacs K, et al. Lymphocytic hypophysis of pregnancy resulting in hypopituitarism: a distinct clinicopathologic entity. Ann Intern Med 1981; 95(2):166–171.

117. Caturegli P, Newschaffer C, Olivi A, et al. Autoimmune hypophysitis. Endocr Rev 2005; 26(5):599–614.

118. Portocarrero CJ, Robinson AG, Taylor AL, et al. Lymphoid hypophysitis. An unusual cause of hyperprolactinemia and enlarged sella turcica. JAMA 1981; 246(16):1811–1812.

119. Thodou E, Asa SL, Kontogeorgos G, et al. Clinical case seminar: lymphocytic hypophysitis: clinicopathological findings. J Clin Endocrinol Metab 1995; 80(8):2302–2311.

120. Leggett DA, Hill PT, Anderson RJ. 'Stalkitis' in a pregnant 32-year-old woman: a rare cause of diabetes insipidus. Australas Radiol 1999; 43(1):104–107.

121. Matta MP, Kany M, Delisle MB, et al. A relapsing remitting lymphocytic hypophysitis. Pituitary 2002; 5(1):37–44.

122. Brandes JC, Cerletty JM. Pregnancy in lymphocytic hypophysitis: case report and review. Wis Med J 1989; 88(11):29–32.

123. Ishihara T, Hino M, Kurahachi H, et al. Long-term clinical course of two cases of lymphocytic adenohypophysitis. Endocr J 1996; 43(4):433–440.

124. Tsur A, Leibowitz G, Samueloff A, et al. Successful pregnancy in a patient with pre-existing lymphocytic hypophysitis. Acta Obstet Gynecol Scand 1996; 75(8):772–774.

125. Leiba S, Schindel B, Weinstein R, et al. Spontaneous postpartum regression of pituitary mass with return of function. Jama 1986; 255(2):230–232.

126. McGrail KM, Beyerl BD, Black PMcL, et al. Lymphocytic adenohypophysitis of pregnancy with complete recovery. Neurosurgery 1987; 20(5):791–793.

127. Kovacs K. Sheehan syndrome. Lancet 2003; 361(9356):520–522.

128. Abs R, Bengtsson BA, Hernberg-Stahl E, et al. GH replacement in 1034 growth hormone deficient hypopituitary adults: demographic and clinical characteristics, dosing and safety. Clin Endocrinol (Oxf) 1999; 50(6):703–713.

129. Kelestimur F. Sheehan's syndrome. Pituitary 2003; 6(4):181–188.

130. Kelestimur F. Hyperprolactinemia in a patient with Sheehan's syndrome. South Med J 1992; 85(10):1008–1010.

131. Stacpoole PW, Kandell TW, Fisher WR. Primary empty sella, hyperprolactinemia, and isolated ACTH deficiency after postpartum hemorrhage. Am J Med 1983; 74(5):905–908.

132. Grimes HG, Brooks MH. Pregnancy in Sheehan's syndrome. Report of a case and review. Obstet Gynecol Surv 1980; 35 (8):481–488.

133. Dejager S, Gerber S, Foubert L, et al. Sheehan's syndrome: differential diagnosis in the acute phase. J Intern Med 1998; 244(3):261–266.

134. Lavallee G, Morcos R, Palardy J, et al. MR of nonhemorrhagic postpartum pituitary apoplexy. AJNR Am J Neuroradiol 1995; 16(9):1939–1941.

135. Vaphiades MS, Simmons D, Archer RL, et al. Sheehan syndrome: a splinter of the mind. Surv Ophthalmol 2003; 48(2):230–233.

136. Dokmetas HS, Kilicli F, Korkmaz S, et al. Characteristic features of 20 patients with Sheehan's syndrome. Gynecol Endocrinol 2006; 22(5):279–283.

137. Jialal I, Desai RK, Rajput MC. An assessment of posterior pituitary function in patients with Sheehan's syndrome. Clin Endocrinol (Oxf) 1987; 27(1):91–95.

138. Kelestimur F. GH deficiency and the degree of hypopituitarism. Clin Endocrinol (Oxf) 1995; 42(4):443–444.

139. Rajatanavin R, Namking M, Himathongkam T, et al. Pituitary function tests in patients with Sheehan's syndrome. J Med Assoc Thai 1988; 71(8):443–450.

140. Kan AK, Calligerous D. A case report of Sheehan syndrome presenting with diabetes insipidus. Aust N Z J Obstet Gynaecol 1998; 38(2):224–226.

141. Sheehan HL, Whitehead R. The neurohypophysis in post-partum hypopituitarism. J Pathol Bacteriol 1963; 85:145–169.

142. Whitehead R. The hypothalamus in post-partum hypopituitarism. J Pathol Bacteriol 1963; 86:55–67.

143. Arnaout MA, Ajlouni K. Plasma vasopressin responses in postpartum hypopituitarism: impaired response to osmotic stimuli. Acta Endocrinol (Copenh) 1992; 127(6):494–498.

144. Iwasaki Y, Oiso Y, Yamauchi K, et al. Neurohypophyseal function in postpartum hypopituitarism: impaired plasma vasopressin response to osmotic stimuli. J Clin Endocrinol Metab 1989; 68 (3):560–565.

145. Hall R, et al. Fertility outcomes in women with hypopituitarism. Clin Endocrinol (Oxf) 2006; 65(1):71–74.

146. Overton CE, Davis CJ, West C, et al. High risk pregnancies in hypopituitary women. Hum Reprod 2002; 17(6):1464–1467.

147. Homburg R, Eshel A, Armar NA, et al. One hundred pregnancies after treatment with pulsatile luteinising hormone releasing hormone to induce ovulation. BMJ 1989; 298(6676):809–812.

148. Minneci PC, Deans KJ, Banks SM, et al. Meta-analysis: the effect of steroids on survival and shock during sepsis depends on the dose. Ann Intern Med 2004; 141(1):47–56.

149. Grinspoon SK, Biller BM. Clinical review 62: Laboratory assessment of adrenal insufficiency. J Clin Endocrinol Metab 1994; 79 (4):923–931.

150. McKenna DS, Wittber GM, Nagaraja HN, et al. The effects of repeat doses of antenatal corticosteroids on maternal adrenal function. Am J Obstet Gynecol 2000; 183(3):669–673.

151. Hurel SJ, Thompson CJ, Watson MJ, et al. The short Synacthen and insulin stress tests in the assessment of the hypothalamic-pituitary-adrenal axis. Clin Endocrinol (Oxf) 1996; 44(2):141–146.

152. Kane KF, Emery P, Sheppard MC, et al. Assessing the hypothalamo-pituitary-adrenal axis in patients on long-term glucocorticoid therapy: the short synacthen versus the insulin tolerance test. QJM 1995; 88(4):263–267.

153. McKenna DS, Fisk AD. The effect of a single course of antenatal corticosteroids on maternal adrenal function at term. J Matern Foetal Neonatal Med 2004; 16(1):33–36.

154. Poon P, Smith JF. The short Synacthen and insulin stress tests in the assessment of the hypothalamic-pituitary-adrenal axis. Clin Endocrinol (Oxf) 1996; 45(2):245.

155. Arlt W, Allolio B. Adrenal insufficiency. Lancet 2003; 361 (9372):1881–1893.

156. Trainer PJ. Corticosteroids and pregnancy. Semin Reprod Med 2002; 20(4):375–380.

157. O'Shaughnessy RW, Hackett KJ. Maternal Addison's disease and foetal growth retardation. A case report. J Reprod Med 1984; 29(10):752–756.

158. Sidhu RK, Hawkins DF. Prescribing in pregnancy. Corticosteroids. Clin Obstet Gynaecol 1981; 8(2):383–404.

159. Albert E, Dalaker K, Jorde R, et al. Addison's disease and pregnancy. Acta Obstet Gynecol Scand 1989; 68(2):185–187.

160. Seaward PG, Guidozzi F, Sonnendecker EW. Addisonian crisis in pregnancy. Case report. Br J Obstet Gynaecol 1989; 96 (11):1348–1350.

161. LaFranchi S. Thyroid hormone in hypopituitarism, Graves' disease, congenital hypothyroidism, and maternal thyroid disease during pregnancy. Growth Horm IGF Res 2006; 16(suppl A): S20–S24.

162. Haddow JE, Palomaki GE, Allan WC, et al. Maternal thyroid deficiency during pregnancy and subsequent neuropsychological development of the child. N Engl J Med 1999; 341(8):549–555.

163. Wiren L, Boguszewski CL, Johannsson G. Growth hormone (GH) replacement therapy in GH-deficient women during pregnancy. Clin Endocrinol (Oxf) 2002; 57(2):235–239.

164. Durr JA. Diabetes insipidus in pregnancy. Am J Kidney Dis 1987; 9(4):276–283.

165. Shehata HA, Okosun H. Neurological disorders in pregnancy. Curr Opin Obstet Gynecol 2004; 16(2):117–122.

166. Kallen BA, Carlsson SS, Bengtsson BK. Diabetes insipidus and use of desmopressin (Minirin) during pregnancy. Eur J Endocrinol 1995; 132(2):144–146.

167. Ray JG. DDAVP use during pregnancy: an analysis of its safety for mother and child. Obstet Gynecol Surv 1998; 53(7):450–455.

168. Durr JA, Lindheimer MD. Diagnosis and management of diabetes insipidus during pregnancy. Endocr Pract 1996; 2 (5):353–361.

169. Kennedy S, Hall PM, Seymour AE, et al. Transient diabetes insipidus and acute fatty liver of pregnancy. Br J Obstet Gynaecol 1994; 101(5):387–391.

170. Krege J, Katz VL, Bowes WA Jr. Transient diabetes insipidus of pregnancy. Obstet Gynecol Surv 1989; 44(11):789–795.

19

Neuro-oncology in pregnancy

Fiona Harris, Sarah J. Jefferies, Rajesh Jena, Katherine E. Burton, Lorraine Muffett, and Neil G. Burnet

INTRODUCTION

This chapter is divided into two main sections. In the first, we will discuss three major tumour types seen in a neuro-oncology practice: gliomas, meningiomas and pituitary tumours. Of these, glioma carries the greatest disease burden, accounts for the majority of tumours and has the most devastating effect on patient population. Discussion of management will therefore centre on this tumour type. In order to make it easier for the reader to understand the considerations involved, we have included a number of clinical scenarios from our own practice. In the second section, an overview is given of the principles underlying radiotherapy (RT), including the acute and late toxicities which may be seen. There are particular clinical situations in which RT is warranted in pregnancy despite potential difficulties. These are discussed and possible solutions are given.

Primary central nervous system (CNS) tumours are rare in the general population. The overall annual incidence is around 7 per 100,000 population, giving approximately 4500 people newly diagnosed with a brain tumour in the United Kingdom each year [4000 in England and Wales (1)], and 3500 deaths [3000 in England and Wales (1,2)]. The incidence has increased by approximately 25% since 1971 (1). Brain and CNS tumours account for only 2% of cancer deaths, but have a huge impact on the affected individual. This can be quantified as the average years of life lost (AYLL), a useful parameter of disease burden (3). For brain and CNS tumours, this equates to just over 20 years of life lost per patient, higher than any other adult cancer (3).

In pregnancy, the overall incidence of any malignancy is 1 per 1000 pregnancies (4), with the predominant tumour types reflecting the overall incidence of tumours in women of child-bearing age, with breast and cervix cancers accounting for just over 50% (4). Brain and CNS tumours are much rarer, with an incidence of less than 1 in 10,000 pregnant women (4,5), perhaps as low as 1 in 20,000 (6) to 1 in 40,000 (7).

Although uncommon, CNS tumours constitute a major management problem because of the practical difficulties involved in treating pregnant patients with RT or chemotherapy, the poor prognosis of some of these tumours and the emotive nature of the situation. There are also legitimate long-term concerns about fetal exposure to ionising radiation and chemotherapy, particularly as DNA-alkylating agents (which form covalent bonds with DNA) are widely used in neuro-oncology. The ethical difficulties involved in the potential conflict between maternal and fetal benefits and risks cannot be overstated, and need to be considered at the outset of the case and discussed with the patient and her family, with input from all of the teams involved in the patient's care (see chapter 9 on ethics). Typically, this must include the obstetric and neuro-oncology teams, but may also involve neurologists, neurosurgeons and palliative care specialists. Achieving the appropriate ethical balance of risk and benefit to both mother and fetus can be extremely challenging (Table 19.1).

HISTOLOGY OF CNS TUMOURS

A neuro-oncology practice comprises a multiplicity of histological tumour types, many of them extremely rare. This diversity in tumour type and behaviour is greater than for any other tumour site in oncology. Nevertheless, there are three major tumour types in CNS (non-surgical) oncology, which account for the majority of cases. Gliomas account for two-thirds of new cases in adults, meningiomas about 10% and pituitary tumours, including craniopharyngioma, another 10% (8). Gliomas are about 1.4 times commoner in men than women, whereas meningiomas are about twice as common in women. These numbers exclude patients with metastases, who in our unit are managed by the appropriate site-specific team. The number of patients with brain metastases is significantly smaller in the pregnant population than in the non-pregnant because of population demographics. A study from the University of California on obstetric emergencies precipitated by malignant brain tumours showed only one patient out of eight had metastatic disease; the remainder had primary gliomas (7).

Gliomas

As gliomas are the most common of the CNS tumours affecting women in pregnancy, as well as by far the most malignant, specific attention will be given to the management of patients with these tumours. A number of case scenarios are described later in the chapter to help illustrate some of the decisions that have to be taken.

Gliomas are neuroepithelial in origin, arising from glial cells which support and nurture neurones. They comprise oligodendrogliomas, astrocytomas and ependymomas, and mixed forms, such as oligoastrocytomas. Pathologically they are graded from I to IV on the WHO system depending on their histological features. The grade relates to the biological behaviour, with grade I being the least aggressive, and grade IV the most malignant. Grade I tumours are most common in childhood, and rarely present in adults. Almost all cerebral grade I tumours seen in adults are in patients under review following treatment as children. Grade IV glioma, the most malignant, is known as glioblastoma. Glioblastoma used to be known as glioblastoma multiforme, but since the WHO 2000 classification, the descriptor 'multiforme' has been dropped, although the abbreviation 'GBM' remains the same. Grade II and III tumours have intermediate behaviour, though should be considered as malignant. Tumours of grades III and IV are often considered together as high-grade gliomas. For high-grade lesions, it is essential for imaging to be considered along with pathology to produce the final 'biological grade', since there is a subset of grade III glioma which behaves as GBM (9) and which may be identified by imaging findings consistent with a higher grade than the pathological determination. This underlines the value of multi-disciplinary team working.

Table 19.1 Issues to be Considered in Relation to Treatment Decisions in a Pregnant Woman

Maternal
Grade and proliferative potential of the tumour
Size, location and invasiveness of the tumour
Efficacy and side effects of treatment(s)
Potential hormonal effects of pregnancy on the tumour
Radiotherapy specific
Anaemia of pregnancy, which decreases oxygen delivery to the
  tumour and reduces effectiveness of RT
Reproducible positioning of the patient over a period of several
  weeks where it may become uncomfortable to be flat and supine
  on a flat table top
Fetal
The stage of pregnancy
Fetal RT or chemotherapy dose
Effect of shielding from RT
Estimation of cancer risk
Fetal assessment and monitoring
Expected effects of maternal ill health on the fetus
How and when the fetus could be delivered
Whether the pregnancy should be terminated
Post-natal care
Combined fetal and maternal
Impact of delaying radiotherapy (after the first few weeks all risks
  reduce as pregnancy progresses)
Legal, ethical and moral issues

Abbreviation: RT, radiation therapy.

The 65% of new adult primary CNS cases which are gliomas are made up of 12% grade II tumours, 9% grade III and 44% GBM. Grouping grade III and GBM tumours together as high grade, over 50% of new cases to the neuro-oncology clinic have a high-grade glioma. The distinction between grade III and GBM tumours is important, because the prognosis is substantially better for those with a grade III tumour (9). For those patients treated with radical, curative intent, the median survival of patients with grade II and III gliomas is around 7 years and 3 years, respectively. The median survival of patients with GBM treated with surgery and RT, however, is only 9 to 12 months (8). The addition of temozolomide chemotherapy has achieved an improvement in median survival of 2.5 months (from 12.1 to 14.6 months in the randomised trial); more importantly, the 2 years survival rate has improved substantially from 10% to 26% (10). Although this improvement is encouraging, the overall outcome remains depressingly poor for patients with GBM.

Of all patients presenting with GBM, about half will be suitable for radical treatment, one-third for palliative treatment and one-sixth for supportive care only (8). It is important to be able to recommend limited treatment or supportive care when appropriate (see clinical scenario 1). Patients treated palliatively have a median survival of around 5 months (8). However, it must always be remembered in managing patients with GBM that the population survival curve invariably has a long tail, representing surprising, and unpredictable, long survival for a few patients.

Neurosurgical biopsy or resection can be undertaken in pregnancy without undue concern for the fetus (11) and indeed histopathological confirmation is a requirement, in order to guide management of the disease. The initial data from the Stupp study showed that patients whose tumours are debulked rather than simply biopsied do better, and pregnancy should not be considered as a contraindication to extensive surgery (10). The most challenging point at which to diagnose a glioma is in early pregnancy, because of the implications for both mother and baby. There is no evidence to suggest that the course of disease in pregnant patients is different to that in the non-pregnant patient, or that response to treatment is altered, so surgery and post-operative RT should proceed in a timely fashion, as per the non-pregnant patient with a high-grade glioma. For patients with low-grade gliomas, that is grade II, a programme of surveillance with regular scans every 6 to 12 months can be commenced. In general, MRI is the imaging modality of choice, but CT is preferred in the first trimester (see below). The dose from a diagnostic CT scan is similar to that from a planning CT. The preference for CT over MRI is because of the theoretical risk to the fetus of exposure to magnetic fields at an early gestational age. Those with grade III or IV tumours, however, require an active management plan from diagnosis. Often the diagnosis may be suspected from the imaging, but histological confirmation of high-grade glioma is essential. Where the appearance is typical of a low-grade glioma, biopsy may be deferred until after delivery.

The relative frequency of GBM, together with the fact that these are particularly devastating cancers, means that these cases dominate the issue of CNS tumours in pregnancy. In our neuro-oncology unit, four patients have presented in pregnancy over a 12-year period (out of approximately 2400 new cases). All had glioma, 1 grade II, 1 grade III (Case 3) and 2 GBM (Cases 1 and 2 below). Of these four patients, two required early intervention during their pregnancies; in one case, this was the direct result of the tumour (Case 1), and had an unsuccessful outcome; in the other case, urgent delivery was carried out by caesarean section due to fetal distress (Case 2). In the major series described by Tewari et al (7), of the eight women who presented with brain tumours during pregnancy, all experienced some degree of significant neurological impairment requiring early delivery, and there were four maternal deaths. A maternal death rate of 50% appears high, and differs from our own experience, but underlines the danger to patients of brain tumours occurring during pregnancy. In another series, only one patient out of seven women required emergency delivery (6).

The management issues surrounding pregnancy in patients previously treated for GBM, although not large in number, are discussed in Case 3, below. The improvements in outcome from the addition of chemotherapy to treatment regimens are likely to lead to this becoming increasingly relevant. Case 4 illustrates a case of a patient with a stable tumour in which RT was initially withheld, achieving a successful outcome to the pregnancy.

As each treatment plan is individualised depending on patient factors, it is difficult to be prescriptive about the course of events for these patients. However, a possible approach to management is shown in Table 19.2 to give some idea of the process leading to a treatment plan.

The current U.K. guidance from the National Institute for Clinical Excellence (NICE) (http://www.nice.org.uk/nicemedia/pdf/TA121guidance.pdf) is that, for GBM, combined concomitant chemo-RT should be considered for all patients of performance status 0 or 1 (Table 19.4). However, at present there are no data available regarding the use of temozolomide in pregnancy, and the manufacturer's current advice is that it should not be used as it has been shown to be teratogenic in rats and rabbits if administered during the period of organogenesis. Since the active moiety from the prodrug is a DNA – alkylating agent, this is to be expected. The alternative chemotherapy regimen often used, PCV, consists of procarbazine, lomustine and vincristine. This is

Table 19.2 Management Guidelines for Patients with Glioma in Pregnancy

Stabilise patient and fetus
- Control epilepsy
- Consider treatment of oedema with dexamethasone
- Analgesia
- Imaging – CT or MRI depending on stage of pregnancy

Oncological review
- Specialist multi-disciplinary team review
- Involvement of obstetric team
- Decision on need for biopsy during pregnancy

Likely low-grade glioma (grade II)
- Defer biopsy until post-partum
- Regular review – minimal imaging if clinical condition stable
- Specialist epilepsy management
- Obstetric planning for delivery

Likely high-grade glioma (grade III and GBM)
- Obtain histological diagnosis
- Specialist multi-disciplinary team review post-biopsy
- Develop treatment plan for mother and fetus
   ○ Oncology and obstetric input
   ○ Patient's informed view
- Resect where possible
   ○ Better outlook and symptom control, reduced steroid requirement
- Expect early radiotherapy
- Defer chemotherapy
- Obstetric planning for delivery

Abbreviation: GBM, glioblastoma.

no longer used as a first-line option in the treatment of GBMs. Procarbazine is a cytostatic agent that has been shown to be teratogenic in animals; lomustine is an alkylating agent and again is contraindicated in pregnancy or breastfeeding; vincristine is an anti-neoplastic agent contraindicated in pregnancy or lactation. This therefore excludes the use of any of our current chemotherapeutic options in the pregnant patient. There are no pharmacokinetic data available for the use of these drugs in the pregnant state, particularly in relation to the increased circulating blood volume in later pregnancy. Chemotherapy doses are calculated on an individual's surface area, by the Dubois formula, body surface area $(m^2) = 0.007184 \times$ (patient height in cm)$^{0.725} \times$ (patient weight in kg)$^{0.425}$ which is unlikely to be accurate in pregnancy.

If a patient with a known glioma relapses whilst pregnant, decisions regarding treatment would have to be made on an individual basis, taking into account the grade of tumour, any previous treatment and the stage of the pregnancy. It may be that, depending on gestation, a decision is made simply to control symptoms, for example, by increasing or altering anticonvulsants, until the post-partum period, and then to instigate definitive treatment.

Meningiomas

Meningiomas are tumours of the meninges, which are twice as common in females as in males. They are generally benign. The incidence increases with age, with the peak being in the seventh and eighth decades, so that most occur after childbearing age. There are three grades of meningioma recognised under the WHO (2007) grading system, grades I to III. Grade III is regarded as malignant meningioma and accounts for about 5% of cases (12).

There is a well-described association between pregnancy and both the presentation and progression of meningioma. It

has been suggested that the increased levels of progesterone in pregnancy may be responsible. Between 60% and 95% of these tumours are positive for progesterone receptors, and there is evidence that peritumoural oedema is associated with progesterone receptor status (13). However, Smith et al (14) looked at multiple possible growth factors associated with meningiomas presenting in pregnancy, and concluded that concentration on progesterone receptors alone, whilst attractive in relation to possible treatment options, was simplistic from the view of pathophysiology. Various immunohistochemical studies have been performed, looking at different growth factor receptors, and the results are conflicting, with some studies suggesting implication of Ki67, and others looking at platelet-derived growth factor, fibroblastic growth factor receptor 2 and epidermal growth factor receptor (14–16).

In pregnancy, most meningiomas are diagnosed on scanning for a neurological symptom, often seizures. In pregnant patients, the best course of action is to control the symptoms with anti-epileptic drugs (see chapter 4) as necessary, and review the situation following delivery. If necessary, neurosurgical intervention is possible (11).

Management of meningioma is primarily surgical. Even if there is a post-operative residuum, the natural history of grade I and II meningiomas is of slow growth over a period of years, in contrast to the growth rate in high-grade gliomas which can be seen in a matter of weeks. Meningiomas can therefore usually be managed expectantly during pregnancy.

A separate problem for women with meningioma is whether or not a subsequent pregnancy might lead to increase in the size of the lesion. If residual tumour is present following surgical resection, then the option of RT post-resection should be considered, in an attempt to reduce the risk of intra-partum tumour growth.

Familial cases tend to be associated with neurofibromatosis type 2, where there is an increased incidence of grade II and III meningiomas, and there may also be multiple meningiomas. Patients with this condition should be managed in the same way as other patients with meningiomas, as they may not cause an issue during pregnancy. Referral for genetic counselling may be appropriate.

Pituitary Adenoma and Craniopharyngioma

Pituitary tumours including craniopharyngioma very rarely present during pregnancy. Their biggest effect, mediated through excess prolactin production or hypothalamic-pituitary axis dysfunction, is to make conception more difficult. Because these syndromes may result in difficulty with conception, they are likely to have been recognised and treated prior to pregnancy. If the patient requires hormone replacement, then endocrine management during the pregnancy is also critical and requires specialist endocrinology input.

As a pituitary tumour's response to RT is measured over a period of many months, the decision regarding RT should be delayed until after the post-partum period.

Very occasionally a patient with a pre-existing adenoma suffers pituitary apoplexy, developing headache, reduced conscious level, loss of vision, cavernous sinus syndrome and panhypopituitarism, sometimes with low blood pressure. This can occur in either the pregnant or non-pregnant state and is due to haemorrhage or infarction within a pre-existing pituitary tumour. Blood is typically seen within the adenoma. Management includes resuscitation, steroid replacement and early neurosurgery if decompression is needed, usually by the trans-sphenoidal route.

CLINICAL CASE STUDIES
Case 1

A 32-year-old woman, P0+0, presented to Accident and Emergency (A&E) with intractable vomiting at 9 weeks' gestation. This was initially thought to be hyperemesis gravidarum, and she was admitted to the prenatal ward, where she was noted to have left hemi-neglect. MRI showed a large infiltrating lesion that involved the whole of the corpus callosum, extended in to the septum pellucidum and infiltrated the adjacent brain. This showed enhancement following the injection of gadolinium, consistent with a high-grade intrinsic lesion (Figs. 19.1 and 19.2). She proceeded to neurosurgical biopsy, which confirmed GBM (grade IV glioma). She deteriorated post-surgery and required admission to a local hospice, and remained there, with little further deterioration in her physical abilities, but with increasing loss of higher mental functions, until she reached 20 weeks. At that stage, ultrasound showed intrauterine growth restriction, with fetal growth below the 5th centile. She commenced a course of palliative RT aimed at delivering 30 Gy (gray) in six fractions. Unfortunately, after four fractions ultrasound confirmed intrauterine death at 22 weeks' gestation. RT was therefore stopped, and she underwent induction of labour. The patient died 4 months later.

Discussion

This patient illustrates one of the more difficult aspects of management in these situations, where the patient's wishes may differ from those of the medical team treating her. At the time of admission to the hospice, her WHO performance status was 4 (Table 19.3), and her cognitive ability was variably impaired. Because of the extensive nature of the tumour, and her rapid physical deterioration, a decision was made to manage her with best supportive care only. It was considered that the potential increase in survival with palliative RT would have been at most a few months, and it was felt that further non-surgical treatment was not in the patient's best interests given the clinical situation and the logistical problems involved in the delivery of RT, the

Table 19.3 WHO (World Health Organisation) Performance Status

0 = Able to carry out all normal activity without restriction.
1 = Restricted in physically strenuous activity but ambulatory and able to carry out light work.
2 = Ambulatory and capable of all self-care but unable to carry out any work; up and about >50% of waking hours.
3 = Capable of only limited self-care; confined to bed or chair >50% of waking hours.
4 = Completely disabled. Cannot carry out any self-care; totally confined to bed or chair.

hospice being geographically separated from the hospital. This decision was made in conjunction with both the patient and her family, and the consequences made clear to all parties. As time went on she remained physically disabled but stable, and the decision changed. In periods of good cognition she had expressed a desire to do everything possible to achieve survival for her and her child. Her family too, given her relatively stable physical condition, were keen to instigate treatment in an attempt to prolong maternal survival to the point at which the baby was viable. It was felt that the intrauterine growth restriction was as a result of the high doses of steroids she had been prescribed (dexamethasone 16 mg) to control symptoms of increased intracranial pressure in combination with opiates. A decision was reached with the medical, obstetric and palliative care teams and the family to commence palliative RT. All parties were aware that the intention of treatment was to prolong maternal survival to allow fetal development to continue to a viable stage, although unfortunately this was not possible.

Case 2

A woman of 29 presented with a seizure at 27 weeks' gestation. MRI demonstrated a large complex deep-seated posterior parietal lesion with peripheral contrast-enhancement and

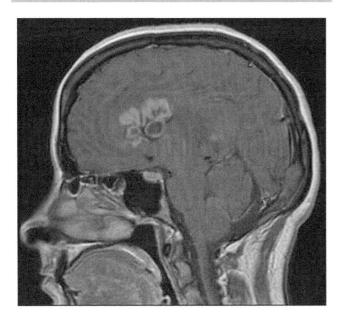

Figure 19.1 Sagittal T1c MRI image of a large infiltrating lesion of the corpus callosum, showing enhancement following the injection of gadolinium, consistent with a high-grade intrinsic lesion.

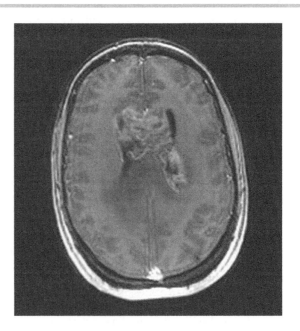

Figure 19.2 Axial T1c MRI image of the same patient as in Figure 19.1, showing contrast-enhancement consistent with a high-grade lesion.

central necrosis, typical of GBM. There was mild obstructive hydrocephalus. She underwent biopsy and third ventriculostomy, and GBM was confirmed. RT was started two and a half weeks later, using a slightly reduced dose per fraction (1.8 Gy rather than 2 Gy typically used for GBM) in the hope of minimising treatment-related oedema. Eight days later at 32 weeks' gestation, the baby developed fetal distress and urgent caesarean section was performed.

Discussion

In this case, the dexamethasone used to control intracranial oedema was considered helpful in achieving a degree of maturation of the fetal lungs. The baby survived and did not have significant neonatal problems. The patient developed relapse of her disease only 4.4 months after completion of treatment, though with palliative treatment she survived a further 15 months from the completion of RT.

Case 3

A woman of 29 was investigated following a generalised tonic-clonic seizure. A small lesion was seen on MRI, though not typical of a neoplasm. The patient was keen for excision, and excision revealed GBM. She was treated with an individualised RT programme, delivering 60 Gy to the tumour with a 20-Gy stereotactic boost, as per the European Organisation for Research and Treatment in Cancer (EORTC) protocol in use at that time, which was investigating the role of standard RT plus high-dose boost versus standard RT to 60 Gy alone in the era before temozolomide. Three years after completion of treatment, she raised the question of whether it might be safe to attempt a pregnancy with a new partner. She was counselled that there should be no additional risk of relapse of the GBM, but that there would be consequences to the child from the loss of a parent if she were to relapse. After careful consideration she decided to proceed. The pregnancy was uneventful, but because of her previous diagnosis, it was decided to deliver the baby by caesarean section because of the concerns about increased intracranial pressure during labour. Mother and baby remained well 2 years on, 5 years from her original diagnosis.

Discussion

As RT can cause late pituitary dysfunction and loss of pituitary hormones, including gonadotrophins, in this case planning included delineation of the hypothalamus and pituitary to minimise the dose of RT to these structures. The aim was to preserve hypothalamic-pituitary axis function, which can be compromised by lower doses of radiation than are used in irradiation of gliomas. In her case this was successful, and conception and pregnancy was completed without the use of exogenous hormones.

Case 4

A 33-year-old woman presented with a 2 to 3 week history of morning headaches followed by a grand mal seizure. She was 20 weeks' gestation in her second pregnancy. CT showed a left parietal lesion (Fig. 19.3), so she underwent stereotactic biopsy. This revealed a WHO grade III (anaplastic) astrocytoma. By the time she was seen in the oncology department, she was at 22 weeks' gestation. Having initially wanted to terminate the pregnancy, she decided after discussion with her oncologist to continue the pregnancy on the understanding that she might require RT prior to delivery. She had been commenced on anti-epileptic medication following her first seizure, and was stable on carbamazepine. Histological features had indicated that this tumour may be at the less aggressive end of the grade III

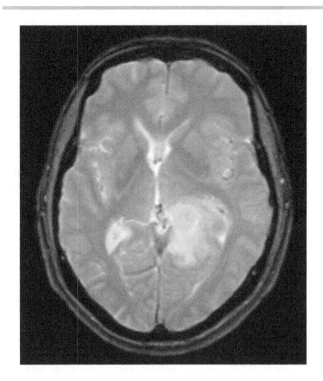

Figure 19.3 CT of a left parietal lesion.

spectrum, with only moderate cellular and nuclear pleomorphism and scanty mitoses, and so a decision was made to plan RT, but to delay it as long as the patient's symptoms were stable. She therefore underwent RT planning as described below, and fetal dose estimations were carried out using a phantom arrangement (17). She remained clinically well, and an MRI performed 8 weeks following diagnosis at 32 weeks' gestation showed stable disease, so no treatment was instigated. The baby was delivered by elective caesarean section at 38 weeks. She commenced RT 2 weeks post-partum. She remained well for 4 years following treatment, when she relapsed. Palliative treatment was instigated and she died six and a half years after giving birth to her son.

Discussion

This indicates the importance of multi-disciplinary working and personalisation of treatment plans. In this instance, treatment was safely deferred because of good prognostic indicators. With active surveillance, a positive outcome was achieved in respect of both the pregnancy and maternal health. In a different setting the pregnancy may have been terminated. The delay in treatment was very unlikely to have resulted in any harm coming to either mother or child, which is the guiding factor behind all treatment decisions.

MANAGEMENT PRINCIPLES

Management is multi-disciplinary in nature, requiring input from neurosurgeons, oncologists, pathologists and radiologists, palliative care physicians, endocrinologists, obstetricians and neonatologists.

Surgery

As noted above, whether a histological diagnosis is required during a pregnancy depends largely on the patient's condition and the likely grade of tumour. In the setting of a presumed low-grade tumour, biopsy may be deferred until conclusion of the pregnancy. Where the imaging suggests high-grade lesions, and modern imaging is relatively good at distinguishing low from high grade, it is advisable to obtain histological confirmation. In cases of likely high-grade gliomas this is important because of the poor prognosis that the diagnosis of high-grade glioma, particularly GBM, has for the patient.

There is good evidence that debulking of high-grade gliomas improves the prognosis (10,18). This is only appropriate for patients whose overall management strategy is radical in intent and would rarely apply to patients in the palliative setting. Unfortunately, a substantial proportion of gliomas arise in deep-seated structures which may preclude surgical debulking.

Radiotherapy

Timing of RT

The timing of RT with respect to the pregnancy may be made difficult because of the physiological anaemia of pregnancy. RT is known to be more effective in the presence of oxygen (19,20), and there is good direct and indirect evidence that GBMs are severely hypoxic in vivo (21–23). Patients with lower haemoglobin levels have been shown in some tumour types to have lower rates of local tumour control (24,25). Tumour resistance to RT in anaemic patients can, at least partially, be prevented or overcome by correction of anaemia, resulting in better locoregional tumour control and overall survival (26). It is therefore our general policy to maintain haemoglobin levels greater than 12 g/dL for the duration of RT through the use of regular transfusion. Regular transfusion can be used in the pregnant state too, if the decision is made to go ahead with RT. For a pregnant patient with a lower than usual haemoglobin, this may constitute another problem in achieving the maximum possible efficacy from a course of RT and so is part of the thinking behind the strategy of delaying treatment until successful completion of a pregnancy if possible, as outlined in Case 4 above. Erythropoeitin (EPO) was used in some patients having radical chemo-RT for head and neck tumours, but the control rate was poorer than in those not given EPO, so its use was dicontinued. EPO is also associated with an increased risk of thromboembolic events and hypertension, although such effects are not common in reports of EPO use in pregnant women treated for anaemia.

Imaging for RT Planning

Modern RT planning for CNS tumours benefits from a combination of both CT and MR imaging. CT provides clear definition of the bony limits of the tumour and provides tissue density data for use in RT dose calculations. MR provides the best visualisation of the tumour and other normal structures within the cranium. The two modalities are co-registered electronically for the purpose of target volume definition.

The fetal dose associated with the planning CT head scan is less than 0.005 mGy, and is therefore negligible within the setting of a planned course of RT. MR imaging carries no ionising radiation dose but there are concerns about exposure of the fetus to magnetic fields during the first trimester of pregnancy. There is some indication that the developing fetal brain may be particularly susceptible to the effects of movement-induced currents: orientation effects are very important to guide the normal growth of neuronal dendrites. It is also possible that very long-lasting changes could be induced by relatively short exposures (27). These conclusions are based on animal studies and it is highly unlikely that a human study

would be performed. In view of this information, however, CT is usually preferred for imaging during the first trimester although avoiding MRI is a relative rather than an absolute strategy.

Target Volume Definition for RT

The concepts behind RT planning for CNS tumours are standard (28) although there are some very specific issues to consider when contemplating RT for a pregnant patient.

Effective RT requires that the patient lie flat and still in a position which is accurately reproducible from one day to the next. In almost all situations the supine position is preferred. However, to lie supine, flat and still on a hard table top in a scanner or treatment machine, is uniquely problematic for a pregnant woman, especially later in pregnancy, both from the point of view of the discomfort involved, and also the implications surrounding impairment of venous return. It may take some time and patience to find an appropriate position, but this will make all subsequent treatments easier to tolerate and administer.

Once the planning images are available, the clinician outlines the gross tumour volume (GTV). For a high-grade glioma, this is defined as the contrast-enhancing area on MRI, excluding post-operative meningeal enhancement. For a low-grade glioma, the GTV is defined as the high signal region seen on T2W MRI.

Because these tumours, particularly GBM, are highly infiltrative, a margin is allowed around the initial volume to account for microscopic disease. This is known as the clinical target volume, or CTV. In high-grade lesions the GTV is increased by around 2.5 cm in all directions of possible tumour spread to generate the CTV (28–30). Since glial tumours cannot breach the intact meninges, these represent natural barriers to spread. In low-grade gliomas the CTV margin is usually around 1.5 cm, with the same anatomical considerations applied. It is noteworthy that these margins, and indeed other details of the RT, such as dose and fraction number, have been determined from large studies, and are relatively constant worldwide. It is unlikely that these margins differ between pregnant and non-pregnant women.

The CTV represents individualised anatomical and pathological RT planning, including both macroscopic tumour (in the GTV) and microscopic infiltration. This is the volume which must be treated adequately to achieve cure. However, a number of uncertainties exist in the process of imaging, planning and delivering RT, and an additional margin must be allowed to account for these. Typically, a margin of 0.5 cm is used to achieve the planning target volume (PTV) (28). It is this final volume that is treated. GBMs are frequently several centimetres in diameter at the time of presentation, so the addition of the CTV leads to a very large volume requiring irradiation. Low-grade tumours are frequently even bigger and although the CTV margin in these patients is a little less, frequently the volume requiring irradiation is extremely large. Typically, over half of the intracranial volume will receive treatment.

This very large volume requiring irradiation has important consequences. In the first instance, RT can cause a degree of swelling within the irradiated volume. This may be greater where a better tumour killing response is seen. Where greater tumour volume remains unresected, patients typically require steroids before commencing RT and will often have to increase the dose of steroid during the course of the treatment. One of the attractions of surgical debulking is to reduce the steroid requirements. The steroid of choice is dexamethasone, used at

Table 19.4 Typical Radiotherapy Dose Details for Treatment of High-Grade Glioma

Radical		
Glioblastoma		
60 Gy	30 fractions	6 wk
Concurrent chemotherapy plus 6 months adjuvant chemotherapy with temozolomide		
Glioma grade III		
54–60 Gy	30 fractions	6 wk
Palliative		
30 Gy	6 fractions	2 wk
35 Gy	10 fractions	2 wk

Notes:
1. The gray (abbreviated Gy) is the SI unit of radiation dose. It describes the energy absorbed by tissue, and is equivalent to joules/kg.
2. The use of concurrent plus adjuvant chemotherapy with temozolomide is based on excellent randomised trial data (10).
3. There is no evidence as yet of value from chemotherapy for patients with grade III glioma, though trials are currently underway to address this question.

doses of up to 16 mg daily, guided by performance status and symptoms.

RT Dose and Fractionation

A total dose of 60 Gy in 30 daily treatments, or fractions, is given for a GBM, 54 to 60 Gy in 30 fractions for grade III gliomas, and around 54 Gy in 30 fractions is typical for low-grade glioma (Table 19.4). The dose is given in daily divided fractions because this provides a therapeutic gain, allowing a greater dose to the tumour whilst limiting the damage to normal tissues. Patients are treated 5 days/wk.

RT Treatment Plan Details

Full details of the RT planning can be found elsewhere (28). However, the introduction of 'conformal' RT techniques which allow the radiation high-dose volume to conform closely to the target volume has been extremely valuable. By shaping each field individually to match the cross-section of the target 'seen'

by the beam, the volume of normal brain irradiated has been reduced, with a consequent reduction in side effects.

In pregnancy it is worthwhile developing a treatment plan using beams that are coplanar with an axial plane through the head. This minimises radiation dose to the abdomen. A beam of energy of around 6 MV is also appropriate, and beams of greater than 10 MV should be avoided to minimise neutron contamination which can contribute to scattered dose (see below).

These planning techniques, combined with modern imaging, especially MRI, allow the delineation of critical normal structures, such as the optic apparatus, brainstem and hypothalamus and pituitary, and the preparation of a treatment plan which can limit dose to these structures. See clinical scenario 3 for the context of hypothalamic-pituitary axis RT dose and function.

RT Side Effects

Side effects from RT are divided into acute and late onset. The former including fatigue, skin reddening in the treatment areas and hair loss in the beam portals, and transient deterioration of symptoms secondary to treatment-induced cerebral oedema. Late effects include pituitary dysfunction, with progressive failure of pituitary hormones, cataract formation from irradiation of the lens and cognitive decline. Other side effects are dependent on the dose received by specific structures, and are predictable following the planning process.

Factors Contributing to Radiation Dose

Total radiation dose is made up of the dose from the primary beam but there is also a contribution, secondary dose, consisting of scatter from metal objects within the beam, for example, the multi-leaf collimators used to shape each field (Fig. 19.4) and also from the linear accelerator itself and the room in which it is housed. It is this secondary radiation that contributes most significantly to fetal dose, as the uterus will not be in the primary beam. The American Association of Physicists in Medicine (AAPM) has shown that leakage (a descriptive term for the amount of radiation outwith the primary beam which leaks from the tube head of the linear accelerator) is also a

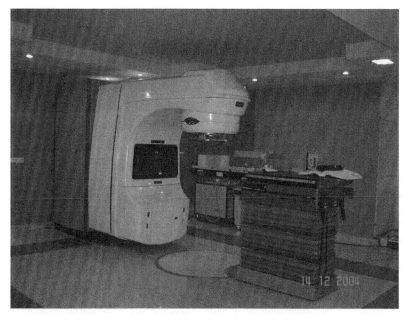

Figure 19.4 Typical linear accelerator.

significant factor in dose outwith the primary beam. A careful choice of linear accelerator is needed since the amount of leakage radiation is dependant on the type of machine (31).

Film badge assessments can be used to establish the energy of scattered radiation, and hence indicate that additional abdominal shielding is worthwhile and can be achieved practically. Although leakage radiation is of high energy, scattered radiation is the main contributor to fetal dose, and this may be of relatively low energy, in the range 208 to 622 keV. A lead shield of about 1 cm over the abdomen could significantly reduce fetal dose. One solution could be the use of X-ray fluoroscopy coats (lead aprons), although alternative structures can be used. In some reports (32) customised bridge structures have been described to carry shielding safely.

RISK OF FETAL DAMAGE RESULTING FROM RADIATION EXPOSURE

There are two major concerns underlying treatment decisions in the types of scenario described above; the risk of damage to the fetus in utero resulting in birth defects, and of cancer induction in later life. Data from survivors of the atomic bombs at Nagasaki and Hiroshima, from children exposed in utero to diagnostic X rays and those exposed in utero following the Chernobyl accident have given some estimates of the risk of exposure of pregnant women, and the consequences to their children (33). The expected radiation effects differ at different time points during pregnancy, and include prenatal death, malformations, developmental delay and cancer induction.

Prenatal Exposure

In the immediate post-conception period, significant exposure is likely to result in failure of implantation. In the period from 3 to 8 weeks, that is organogenesis, exposure may lead to malformation. Between 8 and 25 weeks there may be developmental delay or a loss of IQ, as the developing CNS is susceptible to irradiation. Threshold levels for acquisition of these abnormalities have been determined. Below 8 weeks, malformations can occur above a threshold dose of 0.1 to 0.2 Gy. In the period from 8 to 15 weeks, IQ may be reduced by 21 points for each 1 Gy of exposure, and a fetal dose of 0.1 Gy can result in a verifiable reduction in IQ. The risk of severe developmental delay is approximately 40% following a fetal dose of 1 Gy. From 16 to 25 weeks' gestation, a similar situation prevails, but with a smaller loss of IQ of 13 points per 1 Gy exposure. From 25 weeks until term, the effects of all doses are much less obvious. The threshold for radiation-related severe developmental delay for a fetus of 8 to 15 weeks' gestation is 0.06 Gy, and of 16 to 25 weeks age is 0.28 Gy (34). This very low level shows the importance of avoiding exposure in the first trimester.

Carcinogenesis

With radiation exposure at any point during pregnancy there is an increased risk of childhood leukaemias and solid tumours. The relative risk of carcinogenesis following a prenatal exposure of 0.01 Gy is 1.4 (35). Given that the spontaneous incidence of tumours is 2 to 3 per 1000, this increases the overall risk to 3 to 4 per 1000.

It is important always to take the clinical scenario into account. In the setting of a sufficiently advanced pregnancy to allow the risks of major malformation to be put to one side, the most significant concern must be of carcinogenesis. In clinical scenario 4, the pregnancy was sufficiently advanced to avoid

malformation, severe developmental delay and intrauterine death. Heritable disease caused by radiation exposure has a lower risk than cancer, about 1 in 42,000/cGy (34). The cancer risk up to age 15 years attributable to radiation is 1 in 1700/cGy, and around half of these will be fatal (i.e., 1 in 3300/cGy). An estimated dose of 2.2 cGy would double the risk of fatal cancer by age 15 (17). This should be set against the overall U.K. risk of cancer up to age 15 years, which is 1 in 650. However, this translates into an excess lifetime fatal cancer risk of only 0.5% (36). With the linear accelerator chosen in the above case (17) the estimated maximum dose to the fetus was 2.2 cGy, but only 0.7 cGy at the centre of the uterus. This gives some idea of the likely level of exposure of the fetus, putting into context the doses above. With the use of abdominal shielding as described above, these doses, and therefore the cancer risks, can be halved (32,37). This would reduce the fatal cancer risk to 1 in 3000 for an exposure of 1.1 cGy.

Risk Reduction

Radiation dose diminishes with increasing distance from the radiation source, according to the inverse square law, so that doubling the distance from the source reduces the radiation dose by four times (i.e., 2^2). Accordingly, it is to be expected that the dose received by a fetus from irradiation of the CNS would be small. Dosimetric studies were carried out using phantoms (38), specially constructed devices that act on the treatment beam in a manner similar to human tissue, allowing estimation of dose at specific points. These phantoms were designed to represent a pregnant patient at 4, 12 and 24 weeks' gestation, and measurements of the fetal dose with and without abdominal shielding were made. The authors never recorded a conceptus dose greater than 0.01 Gy without the use of abdominal shielding, throughout a course of treatment designed to deliver a total of 65 Gy to the CNS. Shielding, however, reduced the dose to the fetus by almost three-quarters, if we are using standard UK approach to fractions. This would imply that the risk of damage to a fetus from irradiation of the mother in this situation is minimal, but can be reduced even further with the use of a custom lead shielding device. Estimates of dose can be carried out prior to commencement of treatment to confirm the suitability of the set-up.

CONCLUSIONS

The management of CNS or other tumours during pregnancy invariably requires a multi-disciplinary approach with highly individualised management. There are always tensions in prioritisation, or risks versus benefits, between the mother and the fetus, but with careful planning and a team approach these can be minimised, allowing the best achievable result for both parties.

In considering the need for RT or chemotherapy during pregnancy, it is always appropriate to review the possibility of deferring treatment until after delivery, provided this is safe. In the event that RT is required, this can be done with only slight risk to the fetus from scattered radiation, provided attention is given to the details of the treatment.

REFERENCES

1. Rachet B, Mitry E, Quinn MJ, et al. Survival from brain tumours in England and Wales up to 2001. Survival analysis. Br J Cancer 2008; 99:S98–S101.
2. Cancer Research UK. CancerStats Key Facts: UK Brain and CNS Tumour statistics, 2008. Available at: http://info.cancerresearchuk.org/cancerstats/types/brain/?a=5441.

3. Burnet NG, Jefferies SJ, Benson RJ, et al. Years of life lost (YLL) from cancer is an important measure of population burden – and should be considered when allocating research funds. Br J Cancer 2005; 92(2):241–245.

4. Pavlidis NA. Coexistence of pregnancy and malignancy. Oncologist 2002; 7:279–287.

5. Roelvink NC, Kamphorst W, van Alphen HA, et al. Pregnancy-related primary brain and spinal tumors. Arch Neurol 1987; 44(2):209–215 (review).

6. Isla A, Alvarez F, et al. Brain tumour and pregnancy. Obstet Gynecol 1997; 89:19–23.

7. Tewari KS, Cappuccini F, Asrat T, et al. Obstetric emergencies precipitated by malignant brain tumors. Am J Obstet Gynecol 2000; 182:1215–1221.

8. Burnet NG, Bulusu VR, Jefferies SJ. Management of primary brain tumours. In: Booth S, Bruera E, eds. Palliative Care Consultations in Primary and Metastatic Brain Tumours. Oxford: Oxford University Press, 2004:1–30.

9. Burnet NG, Lynch AG, Jefferies SJ, et al. High grade glioma: imaging combined with pathological grade defines management and predicts prognosis. Radiother Oncol 2007; 85:371–378.

10. Stupp R, Mason WP, et al. European Organisation for Research and Treatment of Cancer Brain Tumor and Radiotherapy Groups; National Cancer Institute of Canada Clinical Trials Group. Radiotherapy plus concomitant and adjuvant temozolomide for glioblastoma. N Engl J Med 2005; 352(10):987–996.

11. Ng J, Kitchen N. Neurosurgery and pregnancy. J Neurol Neurosurg Psychiatry 2008; 79:745–752.

12. CBTRUS: Statistical Report: Primary Brain Tumours in the United States, 1998–2002. Published 2005.

13. Benzel EC, Gelder FB. Correlation between sex hormone binding and peritumoural oedema in intracranial meningiomas. Neurosurgery 1988; 23:169–174.

14. Smith JS, Quiñones-Hinojosa A, Harmon-Smith M, et al. Sex steroid and growth factor profile of a meningioma associated with pregnancy. Can J Neurol Sci 2005; 32(1):122–127.

15. Hatiboglu MA, Cosar M, Iplikcioglu AC, et al. Sex steroid and epidermal growth factor profile of giant meningiomas associated with pregnancy. Surg Neurol 2008; 69(4):356–362; discussion 362–363.

16. Korhonen K, Salminen T, Raitanen J, et al. Female predominance in meningiomas can not be explained by differences in progesterone, estrogen, or androgen receptor expression. J Neurooncol 2006; 80(1):1–7.

17. Haba Y, Twyman N, Thomas SJ, et al. Radiotherapy for glioma during pregnancy: fetal dose estimates, risk assessment and clinical management. Clin Oncol 2004; 16(3):210–214.

18. Bleehen NM, Stenning SP. A Medical Research Council trial of two radiotherapy doses in the treatment of grades 3 and 4 astrocytoma. The Medical Research Council Brain Tumour Working Party. Br J Cancer 1991; 64(4):769–774.

19. Thomlinson RH, Gray LH. The histological structure of some human lung cancers and the possible implications for radiotherapy. Br J Cancer 1955; 9(4):539–549.

20. Horsman MR, Overgaard J. The oxygen effect and tumour microenvironment. In: Steel GG, ed. Basic Clinical Radiobiology. 3rd ed. London: Arnold, 2002.

21. Rampling R, Cruickshank G, Lewis AD, et al. Direct measurement of pO2 distribution and bioreductive enzymes in human malignant brain tumors. Int J Radiat Oncol Biol Phys 1994; 29(3):427–431.

22. Taghian A, DuBois W, Budach W, et al. In vivo radiation sensitivity of glioblastoma multiforme. Int J Radiat Oncol Biol Phys 1995; 32(1):99–104.

23. Burnet NG, Jena R, et al. Mathematical modelling of survival of glioblastoma patients suggests a role for radiotherapy dose escalation and predicts poorer outcome following delay to start treatment. Clin Oncol 2006; 18:93–103.

24. Daly T, Poulsen MG, Denham JW, et al. The effect of anaemia on efficacy and normal tissue toxicity following radiotherapy for locally advanced squamous cell carcinoma of the head and neck. Radiother Oncol 2003; 68(2):113–122.

25. Macdonald G, Hurman DC. Influence of anaemia in patients with head and neck cancer receiving adjuvant postoperative radiotherapy in the Grampian region. Clin Oncol (R Coll Radiol) 2004; 16(1):63–70.

26. Vaupel P, Thews O, Hoeckel M. Treatment resistance of solid tumors: role of hypoxia and anemia. Med Oncol 2001; 18(4):243–259.

27. Independent Advisory Group on Non- Ionising Radiation on behalf of the Health Protection Agency. Static Magnetic Fields (RCE-6). May 2008.

28. Burnet NG, Burton KE, Jefferies SJ. Central nervous system. In: Hoskin PJ, ed. Radiotherapy in Practice - External Beam Therapy. Oxford: Oxford University Press, 2006:295–341.

29. Jena R, Price SJ, Baker C, et al. Diffusion tensor imaging: possible implications for radiotherapy treatment planning of patients with high-grade glioma. Clin Oncol 2005; 17(8):581–590.

30. Price SJ, Jena R, Burnet NG, et al. Improved delineation of glioma margins and regions of infiltration with the use of diffusion tensor imaging: an image-guided biopsy study. AJNR Am J Neuroradiol 2006; 27(9):1969–1974.

31. Sneed PK, Albright NW, Wara WM, et al. Fetal dose estimates for radiotherapy of brain tumors during pregnancy. Int J Radiat Oncol Biol Phys 1995; 32(3):823–830.

32. Mazonakis M, Damilakis J, Varveris H, et al. A method of estimating fetal dose during brain radiation therapy. Int J Radiat Oncol Biol Phys 1999; 44(2):455–459.

33. Valentin J, for the Committee of the IRCP. Biological effects after prenatal irradiation (embryo and fetus): ICRP Publication 90 Approved by the Commission in October 2002. Ann 2003; 33(1-2):5–206.

34. Otake M, Schull WJ, Lee S. Threshold for radiation-related severe mental retardation in prenatally exposed A-bomb survivors: a re-analysis. Int J Radiat Biol 1996; 70(6):755–763.

35. Doll R, Wakeford R. Risk of childhood cancer from fetal irradiation. Br J Radiol 1997; 70:130–139.

36. National Radiological Protection Board (NRPB): Advice on exposure to ionising radiation during pregnancy. Joint guidance from the National Radiological Protection Board, College of Radiographers and Royal College of Radiologists. Chilton: National Radiological Protection Board, 1998; available at: http://www.nrpb.org/publications/misc_publications/advice_during_pregnancy.pdf.

37. Magné N, Marcié S, Pignol JP, et al. Radiotherapy for a solitary brain metastasis during pregnancy: a method for reducing fetal dose. Br J Radiol 2001; 74(883):638–641.

38. Mazonakis M, Damilakis J, Theoharopoulos N, et al. Brain radiotherapy during pregnancy: an analysis of conceptus dose using anthropomorphic phantoms. Br J Radiol 1999; 72(855):274–278.

FURTHER READING

Short SC. Survival from brain tumours in England and Wales up to 2001. Clinical Commentary. Br J Cancer 2008; 99:S102–S103.

20

Pregnancy and movement disorders

Yogini Naidu, Prashanth Reddy, and K. Ray Chaudhuri

INTRODUCTION

Pregnancy is associated with hormonal changes which cause variable responses within the neuropeptide system and receptor status within the brain including striatal areas. A natural consequence of this is the occurrence of movement disorders more frequently or only during pregnancy. These conditions include restless legs syndrome and chorea, among other rarer disorders. The pathophysiology is complex and mostly unclear. The following sections discuss conditions that may arise de novo in pregnancy and those that may be present in women of childbearing age.

RESTLESS LEGS SYNDROME

Restless legs syndrome (RLS) is characterised by an unpleasant sensation in the legs, and occasionally in the arms, that patients describe as creeping or crawling and find extremely unpleasant and sometimes painful (1). Typically, the sensory and motor symptoms of RLS occur at specific times during the day, mostly in the evening and at night. Sleep disruption is common. There is often a family history.

Unifying clinical diagnostic criteria were devised in the late 1990s and are now used worldwide as follows.

Essential Diagnostic Criteria for RLS

1. An urge to move the legs usually accompanied or caused by uncomfortable and unpleasant sensations in the legs (sometimes the urge to move is present without the uncomfortable sensations and sometimes the arms or other body parts are involved in addition to the legs).
2. The urge to move or unpleasant sensations begin or worsen during periods of rest or inactivity, such as lying or sitting.
3. The urge to move or unpleasant sensations are partially or totally relieved by the movement, such as walking or stretching, at least as long as the activity continues.
4. The urge to move or unpleasant sensations are worse in the evening or at night than during the day, or only occur in the evening or night (when symptoms are severe, the worsening at night may not be noticeable but must have been previously present).

RLS has a prevalence of 8% to 12% in the white Western Caucasian population. The prevalence of RLS in pregnant women was first studied by Karl Ekbom in 1945 (2). He found a prevalence of 11.3% among 486 pregnant women (3) (Table 20.1). Several other investigators have studied the prevalence of RLS in pregnant women and describe an overall prevalence of around 20%. The variability of prevalence rates between the various studies (range 11.3–27.3%) is chiefly due to lack of use of the standard diagnostic criteria for RLS except in one study (5). The diagnosis was made using self-completed questionnaires or face-to-face medical interviews. In several studies the minimum threshold of frequency of occurrence of symptoms was not specified, with no mention of geographic area or racial characteristics. Furthermore, the prevalence may have been influenced by when the surveys were conducted during the pregnancy. Using the standard diagnostic criteria, through a structured medical interview on a wide and homogeneous population of women (mean age of 32 years, and mean pregnancy duration of 38 weeks) throughout the course of the entire pregnancy, Manconi et al. reported a prevalence rate of 26% (5).

Natural History

Published studies suggest that the prevalence of RLS may not be uniform during pregnancy and progressively increases starting from the third and fourth month of gestation reaching a plateaux during the third trimester and falling rapidly after delivery (5).

Aetiology of RLS in Pregnancy

The exact aetiology of RLS in pregnancy is not known. However, a few studies have suggested it may be caused by iron or folate deficiency (6,7), both well known to be associated with RLS (8). Plasma iron and folate levels decrease particularly during the second half of pregnancy (9).

The correlation between the rise in oestrogen, progesterone and prolactin, which peak during the third trimester, and the symptom severity of RLS in this trimester also suggests a possible hormonal influence in RLS. Because dopamine strongly inhibits hypothalamic secretion of the prolactin-releasing factor, it is possible that increased prolactin during pregnancy is associated with reduced dopamine levels, thus lowering the RLS symptomatic threshold. This remains speculative (5,10).

Treatment

Since most treatment options have possible effects on the fetus, the foremost medical approach should be the reassurance of the women of the benign nature of the symptoms and their likely disappearance at the end of the pregnancy, with no effects on the development and health of the fetus (5).

Iron and folate supplementations have been recommended in view of the possible association of the condition with low folate and iron stores (9), although this has not been the subject of a clinical trial.

Conservative treatments such as walking, stretching, massaging the affected limbs, applying heat and performing relaxation techniques may also be helpful as has been shown in anecdotal studies in idiopathic RLS. Abstinence from tobacco and alcohol should be reinforced, adequate sleep

Table 20.1 Frequency of Restless Legs Syndrome During Pregnancy

Authors	No. of cases	Prevalence (%)
Ekbom	486	11.3
Jolivet	100	27.3
Ekbom	202	12.4
Goodman et al.	500	19
Suzuki et al. (11)	500	19
Manconi et al.	606	26.6

Source: From Ref. 4.

Table 20.2 Different Drugs Used for RLS Outside Pregnancy (Licensed and Unlicensed)

Dopamine agonists	
Pramipexole	0.125–0.75 mg (salt)/day
Ropinirole	0.25–4 mg/day
Rotigotine	1–4 mg transdermal patch
Levodopa DCI	100–600 mg evening or divided dose
Non-dopaminergic treatments	
Gabapentin	300–1800 mg/day
Carbamazepine	100–600 mg/day
Oxycodone	2.5–25 mg/day
Tramadol	50–100 mg/day
Clonazepam	0.5–2 mg evening dose
Triazolam	0.125–0.25 mg/day
Nitrazepam	2.5–10 mg/day
Clonidine	0.15–0.9 mg/day
Iron sulphate	200 mg twice daily (oral)

Ergot derivatives are no longer recommended in non-pregnant women and should not be used in pregnancy. Refer to text for options in pregnancy.

should be recommended as these may aggravate symptoms of RLS.

Pharmacological therapies licensed for RLS outside pregnancy are dopamine agonists (non-ergot) (Table 20.2). Other options include opiate, benzodiazepines, carbamazepine and gabapentin as in typical RLS (www.eguidelines.co.uk). However, no controlled clinical trials are available to base treatment recommendations for RLS in pregnancy. Benzodiazepines are relatively contraindicated in pregnancy. Dopamine agonists have not been clearly associated with birth defects; however, there is little experience with their use in pregnancy. As studies have failed to show fetal risk with low doses of opiates, drugs such as dihydrocodeine are possibly the safest treatment option in pregnant women who wish to use drug treatments if other measures have failed. High doses can result in neonatal withdrawal syndrome.

McPharland and Pearce reported two severe cases of RLS in pregnancies which were successfully treated with carbamazepine after there was no improvement with benzodiazepines (temazepam and diazepam) and phenobarbital (12). If carbamazepine or other enzyme-inducing medication (e.g., phenytoin, topiramate, phenobarbitone, primidone, oxcarbazepine) is used, giving vitamin K1 10 mg or 20 mg/day to the mother has been recommended in the last 4 weeks of pregnancy to reduce the risk of haemorrhagic disease of the newborn. However, the need for this has been questioned recently as vitamin K given to the baby IM soon after birth is common practice for all babies and this alone is probably sufficient to prevent haemorrhagic disease in the babies of women taking enzyme-inducing anti-epileptic drugs (AEDs).

Because of the lack of adequate information on the management of RLS in pregnant women, pharmacological treatment would be used only during the third trimester, and at the lowest efficacious dosage (13). The majority of pregnant women do not require drug treatment.

PREGNANCY AND CHOREA

Chorea is an involuntary abnormal movement disorder which is characterised by abrupt, brief, non-rhythmic and non-repetitive movement of any limb and it involves proximal and distal muscles. It appears to randomly move from one part of the body to another and it often involves the face leading to non-patterned facial grimaces, tongue movement and grunting noises (14). Chorea can be seen in various conditions and disorder and is caused by imbalance between striatal facilitatory and inhibitory pathways.

Chorea gravidarum (CG) is a rare movement disorder that can develop during pregnancy. The term is given to chorea that occurs during pregnancy characterised by athetosis, the involuntary jerky motion and the inability to maintain stable position of body parts. Previously more common, in the early 1900s it was reported to occur in 1 in 3000 deliveries, a much higher rate than nowadays, partly because of the high prevalence of rheumatic fever (RF) at that time (15).

Chorea with the onset of pregnancy was first described in 1661 by Horstius and is nowadays rare. Before the use of antibiotics for streptococcal pharyngitis, the major cause of CG was RF. According to Willson and Preece's (1932) report, 70% of women who suffered from CG had a previous history of RF or chorea (15). Nowadays approximately 50% of cases are idiopathic. Modern day CG is associated with other diseases such as systemic lupus erythematosus (SLE), Huntington's disease (HD), antiphospholipid syndrome (APLS) and moyamoya disease, a rare disorder of the cerebral vasculature (6,16) (Table 20.1). CG may vary from mild to severe and is now very rare, and was estimated in the 1960s to occur in approximately 1 in 140,000 pregnancies (17). There have been some suggestions that increases in oestrogen and progesterone concentrations in pregnancy may partly be responsible for CG as these hormones may sensitise dopamine receptors at the striatal level and induce chorea (14).

The caudate nucleus plays a key role in the pathogenesis of chorea. In HD, the condition characterised by chorea, there is maximal degeneration in the caudate. The absence of subthalamic nucleus inhibition enhances the motor activity through the motor thalamus and results in abnormal involuntary movement such as chorea. One report of pathological changes at autopsy in CG found perivascular degenerative changes in the caudate nucleus and severe neuronal loss in the caudate nucleus and the putamen, although this may not be a universal finding as all patients in that study suffered from cardiac disease (16). Hormonal changes in pregnancy can, in theory, lead to an enhanced dopaminergic receptor sensitivity which may also increase susceptibility to development of chorea (15).

There is no standard course of treatment for chorea and treatment depends on the type of chorea as well as on the associated disease. Treatments currently used for CG include neuroleptics for symptomatic relief and therapies targeted towards the underlying pathology (18). Oestrogens may stimulate striatal dopamine receptor sensitivity and Donaldson (1982) reported that CG was effectively controlled with haloperidol (17). This potent dopamine antagonist appears to be reasonably safe treatment for moderate to severe CG during the second and third trimesters of pregnancy. The FDA has designated it a category C drug for use in pregnancy, chiefly because of concerns about use in the first trimester. There appears to be no clear adverse fetal effects when used in the second and third trimester.

PREGNANCY AND PARKINSON'S DISEASE

Whilst Parkinson's disease (PD) does not affect a woman's ability to reproduce, pregnancy in PD patients occurs rarely because only a small proportion of cases of PD in women are diagnosed before the age of 50. Consequently, clinical experience with pregnancy in PD is very limited and published evidence consists of a series of case reports.

Many women with PD will have a largely uneventful pregnancy and have a normal full-term vaginal delivery of a healthy infant whilst still being on their anti-parkinsonian medication. However, it has been shown that their PD worsens during the post-partum period and that pregnancy has a long-term exacerbating effect on disease progression (19). In an interview study of 18 women with PD who had a total of 24 pregnancies, Golbe (1987) reported 3 miscarriages, 4 elective abortions, and 17 term pregnancies. Ten of the 17 completed pregnancies were associated with some worsening of motor symptoms of PD (20). Another case study reported a women with PD having a caesarean delivery of a healthy child whilst being on dopamine agonist monotherapy. However, levodopa had to be added post-natally as her condition became progressively worse (21). Dyskinesias may have an adverse effect on pregnancy, particularly disabling diphasic dyskinesias. Diphasic dyskinesias are disabling, accompanying the duration of response to levodopa at onset and termination of effect. Fortunately, these are rare in pregnancy and also rare as a result of the modern trend of using low doses of levodopa.

Studies have reported the use of anti-parkinsonian drugs such as carbidopa/levodopa and amantadine in pregnant patients and have not shown any teratogenicity in humans (19,22). Most of the medications used for PD are categorised as FDA class C due to the lack of human or animal evidence regarding their impact on fetal development. However, the use of amantadine during the first trimester may be associated with embryotoxicity causing miscarriage and fetal malformation (20) and should be avoided. The effects on pregnancy of MAO-B inhibitors (selegiline and rasagiline) and of the non-ergot dopamine agonists are unknown. While there are data on the use of bromocriptine in pregnancy (see chapter 18, 'Pituitary Disease in Pregnancy') and cabergoline (23), the use of these ergot-derived dopamine agonists has been largely superseded by the use of non-ergot-derived dopamine agonists in movement disorders.

The sudden or abrupt cessation of anti-parkinsonian treatment increases the disability of patients and may precipitate a Parkinsonism-hyperpyrexia syndrome although this has not been specifically described in pregnancy.

PREGNANCY AND DYSTONIA

Dystonia is a neurological condition characterised by abnormal muscle contractions, often causing repetitive twisting movements or abnormal postures. It can be classified according to the parts of the body that are affected and can be focal, segmental, multifocal, hemidystonic or generalised (24). Some cases of dystonia can be genetic such as early-onset primary torsion dystonia (DYT1).

As the mean age of onset of dystonia in women is in the mid-twenties, many women may be affected during their reproductive years. There does not appear to be any consistent correlation between the hormonal changes of pregnancy and the severity of dystonia (24), and no clear evidence that the severity of dystonia changes in any consistent way during pregnancy. In a survey of 279 women with dystonia, Gwinn-Hardy et al. (2000) reported no clear worsening of dystonic symptoms in pregnancy (25). Palluzzi et al. (2005) reported no exacerbation of dystonic symptoms in the three women studied during their pregnancy (24).

In patients on treatment with botulinum toxin for craniocervical or other dystonias, the treatment would need to be stopped should the patient become pregnant as botulinum toxin is contraindicated during pregnancy. This may and is likely to aggravate the dystonia and one can only use conservative measures such as pain control during pregnancy. There are no studies of botulinum toxin use for dystonia during pregnancy and this is not recommended. The role of other oral anti-dystonic agents such as trihexyphenydyl, tetrabenazine, baclofen for dystonia during pregnancy has not been explored.

PREGNANCY AND WILSON'S DISEASE

Wilson's disease was originally described by Kinear Wilson in 1912 (26). Wilson's disease is an autosomal recessive disorder with a mutation on chromosome 13 at the site 13q14.3–q21.1 (27). This severe genetic disorder presents in young children and teenagers as liver disease, for example, cirrhosis or acute hepatitis, manifesting between the period of 10 and 13 years old. Young adults present with neuropsychiatric and neurological symptoms. The neuropsychiatric symptoms are usually depression, emotional liability and slow ideation. Neurological symptoms may include tremor dystonia, incoordination, rigidity and dysarthria.

The diagnosis is confirmed by measurement of serum ceruloplasmin, urinary copper excretion and hepatic copper content, as well as the detection of Kayser–Fleischer rings (28,29). Early diagnosis and treatment can potentially reverse the effects of the disorder and prevent permanent brain and liver damage.

Excessive intrauterine copper concentrations may be responsible for the high rate of spontaneous abortions in patients with Wilson's disease and the impairment of fertility, but pregnancy does not have any deleterious effect on the disease (30). Women with Wilson's disease may encounter difficulties in conceiving and this may be linked to cirrhosis (31). Therefore, chelation therapy should be used prior to pregnancy. Antichelating therapy such as penicillamine aims to reduce the level of copper in the body by binding to the copper molecule which is then excreted in the urine. Studies indicate that penicillamine can be continued during pregnancy in low doses and zinc could be taken in conjunction (zinc is also used as an adjunctive treatment for Wilson's disease) (32,33).

CONCLUSION

Movement disorders associated with pregnancy are compounded by the hormonal changes occurring in pregnancy and not enough studies are currently available looking into the aetiology and treatment of these conditions. As most of the disorders discussed above, apart from RLS, are rare during pregnancy, randomised clinical trials are difficult to perform. Information on drug treatment is limited with limited information on risk to the fetus associated with drugs used for movement disorders. Hence, most often a symptomatic approach is prudent and each case needs to be assessed on an individual basis.

REFERENCES

1. Tan EK, Ondo W. Restless legs syndrome: clinical features and treatment. Am J Med Sci 2000; 319(6):397–403.
2. Hedman C, Pohjasvaara T, Tolonen U, et al. Effects of pregnancy on mothers sleep. Sleep Med 2002; 3:37–42.
3. Ekbom KA. Restless legs syndrome. Acta Med Scand 1945; 158:4–122.
4. Ferini-Strambi L, Manconi M. Restless legs syndrome in pregnancy. In: Ondo WG, ed., Restless Legs Syndrome. London and New York: Informa Healthcare, 2007:239–246.
5. Manconi M, Govoni V, De Vito A, et al. Restless legs syndrome and pregnancy. Neurology 2004; 63:1065–1069.
6. Boetz MI, Lambert B. Folate deficiency and Restless legs syndrome in pregnancy. N Engl J Med 1977; 297:670.
7. Lee KA, Zaffke ME, Baratte-Beebe K. Restless legs syndrome and sleep disturbance during pregnancy: role of folate and iron. J Women's Health Gend Med 2001; 10:335–341.
8. O'Keeffe ST, Gavin K, Lavan JN. Iron status and Restless legs syndrome in the elderly. Age Ageing 1994; 23:200.
9. Puolakka J, Janne O, Pakarinen A, et al. Serum ferritin as a measure of iron stores during and after normal pregnancy with and with out iron supplementaion. Acta Obstet Gynaecol Scand Suppl 1980; 95:43–51.
10. Wetter TC, Collado-Seidel V, Oertel H, et al. Endocrine rhythms in patients with restless legs syndrome. J Neurol 2002; 249:146–151.
11. Suzuki K, Ohida T, Sone T, et al. The prevalence of restless legs syndrome among pregnant women in Japan and the relationship between restless legs syndrome and sleep problems. Sleep 2003; 26(6):673–677.
12. McPharland P, Pearce JM. Restless legs syndrome in pregnancy. Case reports. Clin Exp Obstet Gynecol 1990; 17(1):5–6.
13. Early CJ. Clinical practice, restless legs syndrome. N Engl J Med 2003; 348:2103–2109.
14. Ramachandran TS. Chorea Gravidarum. 8 Jan 2007. Available at: http://www.emedicine.com/neuro/topic61.htm#section~References.
15. Willson P, Preece AA. Chorea gravidarum. Arch Intern Med 1932; 49:471–533.
16. Unno S, Iijima M, Osawa M, et al. A case of chorea gravidarum with moyamoya disease. Rinsho Shinkeigaku 2000; 40(4):378–382.
17. Zegart KN, Schwarz RH. Chorea gravidarum. Obstet Gynecol 1968; 32(1):24–27.
18. Dike GL. Chorea gravidarum: a case report and review. MD Med J 1997; 46(8):436–439.
19. Shulman LM, Minagar A, Weiner WJ. The effect of pregnancy in Parkinson's disease. Mov Disord 2001; 15(1):132–135.
20. Golbe LI. Parkinson's disease and pregnancy. Neurology 1987; 37:1245.
21. Mucchiut M, Belgrado E, Cutuli D, et al. Pramipexole-treated Parkinson's disease during pregnancy. Mov Disord 2004; 19(9): 1114–1115.
22. Hagell P, Odin P, Vinge E. Pregnancy in Parkinson's disease: a review of the literature and a case report. Mov Disord 1998; 13(1):34–38.
23. Colao A, Abs R, Bárcena DG, et al. Pregnancy outcomes following cabergoline treatment: extended results from a 12 year observational study. Clin Endocrinol 2008; 68(1):66–71.
24. Paluzzi A, Bain PG, Liu X, et al. Pregnancy in dystonic women with in situ deep brain stimulators. Mov Disord 2005; 21(5):695–698.
25. Gwinn-Hardy KA, Adler CH, Weaver AL, et al. Effect of hormone variations and other factors on symptom severity in women with dystonia. Mayo Clin Proc 2000; 75:235–240.
26. Wilson SAK. Progressive lenticular degeneration: a familial nervous disease associated with cirrhosis of the liver. Brain 1912; 34:295–507.
27. OMIM 277900; Wilson's disease.
28. Ala A, Walker AP, Ashkan K, et al. Wilson's disease. Lancet 2007; 369(9559):397–408 (abstr).
29. Gow PJ, Smallwood RA, Angus PW, et al. Diagnosis of Wilson's disease: an experience over three decades. Gut 2000; 46(3): 415–419 (abstr).
30. Walshe JM. Pregnancy in Wilson's disease. Q J Med 1977; 46(181):73–83 (abstr).
31. Tarnacka B, Rodo M, Cichy S, et al. Procreation ability in Wilson's disease. Acta Neurol Scand 2000; 101(6):395–398 (abstr).
32. Sinha S, Taly AB, Prashanth LK, et al. Successful pregnancies and abortions in symptomatic and asymptomatic Wilson's disease. J Neurol Sci 2004; 217(1):37–40 (abstr).
33. Pinter R, Hogge WA, McPherson E. Infant with severe penicillamine embryopathy born to a woman with Wilson disease. Am J Med Genet A 2004; 128(3):294–298 (abstr).

21

Multiple sclerosis and pregnancy

Peter A. Brex and Pauline Shaw

INTRODUCTION

Multiple sclerosis (MS) is a chronic immune-mediated disease in which patchy damage to the central nervous system (CNS) is caused through a combination of episodes of inflammation and demyelination, a loss of natural repair mechanisms and progressive neurodegeneration. The cause is unknown but is likely to be due to exposure to a combination of environmental factors in a genetically susceptible individual.

The incidence in the United Kingdom is approximately 7/100,000 (1), with a mean age of onset of around 30 years. On average, life expectancy of people with MS is reduced by only a few years and therefore most live with the symptoms for several decades (the U.K. prevalence is approximately 1 in 850). It is more common in women than men (3:1), with both the prevalence and sex ratio increasing over the past century, largely due to a rising incidence in women for reasons that are unknown. Consequently, the disorder frequently affects women of fertile age and the issue of pregnancy and MS is often encountered in clinical practice.

The majority of people with MS present with relapses; episodes of new neurological symptoms lasting for more than 24 hours in the absence of any predisposing causes, such as infection. Typical symptoms include visual loss, diplopia, paraesthesia, weakness or ataxia. These develop over hours or days, plateau for days or weeks and then spontaneously remit, either fully or partially, over weeks or months. The condition then remains static until a further relapse occurs [relapsing-remitting (RR) MS]. The frequency of relapses is highly variable between individuals, with on average 0.5 to 0.7 per year in the fertile female population. In RR MS, disability is caused by the accumulation over time of the residual effects of relapses. In a fifth of people with MS, relapses largely resolve and significant disability does not accrue (benign MS). For the majority, however, relapses become less frequent with time but worsening disability gradually increases [secondary progressive (SP) MS]. By 10 years, half of patients with RR MS will have developed SP MS. Ten to fifteen percent of people with MS will never have relapses and will present in the progressive phase of the condition [primary progressive (PP) MS]; these patients are usually older, with an equal sex ratio of men and women.

The diagnosis of MS is made on the basis of a typical history with supporting clinical signs and characteristic magnetic resonance imaging (MRI) findings in the brain and spinal cord (2). The presence of oligoclonal bands in the cerebrospinal fluid (CSF) (without corresponding bands in the serum) and negative test results for other conditions that can mimic MS may also be necessary to establish the diagnosis.

Disability in MS is most commonly measured using a disability status scale (3) with the higher the number the more disabled the patient. A score of 3 indicates a moderate disability in a fully ambulatory person; 6 indicates the need for unilateral support, such as a cane or stick, to walk 100 m

without stopping; whilst a score of 8 indicates wheelchair dependence, and 10 is death due to MS.

There is no known cure for MS. The management consists of providing education and support, symptomatic treatment with physical therapy and medication, treating relapses that cause distress or limit activity with corticosteroids, and suppressing relapses in patients in whom these are frequent with disease-modifying drugs such as interferon-beta, glatiramer acetate, mitoxantrone, natalizumab and fingolimod. In the United Kingdom, where there is a relatively small number of neurologists compared with some other countries, the specialist nurse takes a central role in the management of MS once the diagnosis has been established, acting as a point of contact, monitoring drug treatments with the neurologist and liaising with the most appropriate health or social care professional when problems arise.

In large clinical trials of selected patients with RR MS, the three available formulations of interferon-beta-1a/b (Betaferon®/Betaseron®, Avonex® and Rebif®) have each been shown to reduce relapse frequency by around a third over 2 years (4–6). Only one study treating patients with SP MS found a beneficial treatment effect of interferon-beta (7), which seemed most effective in the patients who were still having frequent relapses. Glatiramer acetate (Copaxone®) has also been demonstrated to reduce relapse rates by around one-third (8). The monoclonal antibody natalizumab (Tysabri®) reduced the rate of clinical relapses at 1 year by 68% in a clinical trial (9) and is approved for use in the United Kingdom in people with aggressive RR MS. Mitoxantrone (Novantrone®), an antineoplastic drug, has also been demonstrated to reduce relapses by around two-thirds in patients with relapsing MS and is licensed in the United States (but not in Europe where it is also widely used in specialist centres) to treat aggressive relapsing or SP MS (10). Most recently, fingolimod (Gilenya®), a sphingosine-1-phosphate–receptor modulator that prevents lymphocyte egress from lymph nodes, has become licensed in both Europe and the United States as the first oral treatment for MS after clinical trials demonstrated a 54% relative reduction in relapse rate compared to placebo (11).

Other drugs are occasionally used for preventing relapses in MS despite being unlicensed for this indication. These include azathioprine (12), cladribine (13) and immunoglobulin (14–16).

HERITABILITY

Whilst the cause of MS is unknown, a clinically significant heritable component has been demonstrated in epidemiological studies. Around 15% to 20% of people with MS will have an affected relative. Multiple genes are likely to influence the risk of MS, each exerting only modest effects. Loci that are recognised as heritable risk factors for MS have been identified within the major histocompatability complex (MHC) and other areas, most significantly in those genes coding for IL2RA and IL7RA (17).

Women who have MS themselves or whose partners have MS should be counselled that the risk of MS developing in their offspring is 3% to 5%, compared to a 0.2% for an individual who does not have a parent with MS, a 15 to 25 times increased risk. Should both parents have MS, this increases to 29.5%, a 147.5 times increased risk compared to the general population. An adopted child of an affected individual has no greater risk than the general population (18) suggesting that this increased risk in families is due to genetic rather than environmental factors. However, the risk of inheriting MS does appear to be influenced by environmental factors during pregnancy. For example, in the northern hemisphere the risk is increased in children born in spring and reduced in winter (19,20), with this being mirrored in the southern hemisphere (21). The mechanism for this difference remains unclear but the comparatively reduced exposure to sunlight, and thereby vitamin D, during pregnancy has been proposed. The hypothesis that vitamin D deficiency may be a risk factor for MS has also been supported by the finding that vitamin D has immunomodulatory effects and may regulate the MHC (22).

Whilst there is no clear evidence to support the role of vitamin D in reducing the risk of preventing MS in offspring, some expectant mothers who have MS, or whose partner has MS, choose to increase their dietary intake of foods that are high in vitamin D, such as milk, cereal and dark fish, for example, tuna or salmon (within recommended guidelines during pregnancy) or take multivitamins that contain vitamin D, as well as ensuring adequate exposure to sunlight, for example, by regularly going outside around the middle of the day.

CONTRACEPTION AND FERTILITY

Many women with MS do become pregnant and so reliable contraceptive methods should be used if this is not desired, particularly if they are taking medication that may be harmful to a developing child. Contraceptive, either orally or via depot injection, can be used, but in more disabled patients the benefits need to be weighed against the increased risk of venous thrombosis (23). Potential interactions with other medication also need to be considered. Physical disability may limit the ability to use barrier contraceptives, for example, condoms and diaphragms. Intrauterine devices (IUDs) or progestogen-containing IUDs (the Mirena intrauterine system) can be used. Detection of the rare complication of uterine perforation during insertion and migration of an IUD can be hindered by sensory changes (24).

Whether or not fertility is reduced in MS remains unclear (25). Studies are complicated by other reasons why couples, in which one or both partners have MS, may be less likely to have children. Sexual dysfunction is common in men and women with MS. It may occur due to physical causes such as erectile dysfunction, continence issues, sensory disturbance, pain, weakness, fatigue or emotional factors that lead to loss of libido. Testosterone levels may be reduced in men with MS (26), which can affect their fertility. Some people with MS choose to avoid or postpone pregnancy because of concerns about their ability to manage a child due to the unpredictable nature of the condition or because of fears of passing it on.

Medication can also be a factor in the decision about whether to start a family. This may relate to having to stop treatments that give symptomatic relief or fears about the consequences of stopping or delaying the start of disease-modifying drugs. In women, there is no known effect on fertility of interferon-beta and glatiramer acetate, but there may be an increased risk of spontaneous abortion whilst taking interferon-beta. Natalizumab has been shown to reduce female fertility in animal studies, but only when given in higher doses than are used in humans; male fertility has not been shown to be affected. Fingolimod has not been shown to affect fertility in animal studies. Mitoxantrone can reduce female fertility by causing amenorrhea [Fertility and Mitoxantrone in MS (FEMIMS) study; 27]. This can resolve on discontinuation of the drug, but may not do so, especially in women who are over 35 years.

For women with MS who suffer from unexplained infertility, ovulation induction treatments and assisted reproduction technologies, such as in vitro fertilization (IVF), may be used as for the general population, although the safety of the drugs used in these techniques has not been specifically assessed in this group. There have been reports of increased relapse frequency after infertility treatment in MS patients (25,28,29), but on current evidence, women with MS wishing to pursue treatment for infertility should not be discouraged from doing so.

People with MS due to receive treatments that may impair fertility transiently or permanently, for example, mitoxantrone, may wish to store sperm or oocytes and/or ovarian fragments prior to treatment.

EFFECT OF PREGNANCY ON MS
Symptoms

The symptoms of MS vary widely between individuals depending on the areas in the CNS with the greatest burden of disease. Weakness and ataxia are common, but there may be additional troubling symptoms that may need to be specifically enquired about, such as fatigue, reduced cognition and disturbance of the bladder and bowels. These can all worsen during pregnancy because of the growing uterus and hormone changes. Whilst medication is available to treat some of the symptoms of MS, the evidence for their safety during pregnancy is often lacking and so the benefits of medication must always be weighed against the known and unknown risks.

Bladder irritability is a common problem in pregnancy, chiefly as a result of the gravid uterus applying pressure (30). These pressure effects in a healthy pregnant woman are likely to produce symptoms of overactive bladder with 85% of women experiencing frequency and 70% nocturia during pregnancy. Urinary tract infection is also commoner in pregnancy, mainly as a result of the increased residual bladder volume caused by uterine pressure. In pregnant women with MS, the risk of constipation and urinary tract infection is higher still, largely as a result of pressure from a pregnant uterus on a neurogenic bladder and bowel. Women are encouraged to increase fibre in their diet and insure a daily fluid intake of 2 litres. There should be a low threshold for treating presumed urinary tract infections. One or two urinary tract infections in a pregnant woman with a known neurogenic bladder should prompt the consideration of initiating prophylactic antibiotics to prevent recurrence. Drugs commonly used to manage neurogenic bladder symptoms in the non-pregnant woman with MS are not advised during pregnancy. Pregnant women with MS who are experiencing antenatal bladder problems should be reviewed by their obstetrician and/or a member of the urogynaecology team; antenatal pelvic floor exercises may be advised.

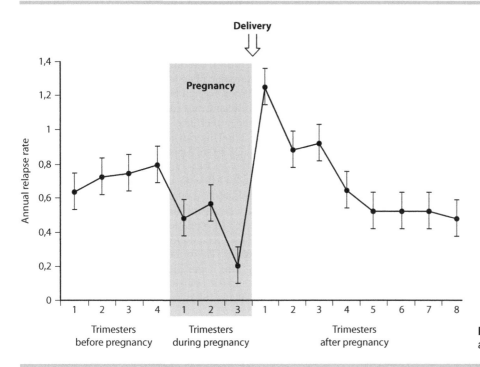

Figure 21.1 Relapse rate before, during and after pregnancy. *Source*: From Ref. 34.

During late pregnancy, women with MS may notice that balance and mobility problems can worsen due to the increasing weight of the uterus and changes in posture. Gentle exercise such as walking, swimming or yoga may be helpful.

Fatigue is a common and troublesome symptom both in people with MS and in pregnant women, and may be a considerable problem in some pregnant women with MS. It is suggested that three factors predispose women to fatigue during pregnancy; physical, psychological and situational factors (31). Physical factors may be due to respiratory and cardiovascular changes during pregnancy. Psychological factors include depression, anxiety and a feeling of change in identity, whilst the situation factors could be living environment, employment status or socioeconomic status. It is important to reinforce to pregnant mothers with MS that it is usual to feel fatigued and to encourage them to take regular rest and learn relaxation techniques. Practical tips to help conserve energy may be the use of internet shopping, sharing household chores with partners and other family members, and raising awareness of fatigue during pregnancy to families and employers to gain understanding and support. Medication for fatigue, for example, amantadine or modafanil, should be avoided during pregnancy.

Relapses

There are obvious difficulties in studying the effects of pregnancy on MS relapses. Women with MS who become pregnant tend to be younger and less disabled than the general MS population; retrospective studies are subject to recall bias which can alter the number and the temporal location of relapses and may lead to false associations; and hospital-based studies are more likely to detect only the more severe relapses or exclude more severely disabled patients who may have difficulty attending clinics.

The effect of pregnancy on the course of MS has been controversial for many years, with some physicians in the past

discouraging people with MS from becoming pregnant believing this would adversely affect the condition (32). Therapeutic abortion was even sometimes recommended. This opinion was largely based on isolated cases of relapses occurring during pregnancy or in the peurperium. By the middle of the 20th century a number of retrospective studies reported that the course of MS stabilises during pregnancy, but that relapses are more likely in the months immediately post-partum.

The Pregnancy in Multiple Sclerosis (PRIMS) study is the largest prospective study of the effects of pregnancy on MS conducted to date (33). It is a multi-centre European study of 254 women during 269 pregnancies that compared relapse activity during each trimester with the pre-pregnancy year. Relapse rate was determined retrospectively in 48% cases. Fatigue alone was not considered evidence of a relapse. The study took place before disease-modifying treatments for MS became widely available. The results support the earlier observations that there is a significant reduction in the relapse rate during pregnancy, most marked in the third trimester [during which the mean annualised relapse rate (ARR) fell from 0.7 to 0.2] followed by a marked increase in the 3 months post-partum (to 1.2). Thereafter, the ARR rate fell slightly but did not differ significantly from the pre-pregnancy year (Fig. 21.1). Despite the increased risk in the 3 months post-partum, 72% of women did not experience any relapses during this period (34).

The risk of relapse in the 3 months post-partum was greater in women who had an increased relapse rate in the pre-pregnancy year, in those who had increased relapse rate during pregnancy and for those with a higher level of disability when becoming pregnant. However, a model incorporating these factors could not reliably predict which women would have a post-partum relapse (Fig. 21.2). In this study, the occurrence of a post-partum relapse was not related to breast-feeding, epidural analgesia, age at MS onset, age at pregnancy onset, disease duration, total number of relapses before

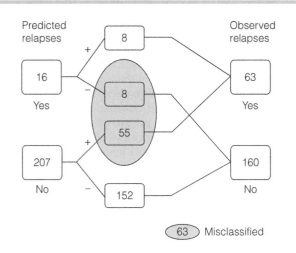

Figure 21.2 Individual prediction of the presence or absence of a relapse in the 3-month period after delivery among 223 women with multiple sclerosis, according to the best multivariate model. *Source*: From Ref. 34.

pregnancy, number of previous pregnancies or child gender. The women in the PRIMS study largely had little in the way of disability (mean EDSS 1.3) and 94% had RR MS with mean disease duration of only 5.5 years. Caution therefore should be taken in extrapolating these results to guide the management of more disabled patients or those with SP MS in whom the effects of pregnancy have been less well studied.

The finding of a reduction in disease activity during pregnancy with an increase post-partum has also been confirmed in studies using MRI as a marker of MS disease activity (35,36).

The immunopathology of MS is complex and is likely to be heterogeneous with different mechanisms in different patients (37). Most MS relapses are due to activated T cells crossing the blood-brain barrier. During pregnancy, cell-mediated immunity is modulated to prevent maternal rejection of the developing fetus, and this is thought to be one of the mechanisms responsible for the reduced relapse rate. In rare cases, women experience an increase in relapse activity during pregnancy. This may be due to these patients having a humeral (antibody-mediated) mechanism causing their MS, as described in a sub-group of MS lesions by Lucchinetti and colleagues; worsening of disease activity during pregnancy is seen in antibody-mediated autoimmune diseases, such as neuromyelitis optica (Devic's disease) (38).

There are reports of the onset of MS during pregnancy (39,40) and when this occurs establishing the diagnosis can be very challenging because of the wider differential diagnosis during pregnancy and the reluctance to perform some investigations, for example MRI scanning, in the first trimester.

Treatment of Relapses
There are no specific studies of relapse management during pregnancy. High-dose steroids, for example, 0.5 to 1 g methylprednisolone per day for 3 to 5 days, are the treatment of choice and can be administered intravenously or orally. The benefits of steroids have only been demonstrated in the short term; there is protective effect against the disease getting worse or remaining stable within the first 5 weeks of treatment (41). No benefit has been demonstrated in the longer term (>6 month) in non-

pregnant patient. Treatment should therefore be reserved for relapses causing distress or limiting activities.

Methylprednisolone crosses the placenta and its use should be avoided in the first trimester as much as possible due to possible teratogenic effects, specifically cleft palate and cataracts. Thereafter, it appears to have little effect on the developing fetus and so is the recommended treatment in pregnant women in the second and third trimesters (42). Treatment with steroids late in pregnancy has been associated with an increased risk of pre-eclampsia, gestational diabetes, venous thrombosis, low birth weight and post-partum adrenal insufficiency and therefore should be used with caution and for as brief a period as necessary.

Immunoglobulin can be given safely during pregnancy. However, whilst there is some evidence of it reducing relapse frequency, the benefits of using it to treat acute relapses is less robust. There have been two case reports suggesting a benefit (43,44) but larger studies have not confirmed this either when given alone (45) or in combination with methylprednisolone (TARIMS trial) (46,47).

Plasma exchange can be of benefit for severe exacerbations of MS that have been resistant to treatment with high-dose steroids (48). There have been no studies in MS of plasma exchange during pregnancy, but it is used during pregnancy to treat other conditions such as myasthenia gravis.

Drug Treatment to Prevent Relapses During Pregnancy
Interferon-beta and glatiramer acetate have not been found to be teratogenic in animal studies, and to date large observational studies in humans have not shown any detrimental outcomes (49–52). Neither interferon-beta nor glatiramer acetate should be initiated in pregnancy, but for those who become pregnant whilst on treatment with interferon-beta continuing use is licensed if the benefit is believed to outweigh risk. However, generally the magnitude of the effect of pregnancy on reducing relapse rate is greater than the effectiveness of these treatments, and if a woman becomes pregnant whilst on treatment in the majority of cases it will be discontinued. Glatiramer acetate is not licensed for use during pregnancy.

The issue of whether or not to discontinue treatment prior to conception is more controversial. It is necessary to discontinue interferon-beta 3 months and glatiramer acetate 1 month prior to conception to ensure that they have been cleared from the body. However, given that for some women it takes several months or even years to conceive, this will leave them untreated during this period. This needs to be carefully discussed prior to conception, so an informed decision can be taken balancing the risks of stopping treatment with continuing it until conception has occurred.

To date no significant adverse outcomes have been reported in patients exposed to natalizumab during pregnancy (53–55). Whilst the numbers of patients exposed is lower than with interferon-beta, by definition these patients have highly active disease and so the risks of discontinuing treatment or continuing until conception will again need to be carefully considered. Once pregnant, Tysabri will usually be discontinued unless it is felt the benefits outweigh any risk. If discontinuing prior to conception, at least 3 months should be allowed to ensure adequate clearance from the body.

Fingolimod is not licensed during pregnancy and women should be advised to discontinue treatment at least 2 months before trying to conceive. It has been demonstrated to be teratogenic in animal studies, causing fetal loss and organ defects. All women taking this treatment should be advised to use contraception.

There are no adequate studies of the effects of mitoxantrone on pregnancy in humans, but in animal studies low fetal birth weight, abnormal fetal renal development and premature delivery have been reported. Treatment should therefore not be given during pregnancy and should be discontinued immediately if pregnancy occurs. If a woman receiving mitoxantrone wishes to become pregnant, she should use contraception for 6 months after discontinuing the drug before trying to conceive.

Immunoglobulin can be infused regularly during the gestational period to reduce relapse rate (56). However, given that it is a blood product, and therefore a potential source of infection, is expensive and relapse rate is generally low during pregnancy even without treatment, it is rarely given in practice.

Disability

The effects of pregnancy on long-term disability are difficult to ascertain because of the slow evolution of the condition in most cases. In studies that have addressed this, the follow-up period has generally been short relative to the chronic nature of the disease. In the PRIMS study, disability measures showed a slow, steady increase throughout the study but pregnancy, delivery and post-partum did not seem to have any impact on disability progression over a 2-year post-partum follow-up period (34). Studies with longer follow-up have also found that women with MS who have children are either no more disabled than those that do not, despite the relatively high risk of post-partum relapses, or may even be less disabled, particularly when pregnancy occurs after the onset of MS (40,57–59).

DELIVERY AND LABOUR

There is no contraindication to either vaginal delivery or caesarean section for women with MS (24). MS mothers who have mobility problems may find it difficult to remain mobile during labour. Weakness of lower limbs and spasticity may hinder the mother's ability to adopt a variety of positions for labour and delivery. Labouring and or delivery in water are a popular option as weak and heavy lower limbs feel supported and the cool water reduces the mother's core temperature, which may have a positive impact on fatigue. In those that do not wish labour or delivery in water, lying on the left side with the upper leg supported may ease delivery.

Dahl and colleagues (60) found a trend towards slower progression of the second stage of labour and an increased risk of forceps delivery in women with MS. Neuromuscular perineal weakness and sensory disturbance combined with spasticity may be contributory. Levels of fatigue also need to be taken into consideration in the labouring women with MS as this will affect the ability of the mother to persevere with labour along with her ability to push.

An increase in caesarean rate has been reported in some (33,60,61) but not all (62,63) studies. This appears to be a result of an increased rate of elective pre-labour caesarean section rather than emergency intervention, suggesting that these problems are generally anticipated (60,64).

For the majority of women with or without MS, pain relief is a necessity during labour. There is no contraindication for women with MS to be given Entonox, Pethidine or to use TENs machines or have epidural anaesthesia. However, for elective or semi-elective caesarean section where there is no immediate urgency to provide analgesia, there are preliminary data that suggest that epidural anaesthesia may be preferable to spinal anaesthesia. Epidural anaesthesia produces a lower concentration of local anaesthesia in the CSF. A study by Bader and colleagues (65) suggested evidence of higher concentrations of anaesthesia in the CSF influencing post-partum relapse rate. Bader and colleagues expressed concerns that regional anaesthesia may expose demyelinated areas of the spinal cord to potential neuro-toxic effects of the local anaesthetic.

There are case reports of mothers with MS with spinal cord involvement developing autonomic dysreflexia (66). This can be provoked during pregnancy, childbirth or in the post-partum period. Symptoms are of elevation in the blood pressure, headache, sweating, cool limbs and anxiety. Hypertensive encephalopathy, stroke and seizures can occur. Eclampsia/pre-eclampsia are an important differential diagnosis of this presentation and may coexist. The management of autonomic dysreflexia involves reducing any avoidable provoking factors, for example, by catheterising the patient or ensuring any catheter in situ is patent, relieving faecal impaction; reducing the blood pressure by sitting the patient up and giving rapid onset, short-acting antihypertensive medication. A patient with autonomic dysreflexia should be closely monitored for at least 2 hours after it has settled to ensure it does not recur and that they do not become too hypotensive as a result of treatment given (67).

Reported effects of the disease on pregnancy outcomes, risk of malformations, fetal birth weight or duration of pregnancy are inconsistent but without any clear increased risks.

Another issue that may arise around the time of delivery is whether mothers should bank umbilical cord blood. Whilst this is not generally available on the National Health Service in the UK, there are commercial companies that provide collection and storage. Umbilical cord blood is a rich source of haemopoietic stem cells and the rational for storage is that these may be able to be used in the future to treat the child should he or she develop MS or certain other diseases. However, there are a number of practical, legal and ethical issues surrounding this practice that need to be considered. Guidance from the Royal College of Obstetricians and Gynaecologists (68) is available (http://www.rcog.org.uk/news/rcog-advice-umbilical-cord-blood-banking-and-storage).

BREASTFEEDING

Some mothers may find breastfeeding difficult due to increased fatigue levels and upper limb weakness. Jacobson (69) suggests the following strategies:

- Set up a particular place or area at home that will be easily accessible and comfortable for nursing.
- Use pillows to help support the positioning of the baby.
- Use a sling to carry the baby which may help prevent fatigue and weakness of upper limbs.
- Use a nursing bra that opens in the front.
- Establish planned rest periods to conserve energy.
- Nurse the baby in a lying position.
- Plan for help with childcare and household tasks.
- Arrange to purchase or hire a breast pump to express milk so the baby can be bottle fed at times allowing the mother to rest.

It is important for the midwife to spend time with the mother with MS in order to establish what position the mother will find best to establish successful breastfeeding. The mother with weak arms may find the side lying position useful as it requires little baby support and involves the use of a number of pillows to support different parts of the mother's body. A pillow support placed under the mother's leg may also help relieve spasticity and promote comfort whist breastfeeding. Mothers who use a wheelchair may find the cradle hold position with the additional use of pillows to support the baby more comfortable.

Breastfeeding should be encouraged for mothers with MS due to the health benefits to both mother and baby. It is important to assure mothers that there is no danger of transferring MS to their child through breast milk and that it offers protection to the child from illness. Drug treatment in breastfeeding mothers should be given only after careful consideration as a caution due to the risks of the drug affecting lactation or being passed on to the infant in the breast milk. The risks will vary depending on the gestational age of the infant at birth.

The Treatment of MS Relapses During Breastfeeding

Disabling relapses which impact on function can be managed with high-dose oral or intravenous methylprednisolone as at other times. Following steroids, it is advised to express and discard breast milk for 8 to 24 hours after a high dose of steroids to reduce the risks of exposure to the infant.

Treatments to Prevent Relapses During Breastfeeding

In women felt to be at high risk of post-partum relapses there is always a dilemma as whether to forego breastfeeding and the consequent health benefits to the mother and infant to enable disease-modifying drug treatment to be restarted. However, studies to date suggest breastfeeding has been associated with a trend towards a lower risk of relapses in the first few months post-partum (33,70,71). Hormonal changes induced by breastfeeding may have a protective effect on relapse rate but it appears that exclusive breastfeeding, that is, without supplemental feeding, may be necessary (72). In the later studies, the apparent benefits of breastfeeding may be attributed, in part, to women with more active MS opting not to breastfeed in order to (re)start treatment with disease-modifying drugs. Interferon-beta, glatiramer acetate and natalizumab are not licensed for use whilst breastfeeding, although in theory the amount of each of the drugs transferred in breast milk is likely to be negligible. However, these drugs may take some time to take effect, and with the early cessation of breastfeeding the likelihood of a relapse in the post-partum period may actually increase (71).

A study in which 1 g of intravenous methylprednisolone was given monthly during the first 6 months of the postpartum period showed a significant reduction in the relapse rate compared to an historical control group. The authors concluded further studies were warranted (73).

Prophylactic administration of intravenous immunoglobulin post-partum has also been studied both against placebo (56) and in a randomised dose comparison study in patients with RR MS [the Gammaglobulin Post Partum (GAMPP) study] (74). Immunoglobulin has been shown to reduce the risk of relapse in the post-partum period (56) without ill effect. The effect was greatest when regular treatment is given throughout pregnancy and the post-partum period.

Given that only one-third of mothers will suffer a relapse in the postpartum period, some of which will be mild, and overall they do not appear to lead to an increase in disability in the long-term, the authors feel that routinely treating women with any of the currently available products throughout the postpartum period is not justified.

The dramatic reduction in relapse frequency that is observed naturally during pregnancy has raised the question as to whether treatment with sex hormones can be given safely and effectively to treat relapses. The Prevention of Post-Partum Relapses with Progestin and Estradiol in Multiple Sclerosis (POPART'MUS) study is a European, multi-centre, randomized, placebo-controlled and double-blind clinical trial, currently ongoing which aims to reduce MS relapses related to the post-partum condition by administrating high doses of progestin with endometrial protective doses of oestradiol (75). Treatment is given immediately after delivery and continuously during the first 3 months post-partum. Should this prove to be positive, it could lead to a new treatment for women with relapsing MS.

CONCLUSIONS

Pregnancy is an important consideration when managing people with MS. It should not be discouraged but needs to be planned. Adequate discussion is needed about the effect of pregnancy on relapses during the course of the pregnancy and during the post-partum period and how they can be managed. The number of treatments for MS is expanding but these may need be interrupted or deferred to allow for pregnancies and breastfeeding due to a lack of safety information. MS should not dictate the method of delivery but sometimes symptoms may impact on labour. Whilst there is an increased risk of MS in children born to parents with this condition, most people with MS have healthy children without a negative long-term impact on the course of their disease.

REFERENCES

1. MacDonald B, Cockerell O, Sander J, et al. The incidence and lifetime prevalence of neurological disorders in a prospective community-based study in the UK. Brain 2000; 123:665–676.
2. Polman CH, Reingold SC, Banwell B, et al. Diagnostic criteria for multiple sclerosis: 2010 Revisions to the McDonald criteria. Ann Neurol 2011; 69:292–302.
3. Kurtzke JF. Rating neurologic impairment in multiple sclerosis: an expanded disability status scale (EDSS). Neurology 1983; 33:1444–1452.
4. The IFNB Multiple Sclerosis Study Group. Interferon beta-1b is effective in relapsing-remitting multiple sclerosis. I. Clinical results of a multicenter, randomized, double-blind, placebo-controlled trial. Neurology 1993; 43:655–661.
5. Jacobs LD, Cookfair DL, Rudick RA, et al. Intramuscular interferon beta-1a for disease progression in relapsing multiple sclerosis. Ann Neurol 1996; 39:285–294.
6. PRISMS (Prevention of Relapses and Disability by Interferon beta-1a Subcutaneously in Multiple Sclerosis) Study Group. Randomised double-blind placebo-controlled study of interferon beta-1a in relapsing/remitting multiple sclerosis. Lancet 1998; 352:1498–1504.
7. European Study Group on interferon beta-1b in secondary progressive MS (EUSPMS). Placebo-controlled multicentre randomised trial of interferon beta-1b in treatment of secondary progressive multiple sclerosis. Lancet 1998; 352:1491–1497.
8. Johnson KP, Brooks BR, Cohen JA, et al. Copolymer 1 reduces relapse rate and improves disability in relapsing-remitting multiple sclerosis: results of a phase III multicenter, double-blind placebo-controlled trial. Neurology 1995; 45:1268–1276.
9. Polman CH, O'Connor PW, Havrdova E, et al. A randomized, placebo-controlled trial of natalizumab for relapsing multiple sclerosis. N Engl J Med 2006; 354:899–910.
10. Hartung HP, Gonsette R, König N, et al. Mitoxantrone in progressive multiple sclerosis: a placebo-controlled, double-blind, randomised, multicentre trial. Lancet 2002; 360:2018–2025.

11. Kappos L, Radue E-W, O'Connor P, et al. Placebo-controlled study of oral fingolimod in relapsing multiple sclerosis. N Engl J Med 2010; 362:387–401.

12. Casetta I, Iuliano G, Filippini G. Azathioprine for multiple sclerosis. J Neurol Neurosurg Psychiatry 2009; 80:131–132.

13. Giovannoni G, Comi G, Cook S, et al. A placebo-controlled trial of oral cladribine for relapsing multiple sclerosis. N Engl J Med 2010; 362:416–426.

14. Fazekas F, Deisenhammer F, Strasser-Fuchs S, et al. Randomised placebo-controlled trial of monthly intravenous immunoglobulin therapy in relapsing-remitting multiple sclerosis. Lancet 1997; 349:589–593.

15. Achiron A, Gabbay U, Gilad R, et al. Intravenous immunoglobulin treatment in multiple sclerosis. Effect on relapses. Neurology 1998; 50:398–402.

16. Fazekas F, Lublin FD, Li D, et al. Intravenous immunoglobulin in relapsing-remitting multiple sclerosis: a dose-finding trial. Neurology 2008; 71:265–271.

17. Hafler DA, Compston A, Sawcer S, et al. Risk alleles for multiple sclerosis identified by a genomewide study. N Engl J Med 2007; 357:851–862.

18. Sadovnick AD, Dircks A, Ebers GC. Genetic counselling in multiple sclerosis: risks to sibs and children of affected individuals. Clin Genet 1999; 56:118–122.

19. Willer CJ, Dyment DA, Sadovnick AD, et al. Timing of birth and risk of multiple sclerosis: population based study. BMJ 2005; 330:120.

20. Salzer J, Svenningsson A, Sundström P. Season of birth and multiple sclerosis in Sweden. Acta Neurol Scand 2010; 121:20–23.

21. Staples J, Ponsonby A, Lim L. Low maternal exposure to ultraviolet radiation in pregnancy, month of birth, and risk of multiple sclerosis in offspring: longitudinal analysis. BMJ 2010; 340:c1640.

22. Ramagopalan SV, Maugeri NJ, Handunnetthi L, et al. Expression of the multiple sclerosis-associated MHC class II allele HLA-DRB1*1501 is regulated by vitamin D. PLos Genet 2009; 5:e1000369.

23. Dwosh E, Guimond C, Sadovnick AD. Reproductive counseling in MS: a guide for healthcare professionals. Int MS J 2003; (3):52–59.

24. Houtchens MK Pregnancy and multiple sclerosis. Semin Neurol 2007; 27:434–441.

25. Cavalla P, Rovei V, Masera S, et al. Fertility in patients with multiple sclerosis: current knowledge and future perspectives. Neurol Sci 2006; 27:231–239.

26. Foster SC, Daniels C, Bourdette DN, et al. Dysregulation of the hypothalamic-pituitary-gonadal axis in experimental autoimmune encephalomyelitis and multiple sclerosis. J Neuroimmunol 2003; 140:78–87.

27. Cocco E, Sardu C, Gallo P, et al. Frequency and risk factors of mitoxantrone-induced amenorrhea in multiple sclerosis: the FEMIMS study. Mult Scler 2008; 14:1225–1233.

28. Laplaud DA, Leray E, Barrière P, et al. Increase in multiple sclerosis relapse rate following in vitro fertilization. Neurology 2006; 66:1280–1281.

29. Hellwig K, Schimrigk S, Beste C, et al. Increase in relapse rate during assisted reproduction technique in patients with multiple sclerosis. Eur Neurol 2008; 61:65–68.

30. Durufle A, Nicolas B, Petrilli S, et al. Effects of pregnancy and childbirth on the incidence of urinary disorders in multiple sclerosis. Clin Exp Obstet Gynecol 2006; 33(4):215–218.

31. Bialobok K, Monga M. Fatigue and work in pregnancy. Curr Opin Obstet Gynecol 2000; 12(6):497–500.

32. Douglass LH, Jorgensen CL. Pregnancy and multiple sclerosis. Am J Obstet Gynaecol 1948; 55:332–336.

33. Confavreux C, Hutchinson M, Hours MM, et al. Rate of pregnancy-related relapse in multiple sclerosis. Pregnancy in Multiple Sclerosis Group. N Engl J Med 1998; 339:285–291.

34. Vukusic S, Hutchinson M, Hours M, et al. Pregnancy and multiple sclerosis (the PRIMS study): clinical predictors of postpartum relapse. Brain 2004; 127:1353–1360.

35. van Walderveen MA, Tas MW, Barkhof F, et al. Magnetic resonance evaluation of disease activity during pregnancy in multiple sclerosis. Neurology 1994; 44:327–329.

36. Paavilainen T, Kurki T, Parkkola R, et al. Magnetic resonance imaging of the brain used to detect early post-partum activation of multiple sclerosis. Eur J Neurol 2007; 14:1216–1221.

37. Lucchinetti C, Brück W, Parisi J, et al. Heterogeneity of multiple sclerosis lesions: implications for the pathogenesis of demyelination. Ann Neurol 2000; 47:707–717.

38. Cornelio DB, Braga RP, Rosa MW, et al. Devic's neuromyelitis optica and pregnancy: distinction from multiple sclerosis is essential. Arch Gynecol Obstet 2009; 280:475–477.

39. Poser S, Poser W. Multiple sclerosis and gestation. Neurology 1983; 33:1422–1427.

40. Runmarker B, Andersen O. Pregnancy is associated with a lower risk of onset and a better prognosis in multiple sclerosis. Brain 1995; 118:253–261.

41. Filippini G, Brusaferri F, Sibley WA, et al. Corticosteroids or ACTH for acute exacerbations in multiple sclerosis. Cochrane Database Syst Rev 2000; (4):CD001331.

42. Sellebjerg F, Barnes D, Filippini G, et al. EFNS guideline on treatment of multiple sclerosis relapses: report of an EFNS task force on treatment of multiple sclerosis relapses. Eur J Neurol 2005; 12:939–946.

43. Soukop W, Tschabitscher H. Gamma globulin therapy in multiple sclerosis. Theoretical considerations and initial clinical experiences with 7S immunoglobulins in MS therapy. Wien Med Wochenschr 1986; 136:477–480 (article in German).

44. Yan J, Richert JR, Sirdofsky MD. High-dose intravenous immunoglobulin for multiple sclerosis. Lancet 1990; 336:692.

45. Roed HG, Langkilde A, Sellebjerg F, et al. A double-blind, randomized trial of IV immunoglobulin treatment in acute optic neuritis. Neurology 2005; 64:804–810.

46. Sorensen PS, Haas J, Sellebjerg F, et al. IV immunoglobulins as add-on treatment to methylprednisolone for acute relapses in MS. Neurology 2004; 63:2028–2033.

47. Visser LH, Beekman R, Tijssen CC, et al. A randomized, double-blind, placebo-controlled pilot study of i.v. immune globulins in combination with i.v. methylprednisolone in the treatment of relapses in patients with MS. Mult Scler 2004; 10:89–91.

48. Weinshenker BG, O'Brien PC, Petterson TM, et al. A randomized trial of plasma exchange in acute central nervous system inflammatory demyelinating disease. Ann Neurol 1999; 46:878–886.

49. Patti F, Cavallaro T, Lo Fermo S, et al. Is in utero early-exposure to interferon beta a risk factor for pregnancy outcomes in multiple sclerosis? J Neurol 2008; 255:1250–1253.

50. Weber-Schoendorfer C, Schaefer C. Multiple sclerosis, immunomodulators, and pregnancy outcome: a prospective observational study. Mult Scler 2009; 15:1037–1042.

51. Salminen HJ, Leggett H, Boggild M. Glatiramer acetate exposure in pregnancy: preliminary safety and birth outcomes. J Neurol 2010; 257:2020–2023.

52. Sandberg-Wollheim M, Alteri E, Moraga MS, et al. Pregnancy outcomes in multiple sclerosis following subcutaneous interferon beta-1a therapy. Mult Scler 2011; 17:423–430.

53. Mahavedan, et al. Natalizumab Use During Pregnancy. Am J Gastroenterol 2008; 103:S449–S450.

54. Cristiano L, Bozic C, Kooijmans M. Preliminary evaluation of pregnancy outcomes from the Tysabri (Natalizumab) Pregnancy Exposure Registry. Mult Scler 2010; 16:P840 (abstr).

55. Hoevenaren IA, de Vries LC, Rijnders RJ, et al. Delivery of healthy babies after natalizumab use for multiple sclerosis: a report of two cases. Acta Neurol Scand 2011; 123:430–433.

56. Achiron A, Kishner I, Dolev M, et al. Effect of intravenous immunoglobulin treatment on pregnancy and postpartum-related relapses in multiple sclerosis. J Neurol 2004; 1133–1137.

57. Weinshenker BG, Hader W, Carriere W, et al. The influence of pregnancy on disability from multiple sclerosis: a population-based study in Middlesex County, Ontario. Neurology 1989; 39:1438–1440.

58. Verdru P, Theys P, D'Hooghe MB, et al. Pregnancy and multiple sclerosis: the influence on long term disability. Clin Neurol Neurosurg 1994; 96:38–41.

59. D'hooghe MB, Nagels G, Uitdehaag BM. Long-term effects of childbirth in MS. J Neurol Neurosurg Psychiatry 2010; 81:38–41.

60. Dahl J, Myhr KM, Dalveit AK, et al. Pregnancy, delivery and birth outcome in women with multiple sclerosis. Neurology 2005; 65:1961–1963.

61. Kelly VM, Nelson LM, Chakravarty EF. Obstetric outcomes in women with multiple sclerosis and epilepsy. Neurology 2009; 73:1831–1836.

62. Worthington J, Jones R, Crawford M, et al. Pregnancy and multiple sclerosis: a 3-year prospective study. J Neurol 1994; 241: 228–233.

63. Mueller BA, Zhang J, Critchlow CW. Birth outcomes and need for hospitalization after delivery among women with multiple sclerosis. Am J Obstet Gynecol 2002; 186:446–452.

64. Dahl, J, Myhr K-M, Daltveit AK, et al. Planned vaginal births in women with multiple sclerosis: delivery and birth outcome. Acta Neurol Scand 2006; 113(S183):51–54.

65. Bader AM, Hunt CO, Datta S, et al. Anaesthesia for the obstetric patient with multiple sclerosis. J Clin Anesth 1988; 1(1):21–24.

66. Bateman AM, Goldish GD. Autonomic dysreflexia in multiple sclerosis. J Spinal Cord Med 2002; 25:40–42.

67. Consortium for Spinal Cord Medicine, 2001. Available at: http://www.pva.org/site/DocServer/AD2.pdf?docID=565.

68. Royal College of Obstetricians and Gynaecologists Scientific Advisory Committee Opinion Paper 2. Umbilical Cord Blood Banking, June 2006.

69. Jacobson P. Multiple sclerosis: a supportive approach for breast-feeding. Mother Baby J 1998; 3:13–17.

70. Nelson LM, Franklin GM, Jones MC. Risk of multiple sclerosis exacerbation during pregnancy and breast-feeding. JAMA 1988; 259:3441–3443.

71. Gulick EE, Halper J. Influence of infant feeding method on postpartum relapse of mothers with MS. Int J MS Care 2002; 4(4):4–12.

72. Langer-Gould A, Huang SM, Gupta R, et al. Exclusive breastfeeding and the risk of postpartum relapses in women with multiple sclerosis. Arch Neurol 2009; 66:958–963.

73. de Seze J, Chapelotte M, Delalande S, et al. Intravenous corticosteroids in the postpartum period for reduction of acute exacerbations in multiple sclerosis. Mult Scler 2004; 10:596–597.

74. Haas J, Hommes O. A dose comparison study of IVIG in postpartum relapsing-remitting multiple sclerosis. Mult Scler 2007; 13:900–908.

75. Vukusic S, Ionescu I, El-Etr M, et al. The Prevention of postpartum relapses with progestin and estradiol in multiple sclerosis (POPART'MUS) trial: rationale, objectives and state of advancement. J Neurol Sci 2009; 286(1–2):114–118.

22

Nutritional deficiencies in pregnancy

Roy A. Sherwood

INTRODUCTION

Nutritional deficiencies associated with neurological symptoms in the mother or fetus are uncommon in the developed world. The most important deficiencies are those of the B vitamins: (thiamine (B1), folate and B12), vitamin D, vitamin E, iodine and iron.

B VITAMINS
Vitamin B1 (Thiamine)

The active form of vitamin B1, thiamine pyrophosphate, is a coenzyme involved in a number of important reactions in intermediary metabolism including formation of acetyl CoA/succinyl CoA, reduced nicotinamide adenine dinucleotide phosphate (NADPH) and in the metabolism of branched-chain amino acids. The earliest feature of deficiency is a peripheral neuropathy (dry beriberi), but if this progresses to a chronic deficiency heart failure ensues leading to oedema (wet beriberi). Most commonly seen in chronic alcoholics, thiamine deficiency can occur in subjects with malnutrition associated with poor nutrient intake. Severe acute deficiency causes the Wernicke–Korsakoff syndrome with encephalopathy and peripheral neuropathy and is a medical emergency. Thiamine administration is usually advised on an empirical basis when the clinical circumstances raise the possibility of thiamine deficiency even in the absence of clinical signs.

Wernicke syndrome is characterised by a confusional state, disturbances of gait and occulomotor abnormalities, although not all features of this triad may be present. The diagnosis is based on the clinical suspicion, exclusion of other causes of encephalopathy, the finding of low whole blood thiamine concentrations, the rapid reversibility of symptoms with administration of thiamine and pathognomonic findings on MRI (Figs. 22.1 and 22.2). Low whole blood thiamine concentrations confirm the diagnosis, although these may not be available in all health care settings. An alternative is to measure the erythrocyte transketolase activity which gives a functional evaluation of vitamin B1 stores.

Wernicke syndrome is well described in association with hyperemesis gravidarum and thyrotoxicosis in pregnancy (1–5) and hyperemesis with dry and wet beriberi has been reported with severe hyperemesis (6).

Nausea and vomiting are common in pregnancy, occurring in up to 90% of women. Hyperemesis gravidarum is an extreme manifestation of this phenomenon resulting in dehydration and ketonuria that requires hospital admission. It is a disabling and potentially life-threatening condition affecting around 0.3% to 2% of pregnant women. The Report on Confidential Enquiries (7) recommended that 'Fluid and electrolyte balance and control of anti-emetic drug therapy in cases of hyperemesis gravidarum require expert management. In all cases where an intravenous infusion is required thiamine should be administered'. Thiamine can be administered orally at a dose of 100 mg/day but is often not tolerated and parenteral

administration in doses of 50 to 300 mg/day together with folic acid (10–20 mg/day) has been recommended to treat Wernicke syndrome in pregnancy (6). The rate of fetal loss in cases of Wernicke syndrome in pregnancy is around 40% (5). Sub-clinical thiamine deficiency is not uncommon in pregnancy; in one study, 25% of pregnant women had low red cell transketolase concentrations (8). Routine supplementation of thiamine in pregnancy is, however, not recommended (9).

Folate

The term folate is given to a group of related compounds including the active forms di- and tetrahydrofolate (Fig. 22.3). These act as donors and acceptors of single carbon groups in reactions involved in the interconversion of certain amino acids and in purine (and thus DNA) synthesis. Folate deficiency due to inadequate intake is rare in the developed world, but can arise due to malabsorption or importantly in states of increased demand such as pregnancy and lactation. It has also been observed during therapy with some anticonvulsant drugs (10). The characteristic feature is a macrocytic, megaloblastic anaemia that can be corrected by folate supplementation. Folate metabolism is interlinked with that of vitamin B12 and the amino acid homocysteine.

The association of folate deficiency with the development of neural tube defects (NTDs) is well established. The teratogenic effect of folate deficiency has been, at least partially, linked to impaired synthesis and methylation of DNA, RNA and synthesis of polyamines (11). During normal pregnancy, maternal folate requirements increase eight- to tenfold. Dietary supplementation (400 µg daily) from the time of conception to at least the 12th week of pregnancy has been shown to reduce the incidence of NTDs up to fourfold (12,13). This has been reinforced by the finding of partial deficiencies of the enzyme methyltetrahydrofolate reductase in some parents of children born with an NTD (14). The U.K.-based National Institute for Health and Clinical Excellence (NICE) (15) advises folic acid supplementation for all women at a dose of 400 µg/day before conception and up to 12 weeks of gestation. Folate supplementation in women with epilepsy contemplating pregnancy is also discussed in chapter 12.

Folate deficiency is treated with folic acid, which, although itself inactive, is metabolised in the body to tetrahydrofolate. Compulsory supplementation of bread with folate has been in place in the United States since 1996 as well as in other countries such as Canada (1998) and Australia (2009). Other countries including the United Kingdom and New Zealand have advocated folate supplementation of bread but have yet to make it compulsory.

Vitamin B12 (Cobalamin)

The cobalamin family of compounds all have a planar, cobalt-containing (corrin) ring and a ribonucleotide set at a right angle and covalently bound to the ring (Fig. 22.4). The major

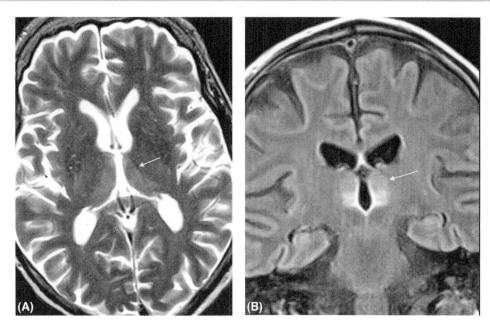

Figure 22.1 Axial T2-weighted image (**A**) and coronal FLAIR image (**B**) show symmetric hyperintensity in the medial thalami (*arrows*). *Source*: Courtesy of Dr Naomi Sibtain.

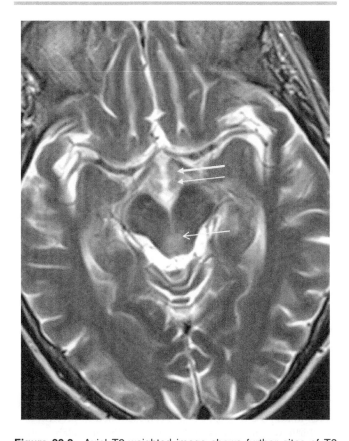

Figure 22.2 Axial T2-weighted image shows further sites of T2 hyperintensity in the hypothalamic region (*thick arrow*), mammillary bodies (*thin arrow*) and peri-aqueductal grey matter of the midbrain (*open arrow*). *Source*: Courtesy of Dr Naomi Sibtain.

Pteroylglutamic acid (folic acid)

Dihydrofolic acid

Tetrahydrofolic acid

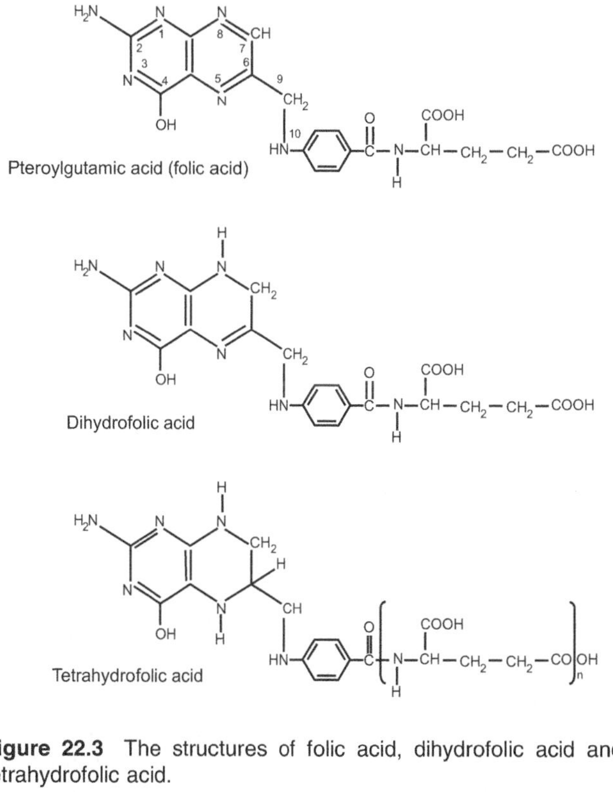

Figure 22.3 The structures of folic acid, dihydrofolic acid and tetrahydrofolic acid.

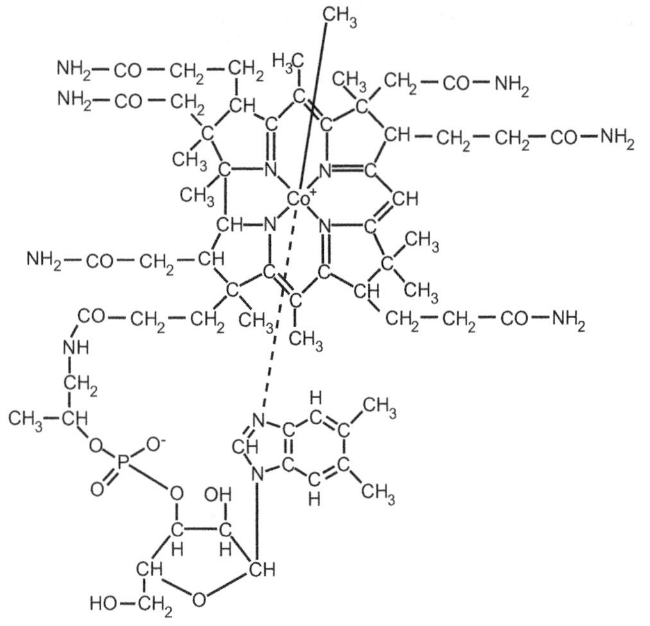

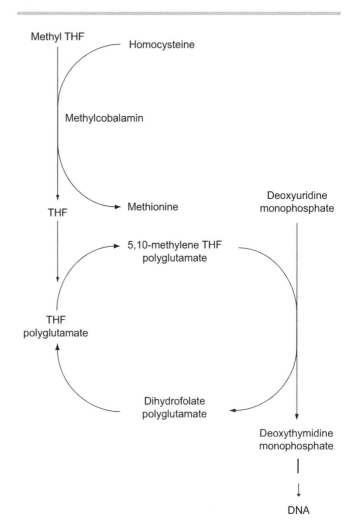

Figure 22.4   Vitamin B12. The major form in the body methylcobalamin is shown.

Figure 22.5   The relationship between folate, B12 and homocysteine metabolism.

form in the circulation is methylcobalamin with the minor forms being hydroxocobalamin and deoxyadenosylcobalamin. The previously mentioned interlinking of vitamin B12 with folate and homocysteine metabolism occurs because vitamin B12 is an essential coenzyme for the conversion of homocysteine and methyltetrahydrofolate to methionine and tetrahydrofolate, making it an essential compound in the formation of DNA (Fig. 22.5). Additionally, deoxyadenosylcobalamin is a coenzyme for methylmalonate CoA mutase which converts methylmalonyl CoA to succinyl CoA. The only dietary sources of vitamin B12 are meat, eggs and milk meaning that vegans are at significant risk of dietary insufficiency. Vitamin B12 deficiency is indicated by a serum B12 concentration less than 150 ng/L (16).

Absorption of vitamin B12 from the lumen of the gut is dependent on the production of intrinsic factor by the parietal cells of the stomach. The complex of intrinsic factor and vitamin B12 is absorbed in the small intestine, that is, jejunum and ileum. Autoantibodies can be produced either to the gastric parietal cell itself or directly against intrinsic factor. These antibodies block the formation of the complex of intrinsic factor and vitamin B12 resulting in failure of absorption and development of the condition pernicious anaemia. In the circulation vitamin B12 is transported by a carrier protein, transcobalamin II. Some analytical methods for measurement of serum B12 concentrations rely on binding of B12 to intrinsic factor to capture the B12 in the sample and are subject to varying degrees of positive interference. For this reason many people consider a serum vitamin B12 concentration falling between 150 and 250 ng/L as a borderline result which does not exclude B12 deficiency. Alternative methods for assessing B12 status are measurement of homocysteine, methylmalonic acid and holotranscobalamin in serum/plasma.

Deficiency of vitamin B12 results in a macrocytic, megaloblastic anaemia, similar to that of folate deficiency, and a neurological disorder, beginning with a peripheral neuropathy and progressing to a subacute combined degeneration of the spinal cord. If untreated, chronic deficiency can result in these neurological changes becoming irreversible. Vitamin B12 and/or folate deficiency result in hyperhomocysteinaemia which is an independent risk factor for cardiovascular and degenerative diseases (17,18).

Vitamin B12 deficiency and the associated hyperhomocysteinaemia in mothers have been associated with the development of an NTD in the fetus (19,20). The effect of maternal vitamin B12 deficiency on the neurodevelopment of infants has been the subject of a recent review (21). Encephalopathy with associated epilepsy in an infant whose mother had pernicious anaemia has been described (22). An Royal College of Obstetricians and Gynaecologists (RCOG) advisory group concluded that there is no evidence from randomised controlled trials to support supplementation of B12 in pregnancy (23).

VITAMIN E

Vitamin E deficiency is rarely seen in healthy adults, due to large stores in adipose tissue, but has been identified in preterm and low birth weight infants and patients with fat malabsorption including cystic fibrosis. Symptoms of deficiency mostly relate to a haemolytic anaemia, but peripheral neuropathy has been reported (24). Rare genetic conditions are recognised in children with a low vitamin E concentration associated with a spinocerebellar disorder, similar to Freidreich's ataxia (25). Vitamin E is

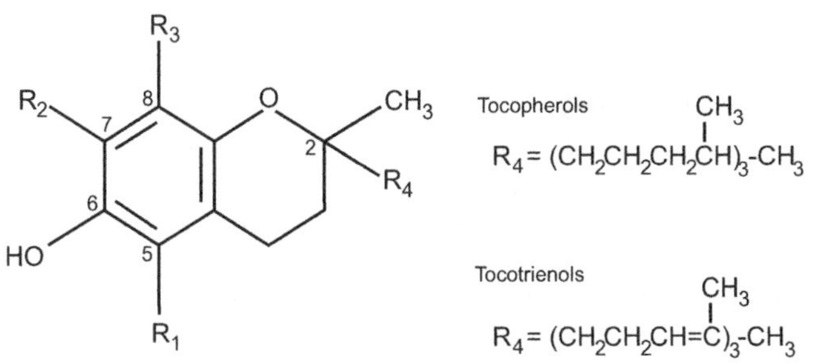

Species	Methyl positions
α	5, 7, 8
β	5, 8
γ	7, 8
δ	8

Figure 22.6 The family of compounds comprising vitamin E.

the name given to a group of lipid-soluble and plant-derived compounds; the tocopherols and tocotrienols (Fig. 22.6). The most biologically active form of vitamin E is the naturally occurring alpha-tocopherol which is present in vegetable oils, nuts, some cereals and some leafy green vegetables. Vitamin E functions as an antioxidant helping to reduce oxidative stress by suppressing free radical activity. Oxidative stress has been linked to a wide range of adult disorders including cancer, cardiovascular disease, inflammatory disorders and neurological diseases. Oxidative stress has also been implicated in the development of pre-eclampsia and with miscarriage and intra-uterine growth retardation (26). Theoretically, therefore, it was thought that supplementation with vitamins with antioxidative properties such as vitamins C and E would reduce the risk of pre-eclampsia. In a meta-analysis of four trials of vitamin E supplementation in combination with other vitamins, Rumbold and Crowther found no evidence that supplementation during pregnancy improved outcomes for either the mothers or babies (27). In the largest study conducted involving 24,100 women receiving supplements of vitamins C and E no reduction in the prevalence of pre-eclampsia was observed and paradoxically there was an increase in the number of low birth weight infants (28). Therefore, based on common evidence vitamin E supplementation in pregnancy cannot be recommended (23).

IRON

Iron deficiency is the most prevalent single-nutrient deficiency in the world (Administration Committee on Coordination/Subcommittee on Nutrition) (29). It is thought to affect more than 2 billion people worldwide with up to 50% of women of reproductive age being iron deficient. In some developing countries it is estimated that up to 80% of pregnant women are at risk of iron deficiency. The overall iron requirement during pregnancy is significantly increased compared to the non-pregnant state despite cessation of menstruation. Expansion of the red blood cell mass and the demands for iron of the placenta and fetus all contribute to the increased requirement for iron which may be up to three- to fourfold that in non-pregnant women, particularly in the second and third trimesters (30). Iron deficiency is considered to be present when the serum ferritin which is an indicator of available iron stores falls to less than 20 μg/L regardless of whether anaemia is present.

The consequences of iron deficiency include fatigue, reduced immune function and neurological symptoms including restless legs syndrome (RLS), idiopathic intracranial hypertension and increased risk of venous sinus thrombosis. Behavioural symptoms associated with iron deficiency include apathy, irritability, hypoactivity and altered cognitive function. Much of the research into the effects of iron deficiency on cognitive function has been carried out in infants but a few studies have investigated iron status in women of reproductive age or during pregnancy (31–33). The emotional and cognitive changes that are caused by iron deficiency during pregnancy may also continue post-partum affecting both infant development and mother-infant interactions (34). The consequences of maternal, and hence, fetal and neonatal, iron deficiency on the neurodevelopment of infants has been reviewed with a particular focus on the hippocampus (35).

RLS is a neurological movement disorder the aetiology of which is poorly understood (see chapter 20). Subjects with RLS have a compelling urge to move their limbs, predominantly the legs, on resting or lying down with the discomfort alleviated by moving the affected limbs or the entire body. There is often a circadian rhythm with increased symptom severity in the evening compared to the morning. An estimated 11% to 27% of pregnant women experience RLS which generally remits post-partum (36). The pathophysiology of RLS is believed to be reduced dopamine concentrations, particularly within the central nervous system (CNS). Dopamine agonists are known to alleviate RLS symptoms. RLS has been associated with iron and folate deficiency, individually or in combination (37). In a prospective trial involving pregnant women with RLS and matched pregnant controls, the serum folate and ferritin concentrations were found to be significantly lower in the RLS cohort compared to controls, although the majority of results fell within the normal reference range (38). Iron and folate are both necessary for the formation of dopamine in the CNS. Iron is required for the formation of tyrosine hydroxylase which is the rate-limiting enzyme in the production of L-dopa which is then decarboxylated to dopamine in the substantia nigra. Folate, in its active form 5-methyltetrahydrofolate, is also required for the formation of tetrahydrobiopterin which itself is a cofactor in the formation of tyrosine hydroxylase. Iron supplementation has been shown to help reduce the symptoms of RLS in end-stage renal disease patients with RLS (39). It would seem prudent to exclude and correct iron deficiency in pregnant women with RLS.

VITAMIN D

Vitamin D is a steroid hormone primarily involved in the regulation of the body's calcium and phosphate metabolism and bone mineralisation. The major circulating form is 25-hydroxycholecalciferol (25-OHVitD) obtained either from the diet or by conversion of 7-dehydrocholesterol in the skin following exposure to UV light. Conversion to the active form takes place in the kidney by further hydroxylation to 1α-25-dihydroxycholecalciferol. Whilst the role of vitamin D in bone metabolism is well known with deficiency leading to osteopaenia and osteomalacia, recent interest has focused on potential roles in the immune system and the brain (40). The relationship between vitamin D and multiple sclerosis is discussed in another chapter (see chapter 21). The detection of the vitamin D receptor and enzymes involved in hydroxylation of vitamin D in the brain suggests a possible role for this hormone in brain development and cognitive function (41).

Vitamin D deficiency in pregnancy has been associated with decreased birth weight and pre-eclampsia.

In recent years, the definition of vitamin D deficiency based on measurement of serum 25-OHVitD has been the subject of much debate. The conventionally accepted definition of a serum 25-OHVitD less than 25 nmol/L (10 µg/L) has been challenged with a variety of alternative cut-offs as high as 75 nmol/L (30 µg/L) being proposed. The general view now is that a serum 25-OHVitD less than 25 nmol/L indicates frank deficiency with values between 25 and 50 nmol/L being suboptimal (42). Vitamin D concentrations are also related to the season, with concentrations being lower in winter, and ethnic origin, with darker skinned subjects tending to lower values even in areas where the level of exposure to the sun is high.

Whilst human and animal studies strongly suggest that vitamin D is involved in brain development, a clear link has yet to be proven. Despite this, it would seem prudent to ensure pregnant or lactating women are vitamin D replete [serum 25-OHVitD > 20 µg/L (50 nmol/L)] and supplementation (1000–2000 IU/day) should be given to women with suboptimal vitamin D status.

The NICE guidelines for antenatal care in 2008 recommended informing women of the importance of maintaining adequate vitamin D stores in those at greatest risk of vitamin D deficiency. These include women of South Asian, African, Caribbean or Middle Eastern origin, women who have limited exposure to sunlight, women who eat a diet particularly low in vitamin D and women with a prepregnancy body mass index above 30 kg/m^2. These women may choose to take vitamin D at a rate of 10 µg/day (15,23). The evidence base for these recommendations is not strong and further research is needed in this area (23).

IODINE

Iodine is an essential mineral for normal thyroid function, mammary gland development and neurological development in the fetus and infant. In the thyroid gland iodine is incorporated into the thyroid hormones triiodothyronine (T3) and thyroxine (T4). Iodine deficiency can result in hypothyroidism with low serum thyroxine, elevated thyroid-stimulating hormone (TSH) and potentially thyroid enlargement (goitre). Frank iodine deficiency is primarily confined to the developing world; however, there is evidence that some countries in Europe and some parts of the United States are marginal in iodine status. The U.S. recommended daily intake (RDI) for iodine is 220 µg in pregnancy and 270 µg in lactation. The National Health and Nutrition Survey (NHANES) in 2001 to 2002 suggested that 36% of women of childbearing age in the United States had inadequate dietary iodine intake based on urine iodine excretion of less than 100 µg/L, with 15% having urine iodine concentrations less than 50 µg/L, at which point thyroid hormone secretion is impaired (43). Mild hypothyroidism secondary to iodine deficiency in pregnant women has been associated with cognitive deficits in their offspring (44). Hearing loss, brain damage and myelination disorders can also occur due to fetal or perinatal hypothyroidism. Maternal iodine deficiency severe enough to result in overt hypothyroidism can lead to gestational hypertension, spontaneous first-trimester abortion and stillbirth (45).

Selenium is a cofactor in the formation of deiodinase selenoenzymes and essential to maintain normal thyroid function. Coexisting iodine and selenium deficiency can exacerbate the development of hypothyroidism. If iodide supplementation is being given then selenium supplements may also be necessary to avoid potential thyroid damage in selenium deficient women (46).

CONCLUSIONS

The association of deficiencies in the B vitamins thiamine, folate and B12, vitamin D, iron and iodine with neurological symptoms in the mother or fetus have been described in this chapter. The potential for a nutritional deficiency should be considered particularly if the mother has a poor diet or other risk factors, investigated using the laboratory tests indicated and supplementation given as appropriate.

REFERENCES

1. Omer SM, Al Kawi MZ, Al Watban J, et al. Acute Wernicke's encephalopathy associated with hyperemesis gravidarum: magnetic resonance imaging findings. J Neuroimaging 1995; 5:251–253.
2. Otsuka F, Tada K, Ogura T, et al. Gestational thyrotoxicosis manifesting as Wernicke's encephalopathy: a case report. Endocrin J 1997; 44:447–452.
3. Gárdián G, Vörös E, Járdánházy T, et al. Wernicke's encephalopathy induced by hyperemesis gravidarum. Acta Neurol Scand 1999; 99:196–198.
4. Togay-Isikay C, Yigit A, Mutluer N. Wernicke's encephalopathy due to hyperemesis gravidarum: an under-recognised condition. Aust N Z J Obstet Gynaecol 2001; 41:453–456.
5. Chiossi G, Neri I, Cavazzuti M, et al. Hyperemesis gravidarum complicated by Wernicke encephalopathy: background, case report, and review of the literature. Obstet Gynecol Surv 2006; 61:255–268.
6. Indraccolo U, Gentile G, Pomili G, et al. Thiamine deficiency and beriberi features in a patient with hyperemesis gravidarum. Nutrition 2005; 21:967–968.
7. Report on Confidential Enquiries into Maternal Deaths in the United Kingdom 1991-1993. London: Stationary Office, 1996.
8. Bakker SJ, ter Maaten JC, Gans RO. Thiamine supplementation to prevent induction of low birth weight by conventional therapy for gestational diabetes mellitus. Med Hypotheses 2000; 55:88–90.
9. Royal College of Obstetricians and Gynaecologists. Scientific advisory committee opinion paper 16. Vitamin supplementation in pregnancy, 2009.
10. Linnebank M, Moskau S, Semmler A, et al. Antiepileptic drugs interact with folate and vitamin B12 serum levels. Ann Neurol 2011; 69:352–359.
11. Heby O. DNA methylation and polyamines in embryonic development and cancer. Int J Dev Biol 1995; 39:737–757.
12. Milunsky A, Jick H, Jick SS, et al. Multivitamin/folic acid supplementation in early pregnancy reduces the prevalence of neural tube defects. J Am Med Assoc 1989; 262:2847–2852.
13. Kalter H. Folic acid and human malformations: a summary and evaluation. Reprod Toxicol 2000; 14:463–476.
14. Botto LD, Yang QH. 5,10-methylenetetrahydrofolate reductase gene variants and congenital anomalies: a HuGE review. Am J Epidemiol 2000; 151:862–877.
15. National Institute for Clinical Excellence (NICE) CG62. Antenatal care: routine care for the healthy pregnant woman, 2008.
16. Cikot RJLM, Steegers-Theunissen RPM, et al. Longitudinal vitamin and homocysteine levels in normal pregnancy. Br J Nutr 2001; 85:49–58.
17. Herrmann W. The importance of hyperhomocysteinemia as a risk factor for diseases: an overview. Clin Chem Lab Med 2001; 39:666–674.
18. Herrmann W, Knapp JP. Hyperhomocysteinemia: a new risk factor for degenerative diseases. Clin Lab 2002; 48:471–481.
19. Steen MT, Boddie AM, Fisher AJ, et al. Neural-tube defects are associated with low concentrations of cobalamin (vitamin B12) in amniotic fluid. Prenat Diagn 1998; 18:545–555.
20. Monson ALB, Bjørke Monson AL, Ueland PM, et al. Determinants of cobalamin status in newborns. Paediatrics 2001; 108:624–630.

21. Dror DK, Allen LH. Effect of vitamin B12 deficiency on neurodevelopment in infants: current knowledge and possible mechanisms. Nutr Rev 2008; 66:250–255.

22. Korenke GC, Hunneman DH, Eber S, et al. Severe encephalopathy with epilepsy in an infant caused by subclinical maternal pernicious anaemia: case report and review of the literature. Eur J Pediatr 2004; 163:196–201.

23. RCOG scientific advisory paper 16. Vitamin supplementation in pregnancy, August 2009.

24. Roberts DCK. Vitamin E. In: Truswell AS, Dreosti IE, English RM, et al. eds. Recommended Nutrient Intakes, Australian Papers. Sydney: Australian Professional Publications, 1990:158–173.

25. Di Donato I, Bianchi S, Federico A. Ataxia with vitamin E deficiency: update of molecular diagnosis. Neurol Sci 2010; 31:511–515.

26. Gagne A, Wei SQ, Fraser WD, et al. Absorption, transport and bioavailability of vitamin E and its role in pregnant women. J Obstet Gynaecol Can 2008; 31:210–217.

27. Rumbold A, Crowther CA. Vitamin E supplementation in pregnancy. Cochrane Database Syst Rev 2005; (2): Art No.: CD004069. DOI: 10.1002/14651858.CD004069.pub2.

28. Poston L, Briley AL, Seed PT, et al. Vitamin C and E in pregnant women at risk for pre-eclampsia (VIP trial): randomised placebo-controlled trial. Lancet 2006; 367:1145–1154.

29. Administration Committee on Coordination, Subcommittee on Nutrition. Fourth Report on the World Nutrition Situation. Geneva, Switzerland: ACC/SCN, 2000.

30. Bothwell TH. Iron requirements in pregnancy and strategies to meet them. Am J Clin Nutr 2000; 72(suppl):257S–264S.

31. Murray-Kolb LE, Beard JL. Iron treatment normalizes cognition function in young adult women. Am J Clin Nutr 2007; 85:778–787.

32. Groner JA, Holtzman NA, Charney E, et al. A randomized trial of oral iron on tests of short-term memory and attention span in young pregnant women. J Adolesc Health Care 1986; 7:44–48.

33. Beard JL, Hendricks MK, Perez EM, et al. Maternal iron deficiency anaemia affects postpartum emotions and cognition. J Nutr 2005; 135:267–272.

34. Perez EM, Hendricks M, Beard JL, et al. Mother-infant interactions, and infant development are altered by maternal iron deficiency anaemia. J Nutr 2005; 135:850–855.

35. Georgieff MK. The role of iron in neurodevelopment: fetal iron deficiency and the developing hippocampus. Biochem Soc Trans 2008; 36:1267–1271.

36. Manconi M, Giovani V, De Vito A, et al. Pregnancy as a risk factor for restless legs syndrome. Sleep Med 2004; 5:305–308.

37. Patrick L. Restless legs syndrome: pathophysiology and the role of iron and folate. Alter Med Rev 2007; 12:101–122.

38. Lee KA, Zaffke ME, Baralte-Beebe K. Restless legs syndrome and sleep disturbance during pregnancy: the role of folate and iron. J Womens Health Gend Based Med 2001; 10:335–341.

39. Earley CJ, Heckler D, Allen RP. Repeated intravenous doses of iron provides effective supplemental treatment of restless legs syndrome. Sleep Med 2005; 6:301–305.

40. McCann JC, Ames BN. Is there convincing biological or behavioural evidence linking vitamin D deficiency to brain dysfunction? FASEB J 2008; 22:982–1001.

41. Buell JS, Dawson-Hughes B. Vitamin D and neurocognitive dysfunction: preventing "D"ecline. Mol Aspects Med 2008; 29:415–422.

42. Hollis BW, Wagner CL. Assessment of dietary vitamin D requirements during pregnancy and lactation. Am J Clin Nutr 2004; 79:717–726.

43. Caldwell KL, Jones R, Hollowell JG. Urinary iodine concentration: United States National Health and Nutrition Examination Survey 2001-2002. Thyroid 2005; 15:692–699.

44. Haddow JE, Palomaki GE, Allan WC, et al. Maternal thyroid deficiency during pregnancy and subsequent neurophysiological development of the child. N Engl J Med 1999; 341:549–555.

45. Dunn JT, Delange F. Damaged reproduction: the most important consequence of iodine deficiency. J Clin Endoc Metab 2001; 86:2360–2363.

46. Zimmerman MB, Kohrle J. The impact of iron and selenium deficiencies on iodine and thyroid metabolism biochemistry and relevance to public health. Thyroid 2002; 12:867–878.

23

Spinal disease and pregnancy

Matthew Crocker and Nicholas Thomas

INTRODUCTION

Spinal pathology is an area that often provokes great anxiety in both patients and the professionals managing them. This relates to sub-specialty nature of spinal expertise within orthopaedic and neurological surgery which means many other surgical and medical disciplines are unaware of the exact implications of particular pathologies, ranging from low back pain to catastrophic spinal cord injury, with the attendant disability and psychological implications.

Pregnancy poses specific challenges when dealing with spinal disease. There may be a concern about exacerbating a pre-existing condition such as back pain or sciatica, or that the pre-existing condition alters the management of the pregnant mother, particularly during childbirth with respect to the type of delivery and the safety of epidural or spinal anaesthesia.

There are also some conditions that initially manifest, either by coincidence or association, during a pregnancy. Most of the common problems may be managed safely with a basic understanding of the underlying condition and the difficulties posed. In this chapter, we discuss the common and unusual spinal disorders impacting on pregnancy and childbirth, and consider the evidence and rationale for proposed management strategies.

LOW BACK PAIN

Low back pain is one of the most common reasons for medical consultation in the developed world, and represents a vast socioeconomic problem. It is frequently encountered in the context of pregnancy, either as an exacerbation of a pre-existing problem or de novo [1].

It is important to appreciate the basic biomechanics of the lumbar spine. Movement between lumbar vertebrae is primarily governed by the intervertebral disc, which allows pivoting of the adjacent endplates about its centre, whilst transferring vertical load between segments. This motion is in turn governed by the facet joints: paired planar synovial joints of the posterior elements. There are a range of ligaments supporting the spine between segments, and paraspinal muscles that stabilise and extend the spine, with flexion subserved primarily by the anterior abdominal wall musculature.

Low back pain has a multiplicity of underlying causes relating to muscular and ligamentous dysfunction, bony, facet joint and capsular pathology and disc degeneration. These changes may be seen in the context of normal or abnormal spinal alignment (scoliosis, kyphosis, exaggerated lordosis or spondylolisthesis). The vast majority of patients with low back pain suffer a relapsing and remitting course and are managed with a variety of conservative approaches based on lifestyle modification (cessation of smoking, weight reduction and exercise), analgesia and core muscle stabilisation exercises. Relatively few patients come to the attention of chronic pain services or spinal surgery. The surgical management of low back pain remains contentious and good-quality randomised data for most low back pain treatment strategies are not available.

There is clear evidence that women with pre-existing low back pain are at risk of exacerbation during pregnancy [2–4]. A number of causative factors are likely, including hormonally mediated pelvic and lumbar ligamentous laxity [5]. Any pre-existing spondylolisthesis or instability is particularly likely to be exacerbated with resultant pain (Fig. 23.1).

A second factor increasing the likelihood of low back pain is that most women will gain weight during the course of a pregnancy. Whilst obesity itself is considered a predisposing factor to mechanical low back pain, the particular distribution of the weight gain in pregnancy, as a consequence of uterine and fetal enlargement, results in an increase in the lumbar lordosis, with shortening of the interspinous ligaments and potentially additional stress placed upon the facet joints.

In addition, there are enforced lifestyle changes during the latter stages of pregnancy such as reduced physical activity that may interfere with the physical coping strategies developed by a long-standing sufferer of low back pain. The resultant muscular deconditioning may lead to an exacerbation of low back pain.

Treatment includes exercise, especially in the earlier stages of pregnancy when this is easiest which serves not only to reduce any excessive weight gain but also to promote muscular conditioning [6].

Sufferers of low back pain in pregnancy should be encouraged by the finding that the majority of low back pain exacerbations during pregnancy will improve following delivery. The number of sufferers experiencing a permanent worsening of their symptoms as a consequence of their pregnancy probably is lower than 10% [2].

SCIATICA

Sciatica is a radicular pain syndrome, typically related to pathology affecting one or more of the roots contributing to the sciatica nerve. L5 and S1 are the most commonly affected roots, hence most sciatica pain is felt below the knee, either anterolaterally or posteriorly. Radicular syndromes typically involve pain at the earlier stages, with sensory and subsequently motor impairment being later features. Radicular syndromes of the higher lumbar roots may cause more proximal symptoms including thigh pain or sensory disturbance, and weakness of knee extension. Disc degeneration is a multifactorial process associated with long periods of driving vehicles, and tall stature, and has been proposed as associated with many other factors although none are conclusively proven [7]. There may be risk factors associated with collagen type IX polymorphisms [8].

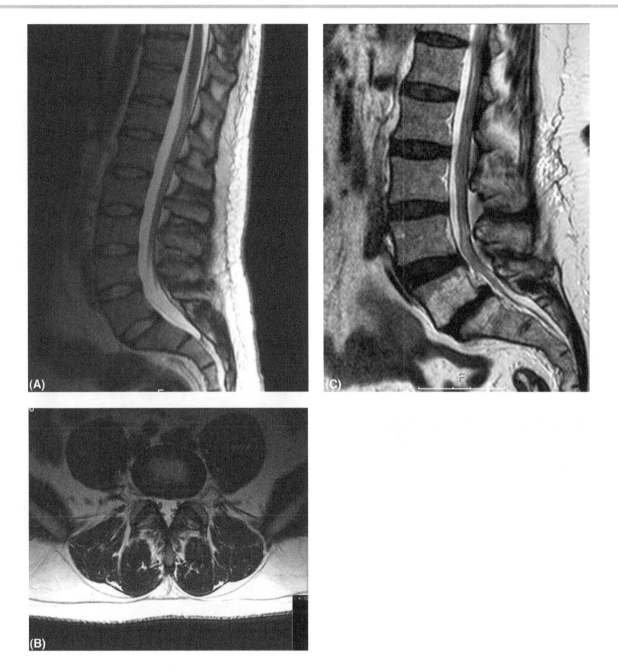

Figure 23.1 (**A**) Normal sagittal and (**B**) axial T2-weighted MRI of lumbar spine. (**C**) T2 sagittal MRI showing L5/S1 spondylolisthesis with associated L5/S1 disc degeneration and vertebral body endplate changes.

The most common cause of sciatica in or out of pregnancy is a posterolateral disc prolapse at one of the two lower lumbar disc levels, L4/5 and L5/S1 (Fig. 23.2). The management of sciatica due to disc prolapse may therefore be considered the same in pregnancy as at other times, modified by the few pregnancy-specific conditions that may also cause sciatica.

Patients with sciatica relating to a disc prolapse should be reassured that an acute episode of sciatica usually resolves with conservative treatment. Even radiologically large disc protrusions may settle with conservative management (Fig. 23.3). Gentle activity within the limits of discomfort in the initial period can be followed by increased mobilisation with simple analgesia and physiotherapy advice.

Surgery should be reserved for patients with pain refractory to conservative treatment after 6 weeks, those with a progressive neurological deficit, usually motor, and for patients with partial or complete cauda equina syndrome, where surgery may reduce the chances of a permanent neurological deficit. Cauda equina syndrome most commonly occurs due to central disc prolapse at L4/5 or L5/S1. It is characterised by severe low back pain, bilateral sciatica, sensorimotor loss in the L5 and/or S1 distributions (shin, calf, buttock; weakness of ankle dorsi- or plantarflexion) and

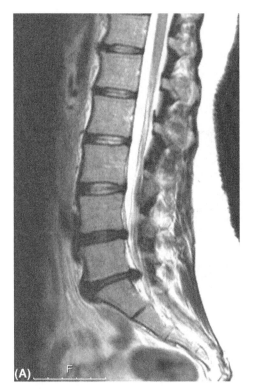

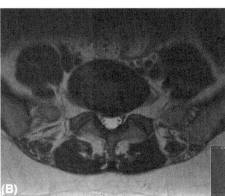

Figure 23.2 (**A**) T2 sagittal MRI showing degenerate disc disease at L4/5 and L5/S1 with disc prolapse at L5/S1. (**B**) Axial T2 sequence showing posterolateral disc protrusion accounting for right S1 distribution sciatic.

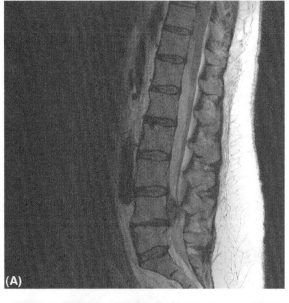

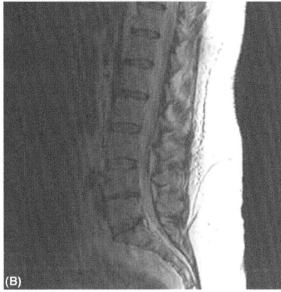

Figure 23.3 (**A**) T2 sagittal MRI showing massive posteriorly extruded disc fragment from L4/5 disc extending rostrally behind body of L4 vertebra with associated effacement of epidural space and CSF in a pregnant patient with minimal symptoms of nerve root compression (pain and mild sensory loss only). (**B**) T2 sagittal MRI of the same patient 6 months later after conservative treatment showing near complete radiological resolution of disc prolapse.

perineal sensory loss with painless urinary retention, or hesitancy in the earlier stages. As a syndrome, some features are not invariably present although perineal sensory loss and sphincter disturbance are key. Treatment is expeditious surgical discectomy after imaging confirms the clinical diagnosis. Whilst there remains some debate about the timing of surgery in a patient with cauda equina syndrome, it is clear that expeditious neural decompression before a full-blown deficit of insensate urinary incontinence, faecal incontinence and perineal sensory loss carries the best chance of avoiding a permanent neurological deficit (9). All such patients should undergo MRI to confirm the diagnosis (Fig. 23.4). The safety of MRI scanning in pregnancy is considered elsewhere in this book, but clearly in a patient with suspected cauda equina syndrome the putative risks are surpassed by clinical need.

A pregnant patient poses special challenges for the spinal surgeon. The prone position, particularly in late pregnancy, requires great care to avoid undue abdominal pressure, and venous engorgement even with optimal positioning may result in less desirable operative conditions. A higher threshold than usual for surgical intervention for disc prolapse should therefore be maintained with the pregnant patient.

Should the patient's pain be refractory to conventional analgesics, more aggressive use may be made of non-surgical interventions to offer temporary relief of symptoms. This

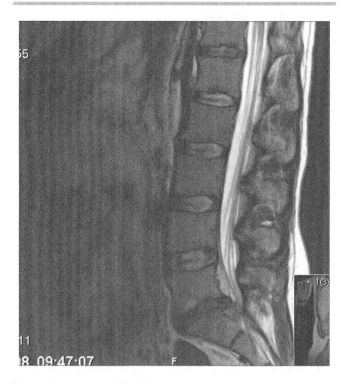

Figure 23.4 Sagittal T2 MRI of a patient at 30 weeks' gestation presenting with cauda equina syndrome, showing large disc prolapse causing severe cauda equina compression at L5/S1. The fetus is clearly demonstrated anterior to the lumbar spine despite motion artefact.

may involve the use of radiologically guided injections, although X ray and CT-guided procedures are relatively contraindicated in pregnancy. Ultrasound guidance is less commonly used but ideally suited to this purpose with comparable targeting results. There is strong evidence to support caudal epidural steroid injections which may be performed 'freehand', for pregnant patients who have severe exacerbations of low back pain or sciatica. This may allow a delay in definitive intervention until after delivery if symptoms persist (10).

As symptoms of sciatica are typically exacerbated by straining and coughing, there may be a concern that valsalva manoeuvres during pushing in labour will worsen disc prolapse and the attendant neurological problems. There are no clear data to suggest that there is a significant chance of a normal vaginal delivery resulting in a rapidly increasing size disc herniation and subsequent cauda equina syndrome. However information about this problem is sparse. In a case series of five women with confirmed lumbar disc prolapse (out of 48,760 consecutive deliveries) all five women were delivered by caesarean because of this concern (11). Despite the lack of evidence to inform such concerns, the marked inconvenience of severe sciatica, and concerns about its exacerbation during childbirth, and the implications for the woman in the post-natal period seem to have resulted in a cautious approach resulting in a trend towards caesarean section in such patients. Whether the mobility restrictions inevitable after a caesarean section are acceptable to avoid the clearly small risks of exacerbation of sciatica following vaginal delivery is in the authors' opinions questionable.

Should cauda equina syndrome due to disc prolapse occur during pregnancy, it must be treated urgently. In later pregnancy, this may involve an unscheduled caesarean section followed directly by lumbar discectomy in the prone position, under the same anaesthetic (12). If the pregnancy is not to be delivered prior to discectomy, utmost care must be taken with positioning of the patient as will be discussed later.

There are several reports of pregnant patients with typical sciatica symptoms as a consequence of epidural venous plexus engorgement (13). This has been seen in association with advanced pregnancy, as well as with inferior vena cava thrombosis and malignancy. The diagnosis is established on MRI. If found in combination with deep vein thrombosis, treatment must include low–molecular weight heparin. The symptoms usually improve after delivery. Neurological deficit as a consequence of epidural venous dilatation is reported, but is exceptionally rare (14).

SPINAL CORD INJURY IN PREGNANCY

Trauma accounts for 15% of non-obstetric maternal deaths, and 15% of spinal cord injuries (SCIs) occur in women of reproductive age, so the correct management of the pregnant patient with SCI is important (15). It falls into two main categories: the acutely injured patient already pregnant and the patient with long-standing SCI who wishes to become pregnant or is pregnant.

Patients with acute SCI are frequently multiply injured. Priority must be given to stabilising the spine in order to prevent the development or the exacerbation of a neurological injury, and also to the management of the attendant physiological disturbances due to the injury.

The unstable cervical spine is conventionally immobilised in anatomical alignment, either by the use of a cervical spine collar with head blocks or manually during the immediate resuscitation phase. Use of external supports to immobilise the thoracic or lumbar spine is rarely possible and hence such patients are maintained on flat bed rest, and turned passively with enough staff to maintain longitudinal alignment (log-rolling). This approach must be tailored to the gravid patient to prevent undue compression of the vena cava. Provided that anatomical alignment of the spine is maintained, the left lateral position with appropriate padding should be adequate. A cervical collar may be used in the lateral position, although clearly conventional head blocks will not be appropriate (Fig. 23.5). For thoracolumbar injuries appropriate bolsters or padding should be used. Care should be taken to ensure they do not compress or slip gradually allowing the patient's position to change.

Stabilisation of the injured spine frequently requires internal fixation, although rigid cervical external fixators ('halo' traction devices) may be employed. The timing of such stabilisation is frequently deferred for a matter of hours or days to allow physiological stabilisation of the patient.

The specific initial consequences of SCI for the pregnant patient may be severe. Autonomic dysfunction with acute SCI, or spinal shock, typically results in loss of sympathetic vasomotor tone with varying degree of bradycardia and hypotension. The correct management after exclusion of occult sources of blood loss is to ensure adequate volume replacement followed by judicious use of vasopressors. In the non-pregnant patient, the blood pressure required is simply one sufficient to maintain cerebral and renal perfusion'

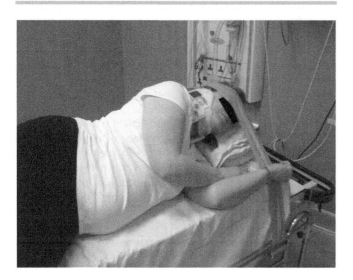

Figure 23.5 Use of a rigid cervical collar in a pregnant patient in the left lateral position for cervical spine immobilisation. The conventional blocks are not used but extensive elastoplast and padding assist immobilisation.

hence, a certain element of hypotension is permitted. In the pregnant patient, uterine perfusion and fetal oxygenation must be maintained and hence normotension or only mild hypotension should be the aim. The choice of vasopressors is a matter of debate, although noradrenaline, typically 'first line' for standard management of spinal shock, is usually avoided in pregnancy and preference is given to dobutamine or dopamine.

The nursing position of the pregnant SCI patient is important. In the later stages of pregnancy, the pelvic venous stasis provoked by the supine position makes the right lateral position preferable. This is reasonable to apply to the SCI patient, as long as spinal alignment is maintained. This will require a well-fitting cervical collar in the context of cervical or cervicothoracic injuries; for thoracolumbar injuries appropriate bolsters or padding should be used. Care should be taken to ensure they do not compress or slip gradually allowing the patient's position to change.

Pregnancy and labour in the patient with an established SCI pose other challenges (16). Vaginal delivery should be preferred where possible (16). Patients with an injury above the level of T6 will risk acute autonomic hyperreflexia as a consequence of uterine contractions: induction of labour with oxytocin may exacerbate this risk. Autonomic hyperreflexia will typically manifest as hypertension and tachycardia in such patients and is an indication for prophylactic epidural anaesthesia, despite the fact that the SCI may make the labour itself painless (16).

The delivery in the SCI patient will be more challenging by virtue of the loss of sensory feedback to the mother. The ability to bear down and push may be lost along with abdominal muscle tone as a result of the original injury. Forceps or ventouse vacuum extraction may be needed. Episiotomy should be avoided if possible in the SCI patient due to chronic atrophy of the pelvic floor. Lack of perineal sensation in these patients places them at relatively high risk of perineal dehiscence (17).

ANAESTHETIC CONSIDERATIONS IN SPINAL DISEASE

Given the high proportion of pregnant patients with suspected lumbar degenerative disease, there will inevitably be concerns over the administration of regional anaesthesia to these patients, either due to worries of an attenuated epidural space due to disc prolapse within the spinal canal or loss of intervertebral height and ligamentous thickening, making the spinal epidural space more difficult to access (18). Delivery of combined spinal/epidural anaesthesia to these patients is possible but may be challenging for anatomical reasons (19). Accurate placement, particularly of epidural catheters, requires a good understanding of the normal and abnormal anatomical variations. Of factors influencing success of epidural catheter placement, palpability of the spinous processes is the strongest predictive factor, emphasising the importance of anatomical knowledge (20).

Back pain itself without major radicular symptoms is not a contraindication to epidural anaesthesia. A routine epidural anaesthetic should not exacerbate pre-existing back pain unless there is an unusual complication such as infection or haemorrhage. The suspicion of a degenerate disc should not preclude successful passage of spinal or epidural anaesthesia. What may make epidural anaesthesia more difficult is the presence of long-standing degenerative spinal disease and associated spinal stenosis (18). In this context, the progressive thickening of the ligamentum flavum and facet joint hypertrophy combine to cause narrowing of the spinal canal (Fig. 23.6). In addition, loss of disc height results in reduction of the interlaminar space; together with calcification of the

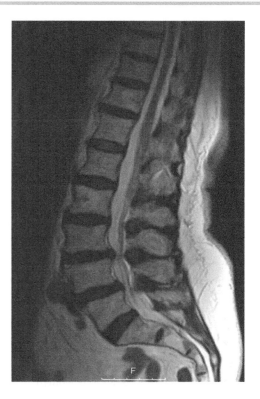

Figure 23.6 Sagittal T2 MRI showing multilevel lumbar spondylosis with loss of disc height, thickening of facet joints and ligamentum flavum and attenuation of the epidural space and CSF, causing spinal stenosis from L5 to L3.

interlaminar ligaments this may make the epidural space difficult or impossible to access. The epidural space, usually filled with fat, is obliterated first and this will increase the prospects of dural puncture or inability to pass the epidural catheter. Fortunately, spinal stenosis is generally seen in the older patient group, and is rarely seen to a significant degree clinically or radiologically in patients under the age of 50. However, a slightly older patient with a long history of low back pain and possibly leg pain or numbness on standing or walking may present a technical challenge for the obstetric anaesthetist.

Patients with back pain and sciatica will similarly make the anaesthetist cautious about spinal or epidural anaesthesia. Careful enquiry into the patient's symptoms is required. There is unlikely to be major spinal canal compromise (and hence difficulty with spinal/epidural delivery) unless there is suspicion of a large central disc prolapse. This will be suspected by a history of sciatica, possibly with a major exacerbation of back pain, with bilateral leg symptoms and possibly perineal symptoms, such as sensory or sphincter disturbance. Such patients will warrant urgent investigation of their symptoms per se either before labour if it is not imminent, or shortly afterwards.

The obstetric anaesthetist will occasionally see women who have undergone previous spinal surgery. Details of the surgery performed should be obtained and these women should be seen before they present in labour and a plan for anaesthetic management should be made (21).

Non-instrumented spinal surgery (simple laminectomy or discectomy) aims to increase the available potential space for the lumbar dura, cerebrospinal fluid (CSF) and nerve roots. As such, intradural administration of spinal anaesthesia should be straightforward. The anatomical landmarks may be lost, as part of the surgery, which may involve removal of the spinous process in the midline or the laminae laterally. The need to puncture scar tissue with the spinal needle may lead to a loss of the 'tissue feedback' that usually guides the anaesthetist. Passage of an epidural catheter in such patients may also be much harder due to scar tissue between the dura and the overlying structures. If the previous surgery was a more minimal operation such as a micro-discectomy (spinous process left intact) then scarring in the midline may be minimal and catheter passage may be routine. If the operation involved a full laminectomy (spinous process and both laminae removed), then scar tissue may make not only catheter passage difficult but also makes free flow of the anaesthetic agents past the nerve roots more problematic (Fig. 23.7).

These issues have been well reported. The largest series of 18 patients with a history of spinal surgery requesting regional anaesthesia for labour reported that half were technically difficult, but that continuous analgesia was achieved in 20 of 21 attempts (22). The commonest problem was of a patchy block, presumably reflecting uneven flow of anaesthetic past epidural scarring and adhesions.

If the previous surgery was at the level of L5/S1 or L4/5 then the level immediately above may be used. As the normal spinal cord terminates at T12/L1, moving the site of epidural insertion more rostrally than L3/4 may increase the prospects of neurological injury and is not recommended. Rarely a patient with an occult low-lying cord will present to the obstetric anaesthetist (Fig. 23.8). This may be suspected from cutaneous stigmata of an associated spina bifida, but may be completely concealed (Fig. 23.8A). The presence of

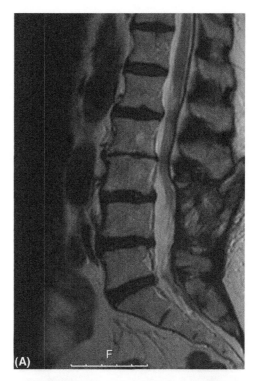

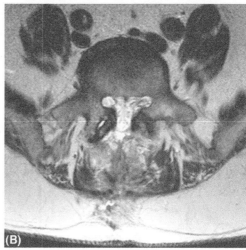

Figure 23.7 (A) Sagittal and (B) axial T2 MRI showing postoperative appearances following L3/4 and L4/5 laminectomy for spinal stenosis. The spinous process in the midline and both laminae are removed.

a typical hairy patch or sacral dimple, with or without palpable bony anatomy, should alert to underlying abnormal anatomy, encourage caution and a consideration of alternative analgesia (23).

The few patients that have undergone instrumented spinal surgery (pedicle screw fixation or stabilisation) are unlikely to cause more problems than those who have had simple decompressive surgery. The exception is the use of linkage bars from one side of the fusion construct to the other, where the passage of a spinal needle or catheter through the midline towards the dura may encounter metal resistance. Should this be found, redirection a few millimetres rostrally

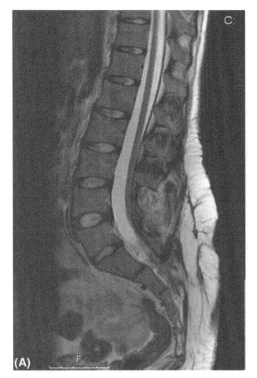

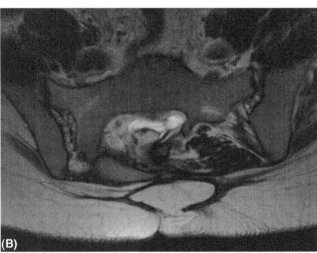

Figure 23.8 (**A**) Sagittal and (**B**) axial T2 MRI showing low-lying cord terminating opposite L5 with a sacral lipomyelomeningocoele. This is part of the spectrum of neural tube defects, or spina bifida. There is agenesis of the posterior elements (laminae and spinous processes).

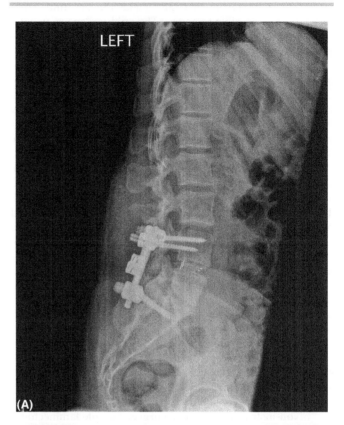

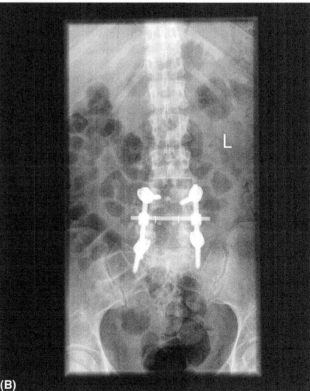

or caudally should be adequate to find the spinal or epidural space as the linkage bars are only a few millimetres wide. An antenatal X ray would show this clearly but is understandably seldom preferred in pregnancy. Post-operative X rays from the original spinal surgery may be available and should be sought (Fig. 23.9).

Failed conventional epidural anaesthesia in a patient who had previously undergone lumbar instrumentation with Harrington rods is reported (24). In this case, a caudal epidural infusion via the sacral hiatus was administered without complication and with good analgesic effects.

Figure 23.9 (**A**) Lateral and (**B**) anteroposterior X rays showing pedicle screw fixation from L4 to S1 and L4/5 interbody cages visible as radio-opaque dots (there are no L5 screws in this construct). A transverse linkage bar is seen on the AP film.

SPINAL TUMOURS IN PREGNANCY

Although the most common spinal tumours are bony metastases from an extraspinal primary malignancy, these are seldom encountered in pregnancy. More likely, but still uncommon, is the patient with an occult spinal tumour, typically benign, that presents during the pregnancy. This may be by chance, or due to hormonally mediated growth of the tumour aggravated by the pregnancy.

Tumours with known hormonal responsiveness include neurofibromata, seen sporadically, or in patients with neurofibromatosis types 1 (NF1, principally cutaneous) and 2 [NF2, marked central nervous system (CNS) involvement]. Patients with NF2 frequently have multiple spinal neurofibromata that may present with radicular or myelopathic symptoms, or may be asymptomatic (Fig. 23.10). NF2 is a clinical diagnosis and may be sporadic or familial. Dermal neurofibromata in both NF1 and NF2 are known to enlarge during pregnancy (25). A low index of suspicion of enlargement in these patients should be maintained, with repeated imaging if in doubt.

The diagnosis of NF2 is typically made around the age of 20. Therefore, the absence of a history of neurofibromatosis does not necessarily exclude the disease. Administration of spinal anaesthesia in women with NF2 is probably contra-indicated unless imaging studies (CT or MRI) have specifically excluded the likely presence of multiple spinal neurofibromata in such women (26,27). There are reports of occult intradural tumours presenting as challenging and complicated spinal anaesthetics but such cases are very rare (28).

Tumours reported as presenting with rapidly progressive neurological deficit in pregnancy include vertebral body haemangiomas. These are usually found as asymptomatic lesions on MRI in non-pregnant patients. They may rarely enlarge to cause neurological compression. The literature suggests that spinal cord compression from vertebral body haemangiomas presenting in pregnancy may be of more acute onset than in non-pregnant women (29). Surgery may be advised in these patients if there has been rapid neurological decline prior to 32 weeks' gestation. Cautious observation after 32 weeks to delivery has been recommended, in view of the fact that a stable deficit is likely to get better following surgery even if it is delayed for a short period.

Given the lack of large series of such patients a common sense view should be applied. Those tumours presenting in coincidence during pregnancy that have benign features on imaging should be managed conservatively if possible, with indications for surgery remaining as usual: progressive neurological deficit, deformity or intractable pain. There should be a higher threshold for surgery given the usual preference to perform spinal surgery in the prone position. Those tumours suspected to be developing under hormonal influence should be treated surgically only when absolutely necessary, as the expectation is that they will regress after delivery.

MISCELLANEOUS SPINAL CONDITIONS

Ankylosing spondylitis (AS) is one of the seronegative spondyloarthropathies, with a male preponderance of 3:1, associated with the HLA B27 genotype. It is characterised by progressive inflammatory calcification of the intervertebral soft tissues and ligaments and stiffness of the spine as a result (Fig. 23.11). Pathological fractures may occur, and in the end stages of the disease ventilation may be severely impaired due to reduced chest wall excursion. It is not subject to exacerbation by pregnancy (30). Neuraxial anaesthesia is very challenging in patients with AS and in a series of 81 subjects epidural anaesthesia proved impossible in all cases (31). For the parturient with AS, attention must be given during labour to positioning

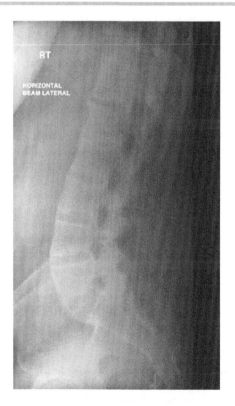

Figure 23.11 Lateral X ray of the lumbar spine of a patient with severe ankylosing spondylitis. There is severe calcification and likely associated fusion across the disc spaces and throughout the posterior elements including the laminae and facet joints.

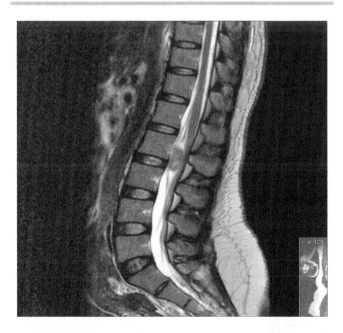

Figure 23.10 Sagittal T2 MRI showing large lumbar neurofibroma filling the spinal canal and attenuating the epidural space at L2/3.

and support of fixed deformities of the spine. Antenatal anaesthetic review is important.

Spina bifida is a congenital failure of neural tube closure which represents a spectrum of disease that may be obvious from the time of birth of the patient or completely occult throughout life (Figs. 8B and 8C). In its most severe manifestation there is complete neurological dysfunction below the level of the defect, typically including flaccid paralysis of the distal lower limbs, absent sensation and sphincter function. A patient with a previously identified defect should be routinely identified as such before labour and an alternative to neuraxial anaesthesia almost certainly sought. If there has been previous surgery in childhood to repair such a defect then regional anaesthesia in this level may be difficult and preference may be for general anaesthesia and caesarean section delivery, although the epidural technique may still be tried and used successfully (32).

POSITIONING THE PREGNANT PATIENT FOR SPINAL SURGERY

Should spinal surgery be indicated during the later stages of pregnancy, consideration to positioning of the patient is important. Conventional spinal surgery is typically performed in the prone position with a variety of padding options to support the torso. These typically have a longitudinal central defect to prevent abdominal compression. This is most important during prone positioning of the pregnant patient. The amount of cushioning material provided should be sufficient that it does not gradually compress and reduce the support provided during the surgery. A report of 10 pregnant patients undergoing spinal surgery recommended the prone position in the first trimester, and the left lateral decubitus positions for second and third trimester, to avoid vena cava compression (33).

This recommendation requires a rare familiarity with spinal surgery in the lateral position (Fig. 23.12). Prone position surgery requires continuous fetal monitoring given the concerns over abdominal pressure. Should the surgeon be familiar with surgery in the lateral position, this may be appropriate; however, the prone position will be almost universally preferred (Fig. 23.13). In this case as has been discussed, pressure on the abdomen must be at an absolute minimum to prevent venous stasis and consequent intraoperative venous bleeding, as well as for the well-being of the fetus (34).

Spinal surgery is occasionally performed under local anaesthetic in the lateral position, but such operations are typically confined to more simple decompressive surgery rather than microscopic or instrumented spinal surgery, and it is unlikely that they would be appropriate for the surgery that might be needed in a woman of childbearing age.

SPINAL COMPLICATIONS OF ANAESTHESIA

Spinal complications of regional anaesthesia are undoubtedly unusual but are always discussed as part of the counselling prior to administration. The common risk of epidural/spinal anaesthesia is persistent dural puncture headache. Less common complications include infection and risk of spinal epidural or subdural haematoma (35,36). The patient with preexisting spinal pathology should be informed that the risks are probably increased by the premorbid condition, but this increase cannot be quantified exactly because of the lack of epidemiological data in such patients. However, it is appropriate to quote an increased risk of persistent low-pressure

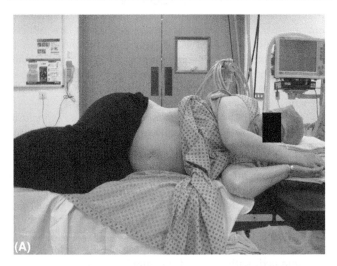

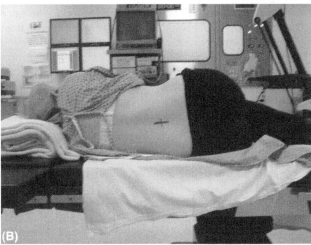

Figure 23.12   (A, B) Positioning of the pregnant patient in the left lateral position for spinal surgery.

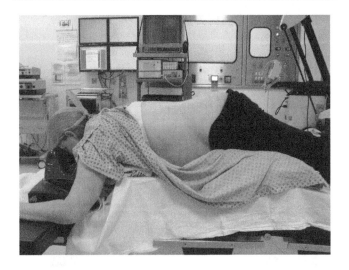

Figure 23.13   Positioning of the pregnant patient prone on the Montreal mattress with appropriate chest and pelvic padding to minimise abdominal compression.

headaches in patients that have undergone previous lumbar surgery on account of the presence of scar tissue, and similarly a much higher incidence of both failure to pass an epidural catheter and inadequate block in patients who have undergone previous surgery in this region.

ACKNOWLEDGEMENTS
Drs Jackie Harvey and Philip Rich for assistance with figures.

REFERENCES

1. Mogren IM, Pohjanen AI. Low back pain and pelvic pain during pregnancy: prevalence and risk factors. Spine 2005; 30(8):983–991.
2. Kristiansson P, Svärdsudd K, von Schoultz B. Back pain during pregnancy: a prospective study. Spine 1996; 21(6):702–709.
3. Wang SM, Dezinno P, Maranets I, et al. Low back pain during pregnancy: prevalence, risk factors, and outcomes. Obstet Gynecol 2004; 104(1):65–70.
4. Padua L, Caliandro P, Aprile I, et al. Back pain in pregnancy: 1-year follow-up of untreated cases. Eur Spine J 2005; 14(2):151–154.
5. Chan YL, Lam WW, Lau TK, et al. Back pain in pregnancy: magnetic resonance imaging correlation. Clin Radiol 2002; 57 (12):1109–1112.
6. Ostgaard HC, Zetherström G, Roos-Hansson E. Back pain in relation to pregnancy: a 6-year follow-up. Spine 1997; 22(24):2945–2950.
7. Leclerc A, Tubach F, Landre MF, et al. Personal and occupational predictors of sciatica in the GAZEL cohort. Occup Med (Lond) 2003; 53(6):384–391.
8. Ala-Kokko L. Genetic risk factors for lumbar disc disease. Ann Med 2002; 34(1):42–47.
9. DeLong WB, Polissar N, Neradilek B. Timing of surgery in cauda equina syndrome with urinary retention: meta-analysis of observational studies. J Neurosurg Spine 2008; 8(4):305–320.
10. Boswell MV, Shah RV, Everett CR, et al. Interventional techniques in the management of chronic spinal pain: evidence-based practice guidelines. Pain Physician 2005; 8(1):1–47.
11. LaBan MM, Perrin JC, Latimer FR. Pregnancy and the herniated lumbar disc. Arch Phys Med Rehabil 1983; 64(7):319–321.
12. Al-Areibi A, Coveney L, Singh S, et al. Case report: anesthetic management for sequential cesarean delivery and laminectomy. Can J Anaesth 2007; 54(6):471–474.
13. Paksoy Y, Gormus N. Epidural venous plexus enlargements presenting with radiculopathy and back pain in patients with inferior vena cava obstruction or occlusion. Spine 2004; 29(21):2419–2424.
14. Pennekamp PH, Gemünd M, Kraft CN, et al. Epidural varicosis as a rare cause of acute radiculopathy with complete foot paresis – case report and literature review. Z Orthop Ihre Grenzgeb 2007; 145(1):55–60.
15. Gilson GJ, Miller AC, Clevenger FW, et al. Acute spinal cord injury and neurogenic shock in pregnancy. Obstet Gynecol Surv 1995; 50(7):556–560.
16. Charlifue SW, Gerhart KA, Menter RR, et al. Sexual issues of women with spinal cord injuries. Paraplegia 1992; 30(3):192–199.
17. Verduyn WH. Pregnancy and delivery in tetraplegic women. J Spinal Cord Med 1997; 20(3):371–374.
18. Vercauteren M, Heytens L. Anaesthetic considerations for patients with a pre-existing neurological deficit: are neuraxial techniques safe? Acta Anaesthesiol Scand 2007; 51(7):831–838.
19. Kuczkowski KM, Zuniga G. Obstetric anesthesia and previous back surgery: an issue? Or not? Rev Esp Anestesiol Reanim 2007; 54(10):632–633.
20. Palencia M, Guasch E, Navas D, et al. Difficulty of epidural puncture for obstetric analgesia: risk factors. Rev Esp Anestesiol Reanim 2006; 53(3):139–144.
21. Fernández Torres B, Fontán Atalaya IM, López Millán JM, et al. Obstetric analgesia for a patient with a history of 3 previous operations on the spine. Rev Esp Anestesiol Reanim 2006; 53(7):446–449.
22. Daley MD, Rolbin SH, Hew EM, et al. Epidural anesthesia for obstetrics after spinal surgery. Reg Anesth 1990; 15(6):280–284.
23. Ahmad FU, Pandey P, Sharma BS, et al. Foot drop after spinal anesthesia in a patient with a low-lying cord. Int J Obstet Anesth 2006; 15(3):233–236.
24. Moeller-Bertram T, Kuczkowski KM, Ahadian F. Labor analgesia in a parturient with prior Harrington rod instrumentation: is caudal epidural an option? Ann Fr Anesth Reanim 2004; 23(9):925–926.
25. Roth TM, Petty EM, Barald KF. The role of steroid hormones in the NF1 phenotype: focus on pregnancy. Am J Med Genet A 2008; 146A(12):1624–1633.
26. Sakai T, Vallejo MC, Shannon KT. A parturient with neurofibromatosis type 2: anesthetic and obstetric considerations for delivery. Int J Obstet Anesth 2005; 14:332–335.
27. Dounas M, Mercier FJ, Lhuissier C, et al. Epidural analgesia for labour in a parturient with neurofibromatosis. Can J Anaesth 1995; 42(5 pt 1):420–422; discussion 422–424.
28. Jaeger M, Rickels E, Schmidt A, et al. Lumbar ependymoma presenting with paraplegia following attempted spinal anaesthesia. Br J Anaesth 2002; 88(3):438–440.
29. Chi JH, Manley GT, Chou D. Pregnancy-related vertebral hemangioma. Case report, review of the literature, and management algorithm. Neurosurg Focus 2005; 19(3):E7.
30. Gromnica-Ihle E, Ostensen M. Pregnancy in patients with rheumatoid arthritis and inflammatory spondylarthropathies. Z Rheumatol 2006; 65(3):209–212, 214–216.
31. Schelew BL, Vaghadia H. Ankylosing spondylitis and neuraxial anaesthesia – a 10 year review. Can J Anaesth 1996; 43(1):65–68.
32. Altamimi Y, Pavy TJ. Epidural analgesia for labour in a patient with a neural tube defect. Anaesth Intensive Care 2006; 34(6): 816–819.
33. Han IH, Kuh SU, Kim JH, et al. Clinical approach and surgical strategy for spinal diseases in pregnant women: a report of ten cases. Spine 2008; 33(17):E614–E619.
34. Brown MD, Levi AD. Surgery for lumbar disc herniation during pregnancy. Spine 2001; 26(4):440–443.
35. Lao TT, Halpern SH, MacDonald D, et al. Spinal subdural haematoma in a parturient after attempted epidural anaesthesia. Can J Anaesth 1993; 40(4):340–345.
36. Van de Velde M, Schepers R, Berends N, et al. Ten years of experience with accidental dural puncture and post-dural puncture headache in a tertiary obstetric anaesthesia department. Int J Obstet Anesth 2008; 17(4):329–335.

24

Neurological disability and pregnancy

David N. Rushton

INTRODUCTION

Pregnancy may be difficult to achieve in women with neurological disability. Maintenance and restoration of sexual function, of which pregnancy is a consequential part, is a goal of neurological rehabilitation (1). In practice, however, professional attention to the sexual problems of people with disabilities (and perhaps in women with disabilities in particular) is often inadequate, delayed or non-existent. When undertaken, an assessment must take sensitive account of a patient's history, personality and social setting. It may be difficult to return to a pre-existing relationship following the acquisition of physical disability. For example, following a brain injury there may be personality change, unstable mood, and fatigability. Following a spinal injury there will be a change or loss in mobility, sexual responses and sensory functions. New sexual and relationship problems may not resolve spontaneously with time, and may become entrenched and unmanageable unless addressed expertly and appropriately in a timely way.

For reasons of space and simplicity, this chapter will consider the interplay of pregnancy and establish neurological disability due to traumatic brain injury (TBI) and spinal cord injury (SCI). Some reference will also be made to multiple sclerosis (MS) as a condition which can affect both the brain and spinal cord, but this condition will be more comprehensively discussed in chapter 10.

Pregnancy and its consequences introduce stressful changes on body, mind and social setting, regardless of disability. It is therefore important if possible to ensure that any disabled person planning pregnancy has been rehabilitated as far as possible so as to minimise the possibility of physical, psychological or social decompensation and breakdown. Of course, this is not always possible because pregnancy is not always planned.

PRE-CONCEPTION CONSIDERATIONS
Medications

Women of childbearing age who are disabled are more likely to need to take medications, often multiple, in comparison with able-bodied women. Certain drugs that are commonly used by people with brain or SCI disease may be harmful at conception or in early pregnancy. Some, such as many of the anti-epileptic drugs, are known to be teratogenic, while most newer drugs are avoided if possible because of lack of adequate information about possible adverse effects. Again, some drugs should be avoided at term and during delivery, while others should be avoided while breastfeeding. Aspirant mothers are usually advised that most drugs (other than vitamin supplements and folic acid) are to be avoided while trying to conceive, unless the benefit clearly outweighs the risk. How should aspirant disabled mothers respond to this dictum?

They may be well aware of the benefits, but how are they to evaluate the risks? Many drugs are too new for the necessary long experience to have accumulated in the literature, or are not widely used by women of childbearing age.

Where there is a choice of drugs, widely used for common conditions and with well-established risks (and severe consequences if stopped), the patient should seek expert medical advice as to the safest course. This is the case for anti-epileptic drugs, although the problem there is that the newest drugs, which may theoretically have the safest profile and the fewest side effects, necessarily have the least accumulated experience. For a full discussion of the choice of anti-epileptic drugs in conception and pregnancy, see chapter 12.

Many people with severe disability, whether cerebral or spinal, suffer from significant or severe spasticity, and require antispastic medication, usually with baclofen or tizanidine, sometimes with diazepam or dantrolene in addition. When spasticity is severe and widespread, an intrathecal baclofen pump may offer the best control of spasticity. Baclofen has been associated with fetal malformations (principally impairments of ossification) in animal tests (rats and rabbits), but the threshold doses are huge (20–40 mg/kg/day) when compared with the typical human clinical dose levels for oral baclofen (0.5–2 mg/kg/day). The clinical dose range for intrathecal baclofen is far lower still (typically, 2–20 μg/kg/day). However, there are no published human studies, only the occasional case report (2–4) of its use in pregnancy.

Fertility

Following TBI or SCI, it is common for menses to cease for several months. In the absence of anterior pituitary damage, the menstrual cycle then usually recovers spontaneously. However, deficient hypothalamic/pituitary function is common following TBI (see below).

In SCI, ovulatory cycles are usually re-established within 6 to 9 months, and cyclical dysmenorrhoea is not uncommon. Basal body temperature charting may be unreliable for contraception (5). There is an ongoing increased risk of deep vein thrombosis following SCI, so women are generally advised to avoid the combined contraceptive pill. Intrauterine contraceptive devices are often avoided in women with SCI because of worsening of dysmenorrhoea, but the progestogen containing intrauterine coil may be appropriate as it reduces the heaviness and pain of periods. Depot progestogens may cause a fall in bone density so they should be used with caution in women who are immobile and are already at risk of osteoporosis.

Sexual Dysfunction

Loss or changes in libido are usual following TBI, and are often associated with other relationship and family problems (6). In TBI, the change may or may not be associated with depression, personality change, irritability, fatigue or sleep disturbance, all of which are common and may be persistent.

In SCI, libido may be affected by change in body image, sensory impairments, loss of sexual pleasure, pelvic and lower limb weakness, incontinence (and fear of incontinence), pain, loss of vaginal lubrication, uncertainty about technique, partner ignorance and fear of (AD) (also referred to as autonomic hyperreflexia). Expert counselling involving both members of the couple is often needed.

Counselling

Both SCI and TBI often are followed by major changes in medical status, lifestyle, occupation, housing, social and financial position, mood, health and self-image. Plans for a family may be changed or deferred, and the necessary adjustments may be helped by psychological counselling support. This is quite apart from specific medical advice on particular difficulties, risks and precautions around conception, pregnancy, delivery, breastfeeding and childcare in the presence of disability.

Medical, nursing and therapy advisers should be aware that a woman with established disability has a good working knowledge of her own abilities, limitations and adaptive strategies. Her immediate family members may be equally aware, and her living environment may or may not be fully adapted to her needs. If a woman who is considering pregnancy comes seeking medical advice as to the risks and procedures, it is likely that an exchange of information in both directions will be appropriate. A rigid or didactic approach is unlikely to be successful.

Decision-Making

Disabled people expect and need to be able to make their own life choices, rather than their role being defined by their medical condition or impairments. This applies in the decisions around starting a family, as much as it does in other major areas. Nevertheless, there is still a lot of prejudice and assumption in society (and in families) as to what disabled people can and cannot do, and counselling may need to address this, to enable a right decision. A 'rehabilitation' approach enables both the impairment-based difficulties and the social difficulties to be properly dealt with.

PREGNANCY AND DELIVERY
Acute Brain Injury and Persisting Vegetative State

Severe brain injury sustained during pregnancy often is followed by spontaneous miscarriage, presumably attributable to one or more of circulatory, hormonal, nutritional, metabolic or electrolyte disturbances. However, there are occasional case reports of brain injury sustained in pregnancy, resulting in persisting vegetative state but followed by spontaneous vaginal delivery at or near term (7).

The approach here is also necessarily much more medical, since the patient will not have been rehabilitated, and may not even be medically stable. The sort of circumstances which may arise are illustrated in the following example.

Patient F, aged 33, in the second trimester of her third pregnancy, suffered a basilar infarction whilst on holiday. She was airlifted home after 3 weeks, and transferred for rehabilitation. She was initially almost 'locked-in', with anarthria and tetraplegia. Once a channel of

communication was established (initially by eye movements, subsequently adding head movements), F made it clear that she wished to continue with the pregnancy, and to continue to be a mother to her family, to the best of her ability. A healthy baby was delivered by caesarian section near to term, by which time F had recovered the ability to swallow (but remained anarthric), and some movement of all four limbs. Initially her sister cared for the children during F's prolonged (over a year) period of inpatient rehabilitation, with the full involvement of other family members and social agencies.

Ten years later, F remains dysarthric and a wheelchair user, but has regained an active and successful role as mother to her family. She has since had a fourth child.

There has been a case series reported (8) detailing cerebral palsy seen in children born to women who suffered traumatic injuries (not necessarily involving the abdomen) during pregnancy. It is suggested that in such cases the fetal insult may be due to a reduction in placental blood flow secondary to maternal hypotension or fat embolism.

Post-traumatic hypopituitarism (PTHP) is not uncommon in the recovery phase following TBI (9). Mechanisms include axonal shearing, vascular damage, hypoxia, haematoma, or basal skull fracture with mechanical injury to the pituitary gland, pituitary stalk, or hypothalamus. Acute responses can be adaptive or traumatic. Pituitary-adrenal insufficiency and pituitary disturbances of fluid balance [either diabetes insipidus or inappropriate antidiuretic hormone (ADH) secretion] may threaten medical stability during the post-acute phase. Hypogonadism and hyperprolactinaemia commonly persist for 3 to 6 months following TBI.

Long-term PTHP is less common, being more often associated with more severe trauma. In the longer term, the somatotrophic and gonadotrophic axes are found to be more vulnerable to the effects of TBI than the thyrotrophic, corticotrophic and posterior pituitary axes (10). Persisting features suggesting hypogonadism in women (such as persisting amenorrhoea, loss of libido, or infertility) following TBI should therefore be investigated, particularly if pregnancy is desired. For women with long-term PTHP, hormone replacement therapy is indicated to prevent climacteric symptoms and premature bone loss, and gonadotropin treatment may be needed to achieve pregnancy.

Spinal Cord Injury or Disease

It is recommended that specialist spinal services be involved when a spinal patient is admitted to an acute hospital for any reason (11). Pregnancy and delivery should therefore be conducted in hospital, with involvement of both the obstetric and the spinal team. Most issues can then be satisfactorily handled. Many of the supposed increased risks need only awareness and appropriate preparation, for example with the provision of a suitable mattress (12).

There is an increase in the incidence of urinary tract infections and urinary incontinence during pregnancy in SCI, just as there is in the able-bodied pregnant population. Pressure sores are prevented by good nursing management, and urinary tract infections are treated when they occur. If urinary tract infections are recurrent during pregnancy then low-dose prophylactic antibiotics may be given, changing the antibiotic type every 8 weeks to avoid the development of drug resistance. Suitable antibiotics include amoxicillin, cephalexin or nitrofurantoin. Nitrofurantoin should be avoided in the last weeks of pregnancy as it is associated with fetal haemolytic anaemia if given within 2 to 3 weeks of delivery. Pregnancy in women with SCI carries an increased risk of anaemia and deep vein thrombosis. The latter can be prevented by using anti-embolism stockings and heparin or low molecular weight heparin. Increased spasticity may be a problem as the pregnancy progresses and may cause difficulty in labour. Respiratory function may be compromised in late pregnancy in women with tetraplegia or high paraplegia who rely on their diaphragm for ventilation. There may be increased difficulty with personal transfers and wheelchair mobility.

Premature delivery and pre-eclampsia are not more common in women who have pre-existing spinal disease. In contrast, blood pressure is often relatively low in women with tetraplegia or high paraplegia, and there may be a relative bradycardia. This may have been identified during the antenatal period. Identifying this as a possible reason for hypotension in labour is important to avoid fluid over-replacement and overload.

The onset of labour in women with paraplegia may be silent as the contractions will be painless, and unattended labour or unplanned delivery away from hospital is a risk. The pregnant women should be instructed that hardening of the uterus and intermittent rising of the uterus in the abdomen may represent uterine contractions. AD may signal the onset of labour.

There may be logistical difficulties in the management of labour in women with paraplegia. Delivery suites often may not be designed to take account of the needs of wheelchair users. Room arrangements for labour therefore need to be carefully planned. A patient with tetraplegia or high paraplegia is not able to push in the second stage of labour and instrumental delivery may be required.

The chief concern during labour, in women with spinal level at T6 or above, is the risk of AD. This is caused by unregulated overactivity of the isolated spinal sympathetic network, causing vasoconstriction and acute hypertension, and can be life-threatening for the mother. Symptoms can include headache, sweating, shivering, anxiety, chest tightness, visual blurring, nasal stuffiness, and pallor or gooseflesh below the lesion, with compensatory flushing above the lesion. Systolic blood pressure rises by 20 to 40 mmHg or more. If AD is severe and prolonged, it may cause cerebral haemorrhage or fatal cardiac arrythmias.

Constipation and urinary infection or retention are common causes of AD, but in pregnancy, labour is the commonest cause. For this reason, it is common to use epidural anaesthesia or caesarian section in spinal deliveries, to prevent AD from occurring. During labour, an indwelling catheter should be used and faecal impaction should be avoided. If AD occurs during labour, a prompt caesarian section is probably the safest course, unless delivery is imminent, in which case instrumental delivery may be performed. Acute hypertension in the pregnant woman can be treated with Nifedipine 10 mg orally or intravenous hydrallazine, labetalol or glyceryl trinitrate. Careful titration of anti-hypertensive agents is essential to avoid maternal hypotension and consequent fetal distress. AD during labour usually resolves after delivery, but may recur due to uterine contractions, bladder distension or constipation. Some advocate leaving an effective epidural in situ for 24 to 48 hours post-delivery (13).

INFANT AND CHILDCARE
Maternal Support
It is very difficult and exhausting for anyone to look after a baby unaided. A disabled mother needs extra consideration and help. People with TBI are often fatigable. If a disabled mother has other children, she will need regular help looking after them, so that she can focus her attention and energy on the new baby. Arranging the necessary help may be undertaken by the mother and her partner, but sometimes (particularly where disabilities are complex) it may require the skills of a case manager to organise, fund and co-ordinate the help needed from health services, social services and perhaps voluntary organisations. A case manager may also be able to arrange peer support and advice from other experienced disabled mothers, which may be extremely valuable.

Handling and Managing a Baby
A mother with hemiplegia may find a baby sling the most convenient way to carry her baby, and it may also help support the baby in position for breastfeeding. If she is a wheelchair user, a lap-belt may assist her to reach out to pick up the baby. The layout of the baby's crib, and nappy changing, needs to be wheelchair accessible. If the mother is immobile, the crib and nappy changing need to be accessible from a single location, which itself needs to position the mother so that she can hold the baby, and breastfeed if desired, using a front-opening nursing bra. These are nowadays designed to be operated one-handed. An extra pillow may help position the baby for breastfeeding.

Breastfeeding (14)
Breastfeeding is an important means of bonding for mother and baby. It is more important when a mother is less able to pick up and handle her baby. Its importance in bonding is also enhanced for the blind mother.

Breastfeeding requires less manual dexterity than bottle feeding, although it can be more time-consuming. For example, upper limb function in tetraplegia below C6 should be adequate for breastfeeding, whereas independent bottle preparation would hardly be practicable. Similarly, one-handed breastfeeding with a plegic or absent upper limb is entirely practicable with pillow support, whereas preparing a bottle feed without assistance would require special equipment.

Traumatic Brain Injury
TBI, in particular, may often cause changes in personality and behaviour such as to make childcare difficult or unsafe. There is a major increase in marital breakdown following TBI (15), and even where the couple stays together there will be changes in parental role and family finances. There may be involvement of social work agencies, and the relationship of children with the injured parent may be damaged, particularly if (as is all too common) there is an ongoing loss of emotional stability and insight (16).

REFERENCES
1. Moffat B. Sexual function. In: Greenwood R, Barnes MP, McMillan TM, et al. eds. Neurological Rehabilitation. Edinburgh, London: Churchill Livingstone, 1993:279–289.
2. Engran N, van de Perre P, Vilain D, et al. Intrathecal Baclofen for severe tetanus in a pregnant woman. Eur J Anaesthesiol 2001; 18:261–263.
3. Delhaas EM, Verhagen J. Pregnancy in a quadriplegic patient treated with continuous intrathecal baclofen infusion to manage her severe spasticity. Case report. Paraplegia 1992; 30:527–528.
4. Munoz FC, Marco DG, Perez AV, et al. Pregnancy outcome in a woman exposed to continuous intrathecal baclofen infusion. Ann Pharmcother 2000; 34:956.
5. Reame NE. A prospective study of the menstrual cycle and spinal cord injury. Am J Phys Med Rehabil 1992; 71:15–21.
6. Lezak M. Brain damage is a family affair. J Clin Exp Neuropsychol 1988; 10:111–123.

7. Ayorinde BT, Scudamore I, Buggy DJ. Anaesthetic management of a pregnant patient in a persistent vegetative state. Br J Anaesth 2000; 85:479–481.

8. Hayes B, Ryan S, Stephenson JBP, et al. Cerebral palsy after maternal trauma in pregnancy. Dev Med Child Neurol 2007; 49:700–706.

9. Bondanelli M, Ambrosio MR, Zatelli MC, et al. Hypopituitarism after traumatic brain injury. Eur J Endocrinol 2005; 152:679–691.

10. Schneider M, Schneider HJ, Stalla GK. Anterior pituitary hormone abnormalities following traumatic brain injury. J Neurotrauma 2005; 22:937–946.

11. RCP (London), BSRM, MASCIP, BASCIS (2008) Chronic Spinal Cord Injury: management of patients in acute hospital settings. National Guidelines. Report, Royal College of Physicians, London.

12. Craig DI. The adaptation to pregnancy of spinal cord injured women. Rehab Nursing 1990; 15:6–9.

13. Kobayashi A, Mizobe T, Tojo H, et al. Autonomic hyperreflexia during labour. Can J Anaesth 1995; 42(12):1134–1136.

14. Riordan J. Breastfeeding and Human Lactation. 3rd ed. Boston: Jones & Bartlett, 2005.

15. Thomsen IV. Late outcome of very severe blunt head trauma: a 10-15 year second follow-up. J Neurol Neurosurg Psychiatry 1984; 47:260–268.

16. Pessar LF, Coad ML, Linn RT, et al. The effects of parental traumatic brain injury on the behaviour of parents and children. Brain Inj 1993; 7:231–240.

25

Peripheral nerve diseases

Robert D. M. Hadden

INTRODUCTION

The commonest disorders of the peripheral nervous system in pregnancy are the mononeuropathies caused by entrapment and compression, particularly during labour (1,2). Alterations of the immune system in pregnancy put the pregnant woman at increased risk of developing rare immune-mediated neuropathies. Treatment of these and of neuropathic pain requires careful consideration of the risks and benefits of treatment. Genetic neuropathies require appropriate genetic counselling.

COMPRESSIVE MONONEUROPATHIES

Peripheral nerves may be damaged by local compression. With increasing duration and pressure this may cause neurapraxia with rapid recovery, focal demyelinating conduction block or axonal (Wallerian) degeneration with slow and incomplete recovery.

Compressive and Entrapment Neuropathy During Pregnancy

Mononeuropathies due to compression (by an external object) or entrapment (by an internal anatomical structure) are more common in pregnancy.

Carpal Tunnel Syndrome
Carpal tunnel syndrome (CTS) is entrapment of the median nerve at the wrist. Symptoms are the same as in the non-pregnant population, namely paraesthesia and pain in the hands, often not well localised to the median nerve territory, and often with no abnormality on examination. The incidence depends on the definition. Eleven to seventeen percent of pregnant women had neurophysiological evidence of CTS, but only half of these ever developed symptoms, and clinically significant CTS may occur in only 0.3% to 2% of pregnant women (3). Risk factors for CTS include age over 30, greater weight gain in pregnancy, and hand or generalised oedema.

CTS may begin at any time in pregnancy (or even commence during lactation), but usually worsens in the third trimester. Most patients improve within 2 weeks after delivery, but approximately half still have some long-term symptoms (4). Risk factors for worse recovery after delivery include onset of symptoms early in pregnancy or before pregnancy, and positive Phalen's test (provocation of symptoms by wrist flexion for a few seconds).

Cochrane systematic reviews of treatment of non-pregnant CTS concluded the following:

1. Local steroid injection is effective for at least 1 month, but is not significantly better than splinting, and a second injection provides no additional benefit (5).
2. Oral steroids, splinting, ultrasound, yoga and carpal bone mobilisation are also beneficial (6).

3. Surgery is more effective than splinting.
4. Minimally invasive CTS surgery is probably no better than standard surgery.

There are no randomised trials of treatment of CTS in pregnancy, and indeed most trials are likely to have excluded pregnant patients. A non-controlled study suggested wrist splinting improved symptoms in pregnancy (7).

An empirical treatment strategy is suggested: do not treat symptoms unless clinically troublesome to the patient. If treatment is required, first use a wrist splint in bed, then if symptoms remain give one local steroid injection, and if symptoms still remain then recommend surgery.

Lateral Cutaneous Nerve of the Thigh (Meralgia Paraesthetica)
Compression or entrapment of the lateral cutaneous nerve of the thigh is characterised by numbness, pain or tingling in the lateral thigh (meralgia paraesthetica). Symptoms do not extend below the knee or significantly medial to the anterior midline of the thigh. The knee reflex is normal and there is no motor weakness. Neurophysiology is unreliable so the diagnosis is clinical. The nerve is most frequently compressed under or within the inguinal ligament or by large tight belts or clothing. In late pregnancy this may be caused by the change in angle between nerve and inguinal ligament caused by increased lumbar lordosis and increased abdominal girth, in combination with an anatomic variant in which the nerve bisects the inguinal ligament (8). A case control study in general practice found the incidence of meralgia paraesthetica in the general population was 4.3 per 10,000 per year. It was significantly more common in pregnancy [odds ratio (OR), 12.0; 95% CI, 1.2–118.0] and in people with CTS (OR, 7.7; 95% CI, 1.9–31.1], yet these risk factors explained only 21% of cases (9). It usually requires no treatment other than reassurance and improves spontaneously following delivery. Rarely, severe cases may require treatment with topical 5% lidocaine patches, capsaicin cream 0.075%, corticosteroid/local anaesthetic injection around the nerve under the inguinal ligament, or oral medications for neuropathic pain.

Femoral nerve. There is a single report of bilateral femoral neuropathy during the third trimester (30–32 weeks, not during labour) with severe pain, but good recovery following caesarean section. Pelvic MRI was normal. The explanation for the bilateral symptoms in this case is uncertain (10).

Lumbosacral (or thoracic) root compression in pregnancy is covered in chapter 23 on spinal disease.

Compressive Neuropathy During Labour

Many different nerves have an increased risk of neuropraxia during labour. In a large prospective study, the total incidence of lower limb nerve palsies post-partum was 0.92% (8). The severity was not specified but symptoms resolved completely after a median 2 months, with only 4% having persistent symptoms (usually only occasional pain) beyond 14 months. The commonest nerve involved was the lateral cutaneous nerve of the thigh, followed by femoral nerve (motor sensory or pure sensory), and less frequently radicular symptoms (L4, L5 or S1 dermatomes) and lesions of the lumbosacral plexus, common peroneal nerve, obturator nerve and sciatic nerve. Most were unilateral except for occasional bilateral involvement of the lateral cutaneous nerve of the thigh or femoral nerve. Logistic regression showed that risk factors for nerve palsy were nulliparity and prolonged second stage of labour, particularly where involving greater time pushing in the lithotomy position with greater hip flexion. It is hypothesised that to avoid nerve palsies, women should be advised to change position frequently during prolonged pushing, avoid prolonged hip flexion/abduction/external rotation, and reduce the active pushing time by allowing the fetus to descend to the perineum and awaiting the urge to push before starting to push.

Non-pregnant patients undergoing surgical procedures in the lithotomy position are at similar risk of many of these palsies, including obturator, lateral cutaneous nerve of the thigh, sciatic and peroneal nerve palsies (11).

Epidural/spinal anaesthesia has not been shown to be a risk factor, but might be expected theoretically to prevent warning sensory symptoms of impending nerve palsy so the woman is less likely to change position, and to prolong the second stage of labour.

Investigation is usually not necessary and most patients do not require treatment other than recognition of the diagnosis, reassurance that it is not a stroke and that it will improve within a few weeks or months with a good outcome, and perhaps physiotherapy. Nerve conduction studies are recommended if there are atypical features, poor recovery, or if medico-legal action is thought to be likely.

There is no evidence as to whether elective Caesarean section should be performed for subsequent pregnancy in a woman with previous obstetric palsy. It is not generally recommended, because the risk of palsy is generally lower for subsequent deliveries, despite a theoretical risk of an underlying anatomic variant. It might be considered if the palsy was severe, or there were no easily avoidable risk factors.

Patients with hereditary neuropathy with predisposition to pressure palsies (HNPP) are theoretically at greater risk of all compression neuropathies secondary to labour, with slower recovery. Neurophysiology in HNPP usually identifies a mild generalised demyelinating neuropathy. The diagnosis may be confirmed by genetic blood test.

The specific syndromes of compressive neuropathy during labour are considered below.

Lateral Cutaneous Nerve of the Thigh (See Also Page 242)
This may be affected during labour by prolonged hip flexion, or occasionally during caesarean section by direct cutting or pressure from a retractor.

Femoral Nerve
Femoral neuropathy causes weakness of knee extension (with or without hip flexion) with reduction of the knee reflex and altered sensation in the anterior thigh and medial calf. If hip flexion is weak, the most likely mechanism of injury is prolonged hip abduction/external rotation causing stretch of the intrapelvic portion of the nerve, which has a poor blood supply and is vulnerable to stretch-induced ischaemia. If hip flexion is not weak, the nerve may have been compressed

under the inguinal ligament due to prolonged hip flexion/abduction/external rotation (8).

Footdrop
The nerve fibres which supply ankle dorsiflexion may be compressed at any of several locations, namely at the L5 root, lumbosacral plexus, sciatic nerve or common peroneal nerve. It may sometimes be difficult to distinguish these clinically. Neurophysiology may be helpful in localisation.

Lumbosacral plexus. The lumbar plexus (lumbosacral trunk) may be compressed between the fetal head or forceps and the bony pelvic brim, affecting fibres from the L4, L5 and sometimes S1 roots. This causes weakness of ankle dorsiflexion, eversion and inversion, but not plantar flexion, and sensory loss in the L5 dermatome often with pain. It is usually unilateral, on the same side as the fetal brow. Risk factors include short stature, large baby, prolonged labour and mid-forceps rotation (12).

Sciatic nerve. Sciatic nerve palsies are often incomplete and often cause more severe abnormality of the common peroneal nerve fibres than the tibial nerve component. A complete lesion would cause weakness of all movements of the ankle and knee flexion, with sensory disturbance of all areas below the knee, sparing the medial calf.

Rare sciatic nerve palsies are reported attributed to compression in the buttock due to the 30° pelvic tilt induced by a wedge placed under the contralateral buttock (to minimise aortocaval compression) during caesarean section (13).

Common peroneal nerve. A common peroneal nerve palsy causes weakness of ankle dorsiflexion and eversion, with normal inversion, and sensory disturbance in the dorsum of the foot and lateral shin. It may be compressed around the knee by prolonged (15–30 minutes) knee flexion during squatting in labour, or prolonged pressure around the knees in the lithotomy position by assistants, the patient or stirrups.

Obturator Nerve
An obturator nerve palsy causes weakness of hip adduction and sensory disturbance in the medial thigh. It may be compressed between the fetal head or forceps and the pelvic bone, with greater risk in the lithotomy position because the nerve is angulated as it leaves the obturator foramen.

Pudendal Nerve and Incontinence
Normal vaginal delivery often causes trauma to the pudendal nerve. In 29% to 80% of women post-partum, there is EMG evidence of denervation and re-innervation in the pelvic floor muscles (14). This is usually asymptomatic or recovers quickly, but in some severe cases causes weakness of pelvic floor striated musculature and urinary stress incontinence or faecal incontinence. This is more likely with a long active second stage of labour and heavier baby. Symptoms may worsen over the following years and with subsequent deliveries. In subsequent pregnancy, elective caesarean section is an option to prevent further damage.

Compression of the lower sacral plexus during difficult vaginal delivery may cause similar symptoms. Specialist neurophysiology showed abnormalities of the S2 to S4 roots, without specific pudendal nerve abnormality or lower limb abnormality, in patients with post-partum perineal sensory disturbance with urinary and/or faecal incontinence and anorgasmia (15).

Post-partum faecal incontinence may be due to direct trauma to the anal sphincter (often at first vaginal delivery), and/or to pudendal nerve injury (often cumulative with subsequent deliveries). In 83 women with post-partum faecal incontinence, neurophysiological assessment (clitoral-anal reflex and external anal sphincter EMG) was abnormal in 38%. Endoanal ultrasound and anal manometry were also performed. Three types of abnormality were found (16). Faecal urgency was associated with pudendal nerve demyelination (delayed reflex), usually after prolonged second stage of labour, and may improve with biofeedback physiotherapy. Severe faecal incontinence usually after difficult forceps delivery was associated with axonal damage (denervation) with poor recovery, sometimes with additional mechanical damage to the sphincter requiring surgery. The most frequent subgroup had marked flatal incontinence with occasional soiling but not major incontinence, gradually worsening over years. These women were often multiparous but with no history of difficult labour: this group had mixed neurophysiology indicating mixed pathology, and usually responded well to dietary advice and biofeedback physiotherapy. A few patients had other medical causes unrelated to labour.

Unfortunately, surgical anal sphincter repair often has poor results when there is unilateral or bilateral pudendal nerve palsy in addition to mechanical sphincter tear (17).

Perinatal Obstetric Brachial Plexus Palsy

The neonate is also vulnerable to compressive neuropathies, of which the commonest and most important is brachial plexus palsy, occurring in 1.5 per 1000 live births (18). The main risk factors are shoulder dystocia, heavier fetal weight and forceps/vacuum delivery with lower risk with twins or caesarean section (18), yet half have no identified risk factor so are not obviously iatrogenic or preventable, and probably have an in utero cause.

The main potentially preventable risk factor is shoulder dystocia (defined as the fetal shoulder becoming stuck behind the pubic symphysis after delivery of the head). After one episode of shoulder dystocia, in the next vaginal delivery there is a 12% risk of recurrent shoulder dystocia, and an overall risk of brachial plexus injury of 2% which rises to 4% if recurrent shoulder dystocia occurs (19). It remains controversial as to whether elective caesarean section is advisable.

Most affected infants make a good spontaneous recovery but a quarter have residual disability (20). The most common type of palsy, affecting only the upper plexus (Erb's palsy, causing proximal upper limb weakness), has a better outcome than palsies involving the whole plexus (20). There are no randomised trials of treatment. Early reconstructive surgery is recommended in those likely to have a poor recovery, especially in those with global palsy or absent biceps function at 3 months (20,21). Secondary reconstructive surgery, often complex and in multiple stages, may benefit some with persistent poor function.

Neonatal radial nerve palsy is occasionally reported.

COMPLICATIONS OF EPIDURAL ANAESTHESIA

This is covered in chapter 7.

AUTOIMMUNE NEUROPATHIES AND IMMUNOLOGICAL CHANGES IN PREGNANCY

Immunological changes occur in pregnancy to prevent immune rejection of the semi-allogenic fetus. These may be driven by hormonal changes which have the effect of suppressing Th1 cytokines and cellular immunity, and enhancing Th2 cytokines and antibody-mediated immunity (22). Therefore,

during pregnancy, autoantibody-mediated (Th2) autoimmune diseases tend to worsen [such as systemic lupus erythematosus (SLE) and multifocal motor neuropathy (MMN)], whereas cell-mediated (Th1) diseases tend to improve but worsen post-partum [such as rheumatoid arthritis and most cases of Guillain–Barré syndrome (GBS) and chronic inflammatory demyelinating polyradiculoneuropathy (CIDP)]. These immune changes also affect a few infective neuropathies.

Bell's Palsy (Idiopathic Facial Palsy)

It was previously thought that Bell's palsy is approximately three times more common in pregnancy (23). However, a recent review and reanalysis of the available epidemiological data suggested the earlier studies were flawed, and found no significant overall increased incidence of Bell's palsy in pregnancy (24). Nevertheless, the incidence does vary at different stages of pregnancy. Of 327 reported cases, 3% occurred in the first trimester, 9% in the second trimester, 75% in the third trimester, and 13% post-partum. The conclusion was that compared with the non-pregnant population, the incidence of Bell's palsy was lower in early pregnancy and higher in the third trimester.

Between 14% and 21% of pregnant patients with acute facial paralysis have aetiologies other than idiopathic Bell's palsy, so investigations including MRI, lumbar puncture and Lyme serology may be considered in atypical cases.

Treatment

Artificial tears or eye ointment should be given to prevent exposure keratitis. A randomised controlled trial of 496 non-pregnant patients showed that outcome was improved by oral corticosteroids (prednisolone 25 mg twice daily for 10 days) but not by aciclovir (25). The proportions of patients who had recovered facial function after 9 months were 94.4% for prednisolone and 81.6% for no prednisolone ($P < 0.001$).

Some reports have suggested the prognosis for recovery of facial power may be worse in pregnant patients, but the evidence for this is weak and may be explained by reluctance to give treatment in pregnancy (24).

Guillain–Barré Syndrome

GBS is the commonest cause of acute neuromuscular paralysis. It is defined clinically as rapidly progressive weakness with areflexia. The autoimmune attack may be directed primarily against either the myelin sheath or the axon, but this does not significantly affect the clinical features, treatment or prognosis.

A population-based epidemiological study in Sweden showed that the incidence of GBS was significantly increased in the first 30 days post-partum (age adjusted rate ratio, 2.93; 95% CI, 1.20–7.11) compared with women not recently pregnant, with no significant difference in the incidence during pregnancy (26).

Exceptionally, the opposite has also been observed. Two cases of GBS improved rapidly post-partum having previously failed to respond to intravenous immunoglobulin (IVIg) and corticosteroids (27). This might be explained by an unusual antibody-mediated mechanism or partial failure of the maternal immunological tolerance toward the fetus.

An extensive review has summarised the 30 previously published case reports of GBS in pregnancy (28). *Campylobacter* was a less frequent antecedent infection than Cytomegalovirus (CMV). CMV in addition may be transmitted to the fetus and cause sensorineural hearing loss, mental retardation and chorioretinitis.

In non-pregnant patients, plasma exchange and IVIg have been shown to be equally beneficial in the treatment of GBS. IVIg is generally preferred, even in pregnancy, because of a lower risk of infection and haemodynamic complications.

Prophylactic anticoagulation with low molecular weight heparin and compression stockings are recommended, as both pregnancy and immobility are risk factors for thromboembolism.

The outcome for the baby is generally good if the maternal condition is stable, and the outcome for the mother is similar to non-pregnant subjects with GBS. Termination of pregnancy does not improve the mother's outcome and is therefore not recommended.

The fetus is not usually directly affected by maternal GBS because GBS is not usually an antibody-mediated disease. There is a single reported case of neonatal GBS: a mother with GBS with serological evidence of CMV and IgM anti-ganglioside GM1 antibodies gave birth to a baby who was initially normal but 10 days later developed demyelinating GBS (29). The mechanism is unclear.

Fears that maternal weakness might hinder labour and increase the need for instrumental delivery are not supported by the evidence. Uterine contraction is not apparently impaired by GBS, with normal spontaneous vaginal deliveries reported in nine women with GBS including one who was tetraplegic and ventilated (28). Therefore, GBS itself is not an indication for caesarean section.

The main anaesthetic risk in GBS is that succinylcholine can provoke hyperkalaemic cardiac arrest, so this drug should be avoided (30).

Following epidural anaesthesia at delivery, one patient with GBS has been reported to have developed sensory-motor block which did not fully recover and left her with prolonged disability (31). This is unexplained but raises the possibility of increased vulnerability of damaged axons. However, here are at least five reports of epidural/spinal anaesthesia in GBS without problems. It would seem wise to give the minimum possible dose.

Multifocal Motor Neuropathy

MMN is hypothesised to be an antibody-mediated disease, most commonly associated with anti-ganglioside GM1 antibodies. Three women with MMN who became pregnant developed increasing weakness and involvement of new muscles. All responded well to IVIg and post-partum returned to their milder pre-pregnancy state (32).

MMN is usually associated with IgM antibodies which do not cross the placenta (33). There is one report of MMN with IgG anti-GM1 antibodies occurring in both mother and neonate, due to transplacental transfer of pathogenic IgG antibodies, with good recovery of the neonate.

Chronic Inflammatory Demyelinating Polyradiculoneuropathy

CIDP is a rare autoimmune neuropathy, which may be thought of as a chronic relapsing form of GBS. In 16 women of childbearing age with CIDP, relapses of CIDP occurred significantly more frequently during the year of pregnancy and 3 months post-partum (0.53 relapses/year) than at other times (0.17 relapses/year) (34). There was a tendency for relapses to occur in the third trimester or immediately post-partum.

Atypically, one case of CIDP which developed in late pregnancy improved rapidly for a week immediately after labour (perhaps due to endogenous corticosteroid secretion or an antibody-mediated pathogenesis) and then worsened again but responded to prednisolone (35).

The three best-proven treatments for CIDP are corticosteroids, IVIg and plasma exchange, but some patients need long-term immunosuppressants.

Epidural and spinal anaesthesia were reported as safe and well tolerated in CIDP (36).

Leprosy

Leprosy is one of the commonest causes of neuropathy in the world, although rare in developed countries. The typical patient has spent many years in India, central Africa or Brazil and has palpably thickened nerves, anaesthetic depigmented patches of skin, often normal reflexes, and loss of sensation particularly in the cooler parts of the body such as the ears, nose, digits and extensor surfaces of joints. The diagnosis is often difficult to make and may require biopsy of nerve or skin.

Leprous neuropathy can relapse or worsen during late pregnancy or lactation even if already treated and apparently cured. This is presumably due to the suppression of cell-mediated immunity (37).

Brachial Plexus Neuropathy (Neuralgic Amyotrophy)

Brachial plexus neuropathy (BPN, also known as neuralgic amyotrophy, Parsonage–Turner syndrome and brachial neuritis) causes acute pain followed by weakness in the proximal upper limb, probably with an autoimmune aetiology. There is usually gradual improvement over months or years, but often some persistent weakness and pain.

Although BPN is overall more common in males than females, acute attacks of both the idiopathic and hereditary forms of BPN are more frequent within the first two weeks post-partum (38). The reason for this is not known, though is likely due to alterations in the immune system. One quarter of all patients have more than one attack, yet five women with a history of a post-partum attack had subsequent deliveries without recurrence of BPN (39). There is no clear evidence that any treatment is beneficial, though non-randomised reports suggest that corticosteroids might shorten the duration of pain.

INHERITED PERIPHERAL NERVE DISEASES

Genetically determined neuropathies include Charcot–Marie–Tooth disease (CMT, also known as hereditary motor and sensory neuropathy), hereditary sensory (and autonomic) neuropathies and multisystem diseases such as familial amyloid polyneuropathies. Each of these categories includes many different mutations and inheritance patterns, but genetic testing is increasingly available, so it is usually possible to identify the mutation in a patient. If a hereditary neuropathy is suspected but a specific genetic mutation has not been detected, the preconception period may be a good time to reassess the diagnosis and consider further genetic testing.

If the genetic cause of the neuropathy has been identified in a parent, preconception counselling and prenatal diagnosis may be helpful, perhaps with a view to offering termination of pregnancy. The various prenatal genetic testing methods available are discussed in chapter 1. However, even when the mutation is known, it may not be possible reliably to predict the eventual severity of disease in the child. In several different genetic neuropathies there are reports of widely differing severity of disability between monozygotic twins. Thus, there are ethical issues in considering termination for a non-fatal condition which in some patients causes only relatively mild disability.

Charcot–Marie–Tooth Disease

The commonest genetic neuropathy is CMT type 1a, due to duplication of the PMP22 gene on chromosome 17. This causes an autosomal-dominant demyelinating neuropathy with full penetrance, usually with onset of symptoms within the first or second decade and progressing to significant disability in later life. The severity of disability is quite variable even within the same family, and some patients only ever develop mild symptoms (40). Deletion of the same gene causes a phenotypically different disease, hereditary neuropathy with liability to pressure palsies (HNPP), which is also common but usually mild and rarely disabling.

Although CMT is usually a chronic slowly progressive condition, subacute exacerbations occasionally occur, presumed due to superadded inflammation (41). In one series of 21 CMT-1 patients, 38% reported worsening weakness during pregnancy, which persisted after delivery in two-thirds of these (42). This observation has not been confirmed, and indeed most CMT experts do not believe CMT patients are at risk of worsening during pregnancy.

A comprehensive epidemiological study of all women with CMT (type unspecified) in the whole of Norway over a period of 35 years described 108 births in 49 women (43). Compared with the normal population, presentation anomalies and post-partum bleeding were twice as common in the CMT women, leading to the more frequent use of forceps, vacuum and emergency ceasarean section. Post-partum bleeding was hypothesised to be due to uterine denervation.

SAFETY OF DRUGS USED FOR THE TREATMENT OF PERIPHERAL NERVE DISEASES IN PREGNANCY

Some neuropathies are treated with drugs that are potentially harmful in pregnancy. This mainly includes immunomodulatory or immunosuppressive drugs for the inflammatory neuropathies, as well as drugs used for neuropathic pain.

See Editorial Note on page viii concerning the United States Food and Drug Administration (FDA) categories for the risk of drugs used in pregnancy.

Immunosuppressants

Acute Immunomodulatory Treatments

GBS and other acute immune-mediated neuropathies are usually treated with IVIg or plasma exchange. There is no evidence to suggest that the benefit or risk of complications from either treatment is different in pregnant patients compared with the non-pregnant.

Intravenous immunoglobulin (FDA category C) is a preparation of purified polyclonal normal immunoglobulin derived from a large number of human donors, which is effective in treatment of a large number of autoimmune diseases (44). The most important adverse effects of potential relevance to pregnancy are thrombosis due to raised plasma viscosity and rare anaphylactic reaction. Nevertheless, IVIg is generally thought to be reasonably safe in pregnancy, and indeed was previously used for treatment of recurrent spontaneous abortion (45).

Plasma exchange seems to have no significantly greater risks in the pregnant than the non-pregnant patient (46). Theoretically, it might induce premature delivery by altering maternal concentrations of circulating hormones such as oestrogen and progesterone, although this effect has never been proven.

Corticosteroids (FDA category C) may exacerbate maternal hypertension, pre-eclampsia and diabetes. There may be an increased risk of premature rupture of membranes in women with SLE or anti-phospholipid antibodies (47). A meta-analysis found a threefold increase in the risk of cleft lip/palate when corticosteroids were given during the first trimester, but the absolute risk was still low (3/1000) and there was no increased incidence of any other abnormality (48). Overall, most experts consider corticosteroids to be reasonably safe in pregnancy (49). Breastfeeding is probably safe, though mothers taking high-dose prednisolone (over 40 mg) may consider expressing and discarding milk for 4 hours after each dose (50).

Chronic Immunosuppressive Drugs

These are most likely to be of relevance if a woman with a chronic neuropathy such as CIDP is already taking such medication and then becomes pregnant or plans to become pregnant. Advice should be given prior to conception. Azathioprine and ciclosporin A may be continued in pregnancy if the benefit is thought to outweigh risk but the others such as cyclophosphamide or methotrexate should be stopped (49).

- **Azathioprine**: Although the FDA classifies this as category D, accumulated experience suggests azathioprine is probably safe in pregnancy at a dose of up to 2 mg/kg/day, if the benefit is felt to outweigh the risk.
- **Ciclosporin A** (FDA category C): Despite some reports of hypertension, prematurity and low birth weight, the overall risk in pregnancy is probably low and it may be continued in pregnancy at the lowest effective dose (49).
- **Cyclophosphamide** (FDA category D): It is teratogenic and should be avoided in pregnancy. It is gonadotoxic and can impair future fertility in both sexes. A gonadotropin-releasing hormone analogue (leuprolide acetate) given during cyclophosphamide treatment for SLE was reported to have reduced subsequent premature ovarian failure from 30% to 5% (51). However, whether GNRH agonists or antagonists have a beneficial effect on fertility after cyclophosphamide treatment remains uncertain and is the subject of a number of ongoing trials.
- **Methotrexate** (FDA category X): Methotrexate is a folate antagonist and can cause neural tube defects and multiple other malformations. It should be avoided in pregnancy and for 3 months before trying to conceive. Women should continue folic acid supplements at a dose of 400 µg daily. Methotrexate does not seem to affect future fertility.
- **Mycophenolate mofetil** (FDA category was changed in 2007 from C to D): This is teratogenic in humans with a high risk of fetal malformations and fetal loss, so is not recommended in pregnancy and should be stopped at least 6 weeks before planned conception.

Breastfeeding is generally not recommended for women taking cyclophosphamide, ciclosporin A or methotrexate, but a consensus view is developing that it is probably safe with azathioprine use (49). In a recent study of 10 breastfeeding women taking azathioprine, there were no clinical or haematological effects in the neonates. Metabolites of azathioprine were undetectable in breast milk from all but one of the women, at a concentration 10 times lower than the therapeutic serum level, and undetectable in blood from all neonates (52). The authors concluded that breastfeeding should not routinely be withheld in infants of mothers receiving azathioprine if the immediate benefits outweigh the risks.

Drugs for Chronic Neuropathic Pain

Peripheral neuropathies often cause neuropathic pain due to spontaneous ectopic impulses arising in the pathological nerves. This is usually treated with drugs that affect ion channels in the axonal membrane or modulate neurotransmission in the central nervous system.

Opioids (tramadol is FDA category C) are relatively safe but may affect the neonate by respiratory suppression and temporary withdrawal effects (53). Tricyclic antidepressants (amitriptyline is FDA category C) are relatively safe (54) but may cause neonatal tachycardia and irritability. Gabapentin (FDA category C) seems relatively safe (55), but there is little information on pregabalin (FDA category C) (see also chapter 12 on epilepsy).

Topical drugs such as lidocaine patches and capsaicin cream have minimal systemic absorption, so are useful in focal pain syndromes and are safe in pregnancy.

METABOLIC AND TOXIC POLYNEUROPATHIES

Hyperemesis gravidarum may lead to polyneuropathy and/or Wernicke's encephalopathy, usually due to thiamine deficiency, with variable recovery (56). Chronically malnourished or alcoholic women might be at greater risk. Treatment is with parenteral thiamine. Tropical myeloneuropathies presenting in pregnancy are also reported in West Africa (57).

Pyridoxine (vitamin B6) is often used for treatment of nausea and vomiting of pregnancy, but excess doses (in some reports as little as 200 mg/day, though usually much more) may *cause* a severe sensory ataxic peripheral neuropathy. However, a prospective study of 192 pregnancies receiving pyridoxine for a mean 9 weeks in the first trimester at a mean dose of 132 mg/day showed no significant adverse effects on mother or fetus compared with pregnant women not receiving pyridoxine (58). There is no evidence that routine supplements are of any benefit for the treatment of nausea and vomiting in pregnancy (59).

Maternal **alcoholism** during pregnancy can cause peripheral neuropathy in the neonate, as well as other congenital abnormalities, including the fetal alcohol syndrome. Nerve conduction tests were abnormal in all of 17 children of alcoholics both in the neonatal period and at 1 year of age (60).

Nitrous Oxide/B12

Inhalation of nitrous oxide (used for mild anaesthesia during labour) if prolonged for several hours can rarely precipitate myeloneuropathy or megaloblastic anaemia in individuals with subclinical vitamin B12 deficiency. In a series of five non-pregnant patients with unrecognised vitamin B12 deficiency, inhalation of nitrous oxide for between 1½ and 3½ hours during surgery provoked subacute combined degeneration of the cord (numbness, weakness and difficulty walking) commencing 2 to 6 weeks later, which greatly improved or normalised after vitamin B12 injections (61).

Diabetes and Autonomic Neuropathy

During normal pregnancy, sympathetic activity is increased and parasympathetic activity is reduced, generally without causing clinical symptoms. These changes are exaggerated in pre-eclampsia (62).

Autonomic neuropathy may occur in patients with diabetes. Diabetic gastroparesis may cause major problems with vomiting during pregnancy and is a relative contraindication to pregnancy. In women with diabetes it may be worth screening for gastroparesis before conception (63,64).

REFERENCES

1. Sax TW, Rosenbaum RB. Neuromuscular disorders in pregnancy. Muscle Nerve 2006; 34(5):559–571.
2. Beric A. Peripheral nerve disorders in pregnancy. Adv Neurol 1994; 64:179–192.
3. Stolp-Smith KA, Pascoe MK, Ogburn PL Jr. Carpal tunnel syndrome in pregnancy: frequency, severity, and prognosis. Arch Phys Med Rehabil 1998; 79(10):1285–1287.
4. Mondelli M, Rossi S, Monti E, et al. Long term follow-up of carpal tunnel syndrome during pregnancy: a cohort study and review of the literature. Electromyogr Clin Neurophysiol 2007; 47(6): 259–271.
5. Marshall S, Tardif G, Ashworth N. Local corticosteroid injection for carpal tunnel syndrome. Cochrane Database Syst Rev 2007; (2):CD001554.
6. O'Connor D, Marshall S, Massy-Westropp N. Non-surgical treatment (other than steroid injection) for carpal tunnel syndrome. Cochrane Database Syst Rev 2003; (1):CD003219.
7. Courts RB. Splinting for symptoms of carpal tunnel syndrome during pregnancy. J Hand Ther 1995; 8(1):31–34.
8. Wong CA, Scavone BM, Dugan S, et al. Incidence of postpartum lumbosacral spine and lower extremity nerve injuries. Obstet Gynecol 2003; 101(2):279–288.
9. van Slobbe AM, Bohnen AM, Bernsen RM, et al. Incidence rates and determinants in meralgia paresthetica in general practice. J Neurol 2004; 251(3):294–297.
10. Pildner von SS, Kuhler A, Herrmann N, et al. [Pregnancy-associated femoral nerve affection.] Zentralbl Gynakol 2004; 126(5):328–330.
11. Warner MA, Warner DO, Harper CM, et al. Lower extremity neuropathies associated with lithotomy positions. Anesthesiology 2000; 93(4):938–942.
12. Feasby TE, Burton SR, Hahn AF. Obstetrical lumbosacral plexus injury. Muscle Nerve 1992; 15(8):937–940.
13. Roy S, Levine AB, Herbison GJ, et al. Intraoperative positioning during cesarean as a cause of sciatic neuropathy. Obstet Gynecol 2002; 99(4):652–653.
14. Allen RE, Hosker GL, Smith AR, et al. Pelvic floor damage and childbirth: a neurophysiological study. Br J Obstet Gynaecol 1990; 97(9):770–779.
15. Ismael SS, Amarenco G, Bayle B, et al. Postpartum lumbosacral plexopathy limited to autonomic and perineal manifestations: clinical and electrophysiological study of 19 patients. J Neurol Neurosurg Psychiatry 2000; 68(6):771–773.
16. Fitzpatrick M, O'brien C, O'connell PR, et al. Patterns of abnormal pudendal nerve function that are associated with postpartum fecal incontinence. Am J Obstet Gynecol 2003; 189(3):730–735.
17. Sangwan YP, Coller JA, Barrett RC, et al. Unilateral pudendal neuropathy. Impact on outcome of anal sphincter repair. Dis Colon Rectum 1996; 39(6):686–689.
18. Foad SL, Mehlman CT, Ying J. The epidemiology of neonatal brachial plexus palsy in the United States. J Bone Joint Surg Am 2008; 90(6):1258–1264.
19. Bingham J, Chauhan SP, Hayes E, et al. Recurrent shoulder dystocia: a review. Obstet Gynecol Surv 2010; 65(3):183–188.
20. Andersen J, Watt J, Olson J, et al. Perinatal brachial plexus palsy. Paediatr Child Health 2006; 11(2):93–100.
21. Hale HB, Bae DS, Waters PM. Current concepts in the management of brachial plexus birth palsy. J Hand Surg Am 2010; 35(2):322–331.
22. Doria A, Iaccarino L, Arienti S, et al. Th2 immune deviation induced by pregnancy: the two faces of autoimmune rheumatic diseases. Reprod Toxicol 2006; 22(2):234–241.

23. Hilsinger RL, Jr, Adour KK, Doty HE. Idiopathic facial paralysis, pregnancy, and the menstrual cycle. Ann Otol Rhinol Laryngol 1975; 84(4 pt 1):433–442.

24. Vrabec JT, Isaacson B, Van Hook JW. Bell's palsy and pregnancy. Otolaryngol Head Neck Surg 2007; 137(6):858–861.

25. Sullivan FM, Swan IR, Donnan PT, et al. Early treatment with prednisolone or acyclovir in Bell's palsy. N Engl J Med 2007; 357(16):1598–1607.

26. Cheng Q, Jiang GX, Fredrikson S, et al. Increased incidence of Guillain-Barre syndrome postpartum. Epidemiology 1998; 9 (6):601–604.

27. Vaduva C, de SJ, Volatron AC, et al. [Severe Guillain-Barre syndrome and pregnancy: two cases with rapid improvement post-partum.] Rev Neurol (Paris) 2006; 162(3):358–362.

28. Chan LY, Tsui MH, Leung TN. Guillain-Barre syndrome in pregnancy. Acta Obstet Gynecol Scand 2004; 83(4):319–325.

29. Luijckx GJ, Vles J, de Baets M, et al. Guillain-Barré syndrome in mother and newborn child. Lancet 1997; 349:27.

30. Feldman JM. Cardiac arrest after succinylcholine administration in a pregnant patient recovered from Guillain-Barré syndrome. Anesthesiology 1990; 72:942–944.

31. Wiertlewski S, Magot A, Drapier S, et al. Worsening of neurologic symptoms after epidural anesthesia for labor in a Guillain-Barre patient. Anesth Analg 2004; 98(3):825–827, table.

32. Chaudhry V, Escolar DM, Cornblath DR. Worsening of multifocal motor neuropathy during pregnancy. Neurology 2002; 59(1): 139–141.

33. Attarian S, Azulay JP, Chabrol B, et al. Neonatal lower motor neuron syndrome associated with maternal neuropathy with anti-GM1 IgG. Neurology 2004; 63(2):379–381.

34. McCombe PA, McManis PG, Frith JA, et al. Chronic inflammatory demyelinating polyradiculoneuropathy associated with pregnancy. Ann Neurol 1987; 21:102–104.

35. Kawada N, Nakayama S, Naitoh Y, et al. [Rapid spontaneous postpartum remission in a case of chronic inflammatory demyelinating polyradiculoneuropathy associated with pregnancy]. Rinsho Shinkeigaku 1992; 32(1):78–80.

36. Velickovic IA, Leicht CH. Patient-controlled epidural analgesia for labor and delivery in a parturient with chronic inflammatory demyelinating polyneuropathy. Reg Anesth Pain Med 2002; 27(2):217–219.

37. Duncan ME. Pregnancy and leprosy neuropathy. Indian J Lepr 1996; 68(1):23–34.

38. van Alfen N, van Engelen BG. The clinical spectrum of neuralgic amyotrophy in 246 cases. Brain 2006; 129(pt 2):438–450.

39. Lederman RJ, Wilbourn AJ. Postpartum neuralgic amyotrophy. Neurology 1996; 47(5):1213–1219.

40. Birouk N, Gouider R, Le GE, et al. Charcot-Marie-Tooth disease type 1A with 17p11.2 duplication. Clinical and electrophysiological phenotype study and factors influencing disease severity in 119 cases. Brain 1997; 120(pt 5):813–823.

41. Ginsberg L, Malik O, Kenton AR, et al. Coexistent hereditary and inflammatory neuropathy. Brain 2004; 127(pt 1):193–202.

42. Rudnik-Schöneborn S, Röhrig D, Nicholson G, et al. Pregnancy and delivery in Charcot-Marie-Tooth disease type 1. Neurology 1993; 43:2011–2016.

43. Hoff JM, Gilhus NE, Daltveit AK. Pregnancies and deliveries in patients with Charcot-Marie-Tooth disease. Neurology 2005; 64(3):459–462.

44. Gold R, Stangel M, Dalakas MC. Drug Insight: the use of intravenous immunoglobulin in neurology–therapeutic considerations and practical issues. Nat Clin Pract Neurol 2007; 3(1):36–44.

45. Perricone R, De CC, Kroegler B, et al. Intravenous immunoglobulin therapy in pregnant patients affected with systemic lupus erythematosus and recurrent spontaneous abortion. Rheumatology (Oxford) 2008; 47(5):646–651.

46. Watson WJ, Katz VL, Bowes WA Jr. Plasmapheresis during pregnancy. Obstet Gynecol 1990; 76(3 pt 1):451–457.

47. Cowchock FS, Reece EA, Balaban D, et al. Repeated fetal losses associated with antiphospholipid antibodies: a collaborative randomized trial comparing prednisone with low-dose heparin treatment. Am J Obstet Gynecol 1992; 166(5):1318–1323.

48. Park-Wyllie L, Mazzotta P, Pastuszak A, et al. Birth defects after maternal exposure to corticosteroids: prospective cohort study and meta-analysis of epidemiological studies. Teratology 2000; 62(6):385–392.

49. Ostensen M, Khamashta M, Lockshin M, et al. Anti-inflammatory and immunosuppressive drugs and reproduction. Arthritis Res Ther 2006; 8(3):209.

50. Ost L, Wettrell G, Bjorkhem I, et al. Prednisolone excretion in human milk. J Pediatr 1985; 106(6):1008–1011.

51. Somers EC, Marder W, Christman GM, et al. Use of a gonadotropin-releasing hormone analog for protection against premature ovarian failure during cyclophosphamide therapy in women with severe lupus. Arthritis Rheum 2005; 52(9):2761–2767.

52. Sau A, Clarke S, Bass J, et al. Azathioprine and breastfeeding: is it safe? BJOG 2007; 114(4):498–501.

53. Hadi I, da SO, Natale R, et al. Opioids in the parturient with chronic nonmalignant pain: a retrospective review. J Opioid Manag 2006; 2(1):31–34.

54. Kallen B. The safety of antidepressant drugs during pregnancy. Expert Opin Drug Saf 2007; 6(4):357–370.

55. Montouris G. Gabapentin exposure in human pregnancy: results from the Gabapentin Pregnancy Registry. Epilepsy Behav 2003; 4(3):310–317.

56. Nel JT, van Heyningen CF, van Eeden SF, et al. Thiamine deficiency-induced gestational polyneuropathy and encephalopathy. A case report. S Afr Med J 1985; 67(15):600–603.

57. Thiam A, Bd-Ali G, Ndiaye MM, et al. [Polyneuropathies of pregnancy. Clinical neurophysiological, and anatomo-pathological study apropos of 38 cases collected at the Neurology Clinic of the the Fann University Hospital Center.] Dakar Med 1996; 41(1):47–54.

58. Shrim A, Boskovic R, Maltepe C, et al. Pregnancy outcome following use of large doses of vitamin B6 in the first trimester. J Obstet Gynaecol 2006; 26(8):749–751.

59. Thaver D, Saeed MA, Bhutta ZA. Pyridoxine (vitamin B6) supplementation in pregnancy. Cochrane Database Syst Rev 2006; (2):CD000179.

60. Avaria ML, Mills JL, Kleinsteuber K, et al. Peripheral nerve conduction abnormalities in children exposed to alcohol in utero. J Pediatr 2004; 144(3):338–343.

61. Flippo TS, Holder WD Jr. Neurologic degeneration associated with nitrous oxide anesthesia in patients with vitamin B12 deficiency. Arch Surg 1993; 128(12):1391–1395.

62. Yang CC, Chao TC, Kuo TB, et al. Preeclamptic pregnancy is associated with increased sympathetic and decreased parasympathetic control of HR. Am J Physiol Heart Circ Physiol 2000; 278(4):H1269–H1273.

63. MacLeod AF, Smith SA, Sonksen PH, et al. The problem of autonomic neuropathy in diabetic pregnancy. Diabet Med 1990; 7(1):80–82.

64. Hagay Z, Weissman A. Management of diabetic pregnancy complicated by coronary artery disease and neuropathy. Obstet Gynecol Clin North Am 1996; 23(1):205–220.

26

Muscle disease and myasthenia in pregnancy

Fiona Norwood

INTRODUCTION

This chapter encompasses those conditions that are primary disorders of skeletal muscle or that affect the neuromuscular junction. A brief overview of each area is given, followed by the interactions with pregnancy of a number of illustrative disorders. Both the effects of muscle disease on the pregnant mother and fetus and the effects of pregnancy on the mother's muscle condition need to be considered. At present, there is a lack of knowledge in this field, particularly for the genetic muscle conditions (1), and studies are needed to address this and to inform and improve standards of care in the future.

GENETIC MUSCLE DISEASE

Muscle diseases may be genetic or acquired. Genetic muscle disease comprises a large and increasing number of recognised conditions (2). It is complex in its range of disease types, including age of onset, distribution of weakness, progression and associated cardiac and respiratory complications. Great progress in classification has been made in recent years through elucidation of the underlying genetic defects (Table 26.1); improved understanding of protein functions and cellular interactions should follow. At present, there are no curative treatments for genetic muscle diseases. Recently there has been publicity about gene therapy efforts for Duchenne muscular dystrophy (DMD), for example, exon 51 skipping dose-escalation trials (3,4), but this is still experimental and the potential introduction of curative treatments for even the most common genetic muscle diseases is likely to be many years away.

Survival of patients with genetic muscle conditions has in general improved markedly in the last three decades, but this has been due to diligent supportive care, led through work in DMD for whom a Standards of Care document sets out expertise in various areas (5,6). Hopefully, these insights will be extrapolated to other conditions as well. Examples include physiotherapy to prevent limb contracture formation and, in particular, the institution of non-invasive respiratory support. Thus, the average life expectancy for patients with DMD is now into their 30s (7). This increased survival has impacted on the adult muscle clinic as those patients who previously would not have survived childhood are coming through and may have the potential to become pregnant.

Examination of the prevalence of the respective muscle conditions is informative as to which conditions are likely to present in pregnancy. Some are quite common, whereas others occur literally once in a million. A population study of the paediatric and adult muscle clinic of the north east of England (8) showed that almost one-third of the patients had myotonic dystrophy type 1 (DM1), 20% a disorder of the dystrophin gene (such as DMD), 10% facioscapulohumeral dystrophy (FSHD) and 5% limb girdle muscular dystrophy (LGMD). Mitochondrial disorders were studied by another group and

a prevalence of 9.2 per 100,000 is described, although this included all mitochondrial conditions and not just those affecting muscle (9). A few of the more frequent conditions have allowed a degree of study of their impact on pregnancy but still numbers are relatively small. For the rarer conditions, occasional case reports appear but contribute little to a systematic study of this area.

The myotonic dystrophies are the most studied. Both DM1 and DM2 (10) are autosomal-dominant, repeat expansion disorders with multisystem features, although in general DM1 is more severe than DM2, especially given that DM1 has a congenital form. The most prominent neuromuscular aspects are distal muscle weakness and myotonia.

An early study (11,12) observed that the rate of obstetric complications in myotonic dystrophy pregnancies was increased. Both polyhydramnios and preterm labour were of increased incidence in those pregnancies in which the fetus was affected by DM1. Eight (31%) patients experienced a worsening of their symptoms, with persistence of this in five of the new mothers. A retrospective study of 31 DM1 patients and literature review (13) commented that often the first indication of maternal disease was a severely affected child, in keeping with clinical observation. Miscarriages were not increased but again preterm labour was, especially when fetuses were affected with congenital DM1. Again, polyhydramnios was also more common. The number of operative deliveries was increased due to problems in labour. Perinatal mortality was raised but mainly due to babies with congenital DM1.

DM2 has also been studied in Germany where it is much more common than in the United Kingdom (14). This study suggested that pregnancy and DM2 have unfavourable influences on each other and that symptoms improved after delivery, although the risk was higher for those women who developed symptoms of DM2 before or during pregnancy. Stillbirths or neonatal deaths were not seen in this study, which is different from DM1 pregnancies (11,12).

Facioscapulohumeral muscular dystrophy (FSHD) is a fairly common muscular dystrophy in which there is predominant weakness of scapular and humeral muscles. Facial muscle weakness may be present to varying degrees, in some being obvious but in others impossible to detect. The genetic basis for the condition was elucidated recently after a long search and confirms a complex genetic mechanism (15). Ciafaloni performed a retrospective study of 105 pregnancies in FSHD women and found that most pregnancies were completed successfully, although the rates of caesarian and operative deliveries were a little higher than the national average (16). Low birth weight was more frequent than expected but pregnancy complications such as pre-eclampsia were not. Twenty-four percent of the pregnancies were reported to result in worsening of the mother's muscle weakness and most did not improve subsequently.

Table 26.1 Abbreviated Classification of Genetic Muscle Conditions

Disease group
Muscular dystrophies
Dystrophinopathies [Duchenne (DMD) and Becker muscular dystrophy (BMD)]
Facioscapulohumeral muscular dystrophy (FSHD)
Limb girdle muscular dystrophies (LGMDs)
LGMD1A-G (autosomal dominant)
LGMD2A-O (autosomal recessive)
X-linked Emery–Dreifuss muscular dystrophy (EDMD-X)
Oculopharyngeal muscular dystrophy (OPMD)
Congenital muscular dystrophy (CMD)
MDC1A
Rigid spine muscular dystrophy
Congenital myopathies
Nemaline myopathy
Central core disease
Collagen VI–related disorders
Bethlem myopathy
Ullrich congenital muscular dystrophy
Distal myopathies
Myofibrillar myopathies
Myotonic syndromes
Myotonic dystrophies 1 and 2 (DM1 and DM2)
Myotonia congenita

A systematic review of mitochondrial disease in pregnancy identified only 10 case reports (17). No cohort studies were found. Problems included threatened preterm labour, pre-eclampsia and magnesium sulphate toxicity, but again it is not possible to generalise, especially given the wide spectrum of clinical manifestations of mitochondrial conditions.

A number of other papers describe outcomes in pregnancies of women with a variety of genetic muscle conditions, some well defined and others with less clear diagnoses. Often this is the case as the passage of time has allowed a definite diagnosis to be identified subsequently whereas the particular condition may not even have been described at the time. It is difficult to draw firm conclusions from these heterogeneous studies. For example, in the highly complex group of limb girdle muscular dystrophies, many patients in the pregnancy outcome reports are not fully characterised. However, the data may well be useful if reanalysed in the light of current knowledge and gathered into larger series.

ACQUIRED MUSCLE DISEASE

This group includes the inflammatory myopathies of which polymyositis and dermatomyositis are rare and less common than previously supposed (18). An estimated combined prevalence of polymyositis and dermatomyositis is only 21.5 per 100,000 (19). This clarification is mainly due to improved diagnostic accuracy with more modern diagnostic tests and criteria. Inclusion body myositis (IBM) is relatively more common in later life (20), but does not occur, other than in possible exceptional cases, in women of childbearing age.

Thus, typical presenting symptoms may be insidious or explosive and comprise muscle pain and weakness mainly in a proximal distribution. Occasionally, presentation can be so severe that critical care support is required due to bulbar and respiratory muscle failure. Treatment is with immunosuppression and is usually needed lifelong, although occasional remissions do occur. Control of symptoms through immunosuppression in these diseases may be very difficult and is

further complicated in women of childbearing age, as in myasthenia gravis (see below), due to potential side effects and teratogenicity of agents.

Only one small case series of women who have undergone pregnancy with active polymyositis or dermatomyositis exists (21). This series describes four cases, two of whom had active disease and had a poor outcome. The authors comment that the outcome of the pregnancy reflects the status of the maternal disease.

Other acquired muscle problems include disorders that affect muscle secondarily, particularly due to endocrine dysfunction. For example, thyroid under- or overactivity are fairly common in this age group and can lead to marked muscle weakness as part of the constellation of symptoms. Correction of the thyroid status should return muscle function to normal. Other conditions such as potassium level alterations, perhaps from hyperemesis, can also produce a secondary, temporary weakness. These conditions are covered elsewhere in this book.

RECOMMENDATIONS

Recommendations for the management of pregnancies in women with genetic and acquired muscle disease were developed at the European Neuromuscular Centre workshop held in 2010 (22). These encompassed the entire extent of the pregnancy process from preconception planning, care in each stage of pregnancy, specific recommendations for particular aspects of certain muscle conditions such as cardiac or respiratory disease and resources for the new mother to care for her baby.

MYASTHENIA GRAVIS AND OTHER MYASTHENIC SYNDROMES

Myasthenia gravis (MG) is an acquired autoimmune disorder in which signal transmission across the neuromuscular junction is adversely affected. This occurs through more than one mechanism but the main issue is the production of antibodies against the acetylcholine receptor (AChR) on the post-synaptic membrane. These antibodies block acetylcholine transmission across the cleft and the result is a reduction in muscle action potential amplitude. In addition there is muscle endplate damage and this can result in muscle atrophy in the longer term if the condition is not treated adequately.

Clinically, patients with MG present with fatigable weakness affecting any or all of eyelid, extraocular, bulbar, neck, limb and respiratory muscles. The initial presentation may be gradual, intermittent or rapid, and frequently diagnosis may be delayed due to the non-specific nature of symptoms. Although clinical judgement is critical, help with confirmation of the diagnosis is through the detection of serum acetylcholine receptor antibodies, muscle action potential decrement on repetitive stimulation EMG or instability on single-fibre EMG and/or through the use of response to symptomatic treatments such as in the traditional *Tensilon* (edrophonium) test.

The prevalence of MG varies geographically between 15 and 179 per million. It appears to be more common in younger women and older men, with the presence of a thymoma associated mainly in the latter but screened for in all. Even if there is no thymoma, the presence of thymic hyperplasia is important as it indicates that surgical removal of the thymus in selected patients may induce a remission or reduction in the long-term immunosuppression needed to control the condition. Whether or not this will turn out to be the case is under investigation in an international multicentre trial which is ongoing. The MGTX trial (https://mgtx.soph.uab.edu/MGTX/) aims to compare overall prednisone dose between those non-thymomatous patients receiving thymectomy or not. Nevertheless, thymectomy has been used for many decades although its use varies by country, as does the exact surgical procedure itself. There is presently a trend towards less invasive surgery, particularly in Europe, although some thoracic surgeons have concerns that this may lead to incomplete removal of thymic tissue and thus less-effective disease control. This is pertinent as a number of the studies on MG in pregnancy indicate a large number of thymectomy operations performed during pregnancy itself, although there may be a delay of 6 to 12 months before the beneficial effect is seen.

Drug treatment for MG is divided into symptomatic treatment with anticholinesterases and disease modification with immunosuppression. Anticholinesterases such as pyridostigmine increase the amount of acetylcholine in the synaptic cleft and thus boost signal strength. However, few patients manage for longer than weeks or months with anticholinesterases alone. The introduction of immunosuppression begins with corticosteroids, usually through a relatively slow upward titration, and may produce symptomatic improvement in a few weeks. Steroid dose modulation and consideration of whether or not to introduce a steroid-sparing agent may be relatively straightforward or very complex depending on the individual situation.

Steroid-sparing agents that may be used in the treatment of MG include azathioprine, methotrexate, mycophenolate mofetil (MMF) or cyclosporin. Azathioprine is the only one for which there is trial evidence of efficacy, with reduction in steroid dose at between 12 and 15 months (23). This delay can be very difficult in the clinical situation particularly if steroid doses have to remain high in the interim to maintain disease control. However, azathioprine is considered, especially in obstetric circles, to be a safe drug in pregnancy and is used in a wide variety of other autoimmune conditions with relative impunity. Methotrexate is absolutely contraindicated in pregnancy and so is reserved for older patients when it may be very useful. MMF has been the subject of controversial trials (24–27) and its efficacy remains uncertain. However, it has been used personally and anecdotally by others in a number of patients with good effect. Its onset of action has been said to be relatively quick at 3 months but the more recent trials were unclear on this point too. Furthermore, recent discussion has focussed on the potential teratogenicity of MMF and so now its use in pregnancy should be considered only in certain clinical situations. Cyclosporin is used infrequently and many patients are not keen given its potential side-effect profile.

Patients may have relapses in disease control due to changes in drug treatment, infections or other factors of which pregnancy may be one, as discussed below. In the situation of a severe myasthenic crisis, urgent treatment may be required. This comprises supportive care in the first instance, removal or treatment of exacerbating factors and administration of intravenous immunoglobulin or plasma exchange. Both of these latter interventions are relatively safe in pregnant women provided that they are given with care. There is a theoretical increased risk of thromboembolism with immunoglobulin and so patients should be warned of this. For those patients undergoing plasma exchange, they should be closely supervised for any haemodynamic problems, especially in the later stages of pregnancy.

Several authors have addressed the topic of the course of myasthenia gravis in pregnancy. Early work (28) reviewed 322 in 225 women and noted relapse in 41%, remission in 29% and

no change in the remainder; 29.8% had exacerbations in the puerperium. Another study examined 64 pregnancies in 47 women (29). Forty-four had had thymectomy prior to conception. Myasthenia relapsed in pregnancy in 17% not on treatment; in those on treatment, it improved in 39% and worsened in 19%. Their figure for neonatal myasthenia was 9%. The authors concluded that MG is highly variable during gestation, it can vary in subsequent pregnancies and there is no effect on the long-term outcome.

Hoff produced a few studies based on the birth registry in Norway. The first (30) reviewed data on 127 births in 79 women. Thymectomy had been performed prior to 35.4% of births. There were higher than expected figures for complications during delivery, interventions during birth, and the caesarian rate was doubled. A subsequent paper examined data on 49 births in 37 mothers in whom MG was asymptomatic or in remission (31). A higher incidence of protracted labour and increased perinatal mortality was found. A further 73 mothers with 135 births (32) showed that the risk of neonatal MG was halved if the mother had had a thymectomy. However, for those mothers themselves, there was no difference in deterioration of the MG during pregnancy, use of medication, complications or interventions during pregnancy and delivery. Only one mother was managed on corticosteroids and three needed crisis management. Another study from Taiwan (33) in 163 women did not find any adverse effect on the fetus, nor any benefit from thymectomy. Caesarian births were more frequent but not significantly so.

Neonatal MG may occur through placental transmission of maternal acetylcholine receptor antibodies that are specific for the fetal isoform. The fetus may be affected by a variable degree of myasthenic weakness. This does not appear immediately after delivery but tends to manifest several hours later. Thus, there is a need for vigilance in the neonatal/post-natal setting to monitor for deterioration. Supportive care may be all that is needed, but if the infant is markedly weak then use of anticholinesterases may be helpful. This should be done in conjunction with a paediatric neuromuscular specialist. The syndrome may persist for days or weeks but eventually the maternal antibodies are cleared and the baby restored to normal strength and no longer needing treatment.

A much rarer condition is fetal arthrogryposis multiplex complex (APC), a severe condition also caused through maternal fetal acetylcholine receptor antibodies. The resulting reduction in fetal movements leads to limb contracture formation and other problems. The prognosis from this condition is poor and usually fatal. Unfortunately, it may recur in subsequent pregnancies.

Other myasthenic syndromes may occur in women of childbearing age. Lambert Eaton myasthenic syndrome (LEMS) is another autoimmune disorder, in this case due to antibodies directed against the voltage-gated calcium channels. It is much rarer than MG although the exact prevalence is unknown at present. Symptoms may be similar to MG in some respects with weakness of extraocular and proximal muscles, but there may also be autonomic symptoms. In a proportion of cases it is paraneoplastic rather than autoimmune and underlying neoplasia should be sought in all. Treatment is with symptomatic treatments, including 3,4-diaminopyridine (3,4-DAP) which acts at the pre-synaptic junction, as well as pyridostigmine on occasion. Immunosuppression may be needed with the range of agents similar to those used for MG.

Congenital myasthenic syndromes (CMS) are not autoimmune but genetic in origin. Their classification is based on the underlying defect in the respective protein. New conditions are being described and the phenotypic range expanding. It is important to establish the exact diagnosis for two main reasons: first to avoid the use of immunosuppression in conditions that will not respond to this, and second to be able to inform the patient of the mode of inheritance of the condition.

SUMMARY AND CONCLUSIONS

This chapter has provided a flavour of the issues in a wide variety of conditions, some of which are mild and might be expected to affect pregnancy little, if at all, ranging to the other end of the spectrum where achieving a successful pregnancy stretches cardiorespiratory support and medical expertise to their limits.

    The optimal management of all patients, whether they are affected by a progressive chronic muscle disease or by a fluctuating degree of muscle strength in myasthenia, needs close coordination of multispecialty and multidisciplinary management.

    Thus, for both muscle disease and myasthenia, there is the opportunity for further work to be carried out in a structured and systematic way to build up the body of knowledge in this area. Work is underway and should contribute to the standards of care for these women in future years.

REFERENCES

1. Argov Z, de Visser M. What we do not know about pregnancy in hereditary neuromuscular disorders. Neuromuscul Disord 2009; 19(10):675–679.
2. Kaplan JC. Gene Table of Neuromuscular Disorders (online resource), 2011. Available at: http://www.musclegenetable.org/.
3. Cirak S, Arechavala-Gomeza V, Guglieri M, et al. Exon skipping and dystrophin restoration in patients with Duchenne muscular dystrophy after systemic phosphorodiamidate morpholino oligomer treatment: an open-label, phase 2, dose-escalation study. Lancet 2011; 378(9791):595–605 [Epub 23 Jul 2011].
4. Goemans NM, Tulinius M, van den Akker JT, et al. Systemic administration of PRO051 in Duchenne's muscular dystrophy. N Engl J Med 2011; 364(16):1513–1522 [Epub 23 Mar 2011].
5. Bushby K, Finkel R, Birnkrant DJ, et al. Diagnosis and management of Duchenne muscular dystrophy, part 1: diagnosis, and pharmacological and psychosocial management. Lancet Neurol 2010; 9(1):77–93.
6. Bushby K, Finkel R, Birnkrant DJ, et al. Diagnosis and management of Duchenne muscular dystrophy, part 2: implementation of multidisciplinary care. Lancet Neurol 2010; 9(2):177–189. Erratum in: Lancet Neurol 2010; 9(3):237.
7. Eagle M, Baudouin SV, Chandler C, et al. Survival in **Duchenne** muscular dystrophy: improvements in life expectancy since 1967 and the impact of home nocturnal ventilation. Neuromuscul Disord 2002; 12(10):926–929.
8. Norwood FL, Harling C, Chinnery PF, et al. Prevalence of genetic muscle disease in Northern England: in-depth analysis of a muscle clinic population. Brain 2009; 132(pt 11):3175–3186 [Epub 18 Sep 2009].
9. Schaefer AM, McFarland R, Blakely EL, et al. Prevalence of mitochondrial DNA disease in adults. Ann Neurol 2008; 63(1):35–39.
10. Day JW, Ricker K, Jacobsen JF, et al. Myotonic dystrophy type 2. Molecular, diagnostic and clinical spectrum. Neurology 2003; 60:657–664.
11. Rudnik-Schoneborn S, Nicholson GA, Morgan G, et al. Different patterns of obstetric complications in myotonic dystrophy in relation to the disease status of the fetus. Am J Med Genet 1981; 80(4):314–321.
12. Rudnik-Schoneborn S, Röhrig D, Zerres K, et al. Increased risk for abnormal placentation in women affected by myotonic dystrophy. J Perinat Med 1998; 26(3):192–195.
13. Rudnik-Schoneborn S, Zerres K. Outcome in pregnancies complicated by myotonic dystrophy: a study of 31 patients and review of the literature. Eur J Obstet Gynecol Reprod Biol 2004; 114:44–53.
14. Rudnik-Schoneborn S, Schneider-Gold C, Raabe U, et al. Outcome and effect of pregnancy in myotonic dystrophy type 2. Neurology 2006; 66:579–580.
15. Lemmers RJLF, van der Vliet PJ, Klooster R, et al. A unifying genetic model for facioscapulohumeral muscular dystrophy. Science 2010; 329(5999):1650–1653.
16. Ciafaloni E, Pressman EK, Loi AM, et al. Pregnancy and birth outcomes in women with facioscapulohumeral muscular dystrophy. Neurology 2006; 67:1887–1889.
17. Say RE, Whittaker RG, Turnbull HG, et al. Mitochondrial disease in pregnancy: a systematic review. Obstet Med 2011; 4(3):90–94.
18. van der Meulen MF, Bronner IM, Hoogendijk JE, et al. Polymyositis: an overdiagnosed entity. Neurology 2003; 61(3):316–321.
19. Bernatsky S, Joseph L, Pineau CA, et al. Estimating the prevalence of polymyositis and dermatomyositis from administrative data: age, sex and regional differences. Ann Rheum Dis 2009; 68:1192–1196.
20. Phillips BA, Zilko PJ, Mastaglia FL, et al. Prevalence of sporadic inclusion body myositis in Western Australia. Muscle Nerve 2000; 23:970–972.
21. Silva CA, Sultan SM, Isenberg DA, et al. Pregnancy outcome in adult-onset idiopathic inflammatory myopathy. Rheumatology 2003; 42:1168–1172.
22. Norwood F, Rudnik-Schoneborn S. 179th ENMC international workshop: Pregnancy in women with neuromuscular disorders 5-7 November 2010, Naarden, The Netherlands. Neuromuscul Disord 2011, Jul 9 [Epub ahead of print].
23. Palace J, Newsom-Davis J, Lecky B. A randomized double-blind trial of prednisolone alone or with azathioprine in myasthenia gravis. Myasthenia Gravis Study Group. Neurology 1998; 50(6): 1778–1783.
24. Meriggioli MN, Ciafaloni E, Al-Hayk KA, et al. Mycophenolate mofetil for myasthenia gravis. An analysis of efficacy, safety and tolerability. Neurology 2003; 61:1438–1440.
25. Sanders D, McDermott M, Thornton C, et al. A trial of mycophenolate mofetil with prednisone as initial immunotherapy in myasthenia gravis. Neurology 2008; 71:394–399.
26. Sanders D, Hart IK, Mantegazza R, et al. An international, phase III, randomized trial of mycophenolate mofetil in myasthenia gravis. Neurology 2008; 71:400–406.
27. Benatar M, Rowland LP. The muddle of mycophenolate mofetil in myasthenia. Neurology 2008; 71:390–391.
28. Plauche WC. Myasthenia gravis in mothers and their newborns. Clin Obset Gynecol 1991; 34(1):82–99.
29. Batocchi AP, Majolini L, Evoli A, et al. Course and treatment of myasthenia gravis during pregnancy. Neurology 1999; 52: 447–452.
30. Hoff JM, Daltveit AK, Gilhus NE. Myasthenia gravis. Consequences for pregnancy, delivery and the newborn. Neurology 2003; 61:1362–1366.
31. Hoff JM, Daltveit AK, Gilhus NE, et al. Asymptomatic myasthenia gravis influences pregnancy and birth. Eur J Neurol 2004; 11:559–562.
32. Hoff JM, Daltveit AK, Gilhus NE, et al. Myasthenia gravis in pregnancy and birth: identifying risk factors, optimising care. Eur J Neurol 2007; 14:38–43.
33. Wen J-C, Liu TC, Chen YH, et al. No increased risk of adverse pregnancy outcomes for women with myasthenia gravis: a nationwide population-based study. Eur J Neurol 2009; 16:889–894.

Index

Page numbers followed by f and t indicate figures and tables, respectively.